MYOFASCIAL PAIN AND FIBROMYALGIA
Trigger Point Management

Myofascial Pain and Fibromyalgia

Trigger Point Management

Edward S. Rachlin, M.D., F.A.C.S.
Assistant Clinical Professor of Orthopedic Surgery
UMDNJ–Robert Wood Johnson School of Medicine
New Brunswick, New Jersey

Assistant Clinical Professor of Anesthesiology
Pain Management Center
Director of Myofascial Pain Program
UMDNJ–New Jersey School of Medicine
Newark, New Jersey

Visiting Assistant Professor of Rehabilitation Medicine
Albert Einstein College of Medicine of Yeshiva University
New York, New York

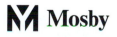 Mosby

St. Louis Baltimore Boston Chicago London Madrid Philadelphia Sydney Toronto

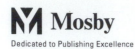

Dedicated to Publishing Excellence

Publisher: *George Stamathis*
Editor: *Robert Hurley*
Associate Developmental Editor: *Lauranne Billus*
Assistant Director/Production, Editing, Design: *Frances Perveiler*
Project Manager: *Nancy C. Baker*
Proofroom Manager: *Barbara M. Kelly*
Designer: *Nancy C. Baker*
Manufacturing Supervisor: *John Babrick*

Printed in the United States of America
Composition by Clarinda
Printing/binding by Maple-Vail/York

Mosby–Year Book, Inc.
11830 Westline Industrial Drive
St. Louis, Missouri 63146

Library of Congress Cataloging in Publication Data
Myofascial pain and fibromyalgia: Trigger Point
  Management / [edited by] Edward S. Rachlin.
      p.   cm.
    Includes bibliographical references and index.
    ISBN 0-8016-6817-4
    1. Myofascial pain syndromes.   2. Fibromyalgia.   I. Rachlin,
  Edward S.
    [DNLM: 1. Myofascial Pain Syndromes—diagnosis.   2. Myofascial
  Pain Syndromes—therapy.   3. Fibromyalgia—diagnosis.
  4. Fibromyalgia—therapy.   WE 500 D536 1993]
  RC925.5.D525   1993
  616.7′4—dc20
  DNLM/DLC   93-36499
  for Library of Congress   CIP

NOTICE
    Every effort has been made to ensure that the drug dosage schedules herein are accurate and in accord with the standards accepted at the time of publication. However, as new research and experience broaden our knowledge, changes in treatment and drug therapy occur. Therefore, the reader is advised to check the product information sheet included in the package of each drug he plans to administer to be certain that changes have not been made in the recommended dose or in the contraindications. This is of particular importance in regard to new or infrequently used drugs.

3   4   5   6   7   8   9   0   98   97   96   95

To my family with love: my wife, Barbara, and my children,
Katherine, Isabel, and John

To Dr. S. William Kalb, a devoted physician, an inspiration, my father-in-law

To Dr. Hans Kraus, friend and mentor

Contributors

Elsayed Abdel-Moty, Ph.D.
Assistant Professor
University of Miami
Supervisor of Ergonomics
Comprehensive Pain and Rehabilitation Center
South Shore Hospital and Medical Center
Miami Beach, Florida

Harold V. Cohen, D.D.S.
Clinical Associate Professor
Center for TMJ Disorders and Oral Facial Pain
  Management
University of Medicine and Dentistry of New
  Jersey
New Jersey Dental School
Robert Wood Johnson University Hospital
New Brunswick, New Jersey

Andrew A. Fischer, M.D., Ph.D.
Associate Clinical Professor of Rehabilitation
  Medicine
Mt. Sinai School of Medicine
City University of New York
Chief of Physical Medicine and Rehabilitation
  Service
Veterans Affairs Medical Center
Bronx, New York

Roy C. Grzesiak, Ph.D.
Assistant Professor and Co-Director
Pain Management Center, Department of
  Anesthesiology
Clinical Assistant Professor
Department of Psychiatry
University of Medicine and Dentistry of New
  Jersey
New Jersey Medical School
Newark, New Jersey

Joseph Kahn, Ph.D., P.T.
Clinical Assistant Professor
State University of New York at Stony Brook
Stony Brook, New York
Adjunct Associate Professor
Touro College
Dix Hills, New York

Tarek M. Khalil, Ph.D., P.E.
Professor and Chairman
Department of Industrial Engineering
University of Miami
Coral Gables, Florida

Hans Kraus, M.D.
Former Associate Professor
Department of Rehabilitation Medicine
New York University
New York, New York

**Glenn A. McCain, M.D., F.R.C.P.,
  F.A.C.P.**
Director, Fibromyalgia Treatment Program
Presbyterian Hospital
Charlotte, North Carolina

Brian Miller, P.T.
Community Physical Therapy
Marquette, Michigan

Matthew Monsein, M.D.
Medical Director, Chronic Pain Clinic
Abbot-Northwestern Hospital
Minneapolis, Minnesota

Richard A. Pertes, D.D.S.
Clinical Associate Professor and Director
Center for TMJ Disorders and Orofacial Pain
  Management
UMDNJ–New Jersey Dental School
Newark, New Jersey

Edward S. Rachlin
*Assistant Clinical Professor of Orthopedic
    Surgery*
*UMDNJ–Robert Wood Johnson School of
    Medicine*
New Brunswick, New York

Isabel Rachlin, P.T.
Physical Therapist
Ithaca, New York

Hubert L. Rosomoff, M.D., D. Med. Sc.
Professor and Chairman
University of Miami
Chief, Department of Neurological Surgery
Jackson Memorial Hospital
Miami, Florida
South Shore Hospital and Medical Center
Miami Beach, Florida

Renee Steele-Rosomoff, B.S.N., M.B.A.
*Adjunct Associate Professor, Department of
    Neurological Surgery*
School of Medicine and School of Nursing
University of Miami
Miami, Florida
Programs Director
South Shore Hospital and Medical Center
Miami Beach, Florida

Lawrence S. Sonkin, M.D., Ph.D.
Clinical Associate Professor
New York Hospital-Cornell Medical Center
Associate Attending Physician
New York Hospital
New York, New York

**Muhammad B. Yunus, M.D., F.A.C.P.,
    F.A.C.R.**
Professor of Medicine
*University of Illinois College of Medicine at
    Peoria*
Peoria, Illinois

Foreword

The vast majority of patients seen in pain management programs have myofascial pain. Yet to most physicians and other health care providers this is a very confusing area in which they have received little training. This book is the state of the art with respect to the etiology, pathophysiology, clinical presentations, laboratory tests, diagnosis and treatment of myofascial pain syndromes, fibromyalgia, and trigger points. It stresses theory as well as technique. It emphasizes the comprehensive interdisciplinary approach to the subject and draws upon experts in physiatry, orthopedic surgery, psychology, physical therapy, rheumatology, endocrinology, dentistry, and industrial engineering. The chapter authors are well known experts who have published extensively in the area of pain management.

The textbook is divided into three parts: Part I presents general considerations preparing the reader with respect to the pathophysiologic mechanisms, the clinical features, the pertinent laboratory tests, and the pharmacologic, non-pharmacologic, and psychological treatment approaches.

Part II is a very important section on trigger point management including theory, background information, and technique. This portion is also designed to be used in the treatment room. In the trigger point management section, with each skeletal muscle the subheadings include the symptoms and referral pain pattern findings on examination, differential diagnosis, anatomy, noninvasive therapy, injection technique of the trigger point, precautions, post-injection follow-up physical therapy program, exercise and home program, as well as corrective and preventive measures. The descriptive illustration of the trigger point injection and the illustrations that show the precise injection of the specific trigger point location in individual skeletal muscles should aid the reader in performing the procedure correctly.

Part III covers physical therapy and rehabilitation including exercise, electrical modalities, therapeutic massage techniques, manual therapy techniques, body mechanics, and ergonomics.

This impressive work will be a very valuable reference and a practical laboratory guide to aid physicians and other health care professionals who treat patients who suffer from the various types of muscle pathology. It also emphasizes the need for further research to clarify our understanding of the relationship between fibromyalgia, myofascial pain syndromes, and our knowledge of referred pain and trigger points. The better we understand this type of skeletal muscle pain, the more rationally we can plan our treatment approach. Dr. Edward Rachlin is to be congratulated for conceptualizing, editing, and writing.

His dedication to the subject matter and patients who suffer from these entities is obvious. He chose equally knowledgeable and dedicated coauthors.

Joel A. DeLisa, M.D.
Professor and Chairman
UMDNJ–New Jersey Medical School
Chief Medical Officer and Medical Director
Kessler Institute for Rehabilitation
Chairman, Physical Medicine and Rehabilitation
Saint Barnabas Medical Center
Newark, New Jersey

Preface

As an orthopedic surgeon and physiatrist, I was asked to speak at a pain management conference. The requested topic was a "How to do it" session for trigger point injection. I was pleased by the awareness of the importance of trigger point pathology in the diagnosis and management of muscle pain. However, I was equally concerned about the limited focus on trigger point injection technique. Therapeutic success depends not only on the technical ability to perform trigger point injections properly and prescribe the necessary follow-up care, but on the recognition and understanding that muscular trigger points represent only one cause of myofascial pain. The management of trigger points requires a thorough knowledge of the multiple and interrelated causes of muscle pain. This includes the diagnoses and management of myofascial pain syndromes and fibromyalgia. The effective treatment of acute and chronic myofascial conditions and the rehabilitation of orthopedic injuries must be based on the accurate diagnosis and understanding of the types of muscle pain that may be present.

Failure to recognize skeletal muscle pathology as a common cause of pain can result in diagnostic errors, poor therapeutic results, and unnecessary surgery. Persistent pain after the treatment of bony or ligamentous injuries often reflects a failure to recognize muscle pathology as the cause of continuing symptoms. Proper conservative care of orthopedic conditions must include the treatment of muscle pathology. A surgical procedure that is indicated and well executed should not be allowed to fail in relieving the patient's symptoms because of the presence of untreated muscle pathology.

This book fulfills the need for an instructional text that provides the current "state of the art" in technique as well as theory in the management of myofascial pain syndromes and fibromyalgia. A comprehensive approach to myofascial pain is emphasized and the appropriate role in the management of trigger points as a cause of muscle pain is clarified.

The complex and multifaceted nature of myofascial pain syndrome and fibromyalgia required an interdisciplinary approach. The treatment of muscle pain is no longer limited to any single discipline. The contributing authors are well known for their research and clinical activities in the field of myofascial pain and fibromyalgia. This book draws on the knowledge and expertise of authorities in the field of rheumatology, physiatry, orthopedic surgery, psychology, endocrinology, physical therapy, dentistry, and industrial engineering.

Dr. Hans Kraus has contributed greatly to the understanding of muscle pain, therapeutic exercise, and trigger points. He has distinguished four types of interrelated pain (muscle tension, muscle spasm, muscle deficiency, and trigger points) and established an effective approach for the treatment of each. An understanding of this concept is essential for therapeutic success.

The text is divided into three parts. Part I, General Considerations, covers the medical and psychological aspects of myofascial pain and fibromyalgia. Diagnosis and treatment are explored from the perspectives of rheumatology, psychology, endocrinology, disability evaluation, and pain management. Dr. Muhammad Yunus and Dr. Glenn A. McCain are well known for their extensive contributions in the field of fibromyalgia. The validity of the concept of fibromyalagia as a recognizable constellation of symptoms and signs was established in 1981 when the first controlled study of the clinical characteristics of this syndrome was published by Dr. Yunus and his colleagues. Dr. Yunus describes clinical features, laboratory tests, diagnosis, and pathophysiological mechanisms of the fibromyalgia and myofascial pain syndromes. Dr. McCain discusses therapeutic modalities and focuses on the proven and unproven value of pharmacological and nonpharmacological treatments. He emphasizes the importance of cardiovascular fitness training in fibromyalgia and outlines an aerobic exercise program for management. Dr. Larry Sonkin is an expert on metabolic and endocrinological conditions which cause and effect muscle pain. His chapter includes a discussion of thyroid management and its relationship to muscle pain.

The majority of patients seen in pain management programs are diagnosed as having myofascial pain. Physicians involved in pain management will find the chapters by Dr. Roy Grzesiak and Dr. Matthew Monsein of particular interest. Dr. Grzesiak's chapter on psychological considerations includes diagnosis, identifying the potentially chronic pain patient, psychological evaluation, relaxation techniques, and therapeutic approaches. Dr. Monsein discusses the disability evaluation of patients with myofascial pain and fibromyalgia, as well as his program for pain management. Dr. Andrew Fischer has written extensively on pressure algometry in the differential diagnosis of muscle pain. In his chapter, Dr. Fischer describes in detail the use of his pressure threshold meter.

In Part II I have provided the theoretical and practical knowledge to enable the practitioner to treat trigger points. Noninvasive and injection techniques are described. Five chapters are devoted to the theory and practice of trigger point management. Some of the subjects discussed include epidemiology, etiology, definition, histopathology, physiology of pain production, history and physical examination for regional myofascial pain syndrome, indications of trigger point injection description of injection technique, complications and contraindications, and reasons for failure in giving trigger point injections.

This text is designed to be used in the treatment room as well as for reference. The specific trigger point management section is unique both in the organization of information and in illustrations. The organization for specific trigger point injections provides concise comprehensive information in outline form to present the reader with the maximum amount of material so that it can be quickly and easily available and understood. Each muscle includes a discussion under specific headings; symptoms and referred pain pattern, findings on examination, differential diagnosis, anatomy, treatment, noninvasive therapy, injection of trigger point, post-injection follow-up program, exercise program, and corrective and preventive measures.

Each muscle is accompanied by an illustration for trigger point injection. In a single diagram one can obtain information which includes the trigger point pain pattern, anatomy of the muscle, position of the patient, and anatomical structures to be avoided. The appendix diagrams aid in diagnosing the trigger points to be treated. The detailed description with photographs of injection technique help the reader visualize the trigger point injection procedure.

Photographs are also used by Dr. Harold Cohen and Dr. Richard Pertes in describing how to perform oral/facial trigger point injections. Of particular interest to physicians and dentists is the differential diagnosis of facial pain, the diagnosis of temporal mandibular joint problems, and trigger point management.

Trigger point management includes a detailed account of the post-trigger point physical therapy program, which is necessary if trigger point injection is to be successful. The program must be followed in its entirety. It is also used as a noninvasive program for trigger point management. The exercise prescription is a vital part of trigger point management. The indicated exercises are prescribed in Part III.

Part III is devoted to physical therapy and rehabilitation. These practical chapters deal with all aspects of physical therapy that apply to myofascial pain and fibromyalgia. Each chapter deals with a specific aspect of physical therapy. Dr. Hans Kraus's chapter on muscle deficiency describes specific exercises which are correlated with the trigger point management and how to prescribe them. His extensive experience has proven his management methods to be most effective. The exercises are well illustrated. Dr. Joseph Kahn, whose expertise is in the area of electrical modalities in physical therapy, describes their use in the treatment of myofascial pain syndrome. Brian Miller and Isabel Rachlin are physical therapists who specialize in manual therapy techniques. Isabel Rachlin describes therapeutic massage techniques for the treatment of myofascial pain syndromes and fibromyalgia. Brian Miller has contributed a comprehensive instructional chapter on the manual therapy options available in the treatment of myofascial pain and dysfunction.

The role of body mechanics and the importance of the work environment in the prevention and treatment of myofascial pain have been extensively researched by Dr. Tarek Khalil and Dr. Hubert Rosomoff. The role of ergonomics in the prevention and treatment of myofascial pain is presented in a comprehensive fashion by Dr. Khalil, Dr. Elsayed Abdul-Moty, Dr. Renee Steele-Rosomoff, and Dr. Hubert Rosomoff.

The resurgence of interest and acknowledgment of the important role of muscle pain has stimulated the need for continued empirical research into the diagnosis and treatment of muscle pain and trigger points. Hopefully, future research will further clarify the relationship between fibromyalgia and myofascial pain syndrome and enhance our knowledge of referred pain patterns and trigger points.

I wish to thank my contributing authors for sharing their expertise and their enthusiasm. Their contributions have enabled this text to be comprehensive and incorporate all the most current and effective methods in the management of myofascial pain syndromes, fibromyalgia, and trigger points.

Edward S. Rachlin, M.D., F.A.C.S.

Acknowledgments

I wish to express my gratitude to all who shaped the content of this text:

To my daughters, Dr. Katherine Rachlin and Isabel Rachlin, to whom I am especially indebted for the long hours they devoted to this project. Their patience and encouragement during our working sessions made my task much easier. Their assistance in organization and editing were essential in the completion of the text.

To Jan Ruvido for her illustrations; Joshua Johnson for his help with photography; Dr. Walter Haas for his help in translation; Dr. Alec Simpson for his useful comments concerning the general surgical aspects of the text; the librarians, Lana Strazhnik and Tina Sharkey, for their efforts in researching the numerous and often difficult to obtain references necessary for the preparation of the text; and the members of my office staff, Susan Schendel, Pat Cubero, Jo Anne Caporaso.

Contents

PART I

GENERAL CONSIDERATIONS

Chapter *1*

Fibromyalgia Syndrome and Myofascial Pain Syndrome: Clinical Features, Laboratory Tests, Diagnosis, and Pathophysiologic Mechanisms

Muhammad B. Yunus, M.D.

FIBROMYALGIA SYNDROME

Definition and Classification of Fibromyalgia

Fibromyalgia is a form of nonarticular rheumatism characterized by widespread musculoskeletal aching and stiffness, as well as tenderness on palpation at characteristic sites, called tender points.[79, 93, 113] Fibromyalgia may be classified as regional, primary, secondary, and concomitant. When unqualified, the term *fibromyalgia* is currently used to include both primary and concomitant varieties (see below).

Regional fibromyalgia has also been called localized fibromyalgia and myofascial pain syndrome, to be described later in this chapter. In regional fibromyalgia, pain symptoms and tender points are limited to a few contiguous anatomic sites. *Primary fibromyalgia* is characterized by widespread musculoskeletal aching and tender points at multiple locations in the absence of a significant underlying or concomitant condition which would partly or fully explain the musculoskeletal symptoms and signs. *Secondary fibromyalgia* is caused by an underlying condition, e.g., active rheumatoid arthritis (RA) and hypothyroidism,[109, 111] and must be differentiated from *concomitant fibromyalgia*, in which the patient has the features of primary fibromyalgia as well as the concomitant presence of another condition. Such a concomitant condition, e.g., osteoarthritis or RA usually affecting a few joints, however, would not explain the widespread musculoskeletal findings and other features of fibromyalgia (such as marked fatigue) in that patient. Recent studies have shown that there are no significant differences between primary fibromyalgia in the absence of a concomitant disease and concomitant fibromyalgia.[93, 103] Thus, the term *fibromyalgia* may be used to include either primary or concomitant fibromyalgia.

Secondary fibromyalgia must be *causally* related to another underlying condition. For example, a patient with severe RA or hypothyroidism may have widespread musculoskeletal aching and multiple tender points, satisfying the criteria for fibromyalgia.[93, 113] Such a patient would have secondary fibromyalgia *if* these fibromyalgia features would remit following the specific treatment of RA or hypothyroidism,[109, 111] without the usual treatment of fibromyalgia.[109] Secondary fibromyalgia with such strict criteria seems quite uncommon and has not been reported in the literature, although we have documented a few such cases. Partial relief of symptoms and tender points would not qualify for secondary fibromyalgia. We have observed a number of fibromyalgia cases who also have hypothyroidism, but an adequate treatment of hypothyroidism made little difference to their pain or tender points, although fatigue improved to an extent; these are examples of concomitant fibromyalgia, and not secondary fibromyalgia.

Terminology

Fibromyalgia has also been described under the term *fibrositis* which was first used by Gowers[38] in relation to lumbago, with a hypothetical assumption that muscles and surrounding connective tissues are inflamed in such cases. However, inflammatory changes have not been documented in fibromyalgia.[25, 106, 113] Since pain is an integral part of fibromyalgia (Gr. *algos*, pain; *ia*, condition), *fibromyalgia* seems to be an appropriate term[93, 94, 109, 111, 113] which further avoids any implication of etiology (such as inflammation) which is currently unknown. Terms such as *myofascial pain* (which has been used to describe localized pain) or *psychogenic rheumatism* should not be confused with fibromyalgia. Several other terms used in the literature, such as *myofasciitis*, *tension myalgia*, and *fibromyositis* also add to the confusion and should be avoided. Patients with psychogenic rheumatism have no consistent pattern of symptoms, lack objective, reproducible physical signs (such as tender points), and have an overt psychiatric problem. The term *psychogenic rheumatism* should particularly be avoided to describe fibromyalgia. Although a subgroup of fibromyalgia patients seen in a referral rheumatology clinic (about 25%–35%) have a significant psychological problem,[46, 109] fibromyalgia features are explicable on a pathophysiologic basis (to be described later), unlike symptoms of psychogenic pain.[2] As will be discussed later, fibromyalgia is not a psychiatric disorder. Since fibromyalgia is a recognizable constellation of symptoms and signs, the term *fibromyalgia syndrome (FMS)* is perhaps the most appropriate one, although the terms *fibromyalgia* and *FMS* will be used interchangeably in this chapter.

Brief History of Fibromyalgia

Aches and pains in the muscles and joints have been described as muscular rheumatism in the European literature since the 17th century.[64] In 1904, Gowers used the term *fibrositis* in an article on lumbago,[38] as mentioned above. However, it was not until the 1960s that the term *fibrositis* was used to describe a well-defined syndrome with *generalized* musculoskeletal aching, tender points at multiple sites, poor sleep, and fatigue.[77, 81] Moldofsky and his associates published the findings of a sleep electroencephalogram (EEG) study in "fibrositis" in 1975,[56] but the validity of the concept of fibromyalgia remained in doubt until 1981 when the first controlled study of the clinical characteristics of this syndrome by a formal protocol was published by Yunus and his colleagues.[113] This study showed that multiple symptoms as well as tender points were significantly more common in fibromyalgia than in an age-, sex- and race-matched normal control group, thus raising fibromyalgia to a recognizable *syndrome* level. A good number of controlled studies on various aspects of fibromyalgia have since been published.[91, 93, 109] The blinded multicenter criteria study incorporating a control group of patients with various types of chronic pain[93] has been very helpful in further validation of the syndrome of fibromyalgia.

Clinical Features of Fibromyalgia Syndrome
Age, Sex, Race, and Prevalence
Fibromyalgia occurs predominantly among females; only 5% to 20% of the patients are males.[35, 93, 109, 113] The most common age at presentation is 40 to 50 years. However, fibromyalgia has been described among juveniles[17, 108] as well as in the elderly.[103] Most fibromyalgia patients described in the literature are whites, probably because of clinic and referral biases. FMS has been described among the Japanese[59] and South African blacks.[50] Age, sex, and race distribution, as well as duration of symptoms, in FMS are shown in Table 1–1. It may be noted that fibromyalgia is a chronic disease with an average symptom duration of 6 to 7 years at the time of presentation in a rheumatology clinic.[109]

The prevalence of FMS in different communities by epidemiologic studies has varied between 1% and 10%,[32, 42, 90] probably due to differences in demographic factors and the methodology used. Future studies employing appropriate methodology will be most useful in determination of the true prevalence of fibromyalgia in the community. An appraisal of the available studies suggests that the prevalence of fibromyalgia in the population, as defined by the ACR criteria,[93] may be about 2% to 4%.[90]

Symptoms
The most common and characteristic symptoms of fibromyalgia are generalized pain, stiffness, fatigue, and poor sleep. Other symptoms include a swollen feeling in soft tissues, and paresthesia. The presence of several associated features has also been well described (Table 1–2).

Pain is the integral and the most common presenting symptom of fibromyalgia. It is usually present in all the four limbs as well as the upper or lower back. Pain in three widespread areas will, however, satisfy the symptom criteria for classification of fibromyalgia,[93] to be described below under Diagnosis

TABLE 1–1.

Age, Sex, Race, and Symptom Duration in Fibromyalgia in Several Selected Series*

	Yunus et al.[111] (n = 113)	Goldenberg[35] (n = 118)	Wolfe et al.[93] (n = 293)	Combined† (n = 524)
Mean age (yr)	40	43	49	44
Females (%)	94	87	89	90
Whites (%)	98	92	93	94
Duration of symptoms (yr)	7	5	NR‡	6

*Modified from Yunus MB, Masi AT: Fibromyalgia, restless legs syndrome, periodic limb movement disorder and psychogenic pain. In McCarty DJ Jr, Koopman WJ, editors: *Arthritis and allied conditions: A textbook of rheumatology*, ed 12, Philadelphia, 1993, Lea & Febiger, pp 1383–1405. Used by permission.
†Results are based on the mean values of the three series.
‡NR = not reported.

TABLE 1–2.

Symptoms in Fibromyalgia Syndrome Based on Several Large Series*

Symptoms†	Frequency (%)	
	Mean‡	Range
Musculoskeletal		
Pain at multiple sites	100	100–100
Stiffness	78	76–84
"Hurt all over"	64	60–69
Swollen feeling in tissues	47	32–64
Nonmusculoskeletal		
General fatigue	86	75–92
Morning fatigue	78	75–80
Poor sleep§	65	56–72
Paresthesia	54	26–74
Associated symptoms		
Self-assessed global anxiety	62	48–72
Headaches	53	44–56
Dysmenorrhea	43	40–45
Irritable bowel symptoms	40	30–53
Self-assessed global depression	34	31–37
Sicca symptoms	15	12–18
Raynaud's phenomenon‖	13	12–18
Female urethral syndrome	12	9–17

*Modified from Yunus MB, Masi AT: Fibromyalgia, restless legs syndrome, periodic limb movement disorder and psychogenic pain. In McCarty DJ Jr, Koopman WJ, editors: *Arthritis and allied conditions: A textbook of rheumatology,* ed 12, Philadelphia, 1993, Lea & Febiger, pp 1383–1405. Used by permission.
†See text for individual references pertaining to various symptoms.
‡Mean values derived from percentage figures reported in multiple studies.
≅Based on the question "Do you sleep well?" or a similar question.
‖Definition specified as "dead white pallor on exposure to cold."

and Differential Diagnosis. About two thirds of the patients state that they "hurt all over," and this symptom has been found to be useful in differentiating fibromyalgia from other conditions.[93, 110, 111] Pain is spontaneously described as aches, soreness, hurting, and pain. Leavitt et al.[47] compared the pain characteristics in 50 patients with FMS and 50 patients with RA using an adapted McGill Pain Questionnaire, and found that pain in fibromyalgia had a greater spatial distribution and involved a greater number of pain descriptors (e.g., radiating, shooting, pressing, pricking, and nagging) as compared with RA.[47]

Common sites of pain or stiffness are low back; neck; shoulder region, including the trapezius muscles; arms; hands; knees; hips; thighs; legs; and feet[109]; however, many other areas, including the temporomandibular[57] and anterior chest[61, 109] regions may be involved. Chest pain in fibromyalgia is sometimes a prominent symptom and may cause confusion with cardiopulmonary disease.[61] The presence of prominent tender points on palpation in the chest wall and other parts of the body (see under Physical Examination, below) suggest fibromyalgia, but does not rule out concomitant cardiopulmonary disease. Metacarpophalangeal and proximal interphalangeal joint areas may also be painful,[103] and may lead to a misdiagnosis of arthritis, particularly if patients also complain of swelling in these areas (see below). Pain in a subgroup of patients is, indeed, predominantly articular, rather than muscular.[65, 89]

We had observed that some patients have predominantly or exclusively one-sided pain.[113] Currently proposed ACR criteria[93] will exclude such unilateral cases, but a study of such patients may provide useful clues regarding a possible pathogenic role of trauma, postural strain, or overuse in initiating or localizing pain in fibromyalgia.

Pain or stiffness is often aggravated by cold or humid weather, anxiety or stress, overuse or overactivity, and poor sleep.[111, 113] Psychological disturbance, as assessed by the Minnesota Multiphasic Personality Inventory (MMPI), is associated with severity of pain (see discussion of psychological factors below). Most patients state that their pain and stiffness are worse in the morning and the evening, but 30% report no consistent pattern.[103]

Stiffness, usually worse in the morning and the evening, is common, but unlike RA, morning stiffness does not correlate with severity of fibromyalgia as determined by degree of pain, number of tender points, or level of fatigue.[111] Most (about 80%), but not all, patients have stiffness. Pain and stiffness sites correlate with each other.

Fatigue is very common in fibromyalgia; moderate or severe fatigue occurs in about 85% of patients.[93] A typical patient describes it by saying that "I am always tired." It is variously described as exhaustion, tiredness, fatigue, and sometimes as a global feeling of generalized weakness. It is aggravated by physical activities, and may cause significant dysfunctions in daily living. Fatigue, rather than pain or stiffness, may be the presenting feature in some patients. Fatigue, like pain, seems to be primarily of central origin (see Pathophysiologic Mechanisms, below), and may be contributed by, or associated with, poor sleep, excessive physical activities, and physical deconditioning, as well as psychological factors.[111]

Poor sleep is also common in fibromyalgia. About 65% of the patients describe their sleep to be poor in response to the question "Do you sleep well?" However, morning fatigue may be a better indicator of the quality of sleep, and is present in about 80%.[109] Poor sleep may be indicated by difficulty in falling asleep, frequent awakening, light sleep, and morning fatigue. In one of our studies,[111] poor sleep was correlated with fatigue as well as mental stress. As stated above, poor sleep may aggravate pain and may contribute to its pathophysiologic mechanism (see below).

Swollen feeling and paresthesia are present in about half the patients.[109] Both symptoms are predominantly present in the extremities, although other anatomic regions may be involved. In some patients, these symptoms are quite severe, but no objective joint swelling or sensory deficits are present on physical examination; however, fingers may look somewhat puffy in an occasional patient (see below). Paresthesias often diffusely involve all the fingers or an extremity, and are described as tingling, pins and needles, or numbness. The etiopathologic mechanisms of these symptoms are unknown, but they do not correlate with the psychological status of a patient.[98, 111] It is, however, possible that both paresthesia and swollen feeling symptoms are related to pain; autonomic disturbance may also play a role. Electromyographic (EMG) and nerve conduction velocity studies are normal in patients with paresthesias (our unpublished data).

Several *associated symptoms and conditions* have been described in fibromyalgia (see Table 1–2). More than one study has shown these to be significantly more common in fibromyalgia than in pain-free normal controls, as well as in those with other chronic pain conditions, such as RA.[18, 93, 110, 111] These include chronic headaches, irritable bowel syndrome, primary dysmenorrhea, and female urethral syndrome. It would appear that these and several other syndromes, including myofascial pain (to be described later), temporomandibular dysfunctional pain,[28] and chronic fatigue[36] form a *dysfunctional spectrum syndrome* with several common features, e.g., predominance in females, lack of pathologic changes in peripheral tissue, and a current lack of a specific laboratory test. It has been proposed that these conditions share a common pathophysiologic mechanism, e.g., a neuroendocrine dysfunction (Fig 1–1), in a genetically susceptible individual.[109]

Other symptoms found to be significantly more common in fibromyalgia than in normal controls include self-assessed global anxiety and depression, as well as sicca symptoms (see Table 1–2). It should be noted, however, that most studies employing appropriate psychological instruments have not found significantly more common anxiety or depression in FMS as compared with other chronic pain patients, although a few have (see discussion of psychological factors, below). The cause of dry mouth in fibromyalgia is not known. This symptom was not related to drugs (such as an antidepressant medication) or to psychological symptoms of anxiety, stress, or depression among our patients.[104, 105] None of our patients with dry mouth had Sjögren's syndrome or other connective tissue disease, either at presentation or on follow-up.[104]

Physical Examination

The most significant finding related to FMS is the presence of *multiple tender points*.[78, 79, 93, 113] The number of tender points present in a patient depends on the method used to elicit this sign, as well as the total number of sites examined. Although a dolorometer has been applied to quantitate the pressure,[18, 93] simple digital pressure can be used reliably with practice. A steady digital pressure of about 4 to 5 kg, approximately at a rate of 1 kg/sec, should first be applied to a control site (such as the forehead). At this pressure, most fibromyalgia patients begin to feel pain (distinct from pressure), and this is the degree of pressure that an examiner should apply digitally in all the examination sites. The pain thus elicited may be graded as mild, moderate, or severe; for moderate or greater pain, a visible physical sign (such as grimacing or withdrawal) should be present. The ACR criteria will be satisfied if mild or greater pain on palpation (as a definition of tender point) is present in 11 of 18 sites (to be discussed later). While the sites to be palpated for tender points in the ACR criteria are 18 (see Fig 1–2), many more sites are tender in fibromyalgia,[93, 103, 110, 113] including the joints.[65, 113] In fact, a small subgroup of patients are diffusely tender all over. It should be noted that while the criteria of Yunus et al.[110, 113] require a fewer number of tender points (such as four or five), ten-

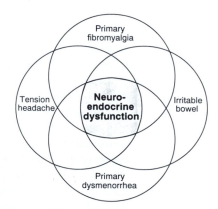

FIG 1–1.   Fibromyalgia, irritable bowel syndrome, tension-type headaches, and primary dysmenorrhea share many overlapping features, e.g., predominant or exclusive female sex, absence of peripheral pathologic findings, and a current lack of any specific laboratory tests. Neuroendocrine dysfunction may be the most important pathogenic factor common to all of these syndromes. (Modified from Yunus MB, Masi AT: Fibromyalgia, restless legs syndrome, periodic limb movement disorder and psychogenic pain. In McCarty DJ Jr, Koopman WJ, editors: *Arthritis and allied conditions: A textbook of rheumatology*, ed 12, Philadelphia, 1993, Lea & Febiger, pp 1383–1405. Used by permission.)

der points in the definition of these criteria require severe pain (with a visible physical sign) on palpation of tender point sites.

Tender points are consistent among the patients when examined by the same as well as by different observers on more than one occasion,[84, 112] and reliably discriminate fibromyalgia patients from normal controls[113] as well as those with other forms of chronic pain.[93]

Other physical signs in fibromyalgia include skin fold tenderness and cutaneous hyperemia. *Skin fold tenderness* is elicited by grasping a fold of skin and subcutaneous tissue by moderate pressure in the tender point examination sites, although such tenderness is globally present in many fibromyalgia patients. *Cutaneous hyperemia* is seen at the tender point examination sites following such an examination. Neither of these physical signs has much diagnostic value, however, since the former strongly correlates with tender point examination[110] and the latter has limited sensitivity and specificity.

Reticular discoloration of skin, first described by Caro as a netlike, mottled, blue or purple discoloration of the skin in the extremities,[20] was present in 15% of patients, but had a high specificity (95%) in the multicenter study.[93] Examination of the joints and the nervous system is essentially normal, despite the fact that many patients complain of subjective joint swelling and of paresthesias, as described before. In some patients, range of motion is somewhat decreased because of pain. As mentioned earlier, some joints (particularly those in the hands and feet) may be tender on palpation. We have occasionally encountered patients who show mild, diffuse puffiness in the fingers (usually with diffuse tenderness) on physical examination. Bone scan studies performed in two such patients were normal. Muscle strength by usual physical examination is normal, although both isokinetic and isometric strengths are significantly decreased as compared with normal controls, when measured with an isokinetic dynamometer.[41] Findings of a concomitant disease (such as osteoarthritis), not related to fibromyalgia, may be present in some patients. Physical findings in FMS are shown in Table 1–3).

Laboratory Tests

Results of the *usual routine laboratory tests,* e.g., complete blood count, erythrocyte sedimentation rate (ESR), chemistry profile (including muscle enzymes), and rheumatoid factor, are normal in FMS.[113] *Antinuclear antibodies* (ANA) are present in about 10% of patients; the frequency of ANA in FMS is not significantly different from that in a control group with similar distribution of age,

TABLE 1–3.

Physical Signs in Fibromyalgia Syndrome

Positive Findings	Negative Findings*
Multiple tender points	Absent joint swelling
Skin fold tenderness	Normal range of motion of the joints
Cutaneous hyperemia	Normal muscle strength†
Reticular skin discoloration	Normal sensory functions
Diffuse puffiness of fingers (rare)	Normal reflexes

*The findings described may be abnormal due to a concomitant disease, e.g., arthritis or neuropathy.
†Reduced maximum voluntary muscle strength by isokinetic dynamometer has been reported.[41]

TABLE 1–4.

Laboratory Tests in Fibromyalgia Syndrome

Abnormal Tests*	Normal Tests†
Sleep EEG studies	Complete blood count
Neuroendocrine tests‡	Erythrocyte sedimentation rate
	Muscle enzymes
	Thyroid function tests
	Rheumatoid factor
	Antinuclear antibodies
	Radiographs; bone scan
	Electromyography
	Muscle biopsy

*No laboratory tests having a satisfactory sensitivity and specificity are currently available in fibromyalgia.
†Several tests listed as normal may be abnormal if a concomitant disease is present, e.g., rheumatoid arthritis or hypothyroidism.
‡See text.

sex, and race.[7, 104] Other tests reported to be normal in FMS include *multiphase skeletal scintigraphy*[100] and *electromyography*[51, 115] (Table 1–4).

Muscle Studies

Our initial uncontrolled muscle biopsy study had shown atrophy of type II fiber and motheaten appearance of type I fiber by histochemistry and myofibrillar lysis with deposition of glycogen and mitochondria by electron microscopy (EM); inflammation was absent by light microscopy.[43] A controlled study by Bengtsson et al.[10] showed no significant differences between patients and controls by histopathologic or histochemical study, with the possible exception of ragged red fiber which was present in the trapezius muscles of 15 (37%) of 41 patients and in none of the ten controls. Since only a few ragged red fibers were seen in each biopsy, the number of the controls studied was small, and the study was not stated to be blinded, the significance of this finding in fibromyalgia is questionable. In their recent preliminary report, Drewes et al.[25] found no ragged red fibers in 50 quadriceps muscle biopsies from 20 fibromyalgia patients as compared with 15 biopsies from ten normal controls, all blindly assessed. EM findings of muscle biopsy in our subsequent controlled and blinded study did not show significant differences between patients and controls.[107] In the above-mentioned study of Drewes et al., however, empty sleeves of basement membrane and many lipofuscin bodies were found by EM in 8 patients as compared with five controls studied.[25] Considering the small numbers of subjects studied, the significance of this finding remains questionable. Moreover, the effects of possible deconditioning on these findings remain unknown. "Rubber band–like" structures described in an earlier report[4] were not confirmed in a recent controlled and blinded study by the same group of investigators.[5]

In 1986, Bengtsson and her colleagues[9] reported a significant decrease in adenosine triphosphate (ATP), adenosine diphosphate, and phosphoryl creatine in trapezius muscles by open biopsy, but similar changes were not significantly different between patients and controls by ^{31}P nuclear magnetic resonance (NMR) spectroscopy, when controls were appropriately matched for physical deconditioning.[73] Muscle oxygenation was found to be significantly low by multipoint oxygen electrode as compared with normal controls in one study,[49] but ischemia of muscles was not reflected in the oxygen uptake ($\dot{V}O_2$) relative to work rate in another preliminary report.[72] Moreover, augmented lactic acidosis on exertion was not found in two reports.[15, 87] It is probable that many of the above-reported changes in the muscles in fibromyalgia are secondary to deconditioning reported in this syndrome.[15] In conclusion, there is little convincing support for significant pathologic changes in muscles in fibromyalgia. Several nonspecific changes which have been described have not been uniformly found by independent investigators and may be secondary to muscle deconditioning. Further blinded studies, employing appropriate controls with a similar deconditioning state as the patients, are indicated.

Sleep Studies

Clinically, most patients with FMS complain of nonrestorative sleep, as described above. The first objective documentation of a sleep anomaly was described by Moldofsky and his colleagues[56] who studied ten fibromyalgia patients (seven females, three males; mean age, 51.9 years) by sleep EEG. Seven patients demonstrated an intrusion of alpha rhythm in their non-rapid eye movement (non-REM) sleep, whereas the other three patients showed an absence of stage 4 as well as stage 3 sleep. In the same study, six healthy volunteers, all men (aged 19–24 years), were deprived of their stage 4 sleep by auditory stimuli. Following deprivation of their stage 4 sleep, the healthy subjects developed musculoskeletal pain and increased tenderness as measured by dolorimetry. Thus, it would appear that nonrestorative sleep may contribute to fibromyalgia features. In subsequent studies, the same group of investigators confirmed the above alpha anomaly during non-REM sleep in six patients with FMS compared with six patients with dysthymic disorder,[39] as well as nine patients with FMS and nine patients with FMS secondary to a febrile illness compared with ten healthy controls having a similar age and sex distribution.[55] Several independent investigators showed a similar sleep anomaly, but others failed to do so in their preliminary reports.[109] Despite its "common sense appeal," an objective sleep anomaly by EEG in FMS is not uniformly demonstrated by independent investigations at this time. The studies mentioned above involve a small sample, and the method of selection (consecutive, random, referral status, etc.) was not clarified. Moreover, it is known that the sleep abnormality reported in FMS is not specific for this condition.[54] For these reasons, as well as the time and cost involved in a sleep EEG study, this procedure cannot be used routinely as a "test" in FMS. It is suggested that a multicenter sleep EEG study with appropriate communications between the investigators be undertaken.

Neuroendocrine Tests

Considering the hypothesis of central pain mechanisms modulated by neurotransmitter and neurohormonal aberrations in FMS,[95] neurobiochemical studies hold promise for useful laboratory tests in this condition. Bennett et al.[14] reported a significantly ($P < .000001$) decreased level of somatomedin C among 70 female fibromyalgia patients compared with 55 healthy controls. In a recent preliminary report, we found that a combination of seven biochemical tests, i.e., plasma histidine, plasma methionine, plasma tryptophan, plasma norepinephrine, plasma isoleucine, plasma leucine, and urinary dopamine, provided a sensitivity of 86% in FMS with a specificity of 77% against normal controls.[99] Neither of the above tests[14, 99] can be reliably used for diagnostic purposes in fibromyalgia at this time without further independent studies employing other control subjects with chronic pain, e.g., RA, osteoarthritis, and regional musculoskeletal pain. The rationale and significance of the above neurohormonal tests is discussed further under Pathophysiologic Mechanisms.

Other Tests

IgG deposition at the dermal-epidermal junction by skin biopsy was found in 19 (53%) of 36 patients with FMS compared with 2 (17%) of only 12 normal controls ($P <.05$) in one study,[21] but in only 4 (11%) of 36 patients in another report.[24] The true prevalence of this nonspecific finding in FMS is unknown. It is not regarded as a true immunologic phenomenon.[21]

Diagnosis and Differential Diagnosis

Fibromyalgia can be easily and reliably diagnosed in most cases by its characteristic symptoms and multiple tender points.[93, 109, 111, 113] The ACR criteria for the *classification* of fibromyalgia include widespread musculoskeletal pain and the presence of mild or greater tenderness in 11 of 18 possible sites (Table 1–5). In clinical practice, not all patients will have 11 tender points or widespread pain as defined in Table 1–5, but may have otherwise characteristic fibromyalgia features. These patients may be diagnosed as having fibromyalgia for the practical purpose of case management. In our observation, the number of ten-

TABLE 1–5.

American College of Rheumatology Criteria for Classification of Fibromyalgia*†

1. History of widespread pain.

   Definition. Pain is considered widespread when all of the following are present: pain in the left side of the body, pain in the right side of the body, pain above the waist, pain below the waist. In addition, axial skeletal pain (cervical spine or anterior chest or thoracic spine or low back) must be present. In this definition, shoulder and buttock pain are considered as pain for each involved side. "Low back" pain is considered lower segment pain. Thus, pain at three widespread sites (e.g., right arm, low back, and left leg) will satisfy the criterion of widespread pain.

2. Pain in 11 of 18 tender point sites on digital palpation (also see Fig. 1–2).

   Definition. Pain (mild or greater) on digital palpation must be present in at least 11 of the following 18 tender point sites:
   Occiput: bilateral, at the suboccipital muscle insertions.
   Low cervical: bilateral, at the anterior aspects of the intertransverse spaces at C5–7.
   Trapezius: bilateral, at the midpoint of the upper border.
   Supraspinatus: bilateral, at origins above the scapula spine near the medial border.
   Second rib: bilateral, at the second costochondral junctions, just lateral to the junctions on upper surfaces.
   Lateral epicondyle: bilateral, 2 cm distal to the epicondyles.
   Gluteal: bilateral, in upper outer quadrants of buttocks in anterior fold of muscle.
   Greater trochanter: bilateral, posterior to the trochanteric prominence.
   Knee: bilateral, at the medial fat pad proximal to the joint line.

   Digital palpation should be performed with an approximate force of 4 kg. For a tender point to be considered "positive" the subject must state that the palpation was painful. "Tender" is not to be considered "painful."

   *From Wolfe F, Smythe HA, Yunus MB, et al: *Arthritis Rheum* 33:160–172, 1990. Used by permission.
   †For classification purposes, patients will be said to have fibromyalgia if both criteria (1 and 2) are satisfied. Widespread pain must have been present for at least 3 months. The presence of a second clinical disorder does not exclude the diagnosis of fibromyalgia.

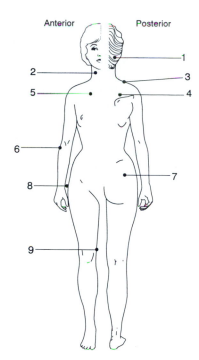

FIG 1–2. Location of nine bilateral tender point sites for the American College of Rheumatology criteria for classification of fibromyalgia (also see Table 1–5). *1* = suboccipital muscle insertions; *2* = cervical, at the anterior aspects of the intertransverse spaces at C5–7; *3* = trapezius, at the midpoint of the upper border; *4* = supraspinatus, at the origin, above the scapular spine near the medial border; *5* = second rib, at the costochondral junction; *6* = lateral epicondyle, 2 cm distal to the epicondyle; *7* = gluteal, in the upper outer quadrant of the buttock; *8* = greater trochanter, just posterior to the trochanteric prominence; *9* = knee, at the medial fat pad proximal to the joint line. (Modified from Yunus MB, Masi AT: Fibromyalgia, restless legs syndrome, periodic limb movement disorder and psychogenic pain. In McCarty DJ Jr, Koopman WJ, editors: *Arthritis and allied conditions: A textbook of rheumatology,* ed 12, Philadelphia, 1993, Lea & Febiger, pp 1383–1405. Used by permission.)

der points found by inexperienced hands tends to be fewer than the number found by examiners who are appropriately trained.

Since FMS has a protean clinical manifestation, it may be confused with a variety of other conditions, including different forms of arthritis, cardiopulmonary disease, and hypothyroidism (Table 1–6). Careful history taking, physical examination, and appropriate laboratory tests will clarify the confusion in most

TABLE 1–6.

Presenting Features of Fibromyalgia With Confounding Diagnoses and Key Points of Differentiation*

Presenting Features	Confounding Diagnosis	Absent in Fibromyalgia†
Joint pain and subjective swelling	Arthritis	Objective joint swelling
Diffuse muscular aching and stiffness	Polymyalgia rheumatica	↑ ESR, ↓ Hb, weight loss
Muscle fatigue, weakness	Myopathy, ↑ muscle enzymes	Objective weakness
Fatigue, sensitivity to cold, muscle pain	Hypothyroidism	↓ T_4, ↑ TSH
Back pain/stiffness	Ankylosing spondylitis	Sacroiliitis
Sciatica-type pain	Disc herniation	Neurologic and radiologic findings
Chest pain	Cardiac or pleural pain	Typical history of cardiac pain, pleural rub, ECG, chest film, or laboratory findings of intrathoracic disease

*From Yunus MB, Masi AT: Fibromyalgia, restless legs syndrome, periodic limb movement disorder and psychogenic pain. In McCarty DJ Jr, Koopman WJ, editors: *Arthritis and allied conditions: A textbook of rheumatology,* ed 12, Philadelphia, 1993, Lea & Febiger, pp 1383–1405. Used by permission.
†ESR = erythrocyte sedimentation rate; Hb = hemoglobin; T_4 = thyroxine; TSH = thyroid-stimulating hormone; ECG = electrocardiogram.

cases. Concomitant presence of diseases should always be remembered. For example, some fibromyalgia patients may have, or will develop, concomitant conditions such as arthritis, spinal stenosis, polymyalgia rheumatica (PMR), and peripheral neuritis. As discussed earlier, fibromyalgia should be diagnosed by its own clinical characteristics. However, concomitant conditions should be appropriately diagnosed and managed. PMR may pose a difficult problem. We have encountered cases of typical PMR with greatly increased ESR who responded satisfactorily to a low-dose corticosteroid preparation, only to develop features of FMS at a later date. Fatigue disproportional to disease activity of PMR, increased number of tender points, a lack of satisfactory response to an increased dose of the corticosteroid preparation, and a normal (or modestly increased) ESR are indicative of a diagnosis of concomitant FMS.

Psychological Factors in Fibromyalgia Syndrome

Psychological status in FMS has been reviewed elsewhere.[37, 97, 109] Only a brief overview is provided here. Several *MMPI* studies have shown that about one third of fibromyalgia patients seen in a rheumatologic clinic have a significant psychological disturbance. *Mental stress*, as measured by Hassles scale and Life Events Inventory, is significantly greater in FMS than in pain-free normal controls as well as in patients with RA. *Anxiety* scores are also significantly elevated in FMS as compared with normal controls,[97, 102] but may be largely explained by the Hassles scores.[85] Overall, the prevalence of *depression* is not significantly increased in FMS, as compared with other chronic pain conditions, e.g., RA.[109] In our blinded interview study of *psychiatric diagnoses* by DSM-III criteria,[1] depression was found to be present in 34% in FMS, 39% in RA, and 26% in normal controls, with no significant differences between the groups. In fact, no significant differences were found between these groups in any lifetime psychiatric diagnoses in this study.

The *relationship between the psychiatric status and clinical features* in fibromyalgia was assessed in one study employing a multivariate approach.[98] It was found that the central features of fibromyalgia (e.g., number of sites of the pain symptom, number of tender points, sleep disturbance, and fatigue), as well as other features of this syndrome (e.g., paresthesia and swollen feeling), were independent of the psychological status. However, pain severity correlated significantly with psychological disturbance,[98] as is the case with other diseases, such as RA.[60]

Finally, it should be noted that virtually all of the studies of psychological status in FMS mentioned above involved patients seen in a rheumatology clinic, with likely referral biases. The only psychological study of patients with FMS seen in a primary care clinic did not show significant differences between fibromyalgia patients and other clinic patients used as controls.[23] It is clear that abnormal psychological status is not a requirement for development of fibromyalgia.[23, 109]

Pathophysiologic Mechanisms

The pathogenesis of FMS is not well understood. It is clear that FMS is not a psychiatric disorder, and as stated above, an abnormal psychiatric status is not necessary for developing fibromyalgia features. FMS is most likely a multifactorial syndrome, of which neuroendocrine aberrations seem most important.[95] Limited data suggest a genetic predisposition[62, 114] which, along with

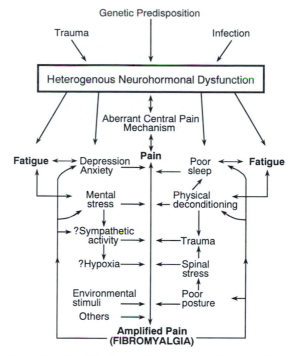

FIG 1–3. Probable pathophysiologic mechanisms in fibromyalgia syndrome (FMS), showing various interacting factors. The most important mechanism in FMS most likely involves neurohormonal dysfunctions. (Modified from Yunus MB: *J Rheumatol* 19:846–850, 1992. Used by permission.)

other stresses (e.g., infection, trauma), may cause a neuroendocrine dysfunction (Fig 1–3). Such a dysfunction alone may cause fibromyalgia in many patients, whereas in others peripheral factors (such as trauma, painful peripheral arthritis, and possible muscle microtrauma from deconditioning) may interact to amplify pain through the mechanism of central nervous system plasticity. Poor sleep, also related to neuroendocrine factors, is likely to be another important interacting factor (see Fig 1–3). Central (neuroendocrine) and peripheral mechanisms are discussed separately below.

Central Mechanisms

Pain is the most important symptom of FMS. The nociceptors (pain receptors) are activated by mechanical, thermal, and chemical stimuli in peripheral tissues. Pain is transmitted by A-deta and C fibers; C fibers utilize substance P (SP) as an important neurotransmitter, although other neurotransmitters may also be involved. The neurotransmitters involved in pain inhibition include serotonin, norepinephrine, γ-aminobutyric acid (GABA), enkephalin, and other less studied neurochemicals.[95, 109] An increased activity of the excitatory neurotransmitter SP or a deficiency of the inhibitory ones may, therefore, cause abnormal pain, may be the case with FMS.

A significantly increased level of SP in the cerebrospinal fluid (CSF) of fibromyalgia patients has been demonstrated as compared with normal controls.[86] A deficiency of serotonin in fibromyalgia found by controlled studies is suggested by low levels of plasma or serum tryptophan (a precursor of serotonin),[66, 101] a decreased transport ratio of plasma tryptophan (an indicator of the brain entry of tryptophan),[101] and a decreased level of CSF 5-hydroxyindoleacetic acid (a metabolite of serotonin).[67] Further, significantly decreased levels of 3-methoxy-4-hydroxyphenethylene glycol (a metabolite of norephinephrine) and homovanillic acid (a metabolite of dopamine) in the CSF of fibromyalgia patients, as compared with CSF values in normal pain-free controls, have also been reported.[67]

Further aberrations of neuroendocrine functions in FMS are supported by an abnormal hypothalamic-pituitary-adrenal axis[30, 52] and low levels of somatomedin C,[14] which reflects an integrated secretion of growth hormone. A decreased level of this hormone was hypothesized because of the fact that much of its secretion occurs during stage 4 sleep, which is disturbed in fibromyalgia.[39, 56] Decreased levels of plasma histidine (a precursor of histamine), methionine (a precursor of S-adenosylmethionine), and of tryptophan, among others in discriminating FMS from normal controls in a multivariate combination[99] also support a neuroendocrine dysfunction, since central neurotransmitter functions have been reported for histamine,[63] S-adenosylmethionine,[19] and serotonin.[16] It has been hypothesized that fibromyalgia results from a complex interaction of more than one neurotransmitter and neurohormone and their receptors, and that these dysfunctions are different from those present in psychiatric disorders.[95, 96] The neurohormonal dysfunctions may be triggered in a genetically predisposed individual by nonspecific stressors, such as physical and psychological trauma, as well as by infection, and by pain itself (see Fig 1–3).

The above-mentioned hypothesis of central pain mechanisms would explain pain and tenderness on palpation even in the absence of pathologic changes in the peripheral tissues, since an abnormally decreased pain threshold caused by neurohormonal changes would be sufficient to cause the pain and tender point features. Many areas of tenderness found in FMS are also tender normally,[113] but the above mechanisms would amplify this phenomenon.

Cognitive dysfunctions observed in some fibromyalgia patients as well as poor sleep are also most likely due to an abnormality in the neuroendocrine functions. Fatigue, an important symptom in fibromyalgia, appears to be predominantly of central origin, aggravated further by muscle deconditioning, poor sleep, and psychological factors. Animal studies suggest that serotonin is a modulator of non-REM sleep as well as pain,[22] but neurotransmitters or neurochemicals involved in cognitive symptoms and fatigue in fibromyalgia have not been specifically studied. It is of interest, however, that the discriminant scores of the seven biochemical variables (including plasma histidine, methionine, tryptophan, and norephinephrine) in our recent study[99] mentioned above correlated ($P < .001$) with fatigue.

Peripheral Mechanisms

Peripheral factors probably play a role in the pathogenesis of FMS in a subgroup of patients. From currently available data mentioned above, muscle biopsy findings do not seem to be significantly abnormal compared with those of appropriately selected normal controls. However, some patients who develop acute localized musculoskeletal pain (e.g., in the neck region) following trauma (e.g., an automobile accident), develop more widespread pain with multiple tender points at a later time. The same phenomenon has been observed in repetitive occupational injuries.[48] It seems that the development of FMS in this group of patients may involve the mechanism of central nervous system (CNS) plasticity through neuroendocrine dysfunctions.[95] Spinal stress[80] and poor posture are probably other forms of indirect trauma that may contribute to pain in FMS.

Bennett[11] proposes that the primary defect in FMS is muscle microtrauma secondary to deconditioning to which patients with this condition may be predisposed. However, current controlled studies do not show significant muscle changes compatible with such trauma or activation of muscle nociceptors. While physical deconditioning may play a role, such deconditioning seems to be secondary to pain or fatigue, or both. Other peripheral factors of possible significance include probable sympathetic overactivity,[6, 13] although it is unclear if this is secondary to a central mechanism or reflective of an effect of chronic pain. Sympathetic function was found to be normal in FMS in a recent study[27] and needs further studies with appropriate pain controls and evaluation of its relationship to psychological factors.

In conclusion, the most important pathophysiologic mechanisms in fibromyalgia involve central mechanisms with aberrant neuroendocrine functions which explain widespread pain and tenderness in multiple tissues (including not just muscles, but also skin, ligaments, and bone), fatigue, poor sleep, and (in a subset of patients) cognitive impairment. There is a lack of convincing evidence for nociceptor-activating pathologic changes in peripheral tissues in chronic FMS, although in a subset of patients such changes following acute trauma may trigger neuroendocrine aberrations in a genetically predisposed individual; this would subsequently cause widespread and chronic musculoskeletal pain and tenderness, as well as other features of FMS, such as fatigue.

Summary

Fibromyalgia syndrome is characterized by *widespread* musculoskeletal pain and *tender points* on palpation at multiple sites. It is a common condition. It seems quite likely that FMS is part of a spectrum of other dysfunctional syndromes ("dysfunctional spectrum syndrome") including, among others, irritable bowel syndrome, chronic headaches, and primary dysmenorrhea. Although significant psychological factors may be present in a minority subgroup of FMS patients, these factors act to aggravate pain, rather than play a primary causative role. There is a lack of convincing evidence for significant pathologic changes in muscles and other peripheral tissues in FMS. The most important pathologic mechanisms in this syndrome involve neuroendocrine dysfunctions.

MYOFASCIAL PAIN SYNDROME

Definition, Terminology, and General Comments

Myofascial pain syndrome (MPS) has been defined as a *regional* pain syndrome accompanied by trigger point(s). A trigger point is stated to have the following characteristics: localized tenderness, presence of a taut band, twitch response, and referred pain on palpation of a trigger point site.[34, 76] MPS has also been called fibromyositis, myofibrositis, myofascitis, myogelosis, and fibrositis.[34] Several authors have failed to distinguish between FMS and MPS, although the generalized vs. regional or localized nature of pain in these two conditions, respectively, seem to be generally accepted.

MPS is a common condition, perhaps more common than FMS, although the prevalence of MPS diagnosed by a validated set of criteria is currently unknown. Based on the strict (and empirical) criteria of regional pain with referral of pain to a specific zone on palpation of a tender spot (a trigger point),

Skootsky and Jaeger[77] found that 16 (9.3%) of 172 patients seen in a university general internal medicine practice had MPS. This prevalence figure was based on both new and follow-up cases which were not separately analyzed.

Regional musculoskeletal pain conditions have been documented in the European literature since the 18th century.[64] The current concept of MPS, however, has been mostly expounded by Travell and Rinzler[82] and by Simons.[74] Although a large number of publications are available on MPS, including a well-known manual,[83] information on this syndrome based on critical research is limited.

Clinical Features

Symptoms

Patients present with *regional pain,* mostly in the neck, shoulders, upper extremities, facial area, low back, and lower extremities. Fricton et al.[34] have quantitated pain and other symptoms among 164 patients diagnosed with MPS of the head and neck regions, based on the criteria of pain and trigger points, as defined above. Eighty-two percent of patients were female and 18% were male, with a mean age of 41.2 years (range, 17–89 years). The mean symptom duration was 7 years for females and 6 years for males. The pain was variously described as pressure (48%), dull (27%), throbbing (26%), sharp (18%), burning (26%), and heavy (14%). Similar to FMS, pain symptoms were aggravated by tension, emotional stress, and exercise, and alleviated by local heat, relaxing, and mild exercise.

Besides pain, several other musculoskeletal and nonmusculoskeletal symptoms were also present, including poor sleep, "swelling," stiff joints, tinnitus, fatigue, paresthesia, nausea, and constipation (Table 1–7). Self-reported depression and anxiety were present in 21% and 18%, respectively. The above-mentioned frequencies of symptoms described by Fricton et al.[34] are useful, but unfortunately they were not compared with a control group.

TABLE 1–7.

Symptoms Reported in Myofascial Pain Syndrome of the Head and Neck (N = 164)*

Symptom	Percent
Musculoskeletal†	
Stiff joints	20
"Swelling"	12
Nonmusculoskeletal	
Poor sleep	42
Tinnitus	42
Ear pain	42
Fatigue	40
Paresthesia	27
Nausea	25
Dizziness	23
Constipation	15
Psychological (by self-report)	
Global depression	21
Global anxiety	18

*Data from Fricton JR, Kroening R, Haley D, et al: *Oral Surg Oral Med Oral Pathol* 60:615–623, 1985.
†Regional musculoskeletal pain was present in 100%.

Signs

The most characteristic physical sign in MPS, by frequently used criteria,[34, 76, 83] is the presence of trigger point(s) as defined above. Diagrams have been published depicting the areas of trigger points and the zones of referred pain on palpation of these points (see Part II, Chapters 7–11).[34, 76, 82, 83] Fricton et al.[34] quantitated the areas of pain with their trigger point locations among their patients seen in a temporomandibular joint (TMJ) and craniofacial clinic. However, the percentage of frequencies of each trigger point location related to a particular area of pain symptom is not known. A large majority of the patients understandably had pain in the jaw (63%) and the TMJ (56%) areas. The corresponding trigger point locations related to these two sites of the pain symptom were superficial masseter, trapezius, digastric, and the medial pterygoid muscles for the jaw pain, and deep masseter, temporalis, and lateral pterygoid muscles for the TMJ pain. It has been suggested that a knowledge of these referral patterns of pain is useful in identifying the "source" (the trigger points) of the presenting pain, so that the trigger points can then be treated appropriately with injection therapy.[34, 83] However, a recent blinded study showed poor interobserver reliability in referral patterns of trigger points among 50 patients with low back pain.[58]

Trigger points have been classified empirically as active and "latent."[76, 83] An *active trigger point* has been defined as an area of tenderness on palpation in the taut band of a muscle, causing referred pain similar to the patient's spontaneous pain complaint. Additionally, a local twitch response should also be visible either on manual palpation of the tender spot or following a needle insertion into this spot. A *latent trigger point* has all of the above characteristics, except for absence of the referred pain similar to the patient's spontaneous pain symptom.[76, 83]

Besides the presence of trigger points, the physical examination in MPS is normal, with an absence of objective joint swelling or neurologic deficits. The range of motion in a joint may be decreased because of pain or a subsequent development of adhesive capsulitis in some patients secondary to trauma. Similarly, the muscle strength may appear to be decreased secondary to pain.

A major problem with the trigger points defined above is that they have not been validated by a blinded and controlled study with normal controls and other patients with chronic pain, such as arthritis. While experimental data support the concept of referred pain,[40, 44] which was reported to be significantly more common in MPS than in normal controls in one study,[92] other findings such as taut band and twitch response are likely to be equally common in healthy pain-free controls. In a recent preliminary study by Wolfe et al.,[92] four experts on MPS examined three groups of subjects (seven with FMS, eight with MPS, and eight pain-free healthy controls) in a blinded manner. Among eight unilateral muscle sites examined by the four MPS experts, local tenderness was found in 82% of examinations, active trigger points in 18%, and latent trigger point in only 2%; while taut band and muscle twitch were found in 50% and 30% respectively, these figures were not significantly different from those found among normal healthy controls or patients with FMS.

In another report, Nice et al.[58] studied intertest reliability of trigger points (defined as hyperirritable areas with referred pain in a predictable zone as described by Travell and Simons[83]) among 12 observers who examined 50 patients with low back pain. Based on low kappa values (.29–.38) and proportion of positive agreements (.43–.52), the authors concluded that examination for trigger points as defined above is unreliable.[58]

Perpetuating Factors

Several perpetuating factors for symptoms and signs of MPS have been suggested. These include mechanical factors, nutritional deficiencies (vitamins B_1, B_6, B_{12}, and folic acid), metabolic and endocrine inadequacies (hypothyroidism, hypoglycemia, hyperuricemia), psychological factors, poor sleep, and chronic infections.[83] While no data are available to support any of these claims, it seems reasonable to suspect that mechanical factors (including trauma and abnormal posture), psychological distress, acute viral or bacterial infections, and non-restorative sleep would aggravate either regional or generalized musculoskeletal pain. No data are currently available to support the notion that vitamin or endocrine deficiencies perpetuate MPS.

Laboratory Tests

Routine laboratory tests, including complete blood count, ESR, and liver and renal function tests, are normal. Routine thyroid function tests or determinations of serum vitamin levels are not recommended. Several tests, as discussed below, have been claimed to be abnormal and will be critically evaluated.

Muscle Biopsy Studies

In a useful review, Simons[75] has described the results of muscle biopsy in regional muscle pain conditions. The findings include fat accumulation, increased sarcolemmal nuclei, fiber changes, and interstitial changes by light microscopy[53]; accumulation of mucinous substance by chemical analysis[3]; and myofibrillar lysis along with capillary changes by EM.[29] These muscle biopsy reports were subsequently evaluated critically by Yunus and Kalyan-Raman,[106] and found to be unreliable because of omission of the criteria used for patient selection, the small number of cases studied, and, above all, a failure to include controls for blinded assessment. It was concluded that no data exist to suggest that muscle biopsy findings are abnormal in MPS.[106]

Electromyographic Studies

Results of several EMG studies in MPS have been reported.[26, 33, 45, 74] Kraft et al.[45] found the clinical areas of muscle spasm to be electrically silent. Motor unit activities were found to be increased in palpable bands in two reports,[33, 74] including one in which clinical twitch responses were elicited on one side but none in the normal contralateral side, which was used as a control site.[33] These results simply reflect the EMG findings of a twitch response in a palpable band which have not been found to be significantly more common in MPS than in normal healthy controls as discussed above.[92] Not surprisingly, EMG recordings from a trigger point, *not* necessarily associated with a twitch response, were normal in another recent study.[26] One may summarize by stating that no consistent EMG abnormalities have been demonstrated in MPS, as compared with controls.

Sleep Studies

Self-reported poor sleep was present in 42% of patients in the study of Fricton et al.[34] Saskin and his colleagues[68] described alpha anomaly in non-REM sleep of 11 female patients with pain related to a motor vehicle accident or work-related trauma; mean duration of the pain symptom was 2.4 years. These findings were similar to those in 11 female patients with FMS. Although not specified, it is likely that some patients in the posttrauma group had MPS.

Thermographic Studies

Bennett[12] and Travell and Simons[83] reviewed the thermographic studies in MPS and found them to be inconsistent, with the findings of both hot and cold spots. In view of a lack of appropriate controls with blindedness, these reports do not provide a reliable conclusion on the status of thermographic findings in MPS. Further well-designed studies in this area are obviously needed.

Diagnosis and Differential Diagnosis

Current criteria suggested by Simons for MPS[76] are shown in Table 1–8. They essentially include regional pain and active trigger point(s) as described earlier, except that the requirement of a twitch response is now listed under Minor criteria. I have previously[96] suggested that acceptable criteria for MPS should be derived from a multicenter controlled and blinded study similar to the ACR criteria study for FMS, including appropriate controls.[93] For a priori case definition, patients with regional pain and tender point(s) (with *or* without referred pain) alone should be included. Subsequently, statistical analyses should be undertaken to examine if MPS patients with additional features of referred pain, taut band, and so forth, are really different from those with regional pain and tender points (without referred pain) alone, and if these additional features significantly improve sensitivity and specificity. No appropriately collected data in a controlled and blinded study are available to demonstrate that patients with tender point(s) *and* referred pain are significantly different from those with only tender points (and no radiation of pain) with regard to their clinical characteristics, treatment response, or long-term prognosis. The criteria should also define "regional pain" and the required symptom duration.

MPS should be differentiated from other causes of local and regional pain, including arthritis, infection, malignancy, and mechanical cases. Patients with systemic symptoms (anorexia, weight loss, fever) and those with positive rheumatologic or neurologic findings should be appropriately investigated. As stated earlier, routine blood tests, urinalysis, and radiographs are normal in uncomplicated "primary" MPS. Adhesive capsulitis, reflex sympathetic dystrophy, and thoracic outlet syndrome[71] should be appropriately ruled out in a patient pre-

---

TABLE 1–8.

Empirical Criteria Suggested for Diagnosis of Myofascial Pain Syndrome (MPS)*

A. Major criteria (active trigger points).
  1. Regional pain complaint.
  2. Taut band palpable in an accessible muscle.
  3. Exquisite spot of tenderness in the taut band.
  4. Pain complaint or altered sensation in the expected distribution of referred pain from the tender spot.
  5. Some restricted range of motion, when measurable.

B. Minor criteria.
  1. Reproduction of clinical pain complaint, or altered sensation, by pressure on the tender spot.
  2. Local twitch response by transverse snapping palpation of, or needle insertion into, the taut band.
  3. Pain alleviation by stretching the involved muscle or injecting the tender spot in it.

For diagnosis of MPS, all the major criteria and at least one of the three minor criteria need to be fulfilled.

*Modified with permission from Simons DG: Muscular pain syndromes. In Fricton JR, Awad EA, editors: *Advances in pain research and therapy*, vol 17, New York, 1990, Raven Press, pp 1–41.

senting with upper extremity pain, which was found to be the most common symptomatic site in MPS in a recent study.[69]

The clinical features of FMS with widespread pain and tender points[93, 111, 113] are different from those in MPS with regional pain and tenderness as described above. Several differences of interest emerged in a direct comparison study of 20 patients with FMS and 19 with MPS.[69] Patients with FMS were older (mean age, 46 years vs. 34.7 years), had greater pain intensity and total tender point ("myalgic") score, and lower pain threshold. The common sites of pain in this study[69] were right upper quadrant, left upper quadrant, left lower quadrant, and axial regions. Interestingly, no significant differences were found in self-reported global sleep quality, anxiety, or depression. However, for inexplicable reasons, three patients with pain "all over" were included in the MPS group, raising the question of "purity" of group classification.

Psychological Factors

Very few well-designed and detailed psychological studies have been carried out in MPS. Fricton et al.[34] have described depression in 21% of patients and anxiety in 18% by self-report, and 23% and 26%, respectively, by "psychological evaluation," the details of which were not provided. Fishbain et al.[31] studied psychiatric diagnoses by DSM-III criteria among 238 patients (132 men and 106 women) with MPS, apparently diagnosed by the criteria of Simons and Travell mentioned earlier. Current major depression was found in 3.8% of men and 4.5% of women. However, the proportion of patients with all forms of depression (including major depression, dysthymic disorder, and cyclothymic disorder) were present in 65% of women and 52% of men. Generalized anxiety disorder was present in 17% of women and 15% of men, whereas conversion disorder was diagnosed in 35% of men and 47% of women.[31] Apart from the question of whether patients with FMS were included (authors also used the term "fibrositis"), this study failed to include an age- and sex-matched normal pain-free group as well as another group with chronic pain (such as arthritis) as desirable controls. Inclusion of a control group with chronic pain in psychological evaluation of MPS or FMS is important in assessing the effects of chronic pain on the psychological status of these groups of patients.[96] Although reliable data are lacking in MPS, it would seem that patients with this condition overall have less psychological distress compared with those diagnosed as having FMS.

Pathophysiologic Mechanisms

Proposed pathophysiologic mechanisms in MPS[34, 83] include release of free calcium through disruption of sarcoplasmic reticulum following micro- or macrotrauma, an interaction of calcium with ATP, and subsequent muscle fiber contraction. This contraction later becomes sustained in a vicious cycle, leading to hypoxia and release of nociceptor-activating substances in the muscles, such as serotonin, bradykinin, and high concentrations of potassium. These noxious substances would further cause inflammation in the interstitial connective tissue, causing further disruption of the calcium pump.[34] The concept of trauma causing disruption of sarcoplasmic reticulum and subsequent changes (including hypoxia) was based on such findings as myofibrillar lysis and endothelial changes by EM,[29] accumulation of mucinous substances,[3] as well as interstitial inflammation,[53] none of which may be regarded reliable because of an absence of appropriate controls in the evaluation of muscle biopsies.[106] Overall, little experimental evidence exists in chronic cases of MPS to suggest elaboration of noxious substances to activate nociceptors.

It seems plausible that certain changes (inflammatory, metabolic) do occur in peripheral tissues in *acute* posttraumatic cases as well as work-related repetitive strain injury (RSI), causing activation of nociceptors.[70] In a genetically predisposed individual, the acute posttraumatic pain would likely become chronic, and perhaps subsequently generalized, through the mechanism of CNS plasticity, involving neuroendocrine aberrations with a dysfunction of various neurotransmitters (serotonin, norepinephrine, endorphins, substance P) as well as hormones of the hypothalamic-pituitary-adrenal axis,[95] as has been discussed above under Fibromyalgia Syndrome. The same mechanisms are also likely to be operative in causing chronic and generalized pain in many cases of RSI.[48] The nontraumatic cases of MPS perhaps represent an earlier and more localized stage of FMS, based on the proposed mechanisms of neurohormonal dysfunction without an initial peripheral cause.[95] However, it seems possible that in some cases which are not related to obvious trauma, various forms of mechanical stresses (poor posture, joint hyperlaxity, leg length discrepancies) would cause similar changes as in RSI on the basis of repetitive muscle overload.

The above-mentioned local and central (neuroendocrine) factors are likely to further interact with psychological factors, poor sleep, muscle deconditioning, various environmental factors (such as cold weather and noise), as well as the pain itself, to cause amplified and sustained chronic pain.[95]

RELATIONSHIP BETWEEN FIBROMYALGIA SYNDROME AND MYOFASCIAL PAIN SYNDROME

Similarities and differences between FMS and MPS are shown in Table 1–9. The relationship between these two syndromes has not been well studied, but they clearly overlap. It may be noted that trigger points with local tender spots and referred pain, said to be a characteristic finding in MPS, is not uncommon

TABLE 1–9.

Comparison of Various Features of Fibromyalgia Syndrome (FMS) and Myofascial Pain Syndrome (MPS) Based on Evaluation of Available Data*

Features	FMS	MPS
Musculoskeletal pain	Widespread	Regional
Tender points	Multiple, widespread	Few, regional
Referred pain	+	++
Taut band	Similar to normal controls	Similar to normal controls
Twitch response	Probably similar to normal controls	Similar to normal controls
Fatigue	++++	++
Poor sleep	++++	++
Paresthesia	+++	++
Headaches	+++	++
Irritable bowel	++	+
Swollen feeling in tissues	++	+

*+ = 24% or less; ++ = 25%–49%; +++ = 50%–74%; ++++ = 75%–100% of patients.

in FMS.[8, 92] An acute case of localized musculoskeletal pain is quite different from FMS, but as an acute case gradually evolves into a chronic form to qualify for a diagnosis of MPS, the resemblance between such a case and that of FMS becomes apparent. As hypothesized above, it seems possible that plastic changes occur in the CNS as pain continues, causing neurohormonal aberrations which lead to chronicity and, in some cases, generalized of pain and FMS, such as fatigue. It is hypothesized that *chronic* MPS represents forme fruste FMS. Many FMS patients give a clear history of initial localized pain with or without preceding trauma, and many patients diagnosed as having MPS may have more generalized pain and tender points on systematic enquiry and examination. Such a hypothesis can be tested in prospective studies of MPS with protocols that include recording of the pain symptom on a human figure and tenderness on palpation in all MPS and FMS sites,[92, 93, 113] along with other characteristic symptoms of FMS (see Table 1–2).

CONCLUSION

Fibromyalgia syndrome is characterized by widespread musculoskeletal pain and tenderness on palpation (tender points), whereas myofascial pain syndrome is a regional pain condition with "trigger points." Currently defined trigger points include localized tender spots, referred pain, and palpable band and twitch response—the reliability and validity of which need to be established by appropriately designed studies. Preliminary studies suggest that palpable bands and twitch responses are equally frequent in MPS, FMS, and pain-free healthy controls. The significance of referred pain in the definition of trigger points is also unknown. A multicenter controlled and blinded study is essential to establish acceptable criteria for MPS.

FMS and MPS share various other symptoms besides pain and tenderness on palpation, including fatigue, poor sleep, paresthesia, and irritable bowel symptoms. These symptoms are more common in FMS, but suggest that these two syndromes overlap, and may share aberrant central pain mechanisms as the most important pathophysiologic basis for maintenance of chronic pain. Peripheral mechanisms, including trauma and mechanical stresses, may be important in initiating symptoms in some cases of MPS and FMS. Further well-designed studies are clearly needed in these painful and common conditions that cause much disability in a large number of our patients.

REFERENCES

1. Ahles TA, Khan SA, Yunus MB, et al: Psychiatric status of primary fibromyalgia and rheumatoid arthritis patients and nonpain controls: A blinded comparison of DSM-III diagnoses, *Am J Psychiatry* 148:1721–1726, 1991.
2. American Psychiatric Association: *Diagnostic and Statistical Manual of Mental Disorders, DSM-III-R*, ed 3 revised, Washington, DC, 1987, American Psychiatric Association, pp 264–266.
3. Awad EA: Interstitial myofibrositis: Hypothesis of the mechanism, *Arch Phys Med Rehabil* 54:449–453, 1973.
4. Bartels EM, Danneskiold-Samsoe B: Histological abnormalities in muscle from patients with certain types of fibrositis, *Lancet* 1:755–757, 1986.

5. Bartels EM, Norregaard J, Harreby M, et al: Single cell morphology in fibromyalgia, *Scand J Rheumatol Suppl* 94:67, 1992.
6. Bengtsson A, Bengtsson M: Regional sympathetic blockade in primary fibromyalgia, *Pain* 33:161–167, 1988.
7. Bengtsson A, Ernerudh J, Vrethem M, et al: Absence of autoantibodies in primary fibromyalgia, *J Rheumatol* 16:1466–1468, 1989.
8. Bengtsson A, Henriksson KG, Jrfeldt L, et al.: Primary fibromyalgia: A clinical and laboratory study of 55 patients, *Scand J Rheumatol* 15:340–347, 1986.
9. Bengtsson A, Henriksson KG, Larsson J: Reduced high-energy phosphate levels in the painful muscles of patients with primary fibromyalgia, *Arthritis Rheum* 29:817–821, 1986.
10. Bengtsson A, Henriksson KG, Larsson J: Muscle biopsy in primary fibromyalgia: Light microscopical and histochemical findings, *Scand J Rheumatol* 15:1–6, 1986.
11. Bennett RM: Beyond fibromyalgia: Ideas on etiology and treatment, *J Rheumatol* 16(suppl 19):185–191, 1989.
12. Bennett RM: Myofascial pain syndromes and the fibromyalgia syndrome: A comparative analysis. In Fricton JR, Awad EA, editors: *Advances in pain research and therapy,* vol 17, New York, 1990, Raven Press, pp 43–65.
13. Bennett RM, Clark SR, Campbell SM, et al: Symptoms of Raynaud's syndrome in patients with fibromyalgia, *Arthritis Rheum* 34:264–269, 1991.
14. Bennett RM, Clark SR, Campbell SM, et al: Low levels of somatomedin C in patients with the fibromyalgia syndrome: A possible link between sleep and muscle pain, *Arthritis Rheum* 35:113–116, 1992.
15. Bennett RM, Clark SR, Goldberg L, et al: Aerobic fitness in patients with fibrositis: A controlled study of respiratory gas exchange and xenon clearance from exercising muscle, *Arthritis Rheum* 32:454–460, 1989.
16. Besson J-M, editor: *Serotonin and pain,* Amsterdam, 1990, Excerpta Medica.
17. Calabro JJ: Fibromyalgia (fibrositis) in children, *Am J Med* 81(suppl):57–59, 1986.
18. Campbell SM, Clark S, Tindal EA, et al: Clinical characteristics of fibrositis: I. A "blinded" controlled study of symptoms and tender points, *Arthritis Rheum* 26:817–824, 1983.
19. Carney MWP, Toone BK, Reynolds EH: S-adenosylmethionine and affective disorder, *Am J Med* 83(suppl 5A):104–106, 1987.
20. Caro XJ: Immunofluorescent detection of IgG at the dermal-epidermal junction in patients with apparent primary fibrositis syndrome, *Arthritis Rheum* 27:1174–1179, 1984.
21. Caro XJ, Wolfe F, Johnston WH, et al: A controlled and blinded study of immunoreactant deposition at the dermal-epidermal junction of patients with primary fibrositis syndrome, *J Rheumatol* 13:1086–1092, 1986.
22. Chase TN, Murphy DJ: Serotonin and central nervous systems function, *Annu Rev Pharmocol* 13:181–197, 1973.
23. Clark S, Campbell SM, Forehand ME, et al: Clinical characteristics of fibrositis. II. A "blinded" controlled study using standard psychological tests, *Arthritis Rheum* 28:132–137, 1985.
24. Dinerman H, Goldenberg DL, Felson DT, et al: A prospective evaluation of 118 patients with fibromyalgia syndrome: Prevalence of Raynaud's phenomenon, sicca syndrome, ANAs, low complement and IG deposition at the dermal epidermal junction, *J Rheumatol* 13:368–373, 1986.
25. Drewes AM, Andreasen A, Schroder HD, et al: Muscle biopsy in fibromyalgia. *Scand J Rheumatol Suppl* 94:20, 1992.
26. Durette MR, Rodriguez AA, Agre JC, et al: Needle electromyographic evaluation of patients with myofascial or fibromyalgic pain, *Am J Phys Med Rehabil* 70:154–156, 1991.
27. Elam M, Johnsson G, Wallin BG: Do patients with primary fibromyalgia have an altered muscle sympathetic nerve activity?, *Pain* 48:371–375, 1992.
28. Erickson PP, Lindman R, Stal P, et al: Symptoms and signs of mandibular dysfunction in primary fibromyalgia syndrome, *Swed Dent J* 12:141–149, 1988.
29. Fassbender HG: *Pathology of rheumatic disease,* New York, 1975, Springer Verlag, pp 304–307.
30. Ferraccioli G, Cavalieri F, Salaffi F, et al: Neuroendocrine findings in primary fibromyalgia and in other chronic rheumatic conditions (rheumatoid arthritis, low back pain), *J Rheumatol* 17:869–873, 1990.

31. Fishbain DA, Goldberg M, Steele R, et al: DSM-III diagnoses of patients with myofascial pain syndrome (fibrositis), *Arch Phys Med Rehabil* 70:433–438, 1989.
32. Forseth KO, Gran JT: The prevalence of fibromyalgia among women aged 20–49 years in Arandal, Norway, *Scand J Rheumatol* 21:74–78, 1992.
33. Fricton JR, Auvinen M, Dykstra D, et al: Myofascial pain syndrome: Electromyographic changes associated with the local twitch response, *Arch Phys Med Rehabil* 66:314–317, 1985.
34. Fricton JR, Kroening R, Haley D, et al: Myofascial pain syndrome of the head and neck: A review of clinical characteristics of 164 patients, *Oral Surg Oral Med Oral Pathol* 60:615–623, 1985.
35. Goldenberg DL: Fibromyalgia syndrome: An emerging but controversial condition, *JAMA* 257:2782–2787, 1987.
36. Goldenberg DL: Fibromyalgia and its relation to chronic fatigue syndrome, viral illness and immune abnormalities, *J Rheumatol* 16(suppl 19):91–93, 1989.
37. Goldenberg DL: Psychological symptoms and psychiatric diagnosis in patients with fibromyalgia, *J Rheumatol* 16(suppl 19):127–130, 1989.
38. Gowers WR: Lumbago: Its lessons and analogues. *Br Med J* 1:117–121, 1904.
39. Gupta MA, Moldofsky H: Dysthymic disorders and rheumatic pain modulation disorder (fibrositis syndrome): A comparison of symptoms and sleep physiology, *Can J Psychiatry* 31:608–616, 1986.
40. Hockaday JM, Whitty CWM: Patterns of referred pain in the normal subject, *Brain* 90:481–496, 1967.
41. Jacobsen S, Wildschiodtz G, Danneskiold-Samsoe B: Isokinetic and isometric muscle strength combined with transcutaneous electrical muscle stimulation in primary fibromyalgia syndrome, *J Rheumatol* 18:1390–1393, 1991.
42. Jacobsson L, Lindgarde F, Manthorpe R: The commonest rheumatic complaints of over six weeks' duration in a twelve-month period in a defined Swedish population, *Scand J Rheumatol* 10:841–844, 1983.
43. Kalyan-Raman UP, Kalyan-Raman K, Yunus MB, et al: Muscle pathology in primary fibromyalgia syndrome: Light microscopic, histochemical and ultrastructural study, *J Rheumatol* 11:808–813, 1984.
44. Kellgren JH: Deep pain sensibility, *Lancet* 1:943–949,1949.
45. Kraft GH, Johnson EW, LaBan MM: The fibrositis syndrome, *Arch Phys Med Rehabil* 49:152–162, 1968.
46. Leavitt F, Katz RS: Is the MMPI invalid for assessing psychological disturbance in pain related organic conditions?, *J Rheumatol* 16:521–526, 1989.
47. Leavitt F, Katz RS, Golden HE, et al: Comparison of pain properties in fibromyalgia patients and rheumatoid arthritis patients, *Arthritis Rheum* 29:775–781, 1986.
48. Littlejohn GO: Fibrositis/fibromyalgia syndrome in the workplace, *Rheum Dis Clin North Am* 15:45–60, 1989.
49. Lund N, Bengtsson A, Thorborg P: Muscle tissue oxygen pressure in primary fibromyalgia, *Scand J Rheumatol* 15:165–173, 1986.
50. Lyddell C, Meyers OL: The prevalence of fibromyalgia in a South African community, *Scand J Rheumatol Suppl* 94:8, 1992.
51. McBroom P, Walsh NE, Dumitro D: Electromyography in primary fibromyalgia syndrome, *Clin J Pain* 4:117–119, 1988.
52. McCain GA: Nonmedicinal treatments in primary fibromyalgia, *Rheum Clin North Am* 15:73–90, 1989.
53. Miehlke K, Schulze G, Eger W: Klinische und experimentelle Untersuchungen zum Fibrositissyndrom, *Z Rheumatol* 19:310–330, 1960.
54. Moldofsky H, Lue FA, Smythe HA: Alpha EEG sleep and morning symptoms in rheumatoid arthritis, *J Rheumatol* 10:373–379, 1983.
55. Moldofsky H, Saskin P, Lue FA: Sleep and symptoms in fibrositis syndrome after a febrile illness, *J Rheumatol* 15:1701–1704, 1988.
56. Moldofsky H, Scarisbrick P, England R, et al: Musculoskeletal symptoms and non-REM sleep disturbance in patients with "fibrositis" syndrome and healthy subjects, *Psychosom Med* 37:341–351, 1975.
57. Müller W: The fibrositis syndrome: Diagnosis, differential diagnosis and pathogenesis, *Scand J Rheumatol Suppl* 65:40–53, 1987.
58. Nice DA, Riddle DL, Lamb RL, et al: Intertester reliability of judgements of the presence of trigger points in patients with low back pain, *Arch Phys Med Rehabil* 73:893–898, 1992.

59. Nishikai M: Fibromyalgia in Japanese, *J Rheumatol* 19:110–114, 1991.
60. Parker J, Frank R, Beck N, et al: Pain in rheumatoid arthritis: Relationship to demographic, medical and psychological factors, *J Rheumatol* 15:433–437, 1988.
61. Pellegrino MJ: Atypical chest pain as an initial presentation of primary fibromyalgia, *Arch Phys Med Rehabil* 71:526–528, 1990.
62. Pellegrino MJ, Waylonis GW, Sommer A: Familial occurrence of primary fibromyalgia, *Arch Phys Med Rehabil* 70:61–63, 1989.
63. Prell GD, Green JP: Histamine as a neuroregulator, *Annu Rev Neurosci* 9:209–254, 1986.
64. Reynolds MD: The development of the concept of fibrositis, *Hist Med Allied Sci* 38:5–35, 1983.
65. Riley PA, Littlejohn GO: Peripheral arthralgic presentation of fibrositis/ fibromyalgia syndrome, *J Rheumatol* 19:281–283, 1992.
66. Russell IJ, Michalek JE, Vipraio GA, et al: Serum amino acids in fibrositis/ fibromyalgia concentration, *J Rheumatol* 16(suppl 19):158–163, 1989.
67. Russell IJ, Vaerøy H, Javors M, et al: Cerebrospinal fluid biogenic amine metabolites in fibromyalgia/fibrositis syndrome and rheumatoid arthritis, *Arthritis Rheum* 35:550–556, 1992.
68. Saskin P, Moldofsky H, Lue FA: Sleep and posttraumatic rheumatic pain modulation disorder (fibrositis syndrome), *Psychosom Med* 48:319–323, 1986.
69. Scudds RA, Trachsel LCE, Luckhurst BJ, et al: A comparative study of pain, sleep quality and pain responsiveness in fibrositis and myofascial pain syndrome *J Rheumatol* 16(suppl 19):120–126, 1989.
70. Sejersted OM: Acute localized muscle pain: Etiology and pathogenesis, *Scand J Rheumatol Suppl* 94:3, 1992.
71. Sheon RP, Moskowitz RW, Goldberg VM: *Soft tissue rheumatic pain,* ed 2, Philadelphia, 1987, Lea & Febiger.
72. Sietsema KE, Cooper DM, Caro XJ: Oxygen utilization during muscular exercise in patients with primary fibromyalgia patients (abstract), *Arthritis Rheum* 33(suppl):S137, 1990.
73. Simms RW, Roy S, Skrinar G, et al: 31P-NMR spectroscopy of muscle in fibromyalgia patients and sedentary controls. *Arthritis Rheum* 34:S189, 1991.
74. Simons DG: Electrogenic nature of palpable bands and "jump sign" associated with myofascial trigger points, *Adv Pain Res Ther* 1:913–918, 1976.
75. Simons DG: Muscle pain syndrome—Part II, *Am J Phys Med* 55:15–42, 1976.
76. Simons DG: Muscular pain syndromes. In Fricton JR, Awad EA, editors: *Advances in pain research and therapy,* vol 17, New York, 1990, Raven Press, pp 1–41.
77. Skootsky SA, Jaeger B, Oye RK: Prevalence of myofascial pain in general internal medicine practice, *West J Med* 151:157–160, 1989.
78. Smythe HA: Non-articular rheumatism and the fibrositis. In McCarty DJ, editor: *Arthritis and allied conditions: A textbook of rheumatolgy,* Philadelphia, 1972, Lea & Febiger, pp 874–884.
79. Smythe HA: Non-articular rheumatism and psychogenic musculoskeletal syndromes. In McCarty DJ, editor: *Arthritis and allied conditions: A textbook of rheumatology,* Philadelphia, 1979, Lea & Febiger, pp 881–891.
80. Smythe HA: Non-articular rheumatism and psychogenic musculoskeletal syndromes. In McCarty DJ Jr, editor: *Arthritis and allied conditions: A textbook of rheumatology,* ed 11, Philadelphia, 1989, Lea & Febiger, pp 1241–1254.
81. Traut EF: Fibrositis, *J Am Geriatr Soc* 16:531–538, 1968.
82. Travell JG, Rinzler SH: The myofascial genesis of pain, *Postgrad Med* 11:425–434, 1952.
83. Travell JG, Simons DG: *Myofascial pain and dysfunction: The trigger point manual,* Baltimore, 1983, Williams & Wilkins.
84. Tunks E, Crook J, Norman G, et al: Tender points in fibromyalgia, *Pain* 34:11–19, 1988.
85. Uveges JM, Parker JC, Smarr KL, et al: Psychological symptoms in primary fibromyalgia syndrome: Relationship to pain, life stress and sleep disturbance, *Arthritis Rheum* 33:1279–1283, 1990.
86. Vaerøy H, Helle R, Forre Ø, et al: Elevated CSF levels of substance P and high incidence of Raynaud's phenomenon in patients with fibromyalgia: New features for diagnosis, *Pain* 32:21–26, 1988.
87. Valen PA, Flory W, Powell M, et al: Forearm ischemic exercise testing and

plasma ATP degradation products in primary fibromyalgia, *Arthritis Rheum* 31:C115, 1988.

88. Wallace DJ: Genitourinary manifestations of fibrositis: An increased association with the female urethral syndrome, *J Rheumatol* 17:238–239, 1990.
89. Wolfe F: The clinical syndrome of fibrositis, *Am J Med* 81:7–14, 1986.
90. Wolfe F: The epidemiology of fibromyalgia, *JMP* (in press).
91. Wolfe F, Hawley DJ, Cathey MA, et al: Fibrositis: Symptom frequency and criteria for diagnosis, *J Rheumatol* 12:1159–1163, 1985.
92. Wolfe F, Simons DG, Fricton J, et al: The fibromyalgia and myofascial pain syndromes: A preliminary study of tender points and trigger points in persons with fibromyalgia, myofascial pain syndrome and no disease, *J Rheumatol* 19:944–951, 1992.
93. Wolfe F, Smythe HA, Yunus MB, et al: The American College of Rheumatology 1990 criteria for classification of fibromyalgia: Report of the Multicenter Criteria Committee, *Arthritis Rheum* 33:160–172, 1990.
94. Yunus MB: Fibromyalgia syndrome: A need for uniform classification, *Compr Ther* 10:841–844, 1983.
95. Yunus MB: Towards a model of pathophysiology of fibromyalgia: aberrant central pain mechanisms with peripheral modulation, *J Rheumatol* 19:846–850, 1992.
96. Yunus MB: Research in fibromyalgia and myofascial pain syndromes: Current status, problems and future directions, *JMP* 1:23–41, 1992.
97. Yunus MB: Psychological factors in fibromyalgia syndrome: An overview, *JMP* (in press).
98. Yunus MB, Ahles TA, Aldag JC, et al: Relationship of clinical features with psychological status in primary fibromyalgia, *Arthritis Rheum* 34:15–21, 1991.
99. Yunus MB, Aldag JC, Dailey JW, et al: Interrelationships of biochemical parameters in classification of fibromyalgia and normal controls, *Arthritis Rheum* 35:S113, 1992.
100. Yunus MB, Berg BC, Masi AT: Multiphase skeletal scintigraphy in primary fibromyalgia syndrome: A blinded study, *J Rheumatol* 16:1466–1468, 1989.
101. Yunus MB, Dailey JW, Aldag JC, et al: Plasma tryptophan and other amino acids in primary fibromyalgia: A controlled study, *J Rheumatol* 19:90–94, 1992.
102. Yunus MB, Dailey JW, Aldag JC, et al: Plasma and urinary catecholamines in primary fibromyalgia: A controlled study, *J Rheumatol* 19:95–97, 1992.
103. Yunus MB, Holt GS, Masi AT, et al: Fibromyalgia syndrome among the elderly: Comparison with younger patients, *J Am Geriatr Soc* 35:987–995, 1988.
104. Yunus MB, Hussey FX, Aldag JC: Antinuclear antibodies and "connective tissue disease features" in fibromyalgia syndrome: A controlled study, *J Rheumatol* (in press).
105. Yunus MB, Hussey FX, Aldag JC, et al: Antinuclear antibodies and connective tissue disease features in primary fibromyalgia (abstract), *Arthritis Rheum* 34:R12, 1991.
106. Yunus MB, Kalyan-Raman UP: Muscle biopsy findings in primary fibromyalgia and other forms of nonarticular rheumatism, *Rheum Dis Clin North Am* 15:115–134, 1989.
107. Yunus MB, Kalyan-Raman UP, Masi AT, et al: Electron microscopic studies of muscle biopsy in primary fibromyalgia syndrome: A controlled and blinded study, *J Rheumatol* 16:97–101, 1989.
108. Yunus MB, Masi AT: Juvenile primary fibromyalgia syndrome, *Arthritis Rheum* 28:138–144, 1985.
109. Yunus MB, Masi AT: Fibromyalgia, restless legs syndrome, periodic limb movement disorder and psychogenic pain. In McCarty DJ Jr, Koopman WJ, editors: *Arthritis and allied conditions: A textbook of rheumatology*, Philadelphia, 1992, Lea & Febiger, pp 1383–1405.
110. Yunus MB, Masi AT, Aldag JC: Preliminary criteria for primary fibromyalgia syndrome (PFS): Multivariate analysis of a consecutive series of PFS, other pain patients, and normal subjects, *Clin Exp Rheumatol* 7:63–69, 1989.
111. Yunus MB, Masi AT, Aldag JC: A controlled study of primary fibromyalgia syndrome: Clinical features and association with other functional syndromes, *J Rheumatol* 16(suppl. 19):62–71, 1989.
112. Yunus MB, Masi AT, Aldag JC: Short-term effects of ibuprofen in primary fibro-

myalgia syndrome: A double blind, placebo controlled trial, *J Rheumatol* 16:527–532, 1989.

113. Yunus MB, Masi AT, Calabro JJ, et al: Primary fibromyalgia (fibrositis): Clinical study of 50 patients with matched normal controls, *Semin Arthritis Rheum* 11:151–171, 1981.
114. Yunus MB, Rawlings KK, Khan MA: A study of multicase families with fibromyalgia with HLA typing, *Arthritis Rheum* 35:S285, 1992.
115. Zidar J, Backman E, Bengtsson A, et al: Quantitative EMG and muscle tension in painful muscles in fibromyalgia, *Pain* 40:249–254, 1990.

Chapter 2

Treatment of Fibromyalgia and Myofascial Pain Syndromes

Glenn A. McCain, M.D.

Fibromyalgia (FMS) and myofascial pain syndromes (MPS) have undergone considerable scrutiny in recent years not only with respect to classification but also in regard to treatment. At present much of the recommended treatment strategy remains empirical and many often-used modalities are essentially unproven. This has fostered the development of many disparate types of therapeutic interventions and no cohesive approach or grand paradigm has emerged to date as the most efficacious. Nevertheless, some important strides have been made in recent years with the result that a body of knowledge has evolved which is based for the most part on firm scientific underpinnings. One such scientific advance has been the development of diagnostic criteria for FMS sanctioned by the American College of Rheumatology[38] (Table 2–1). The development of these criteria has served as an important preamble to the development of successful treatment modalities in that they have enabled investigators to study different types of interventions in a homogeneous patient population. A patient cohort with stable and reproducible clinical characteristics is a prerequisite for any conclusions regarding the efficacy of purportedly helpful interventions. Similarly, observation of patient responses to treatment leads naturally to theories about etiology. Testing of these hypotheses in turn leads to general principles of treatment and eventually to more firmly based concepts of causation and treatment. Diagnostic criteria for MPS have been suggested by one group of investigators (Table 2–2) and are in general use. However, these criteria have not been subjected to testing in the clinical realm and thus remain empirical in nature.[34]

It is the purpose of this chapter to summarize the literature on the treatment of FMS and MPS with special emphasis on those studies which use acceptable scientific methods of investigation. Studies using subexperimental designs and less stringent identification of homogeneous patient populations are not included.

FIBROMYALGIA SYNDROME

The long-term treatment of fibromyalgia remains problematic since the natural history of this condition appears to be one of continuous and unremitting

TABLE 2–1.

The American College of Rheumatology 1990 Criteria for the Classification of Fibromyalgia*†

1. History of widespread pain.

   Definition. Pain is considered widespread when all of the following are present: pain in the left side of the body, pain in the right side of the body, pain above the waist, pain below the waist. In addition, axial skeletal pain (cervical spine or anterior chest or thoracic spine or low back) must be present. In this definition, shoulder and buttock pain are considered as pain for each involved side. Low back pain is considered lower segment pain.

2. Pain in 11 of 18 tender point sites on digital palpation.

   Definition. Pain on digital palpation must be present in at least 11 of the following 18 tender point sites:
   Occiput: bilateral, at the suboccipital muscle insertion.
   Low cervical: bilateral, at the anterior aspect of the intertransverse spaces at C5–7.
   Trapezius: bilateral, at the midpoint of the upper border.
   Supraspinatus: bilateral, at origins above the medial border of the scapular spine.
   Second rib: bilateral, upper surfaces just lateral to the costochondral junctions.
   Lateral epicondyle: bilateral, 2 cm distal to the epicondyles.
   Gluteal: bilateral, in upper outer quandrants of buttocks in anterior fold of muscle.
   Greater trochanter: bilateral, posterior to the trochanteric prominence.
   Knee: bilateral, at the medial fat pad proximal to the joint line.

Digital palpation should be performed with a force of 4 kg.
For a tender point to be considered "positive" the subject must state that the palpation was painful. "Tender" is not to be considered "painful."

*Modified from Wolfe F, Smythe HA, Yunus MB, et al: *Arthritis Rheum* 33:160–172, 1990. Used by permission.
†For classification purposes, patients will be said to have fibromyalgia if both criteria are satisfied. Widespread pain must have been present for at least 3 months. The presence of a second clinical disorder does not exclude the diagnosis of fibromyalgia.

TABLE 2–2.

Clinical Criteria for the Diagnosis of Myofascial Pain*

Major criteria.

1. Regional pain complaint
2. Pain complaint or altered sensation in the expected distribution of referred pain from a myofascial trigger point
3. Taut band palpable in an accessible muscle
4. Exquisite spot tenderness at one point along the length of the taut band
5. Some degree of restricted range of motion, when measurable

Minor criteria.

1. Reproduction of clinical pain complaint, or altered sensation, by pressure on the tender spot
2. Elicitation of a local twitch response, by transverse snapping palpation at the tender spot or by needle insertion into the tender spot in the taut band
3. Pain alleviated by elongating (stretching) the muscle or by injecting the tender spot

*Modified from Simons DG: Muscular pain syndromes. In Fricton JR, Awad EA, editors: *Advances in pain research and treatment*, vol 17, New York, 1990, Raven Press, pp 1–41.

---

pain. One current report has shown that only 5% of patients sustained remission of all symptoms during a 3-year follow-up.[10] Over 60% of patients continued to complain of significant fatigue and nonrestorative sleep despite the fact that over 85% received medication during the study period. Even though some of these therapies have been studied with acceptable scientific rigor, no definitive treatment strategy has emerged. Two studies have asked patients about the effectiveness of their previous treatment regimens. Cathey et al.[6] surveyed medication use in 81 patients during the previous year of their illness. They noted that the average patient used 4.7 drugs during the year and was taking 3.8 medications at year's end. Of the 50% of patients taking amitriptyline or cyclobenzaprine only one third improved sufficiently to report moderate or great improvement. Interestingly, analgesics were reported to be as effective as these two medications. Goldenberg and co-workers[16, 17] have reported similar results after following 87 patients treated over a 3-year period. Their observations indicated that over 50% of patients failed to respond to numerous pharmacologic and nonpharmacologic therapies. This indicates that fibromyalgia patients present difficult treatment problems, and that the average patient will require multiple methods of treatment over the natural course of the disease, often with limited success.

A list of therapies purported to be beneficial in fibromyalgia is shown in Table 2–3. Treatments for fibromyalgia can be divided into those based on pharmacologic and on nonpharmacologic principles.

Pharmacologic Treatments

Acceptable clinical trials have now been completed showing that both amitriptyline[4, 17, 21, 33] and cyclobenzaprine[3, 30, 31] are effective in fibromyalgia. The recommended dose of these drugs (10–50 mg of amitriptyline and 10–30 mg of cyclobenzaprine) is much smaller than the dose used in the treatment of depression. In fact, even low doses of these drugs are often poorly tolerated in fibromyalgia as a result of what seems to be extreme sensitivity to their central nervous system and anticholinergic side effects. Common side effects are drowsiness, agitation, and gastrointestinal upset. Jaeschke et al.[21] have reported

TABLE 2–3.

Treatment of the Fibromyalgia Syndrome*

Proven	Unproven or Ineffective
Medicinal	
Amitriptyline	Imipramine
Cyclobenzaprine	Fenfluramine
	Doxepin
Alprazolam	
Zopiclone	Prednisone
Dothiepin	Naproxen (alone)
S-adenosylmethionine	
Regional sympathetic block	
Nonmedicinal	
Cardiovascular fitness training	TNS
	Interferential current
EMG biofeedback	Local injection
	Postisometric relaxation
Cognitive behavioral therapy	Laser therapy
	Massage
	Hypnosis
	Acupuncture
	Local ice/heat

*TNS = transcutaneous nerve stimulation; EMG = electromyogram.

on amitriptyline using the new method of "N-of-1" trials. About one third of patients who initially were believed eligible for entry into these studies benefited from amitriptyline. This corroborates a clinical observation that amitriptyline may be quite useful in selected patients but that these are usually in the minority. No N-of-1 trials have been reported for cyclobenzaprine. One study has correlated electroencephalographic (EEG) sleep recordings in 12 patients taking cyclobenzaprine in a double-blind, placebo-controlled, crossover design.[31] While improvements were noted in evening fatigue and total sleep time during cyclobenzaprine treatment, present pain intensity, pain thresholds over fibrositic tender points (FTPs), and mood ratings did not change. The most striking finding was that alpha non-rapid eye movement (non-REM) EEG sleep anomaly was unchanged in patients taking cyclobenzaprine.

Alprazolam, a triazalobenzodiazepine, has been approved for the treatment of anxiety and the depression associated with anxiety. Its antidepressant activity is comparable to imipramine, amitriptyline, and doxepin. One report has compared alprazolam alone or in combination with ibuprofen in a placebo-controlled, randomized, double-blind protocol.[32] Over half of the patients treated with alprazolam plus ibuprofen showed a greater than 30% improvement, which was considered clinically significant. The authors remarked on the greater-than-expected dropout rate (>30%) and the fact that, while alprazolam showed good effects at 8 weeks, improvements were slow to occur and required up to 16 weeks of treatment for some patients.

Several other medications have been shown to have little or no effect on the symptoms and signs of fibromyalgia. Imipramine, for example, was found to be ineffective in one report.[39] Doxepin and fenfluramine have also had anecdotal success in treatment but no controlled trials have been carried out specifically studying these compounds. Similarly, phenothiazines have not been well studied but have been shown to be of limited usefulness, because of the unacceptable incidence of side effects.[27] They do, however, lead to a predictable improvement in sleep disturbance. Dothiepin has been reported to be superior to placebo in one study, when given as a single dose of 75 mg at bedtime.[5] Bengtsson et al.[2] have also reported on the beneficial effects of regional sympathetic blockade in fibromyalgia. Anti-inflammatory medications have shown disappointing results in clinical trials. In properly controlled randomized trials prednisone 20 mg/day[7] and naproxen 500 mg/day[17] were no more effective than placebo. A novel compound S-adenosylmethionine (SAMe), which has both antidepressant and anti-inflammatory properties, has been found to be more effective than placebo in one report.[36] Zopiclone, a nonbenzodizepine hypnotic, has been reported to improve subjective sleep complaints but not pain-reporting behavior in FMS.[9]

Nonpharmacologic Treatments

It is apparent from the foregoing discussion that drug therapy alone is often insufficient for patients with fibromyalgia. Medicinal therapies are, therefore, often relegated to an adjunctive role and it is often necessary to include a number of nonmedical modalities of treatment for patients with this disorder. Note that, so far, only a minority of such treatments have been studied using acceptable scientific methods. At present, these treatments are used with little rationale, often haphazardly, and rarely in conjunction with pharmacologic therapies. To date, preliminary evidence exists only for three forms of such treatment: cardiovascular fitness training,[23-26] EMG biofeedback training,[14] and cognitive-behavioral therapy.[29]

Cardiovascular Fitness Training

A recent study reported the effects of cardiovascular fitness training on the manifestations of primary fibromyalgia. Forty-two patients were randomized to a 20-week program of either (1) cardiovascular fitness training or (2) a program of flexibility training.[25] Enhanced cardiovascular fitness was attained in 83% of those randomized to the cardiovascular fitness group. Significant improvements in pain threshold measurements over FTPs were noted in those receiving cardiovascular fitness training when compared with patients treated with flexibility exercises alone. Both physician and patient global assessment scores were also improved in the cardiovascular-treated group. However, no significant differences were found between the groups in present pain intensity scores as measured by visual analog scale, percent total body area involved, or in hours per night or nights per week of disturbed sleep. Psychological profiles were no different in the two groups before and after treatment. The authors concluded that cardiovascular fitness training improved objective and subjective measurements of pain in primary fibromyalgia.

Since the publication of this study cardiovascular training has been felt to be important in the overall treatment of FMS and now constitutes a major portion of most inpatient and outpatient treatment programs. The use of exercise in the clinical setting, however, presents some difficulties. Failure to understand the overall aim of physical exercise as well as the end points of successful treatment is the major pitfall in the design of an exercise program. One additional reason is that exercise is usually administered and supervised by therapists whose expertise is derived from their experience in sports medicine clinics. While it is well recognized that the principles of exercise as they relate to sports injury and sports medicine cannot be imported in their entirety for the treatment of chronic pain patients, particular confusion exists for many therapists when faced with the markedly painful muscles of patients with FMS. Some simple guidelines and caveats should therefore be applied to the difficult problem of how to initiate a well-rounded program of exercise in these patients.

The first and most basic principle is that "hurt does not equal harm." That is, exercise studies like the one alluded to above have shown conclusively that high levels of physical exercise can be achieved in FMS patients with impunity. Patients may complain bitterly after exercising painful muscles but no physical or anatomic harm has been shown to result from such effort. Indeed the reason for inactivity in some patients with FMS is a real fear of worsening of their condition through forceful movement, a cognition erroneously reinforced by the natural occurrence of pain and stiffness in exercising muscles unaccustomed to such activity. The therapist, therefore, must take a different approach to FMS patients, encouraging them to work through initial worsening of pain and reinforcing the "hurt does not equal harm" paradigm.

This brings us to the second principle of the use of exercise in good pain management. The evolution of a successful long-term coping strategy for chronic pain relies on (1) the development of practical physical techniques that reproducibly lead to a diminution in the degree of perceived pain intensity—a concept often referred to as mastery over pain or improved self-efficacy in controlling the painful experience; (2) improvements in self-esteem; and (3) successful social support from significant others who view the patient's pain as real and who support, and thus positively influence, the patient's attempts to deal with it. Physical exercise is useful in obtaining gains in all of the areas listed above. That is, FMS patients who attain high levels of physical exercise commonly report not only an improvement in self-esteem but also a sense of control over the painful experience. Stated another way, the attainment of physical fitness in FMS patients often leads to a decrease in present pain intensity that is the result of mechanisms quite apart from its physiologic effect, although this latter mechanism must not be discounted. Such improvements in function rarely go unnoticed by significant others and may lead to eradication of punishing or overly solicitous responses, behaviors which have been shown to augment the painful state. Exercise, therefore may lead directly to observable improvements in mastery over pain, enhanced self-esteem, and to better social support behaviors by significant others. Improvement in these three dimensions usually results in a more adaptive coping strategy for pain. In this way exercise may be used as a tool to effect known principles of good pain management and as such may be useful in pain therapy programs based on the cognitive-behavioral treatment model.

In summary, the aim of an exercise regimen in the treatment of FMS is to reinforce that hurt does not necessarily mean harm, improve mastery over the painful experience, improve self-esteem, enhance adaptive behaviors in significant others, and finally to provide a physiologic effect which in itself may be reparative to the painful state. How can this be accomplished on the practical level and what constitutes a well-rounded exercise program?

Physical exercise for the FMS patient should consist of a series of maneuvers which lead to enhanced cardiovascular fitness, muscular endurance, and flexibility. Cardiovascular fitness is the easiest to monitor since the end points are more easily identified. Cardiovascular fitness, simply put, is the ability of the cardiovascular system to deliver oxygen to the tissues more efficiently. This means that for any given oxygen requirement the heart pumps more efficiently so that the lowest stoke volume and heart rate are selected. Oxygen is delivered to the tissues at a work level which is lower for the fit person compared with the person less fit. The fit person therefore has a lower resting heart rate, an increased stroke volume, and a less marked increase in these parameters in response to exercise. The result is that the fit person does more work per unit of time at a lower heart rate. This translates into some practical guidelines for the monitoring of cardiovascular fitness in patients with FMS.

It is best to begin with exercise which does not unduly load the joints of the extremities. Jogging or aerobic exercise is not well tolerated for this reason and often leads to interruptions of exercise programs because of tendonitis or other soft tissue inflammatory conditions. I prefer to use bicycle ergometry for this purpose since it is generally better tolerated than other modalities and may be used in the obese patient as well as the older patient. It also has the advantage that patients may follow their own home program of exercise obviating the need for costly supervision. Occasionally water exercise, if monitored by a therapist conversant with cardiovascular exercise principles, may also be useful.

A cardiovascular fitness protocol includes a flow sheet on which the patient records resting heart rate, maximal heart rate achieved during exercise, and the duration of cardiovascular effort in minutes. Resting heart rate is important since this reflects the basal level of fitness of the patient and should decrease over time if true cardiovascular fitness is achieved. This can be used as a reasonable monitor of long-term effectiveness of the exercise program. No change should be expected in this outcome measure before 12 weeks in most patients and improvement may be delayed as long as 20 weeks. This contrasts to a period of 6 weeks in a normal person. Resting heart rates of 55 to 65 beats/min may be targeted for most FMS patients between 20 and 50 years of age. These values reflect excellent cardiovascular fitness levels. After recording resting heart rates patients are instructed to begin exercising usually with a 2-minute warm-up followed by a variable period of exercise on the bicycle ergometer. The period of exercise is low at first and is gradually lengthened until a heart rate of 150 beats/min (HR150) is achieved. Thereafter heart rates are monitored at 5-minute intervals and the period of time spent at a heart rate of 150 beats/min (T150) is recorded. The value of 150 beats/min is an arbitrary one which for most patients in the fibromyalgia age group represents 75% to 80% of aerobic threshold. It is important to emphasize to the patient that exercising above these heart rates provides little additional cardiovascular fitness. These goals are also better tolerated and so improve patient compliance. Most problems arise because patients or therapists are impatient with the pace of exercise. Patient compliance is improved if the progression of time spent at HR150 is attained slowly. I routinely tell patients to increase the length of time spent at HR150 at a rate one third as fast as a normal person. This usually means that true cardiovascular fitness is rarely achieved prior to 20 weeks of exercise. Many patients require longer periods of time to achieve even modest degrees of fitness. A sign that the patient is progressing normally is the observation that it becomes progressively more difficult to attain HR150 in the usual amount of time allotted for exercise. That is, it takes longer to achieve T150 for a given exercise period. This is reflective of increased cardiovascular performance and should not be viewed as a failure of the exercise protocol. An increase in the workload can be achieved by simply increasing the tension on the wheel of the ergometer for a given exercise period or, alternatively, increasing the pace of exercise. Most patients can learn to monitor their heart rates and construct a weekly diary of exercise which includes resting heart rate, HR150, exercise time, and workload (wheel tension). Diaries may be used for physician feedback and as a check on patient compliance.

A well-rounded exercise program must also include a mixture of flexibility and muscular endurance exercises in addition to cardiovascular fitness exercises. Flexibility exercises may be used both before and after cardiovascular and muscular endurance exercises. They are most helpful in preventing injury and promoting maximal contraction of specific muscle groups when done before other exercises, and most helpful in minimizing stiffness when done after other exercises. Most therapists are adept at these kinds of exercises since they constitute a large portion of most athletic training programs. This may also be said for muscular endurance exercises. However, muscular endurance exercises are aimed at repetition of specific tasks and as such are most useful in developing stamina. Indeed, many patients with FMS may respond to these exercises preferentially if stamina is considered inadequate or one of their chief complaints. The only caveat for these two forms of physical exercise is that they must be done slowly and with perseverance. They are most helpful when targeted to specific muscle groups which have been deemed by the therapist to be important in the recovery of identified functions. As such, these exercises can be quite specific for function recovery and may be used as a prelude to more formal work-hardening programs.

EMG Biofeedback Training

Only one controlled study of the effects of biofeedback training in primary fibromyalgia has been reported.[14] This study consisted of an open trial of 15 patients who underwent 15 sessions of EMG biofeedback over a 5-week observation period. Nine patients had improvement in the number of FTPs, present pain intensity as measured by visual analog scores, and morning stiffness. These improvements persisted up to 6 months after EMG biofeedback had ceased. A follow-up study, randomizing a further 12 patients to a similar regimen of EMG biofeedback or sham biofeedback, showed a significant improvement in visual analog pain scores, morning stiffness, and number of FTPs in the true EMG biofeedback group. Again, these differences were significant both at 5 weeks and 5 months after treatment. A recent report by the same authors indicated that EMG biofeedback reduces plasma adrenocorticotropic hormone (ACTH) and β-endorphin levels during treatment, indicating an opioid or neuroendocrine basis, or both, for some of the observed beneficial effects in fibromyalgia.[28]

Cognitive-Behavioral Therapy

Cognitive-behavioral therapy of chronic pain has been proved useful in a number of clinical settings, such as low back pain, headache, temporomandibular joint pain, and rheumatoid arthritis. This multidisciplinary approach has recently been applied to fibromyalgia.[29] Thirty consecutive patients attending a rheumatic diseases unit were assessed 5 months before, at admission to, and at discharge from a 3-week inhospital multidisciplinary cognitive-behavioral treatment program. The program included medical, psychological, social work, physiotherapy, occupational therapy, and nursing interventions based on the cognitive-behavioral model. The primary goal of the program was to assist patients in developing an active, resourceful, self-management approach to coping with their fibromyalgia. Cognitive techniques were used in conjunction with aerobic exercise, physiotherapy, biofeedback training, and relaxation therapy. Outcome measures were primarily psychological in nature and showed significant improvements in perceived pain severity, affective distress (depressed mood, irritability, and tension), and the extent to which pain interfered with normal activities. Sense of control and mastery over life circumstances were also enhanced in comparison to preadmission status. This study provided no follow-up data on how long these good effects persisted, but did show very statistically significant improvements over the short term. No data were provided regarding the effect of cognitive-behavioral therapy on specific disease-related outcome measures like pain threshold over FTPs, pain palpation scores, or degree of morning stiffness. There was an improvement, however, in functional abilities such as time spent out of bed and activity level. Cognitive-behavioral therapy, therefore, may be of benefit to selected patients when administered in the proper setting by trained personnel.

MYOFASCIAL PAIN SYNDROME

Myofascial pain syndrome, like fibromyalgia, can be a chronic disease. Although no long-term studies have been done to determine the natural history of this condition it is accepted that most patients receive multiple modalities of treatment usually over many years with only limited benefit. In one study of 164 patients the mean duration of complaint was 5.8 years for males and 6.9 years for females.[13] In another study of 102 patients with orofacial pain in which 59.8% had MPS, the mean duration of pain was 6.0 years.[12] These studies documented numerous treatment modalities and physician contacts indicating that MPS patients are significant users of health care facilities.[1]

Treatment

Since limited studies have been reported on the outcome of specific modalities of therapy, any discussion on treatment must remain strictly anecdotal. However, some general treatment strategies can be enunciated on empirical grounds and are amenable to future study. Management of MPS must take into account the chronic nature of the disease process and must include measures to eradicate muscular trigger points, prevent their recurrence, and deal with possible aggravating or predisposing factors. This approach necessarily involves treating the whole patient and fits into our current paradigm of multidisciplinary treatment for chronic pain syndromes in general.

Inactivation of trigger points is accomplished through counterstimulation coupled with active and passive stretching which may include postural rehabilitation.[37] The goal is to restore the muscle to normal length, posture, and full range of motion. Preventing the redevelopment of trigger points includes maintenance of an exercise program with concomitant control of predisposing contributing factors. Counterstimulation may be achieved by a number of measures which although widely used have been tested rather poorly in well-controlled studies. These measures include massage, acupressure, ultrasound, moist heat, ice packs, fluorimethane spray, and diathermy. Transcutaneous nerve stimulation, electroacupuncture, and direct current stimulation have also been used (see Chapter 16). Acupuncture and trigger point injections with a local anesthetic, saline, or steroid cause mechanical disruption of trigger points (see Chapter 9). It is generally acknowledged that counterstimulation can provide short-term relief from pain but that long-term management by a regular muscle stretching and strengthening program is also important. Postural contributing factors, whether behavioral or biological, perpetuate trigger points if not corrected.[13, 15, 35] One study of 164 head and neck MPS patients found poor sitting or standing posture in 96%, forward head in 84.7%, rounded shoulders in 82.3%, lower tongue position in 67.7%, abnormal lordosis in 46.3%, scoliosis in 15.9%, and leg length discrepancy in 14% of patients.[13] Muscles held in sustained contraction, either in normal position or in an abnormal shortened position, are more prone to redevelop trigger points. Mechanical abnormalities like spinal scoliosis or leg length discrepancy, therefore, should be corrected with orthoses and other devices whenever possible. Similarly, unusual or repetitive movements in the workplace or at the work station should be simplified to allow for stretching and use of alternative muscle groups (see Chapter 16).

Special care must be taken to address psychological contributing factors such as those associated with litigation and long-term disability which lead to uncertainty about future employability. Loss of self-esteem is the consequence of the anxiety surrounding these issues and should be dealt with through patient education and practical guidance regarding money issues when necessary. Learned illness behaviors which detract from an adaptive coping style are best remedied with a cognitive-behavioral approach. These psychological factors may be the source of the greatest morbidity in both FMS and MPS. Attention to details in

TABLE 2–4.

Treatment of Myofascial Pain: Acute Onset With Rapid Resolution*

Clinical Characteristics	Treatment (3 mo)
Onset less than 2 mo	Fluorimethane spray and stretch (office)
No previous treatment	
Simple psychological/behavioral factors	Home exercises: stretching and posture exercises for affected muscle groups
Few trigger points unilateral	Control of contributing factors
No other symptoms	Reduction of muscle tension habits
Prognosis excellent	Evaluation for other perpetuating factors

*Adapted from Fricton JR: Management of myofascial pain syndrome. In Fricton JR, Awad EA, editors: *Advances in pain research and therapy*, vol 17, New York, 1990, Raven Press. Used by permission.

this area may often yield the most success when return of function is the end point of treatment (see Chapters 4–7).

These principles are outlined in Tables 2–4, 2–5, and 2–6, which give an approach that can be tailored not only to the severity but also to the impact of MPS on the functional abilities of the individual patient. The following paragraphs discuss the evidence for efficacy of two commonly used counterstimulation techniques, namely stretch and spray therapy and trigger point injections.

Stretch and Spray Therapy

Stretch and spray therapy involves passive stretching of a muscle while the simultaneous application of a vapocoolant spray, such as fluorimethane, is administered to the skin overlying an affected muscle. The technique involves directing a fine stream of fluorimethane spray from a calibrated nozzle toward the skin directly overlying the muscle with the trigger point. The spray is directed over the reference zone to which pain radiates on previous palpation of the trigger point. After a few initial sweeps over the reference zone the affected muscle is passively stretched with enough force to elicit pain and discomfort.

TABLE 2–5.

Treatment of Myofascial Pain: Subacute Onset With Good Response*

Clinical Characteristics	Treatment (6 mo)
Onset within 2–6 mo	Fluorimethane spray and stretch (office and home)
Minimal previous treatment	
Some psychological/behavioral factors	Home exercises: stretching and posture exercises for affected muscle groups
Numerous trigger points bilaterally	Stabilization splints for craniofacial pain
No other symptoms	Nonsteroidal anti-inflammatory drugs optional
Prognosis good	Control of contributing factors
	Reduction of tension-producing habits; postural habits; behavioral therapy to include relaxation techniques, biofeedback, pacing skills
	If not successful, use physical therapy, trigger point injections, or accupuncture, or reevaluate perpetuating factors

*Adapted from Fricton JR: Management of myofascial pain syndrome. In Fricton JR, Awad EA, editors: *Advances in pain research and therapy*, vol 17, New York, 1990, Raven Press. Used by permission.

TABLE 2–5.

Treatment of Myofascial Pain: Subacute Onset With Good Response*

Clinical Characteristics	Treatment (6 mo)
Onset within 2–6 mo	Fluorimethane spray and stretch (office and home)
Minimal previous treatment	
Some psychological/behavioral factors	Home exercises: stretching and posture exercises for affected muscle groups
Numerous trigger points bilaterally	Stabilization splints for craniofacial pain
No other symptoms	Nonsteroidal anti-inflammatory drugs optional
Prognosis good	Control of contributing factors
	Reduction of tension-producing habits; postural habits; behavioral therapy to include relaxation techniques, biofeedback, pacing skills
	If not successful, use physical therapy, trigger point injections, or accupuncture, or reevaluate perpetuating factors

*Adapted from Fricton JR: Management of myofascial pain syndrome. In Fricton JR, Awad EA, editors: *Advances in pain research and therapy*, vol 17, New York, 1990, Raven Press. Used by permission.

The muscle is then put on progressive passive stretch while the vapocoolant stream is directed at an acute angle 30 to 50 cm away. The spray is applied in one direction from the trigger point toward its reference zone in slow, even, parallel sweeps over the whole muscle at a rate of about 10 cm/sec. This sequence can be repeated four times with careful attention not to freeze the underlying skin, which may aggravate the trigger point.* The end point is the eradication of pain and point tenderness over the trigger point as well as an improvement in the range of active and passive movement. Despite its great popularity only one study has shown that trigger point tenderness as measured by pressure algometry and visual analog pain-rating scales were reduced after stretch and spray therapy.[19] Referred pain was also reduced after stretch and spray therapy in this study.

Trigger Point Injections

Trigger point injections have been shown to reduce pain, increase range of motion, increase exercise tolerance, and increase circulation of muscles.[8, 18, 20, 22] The pain relief may last from minutes to many months depending on the chronicity and severity of the trigger point. The critical factor in needling is the mechanical disruption of the trigger point rather than the solution used during injection. Therefore, precision in needling of the exact trigger point is the most important factor in trigger point inactivation. Fine et al.[11] used a double-blind, crossover study designed to determine if analgesia after trigger point injection was reversed with naloxone and thus mediated by activation of the endogenous opioid system. Naloxone reversed the short-term analgesic effect of injections compared to placebo suggesting that the antinociceptive ef-

Editor's note: The above description is one method of performing stretch and spray. Techniques may vary according to individual physical therapists and patient requirements. Relaxation techniques should precede stretching. Active range of motion should be emphasized (see Chapter 9).

fects of injection of trigger points is in part mediated by the opioid system. It did not explain the long-term analgesia often seen after such injections.

Trigger point injections with local anesthetic agents are preferred to dry needling or injecting other substances because they are inherently less painful. Local anesthetics such as 3% chlorpromazine (short-acting) and 0.5% procaine (medium-acting), or 1% lidocaine without vasoconstrictors is suggested.[12] Hamerhoff et al.[18] compared injection of bupivacaine, etidocaine, and saline and found the first two anesthetics superior to saline. One study compared dry needling, injection of saline or procaine, and placebo skin injection in a double-blinded design. These authors found that reduction in trigger point tenderness was dependent on penetration of the trigger point with the needle. Reduction of referred pain was greater with injection of either saline or procaine than dry needling or placebo. Only one other study looked at the short- and long-term effects of dry needling of trigger points and found immediate improvement in 86.8% of patients and permanent improvement in 29.8%.[22]

The following considerations are important for trigger point injection (see Chapter 9). The patient must be positioned in a comfortable, relaxed posture so that the location of the exact trigger point can be determined. Proper aseptic skin preparation is required. The needle must be inserted quickly through the skin for maximum comfort and placed directly and precisely within the trigger point within the taut band of muscle at the tip of the needle. The "local twitch response" or contraction of the band containing the trigger point as well as the intensification of dull pain over the muscle or in the zone of reference will indicate when the trigger point has been needled. It is at this point that aspiration and slow injection of the local anesthetic can be accomplished. Repeated probing of the taut band without removal of the needle may isolate satellite trigger points, which can also be injected. Pain relief should be seen within a few minutes. One method of postinjection management attempts immediate full range of manual stretching of the muscle to restore the muscle to normal resting length and to determine whether additional trigger points are present. Shortening activation or a reactive spasm may occasionally occur due to shortening of an antagonist muscle that also contains a trigger point. This may cause a slight increase in pain 2 to 5 hours after injection. Failure to eradicate pain beyond this period can be the result of inexact needling of the isolated trigger point. Trigger point injection should not be attempted in the acute phase after muscle trauma or in patients with bleeding diatheses, allergy to anesthetic agents, or with cellulitis of the injection area (see Chapter 9).

SUMMARY

Treatment strategies for fibromyalgia have a much stronger scientific basis than those used for MPS. This is not only the result of the development of rigorous diagnostic criteria but also because of the use of more powerful study designs. Nevertheless, important advances in our understanding of these conditions have evolved. It is clear that both medicinal and nonmedicinal modalities of therapy will play a role in future treatment of these conditions. Our hope is that well-tested diagnostic criteria for MPS will soon be in general use so that homogeneous patient populations will be studied in the future. It is also our hope that appropriate study designs will be used to test future interventions. It is only through the use of the scientific method that progress in this complex and challenging area of investigation will capture the hearts and minds of now disbelieving physicians and lead to a clearer understanding of these musculo-skeletal pain syndromes.

REFERENCES

1. Aronoff GM, Evans WO, Enders PL: A review of follow-up studies of multidisciplinary pain units, *Pain* 16:1–11, 1983.
2. Bengtsson A, Bengtsson M: Regional sympathetic blockade in primary fibromyalgia (abstract), *Pain* 33:161–167, 1988.
3. Bennett RM, Gatter RA, Campbell SM, et al: A comparison of cyclobenzaprine and placebo in the management of fibrositis, *Arthritis Rheum* 31:1535–1542, 1988.
4. Carette S, McCain GA, Bell DA, et al: Evaluation of amitriptyline in primary fibrositis. A double-blind, placebo-controlled study, *Arthritis Rheum* 29:655–659, 1986.
5. Caruso I, Sarzi Puttini PC, Boccassini L, et al: Double blind study of dothiepin versus placebo in the treatment of primary fibromyalgia syndrome, *J Int Med Res* 15:154–159, 1987.
6. Cathey MA, Wolfe F, Kleinheksel SM, et al: Socioeconomic impact of fibrositis: A study of 81 patients with primary fibrositis, *Am J Med* 81(suppl 3A):78–84, 1986.
7. Clark SR, Tindall EA, Bennett RA: A double-blind crossover trial of prednisone versus placebo in the treatment of fibrositis, *J Rheumatol* 12:980–983, 1985.
8. Dorigo B, Bartoli V, Grisillo D, et al: Fibrositic myofascial pain in inermittent claudication. Effect of anesthetic block of trigger points on exercise tolerance, *Pain* 6:183–190, 1979.
9. Drewes AM, Andreasen A, Jennum P, et al: Zopiclone in the treatment of sleep abnormalities in fibromyalgia, *Scand J Rheumatol* 20:288–293, 1991.
10. Felson DT, Goldenberg DL: The natural history of fibromyalgia, *Arthritis Rheum* 29:1522–1526, 1986.
11. Fine PG, Milano R, Hare BD: The effects of myofascial trigger point injections are naloxone reversible, *Pain* 32:15–20, 1988.
12. Fricton JR: Management of myofascial pain syndrome. In Fricton JR, Awad EA, editors: *Advances in pain research and therapy.* vol 17, New York, 1990, Raven Press, p 325.
13. Fricton JR, Kroening R: Practical differential diagnosis of chronic craniofacial pain, *Oral Surg* 54:628–634, 1982.
14. Furaccioli G, Chirelli L, Scita F, et al: EMG-biofeedback training in fibromyalgia syndrome, *J Rheumatol* 14:820–825, 1987.
15. Glyn JH: Rheumatic pains: Some concepts and hypotheses, *Proc R Soc Med* 64:354–360, 1971.
16. Goldenberg DL: Treatment of fibromyalgia syndrome, *Rheum Dis Clin North Am* 15:61–67, 1989.
17. Goldenberg DL, Felson DT, Dinerman H: A randomized, controlled trial of amitriptyline and naproxen in the treatment of patients with fibromyalgia, *Arthritis Rheum* 29:1371–1377, 1986.
18. Hameroff SR, Crago BR, Blitt CD, et al: Comparison of bupivicaine, etidocaine, and saline for trigger point therapy, *Anesth Analg* 60:752–755, 1981.
19. Jaeger B, Reeves JL: Quantification of changes in myofascial trigger point sensitivity with the pressure algometer following passive stretch, *Pain* 27:203–210, 1986.
20. Jaeger B, Skootsky SA: Male and female chronic pain patients categorized by DSM-III psychiatric criteria, *Pain* 29:263–266, 1987.
21. Jaeschke R, Adachi J, Guyatt G, et al: Clinical usefulness of amitriptyline in fibromyalgia: The results of 23 N-of-1 randomized controlled trials, *J Rheumatol* 18:447–451, 1991.
22. Lewit K: The needle effect in the relief of myofascial pain, *Pain* 6:83–90, 1979.
23. McCain GA: Role of physical fitness training in the fibrositis/fibromyalgia syndrome, *Am J Med* 81 (suppl 3A):73–77, 1986.
24. McCain GA: Non-medicinal treatments in fibromyalgia, *Rheum Dis Clin North Am* 15:73–90, 1989.
25. McCain GA, Bell DA, Mai F, et al: A controlled study of the effects of a super-

vised cardiovascular fitness training program on the manifestations of the primary fibromyalgia syndrome, *Arthritis Rheum* 31:1135–1141, 1988.

26. McCain GA, Bell DA, Mai FM, et al: A controlled study of the effects of a supervised cardiovascular fitness program on the manifestations of the primary fibromyalgia syndrome, *Arthritis Rheum Primary Care Rev* 2:1–15, 1990.
27. Moldofsky H, Warsh JJ: Plasma tryptophan and musculoskeletal pain in non-articular rheumatism, *Pain* 5:65–71, 1978.
28. Molina E, Cecchettin M, Fontana S: Failure of EMG-BF after sham BF training in fibromyalgia, *Fed Proc* 46:1357, 1987.
29. Nielson WR, Walker C, McCain GA: Cognitive behavioural treatment of fibromyalgia syndrome: Preliminary findings, *J Rheumatol* 19:98–103, 1991.
30. Quimby LG, Gratwick GM, Whitney CA, et al: A randomized trial of cyclobenzaprine for the treatment of fibromyalgia, *J Rheumatol* 16(suppl 19):140–143, 1989.
31. Reynolds WJ, Moldofsky H, Saskin P, et al: The effects of cyclobenzaprine on sleep physiology and symptoms in patients with fibromyalgia, *J Rheumatol* 18:452–454, 1991.
32. Russell IJ, Fletcher EM, Michalek JE, et al: Treatment of primary fibrositis/fibromyalgia syndrome with ibuprofen and alprazolam: A double-blind, placebo-controlled study, *Arthritis Rheum* 34:552–560, 1991.
33. Scudds RA, McCain GA, Rollman GB, et al: Improvements in pain responsiveness in patients with fibrositis after successful treatment with amitriptyline, *J Rheumatol* 16(suppl 19):113–119, 1989.
34. Simons D: Muscular pain syndromes. In Fricton JR, Awad EA, editors: *Advances in pain research and therapy.* Volume 17, New York, 1990, Raven Press, p 1.
35. Simons DG, Travell JG: Myofascial origins of low back pain. 1. Principles of diagnosis of treatment, *Postgrad Med* 73:68–77, 1983.
36. Tavoni A, Vitali C, Bombardieri S: Evaluation of S-adenosyl-methionine in primary fibromyalgia, *Am J Med* 83(suppl 5A):107–110, 1987.
37. Travell JG, Simons DG: *Myofascial pain and dysfunction. The trigger point manual,* Baltimore, 1983, Williams & Wilkins.
38. Wolfe F, Smythe HA, Yunus MB, et al: The American College of Rheumatology 1990 criteria for the classification of fibromyalgia. Report of the Multicenter Criteria Committee, *Arthritis Rheum* 33:160–172, 1990.
39. Wysenbeek AJ, Nor F, Lurie T, et al: Imipramine for the treatment of fibrositis: A therapeutic trial, *Ann Rheum Dis* 44:752–753, 1985.

Chapter 3

Myofascial Pain Due to Metabolic Disorders: Diagnosis and Treatment

Lawrence S. Sonkin, M.D., Ph.D.

Myofascial pain occurs in many endocrine disorders and may be the presenting complaint.[24] The patient's initial visit may be to a physiatrist, physiotherapist, orthopedist, temporomandibular joint expert, rheumatologist, or other practitioner who treats myofascial pain and trigger points. Failure to recognize a metabolic cause of the symptoms may result in prolonged, ineffective therapy, visits to a variety of therapists, and occasionally one or more fruitless surgical procedures.

This chapter discusses (1) the chemistry of muscle contraction, and its perturbation by metabolic disorders; (2) the mechanism, detection, and treatment of endocrinologically induced myofascial pain; (3) a rationale for therapeutic trials with thyroid hormones performed on chemically euthyroid patients with generalized myofascial pain and hypothyroid–like symptoms; and (4) data collected by the author over the past 38 years which support Weintraub's recent statement from the National Institutes of Health (NIH): "Thyroid hormone resistance syndrome may affect thousands of unsuspecting Americans."[27]

CHEMISTRY OF STRIATED MUSCLE CONTRACTION

Figure 3–1 is a composite of drawings summarize striated muscle structure and function[1–3, 7] and provide an understanding of endocrinologically induced defects which may cause muscle pain and dysfunction: *(1)* a subcellular myofibril consisting of parallel bands of actin and myosin filaments surrounded by the sarcolemmal reticulum, a pouchlike mesh, that contains ionized calcium; *(3)* a section through sarcolemmal reticulum and filaments. The myofibrils are interconnected by a system of tubules which connects to the cell surface and transmits signals for contraction from the myoneural junction. Connections between the tubular rings and sarcolemma are called triads; *(2)* mitochondria are layered around the surface of the unit. A motor impulse at the cell surface passes via the tubules to the triads, and causes calcium release into the myofibril activating adenosine triphosphatase *(ATPase)* endings on the myosin filaments; *(5)* high energy phosphate is released from adenosine triphosphate *(ATP)* resulting in the formation of contracted actomyosin and a molecule of adenosine

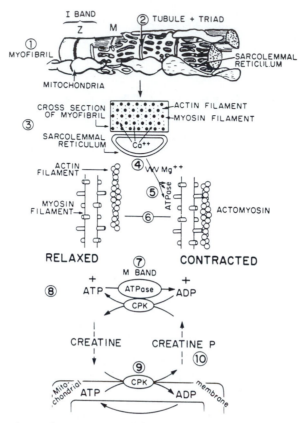

FIG 3–1. Striated muscle structure and function. See text. From Sonkin LS: Endocrine disorders and muscle dysfunction. In Gelb H, editor: *Clinical management of head, neck, and TMJ pain and dysfunction*, Philadelphia, 1985, JB Lippincott. Used by permission.

diphosphate *(ADP)*; *(6)* relaxation occurs with cessation of the myoneural impulse, and calcium flows back into the sarcolemmal reticulum; *(9)* the creatine shuttle of Bessman and Geiger[1] transfers creatine from the intracellular myofibril to its mitochondria for recombination with high energy phosphate by creatine phosphokinase *(CPK)* to re-form creatine phosphate, which is recycled to the myofibril. Sodium and potassium flux at the muscle cell membrane, not shown in the figure, also play an important role in activating muscle contraction and relaxation.

Virtually all endocrine dysfunction may affect the above reactions and cause muscle spasm, trigger points, and myofascial pain. A brief endocrine system review, therefore, is important in the initial history. Observations made during physical examination may initiate further metabolic evaluation, or endocrine referral. Symptoms and signs which suggest further metabolic evaluation are discussed below with their specific endocrine disorders.

SYNDROMES OF THYROIDAL DEFICIENCY

This section addresses several proven and putative forms of thyroidal deficiency including the classic form of hypothyroidism, and emerging peripheral resistance syndromes in patients with normal or inappropriate secretion of thyroid and pituitary hormones.

Hypothyroidism

Hypothyroidism is due to inadequate production of the thyroid hormones, levothyroxine and liothyronine resulting from malfunction in the hypopthalamic-pituitary-thyroid (HPT) axis. It is usually detected by the internist or general practitioner who orders chemical profiles and thyroid function tests as part of a routine laboratory evaluation, and responds rapidly to thyroid hormone replacement in physiologic doses. The patient with severe myofascial complaints may first seek a practitioner who deals with rheumatic or myofascial problems.

In the United States the disease is commonly due to congenital autoimmune thyroiditis, thyroid ablation via surgery or radioactive iodine therapy, and medication with thiouracil or lithium, and rarely from subacute thyroiditis, iodine deficiency, dietary factors, congenital abnormalities in iodination, or pituitary failure.

Chemical Abnormalities in Hypothyroid Muscle. Creatinuria follows initial administration of thyroid to myxedematous patients,[20] and high muscle creatine levels have been demonstrated prior to treatment.[25] Hypothyroidism causes myopathy in most patients,[14] and is manifested by diffuse stiffness, trigger points, weakness, and delayed relaxation of ankle reflexes. Rives and co-workers,[18] however, have determined that the ankle reflex is an unreliable indicator of hypothyroidism. Other chemical abnormalities related to hypothyroid muscle have included elevated serum CPK levels,[3] and muscle acid maltase deficiency with secondary accumulation of muscle glycogen similar to that seen in type II glycogen storage, or Pompe's, disease.[12]

Medical History. The patient should be queried about complaints of fatigue, dry skin and hair, alopecia, peeling or cracking fingernails, Raynaud's disease, puffy eyelids, dryness of eyes and other mucous membranes, nasal congestion, hoarseness, bloating, constipation, cold intolerance, excessive use of clothing or blankets, depression, lack of attention span, infertility, loss of libido, impotence, weight gain, muscle cramps, and fluid retention. Menometrorrhagia is more common than amenorrhea. None of the complaints is specific, but a constellation of these symptoms should raise the question of impaired thyroidal function. The family history may reveal a variety of thyroid problems.

Physical Examination. Hypothyroid patients are often but not always overweight, and may be hypertensive. Skin is dry, sallow, rough, occasionally carotinemic. Hair is dry, dull, and may be thin in the female patient. Eyelids may be puffy, and nasal membranes congested. The voice is hoarse, and has a characteristic timber. The thyroid gland is often enlarged, sometimes nodular, but may not be palpable. Heart rate may be slow. Muscles are stiff, often tender, and occasionally weak. Muscle hypertrophy may be prominent, especially in juvenile myxedema.[4] Trigger points are frequently detected. Delayed relaxation of the ankle jerk and low early-morning subaxillary temperatures have been suggested as diagnostic findings, but are unreliable. Mild cases may be relatively devoid of symptoms and signs. Diffuse muscle tenderness may be the major finding.

Laboratory Diagnosis.   Hypothyroidism is easily demonstrated by low serum thyroxine (T_4), free thyroxine index, and high thyroid-stimulating hormone (TSH) levels. These values may, however, be normal in mild symptomatic hypothyroidism, in which case injection of thyrotropin releasing hormone (TRH) produces an abnormally high secretion of pituitary TSH in 1 hour. Serum creatine kinase (CK) may be elevated.[3]

Therapy.   An adequate dose of a thyroid hormone controls the condition. The current practice of adjusting to a physiologic dose of about 0.112 mg of levothyroxine sodium to normalize the TSH level should control symptoms of patients with true hypothyroidism as defined by failure of the HPT axis, but is ordinarily inadequate for treatment of peripheral resistance syndromes.

Generalized Resistance to Thyroid Hormone (GRTH) With Feedback— the Refetoff Syndrome

In 1967 Refetoff and co-workers[15, 16] identified the first of a succession of kindreds with clinical hypothyroidism, paradoxically elevated serum protein-bound iodine (PBI) (later T_4), inappropriately normal to slightly high serum TSH, deaf-mutism, short stature, bone anomalies, stippled epiphyses, goiter, and incomplete tissue resistance to thyroid hormone. The syndrome was viewed as a rarity for many years. Physiologic doses of T_4 do not control the symptoms, and supraphysiologic doses are required but may not control the symptoms completely. After many years of uncertainty, the cause is now recognized to be genetic point mutation at various sites of one of two chromosomes. Peripheral resistance may coexist with primary disease of the thyroid.[5]

The most recent report from Weintraub's group at the NIH[28] adds four new families, and now recognizes a total of 20 distinct familial point mutations, of which 18 are located in two regions and 18 different sites of the c-erbA gene which encodes the thyroid receptor. Kindreds are identified by the inappropriate elevation of serum T_4, and TSH, a result of a feedback signal from the thyroid-resistant periphery to the HPT axis.

Studies of resistance in bone, brain, liver, and heart in the four recently identified kindreds were variable. The basal metabolic rate (BMR) response to thyroid administration appeared to be affected in all four kindreds, but bone, brain, and heart of different kindreds were differently affected, raising the question whether the term "generalized" is valid. Muscle affinities other than heart were not reported. A connection was noted between affected receptor sites, speech, and possibly dyslexia.

It is questionable whether the syndrome would have been recognized in the absence of the feedback signal. An opinion has been expressed that the feedback signal is an exception rather than the rule in peripheral resistance syndromes, and that there may be a large population of undiagnosed peripheral resistance which does not feed back to the HPT axis. My series of therapeutic trials in symptomatic, chemically euthyroid patients who show no evidence of feedback and frequently respond to thyroid therapy probably contain members of this putative population.

A current paradigm in endocrinology which precludes administration of thyroid to symptomatic patients with normal serum levels of free thyroxine, TSH, and radioiodine (RAI) uptake is questionable. Two subspecialty groups long aware of this fact are physiatrists dealing with intractable generalized myofascial pain and trigger points, and psychiatrists who use triiodothyronine (T_3) to synergize antidepressants in apparently euthyroid patients with rapidly cycling endogenous depression. It seems reasonable in the face of current evidence and uncertainty to give the patient the benefit of the doubt, and offer a therapeutic trial with thyroid, which is innocuous and frequently effective (see below).

Weintraub[27] mentions that pituitary response to thyroid hormone may be normal in GRTH. The observation suggests that determination of the correct thyroid dose by titration of serum levels of pituitary TSH to normal is inappropriate in treatment of peripheral resistance.

Metabolic Insufficiency, Hypometabolism, Peripheral Resistance to T_4

In 1957 Kurland and co-workers[10] reported four patients with symptoms of hypothyroidism, BMR below -20, normal serum cholesterol, PBI, and RAI uptake who were unresponsive to levothyroxine (T_4) but rapidly responsive metabolically and symptomatically to liothyronine (T_3) alone or combined with T_4. Two of the patients were ultimately able to sustain metabolic improvement on T_4 alone. The authors concluded that resistance was due to the inability to deiodinate T_4 to T_3, the biologically active form of the hormone, and named the condition *hypometabolism*. A number of confirmatory anecdotal reports followed, and were well summarized by Keating,[8] who suggested that the controversy over hypermetabolism and metabolic insufficiency be resolved by double-blind studies. Two double-blind trials were reported 2 years later.

Double-blind Studies.   The double-blind trials were done early in the development of the technique, and appear to be flagrant examples of the β error, i.e., acceptance of a null hypothesis when it is, in fact, unproven. Both double-blind studies were done on an inadequate number of patients. One study[11] used 18 patients who complained of fatigue, and had normal PBI and low BMR. They were divided into three groups of six patients which received either levothyroxine, liothyronine, or placebo for an inadequate period of 2 weeks after gradual increase of dose over a 2-week period. No differences in metabolic or symptomatic response were noted on and off therapy.

The second study[21] was done on 19 students, 1 male and 18 females, in a student health service who complained of fatigue and had moderately low BMRs. Administration of liothyronine did not reveal a difference in response of either the treated patients or controls. The report included data on unblinded studies in which there appeared to be a metabolic response, but no statistical studies were reported.

Both studies had inadequate numbers of patients in each group, failed to provide adequate duration of therapy, and failed to select from a high-risk cohort of chemically euthyroid symptomatic patients who had previously manifested symptomatic responses to therapeutic trials in unblinded studies. Despite defects which would void two these double-blind studies in today's state of the art, the chapters on hypometabolism, metabolic insufficiency, and peripheral thyroxine resistance in nongoitrous, chemically euthyroid patients have remained closed. Williams' call[29] 2 years later for additional relevant double-blind studies went unheeded. The rejection ultimately contributed to the premature obsolescence of the BMR, a major test for evaluation of peripheral response to thyroid hormone, although it remains an essential test in studies of GRTH by Refetoff[15] and other workers.

Peripheral Resistance to Thyroid Hormone Without Feedback

In 1952 and 1953 I spent a year of endocrine residency at New York Hospital where measurement of the BMR had been developed 30 years previously. One of the resident's duties was to perform all BMR measurements on the experimental metabolic unit. The test was useful in detecting thyroid dysfunction, and in following treatment with sequential measurements on the same patient, but had shortcomings as a single measurement because of its wide "normal" range. In 1954 I decided to limit the use of the test to therapeutic trials with at least two measurements, one off and one on thyroid replacement using the patient as his or her own control for a minimal period of 3 months, the period in which a placebo effect usually ends. The trials were done on symptomatic patients who were chemically euthyroid. Twelve therapeutic withdrawals, all

TABLE 3–1.

Complaints and Responses to Therapeutic Trials With Thyroid Hormones in Chemically Euthyroid Patients (Total Trials = 174)

Complaint	Total	Positive Responses
Fatigue	88	51
Myofascial pain	63	46
Weight gain	48	18
Dry skin	39	24
Depression	39	20
Thyroid nodules	24	7
Dysmenorrhea	20	5
Cold intolerance	17	13
Hair loss	14	3
Temporomandibular joint syndrome	7	3
Constipation	7	6
Swollen eyelids	6	3
Arthritis	5	1
Infertility	5	2
History of thyroidectomy	5	2
Hoarseness	4	1
Headache	4	3
Flushes	4	0
Fluid retention	3	1
Insomnia	3	1
Stiffness	2	0
Weakness	2	1
Nervousness	2	0
Bloat	2	2
Numbness	1	0
Nasal congestion	1	1
Anemia	1	0
Puffiness	1	1
Impotence	1	0
Menorrhagia	1	1

negative, were done on patients who were taking thyroid without any apparent indication.

Table 3–1 lists the various complaints of patients subjected to 174 therapeutic trials, and the number of therapeutic responses to each complaint. Myofascial pain was the second most common complaint, after fatigue. Of 63 patients with muscle pain, 46 (73%) had symptomatic improvement with thyroid therapy.

Response to therapy was determined by scoring changes in symptoms and signs indexed at the start of the trial. Zero was no change, incomplete improvement was scored 1, and full improvement was scored 2. The scores were then averaged for each patient. Each point plotted on a nomogram (Fig 3–2) was determined by the change in BMR and serum cholesterol in each trial. An average score of less than 1 was plotted as an open circle, and a score of 1 to 2 was plotted as a black dot.

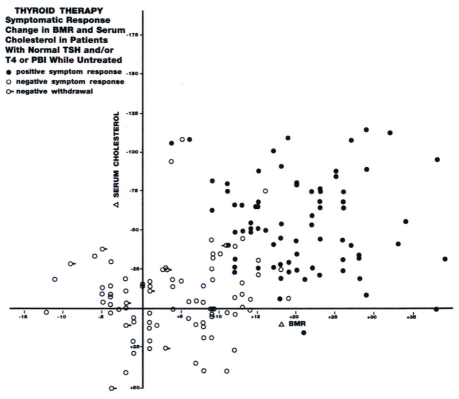

FIG 3–2. Results of 172 therapeutic trials and withdrawals with varying combinations of T_3 and T_4 in patiens with symptoms suggesting possible thyroid hormone deficiency. All patients had normal PBIs or more recently normal TSHs and/or T_4 measurements. None had symptoms of hyperthyroidism produced by therapy. The graph shows a distinct response in BMR and cholesterol in many patients. Furthermore, those with the most clear-cut responses in these two measurements had positive clinical responses (black circles), whereas patients with no significant metabolic response in BMR and cholesterol had no clinical response (open circles). This graph seems to support the validity of using the change in BMR and cholesterol in response to thyroid hormone medication for confirmation of a positive or negative clinical response to treatment in patients who cannot be proved to be thyroid deficient by any other technique. From Sonkin LS: Endocrine disorders and muscle dysfunction. In Gelb H, editor: *Clinical management of head, neck, and TMJ pain and dysfunction*, Philadelphia, 1985, JB Lippincott. Used by permission.

Figure 3–2 is almost identical with one reported by the author in the first 103 therapeutic trials in an abstract submitted to the 1978 meeting of the Endocrine Society[22] concluded:

1. Symptomatic patients found to be chemically euthyroid may be metabolically and symptomatically responsive to therapeutic doses of thyroid hormones "doses now considered supraphysiologic". 2. Sequential BMR and serum cholesterol measurements aid in the evaluation of therapeutic responses to thyroid hormones. 3. The BMR, recently and inappropriately under pressure to be obsoleted remains a source of useful clinical information not currently available from other thyroid tests except serum cholesterol. It also remains a useful tool in the follow up of conventionally hypothyroid and thyrotoxic patients during and after treatment.[22]

The plot of a subgroup who received a fixed dose of 0.2 mg levothyroxine sodium (see Fig 3–3). It showed no difference from that obtained with various higher doses, which, along with Refetoff's observation that patients with peripheral resistance to thyroid require supraphysiologic therapeutic doses, and clinical evaluations, suggests that the responses do not reflect an iatrogenic subclinical thyrotoxic "high."

Response in BMR and serum cholesterol were insignificant in the population who had a negative symptomatic response to therapy *(circles)*, whereas the laboratory responses were unequivocally distributed into the quadrant that identified a positive response *(dots)* with only a slight overlap. The nomograms suggest that paired measurements of oxidative metabolism and serum cholesterol measurements are an effective method for confirming a symptomatic response to thyroid administration, and that properly selected symptomatic, chemically euthyroid patients are metabolically responsive to thyroid administration. This group of patients with symptomatic low metabolism responsive to

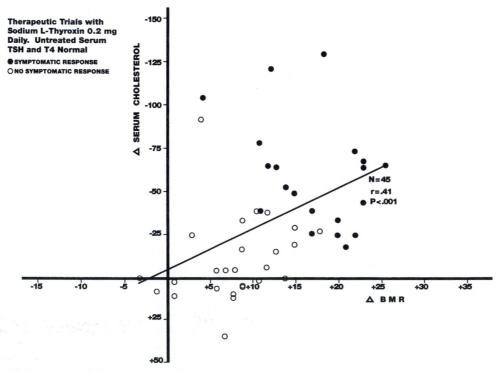

FIG 3–3.

thyroid probably reveals a population of patients with peripheral resistance to thyroid hormone that does not feed back to the HPT axis, and is probably a result of one or more postreceptor defects in the cascade of biochemical reactions that translate hormonal action to the biological action of the cell.

In summary, this discussion challenges currently prevailing concepts that (1) hypothyroidism due to failure of the HPT axis is the sole cause of symptomatic thyroidal insufficiency; (2) preclude therapeutic trials with thyroid hormone in patients with normal blood tests of thyroid hormone production; and (3) proscribe therapeutic doses of thyroid hormones that lower serum TSH below "normal" levels. The following observations offer a broader concept of thyroidal insufficiency.

The Refetoff syndrome of GRTH with a feedback signal to the HPT axis in most cases is being recognized in increasing numbers of kindreds. Over twenty families, comprising over 200 cases, have been identified, and are now being recognized as "the tip of an iceberg."

My observations of metabolic and clinical improvement in patients with symptomatic low metabolism presume peripheral resistance to thyroid at one or more points in a biochemical cascade which translates the hormonal stimulus into the biological action of the cell without a feedback signal to the HPT axis, resulting in normal serum thyroid profiles and normal TSH levels in the symptomatic patient.

The concept of Kurland and co-workers,[10] of metabolic insufficiency as a peripheral resistance syndrome due to inadequate conversion of T_4 to T_3 was rejected as a result of two poorly designed, irrelevant double-blind studies despite reports which support the observations, and warrants further investigation. These observations are summarized in Table 3–2.

HYPERTHYROIDISM

Hyperthyroidism is a common disorder affecting both sexes at any time of life. The medical history and physical examination frequently reveal heat intol-

TABLE 3–2.

Hypothyroidism and Peripheral Resistance to Thyroid Hormones*

	Hypothyroidism	Refetoff Syndrome (GRTH)	Hypometabolism	Symptomatic Low Metabolism
Mechanism	Failure of HPT axis	T_3 receptor gene mutations	Failure peripheral conversion T_4 to T_3	Postreceptor resistance?
Goiter	Yes or no	Yes	No	No
Serum T_4	Low	Inappropriate high	Normal PBI	Normal
Serum TSH	High	Inappropriate high	?	Normal
BMR	Low	Low	Low	Low to normal
Treatment	T_4	T_4	T_3	T_4, T_3, $T_4 + T_3$
Dose	Physiologic c. 0.112 mg daily	Supraphysiologic	Physiologic	Supraphysiologic
Feedback	Yes	Yes	No	No
Proof	Thyroid profile	Gene and receptor probes	Anecdotal	Therapeutic trials
Myofascial pain and trigger points	Yes	?	?	Yes

*HPT = hypothalamic-pituitary-thyroid; T_3 = triiodothyranine; T_4 = thyroxine; TSH = thyroid-stimulating hormone; BMR = basal metabolic rate; PBI = protein-bound iodine.

erance, sweating, weight loss, increased appetite, thinning hair, muscle weakness and occasionally pain, emotional and mental disorders, and sexual dysfunction.

Physical Findings.   Physical findings may reveal goiter; bruit over the neck; proptosis, loss of convergence, lid lag and eyeball lag; fine, warm, moist skin; rapid deep tendon reflexes; muscle wasting; weakness; tenderness; trigger points; fine tremor in the oustretched hands; and tachycardia and cardiac arrhythmias.

Laboratory Findings.   Laboratory findings, usually clear-cut but occasionally occult, include elevation of all components of the thyroid profile, T_3 uptake, T_4 by radioimunoassay (RIA), and calculated free thyroxine index. Additional supportive data will be found in a low pituitary TSH level, high RAI uptake by the thyroid gland, and flat response of the TSH level to an injection of hypothalamic TRH.

Chemical Derangement in Thyrotoxic Myopathy.   This was first demonstrated by Richardson and Shorr,[10, 17] and later confirmed by Thorn and Eder.[25, 26] Shorr et al.[20] demonstrated increased urinary excretion of muscle creatine in thyrotoxic patients which was rapidly abolished by treatment with iodine or thiouracil. Occasionally, an odd form of hyperthyroidism, T_3 thyrotoxicosis, may be confirmed by a normal level of serum T_4, and an elevated level of liothyronine (T_3).

Treatment usually controls or abolishes the condition, and may consist of oral propylthiouracil or methimazole which blocks the formation of T_4 and T_3 in the thyroid gland. Administration to patients with relatively small goiters that shrink during therapy may produce permanent remissions. Relapse may be followed by subtotal thyroidectomy. RAI therapy has become more popular over the years as it has proved to be well tolerated, and free of the risk of surgery, and of agranulocytosis, which occurs in about 0.1% of patients treated with thiouracil. Dosage with RAI and thiouracil varies considerably, and should be determined by an endocrinologist.

The following case report describes a patient with thyrotoxic myopathy.

> A 32-year-old single black woman accountant was referred by her company physician for diagnosis and treatment of suspected hyperthyroidism. Her chief complaints were neck pain, jaw pain while chewing, headaches, and weakness in the knees. The patient reported a 6-month history of muscle soreness, menstrual frequency for a period of 2 years, fatigue on arising, pounding heart, 15-lb weight loss in 1 month, shortness of breath, swollen ankles, nervousness, and tearfulness. She complained of a generalized nocturnal itch for a period of a month.
>
> Positive physical findings included a pulse of 112 beats/min despite 10 mg propranolol orally three times daily; warm, moist excoriated skin; diffuse tenderness; and trigger points in all muscles, mandibles, and ear canals. The thyroid gland was diffusely enlarged to about 50 g, and a systolic murmur was heard over the left lobe.
>
> Abnormally high laboratory values included RAI uptake of 85%; T_4/T_3 conversion ratio, 89%; T_4 RIA, 15.2 µg/dL; T_3 uptake, 65%. Serum cholesterol was low: 95 mg/dL. The patient was treated with 5.63 mCi of ^{131}I on November 10, 1976. Her course following therapy was complicated by staphylococcal tonsillitis. By January 6, 1977 all manifestations of hyperthyroidism had cleared. Her myofascial and jaw pains had subsided completely.

ESTROGENIC INSUFFICIENCY, MENOPAUSE

Menopause

Menopause is a common cause of myofascial pain and trigger points, and a probable cause if the onset of pain, sweats, and flushes occur in approximately the same period. On the other hand, estrogenic insufficiency may be asymptomatic except for a complaint of muscle or joint pain due to drop of the estrogen level. It may occur in the premenopausal woman. The myofascial pain usually clears promptly with a trial of oral or cutaneous estrogen therapy. Symptoms of anxiety, weakness, fatigue, depression, inability to cope, loss of creativity, and libido often improve rapidly with estrogen replacement. Osteoporosis is a source of pain in this group owing to postural changes associated with collapse of vertebrae, and microfractures.

Therapy has changed slightly since the pioneering studies by Ephraim Shorr on the metabolic unit at New York Hospital in the late 1940s and early 1950s. Conjugated estrogens remain the gold standard of treatment. The usual starting dose is 0.625. mg/day orally for 21 days, or estrogen patches containing either 0.05 or 0.1 of estradiol mg applied twice weekly for 3 weeks, followed by 1 week of rest and then resumption of the dosage. Larger doses may be required, supplemented in women with an intact uterus by a progestin such as norethindrone acetate 5 mg or medroxyprogesterone 2.5 to 10.0 mg/day over the last 7 days of estrogen therapy to reverse proliferative changes in the endometrium, and to enhance the onset of endometrial shedding and withdrawal bleeding. Many practitioners administer the progestin for 10 days. Following hysterectomy there appears to be no good rationale for progestin therapy. Other therapeutic modalities include supplemental calcium 1,000 mg/day, vitamin D_2 50,000 units twice weekly, or calcitriol 0.25 µg once daily, human calcitonin 1 vial intramuscularly (IM) daily (unpopular), and etidronate 200 mg twice daily for 2 weeks every 3 months taken orally 2 hours before or after meals with a daily calcium supplement.

Menopausal patients are occasionally resistant to estrogen therapy. The use of "conventional regimens" monitored by including a so-called maturation index with the Papanicolaou smear will not detect resistance. We have routinely used Shorr stain, a sensitive stain devised by Shorr[29] and Cohen.[30] The ultimate composition of the stain as described in the Shorr report is attributed to Dr. Eugene Cohen. It is up to the practitioner or a well-trained technician to prepare the specimen. Once the preparation is made correctly, the specimen can be stained in an office laboratory in about 5 minutes, and read by the practitioner. Shorr identified four levels of function from slides stained on alternate days through the menstrual cycle as atrophic, hypofunctional, cyclical (indicating a normal estrus), and rarely hyperfunctional, in which there appears to be a constant excessive estrogen production. This last condition is unknown to the practitioner who does not employ the Shorr stain, and therefore is generally unrecognized. An atrophic, or hypofunctional smear in an estrogen-resistant, menopausal woman who remains symptomatic on conventional estrogen and progestin doses should initiate a titration to a higher dose.

Symptoms may appear before amenorrhea occurs, due to the fall of estrogen levels as menopause approaches, or recur at any time after onset of menopause. Younger women with primary or secondary amenorrhea, or hypofunctional, acyclical bleeding characterized by low estrogen levels as detected by the Shorr stain may have menopausal and myofascial symptoms. Other menopausal age–related symptoms such as depression, inability to cope, and loss of libido should alert the practitioner to possible need for estrogen replacement.

Male Menopause

Male menopause is much less frequent and of slower onset than in the female. The condition is due to the gradual fall of serum testosterone, and manifests as weakness, depression, and apathy. Myofascial pain and trigger points may be conspicuous. Methyltestosterone 10 to 25 mg/day, or testosterone enanthate 200 mg IM monthly may relieve symptoms.

CUSHING'S DISEASE AND SYNDROME

Both Cushing's disease and Cushing's syndrome are manifested by excessive secretion of cortisol by the adrenal cortex. Cushing's disease is produced by an adrenocorticotropic hormone (ACTH)–secreting tumor of the pituitary with secondary adrenal hyperplasia, whereas Cushing's syndrome is caused by a primary adrenal tumor or ectopic production of ACTH.

Diagnostic Signs

Diagnostic signs include a round, ruddy face; facial hirsutism in the female; centripetal obesity; purple striae on the abdomen; thin skin, which tears and bruises easily; thinning of scalp hair; hypertension; mild diabetes mellitus; polycythemia; mental disorders; bone mineral loss; and spinal fractures. Muscle wasting, weakness, pain, and spasm are characteristic.

Laboratory confirmation includes elevation of A.M. plasma cortisol which cannot be suppressed by an oral dose of 1 mg dexamethasone at bedtime, and elevation of 24-hour urinary free cortisol. Plasma ACTH is high in pituitary disease, and low in primary adrenal disease. Imaging of the pituitary or adrenals by computed tomography (CT) scans or magnetic resonance imaging (MRI) usually reveals the tumor.

Treatment

Treatment of primary adrenal tumors is by surgical removal. Transphenoidal hypophysectomy or pituitary irradiation may be effective for a pituitary tumor. Oral chemotherapy may be effective. Mitotane is the most powerful of the drugs and causes pituitary ablation usually in doses of between 8 and 12 g/day. Aminoglutethimide, a blocker of steroid production from cholesterol, is given in doses increasing to about 2 g/day orally. Oral cyproheptadine, a serotonin blocker, has been effective in a few cases, and recently the antifungal ketoconazole has been found to be effective in some patients.

The physiatrist has an important role in rehabilitation following cure of the hormonal excess, because catabolic effects of the disease may be persistent and disabling. Hemiplegia may occur due to spinal fractures, and muscle damage may be severe.

ADDISON'S DISEASE

Addison's disease, due to primary adrenal insufficiency, may first manifest itself during adrenal crisis, or insidiously through muscle pain, spasm, or knee contractures probably resulting from low serum sodium and elevated potassium.[2] Kraus[9] relates diagnosing a case of Addison's disease when he observed prominent skin pigmentation in a patient with severe muscle pain. Five cases of muscle contractures have been reported by a group of rheumatologists.[19] Once suspected, the condition can be confirmed by manifestations of skin and mucous membrane pigmentation, low blood pressure, postural hypotension, cachexia, weakness, electrolyte abnormalities, high serum ACTH, and failure of serum cortisol to rise 1 hour after an injection of synthetic ACTH. Detection in the black patient may be especially difficult, but a careful history usually reveals that the patient has become darker during the course of the disease.

PITUITARY-ADRENAL INSUFFICIENCY

Pituitary-adrenal insufficiency is usually due to atrophy of adrenal glands secondary to a pituitary tumor, infarction, or hemorrhage. The patient may appear in the office of a practitioner other than an internist or endocrinologist because of myofascial pain and trigger points. Males often present with a eunuchoid appearance, thin facial hair, sallowness, poor muscle development, weakness, loss of libido, testicular atrophy, and sometimes a high-pitched voice. Hyperpigmentation is absent.

An obtunded 60-year-old retired white man was admitted to the surgical service of the New York Hospital emergency room in December 1952 for a second episode of acute abdominal pain which extended to the flanks and back. A provisional diagnosis of acute pancreatitis was made despite the fact that it could not be confirmed by an exhaustive clinical, chemical, and radiologic evaluation during the previous hospitalization. The chief medical resident, while leaving the hospital via the emergency room, glanced at the semicomatose patient, recognized the appearance of panhypopituitarism, and suggested the possibility of pituitary-adrenal crisis and pain due to muscle spasm related to hyponatremia. A stat serum sodium determination of 109 mg/dL (normal 131–145) proved him to be correct. The patient was admitted to the endocrine service where he was treated with 5 mg of desoxycorticosterone acetate (DOCA) in oil IM, every 6 hours, and a 0.9% saline solution was administered intravenously (IV). The patient rapidly regained consciousness, and the myofascial abdominal and flank pain subsided. In view of the fact that pituitary-adrenal insufficiency may not cause salt loss, but may cause low serum sodium due to delayed excretion of a water load, the endocrine staff decided to do the then conventional test for adrenal insufficiency, salt withdrawal. Steroid therapy was discontinued, and his salt intake was reduced to 1 g/day. In 24 hours he became too weak to stand, blood pressure dropped to 100/50 mm Hg, serum sodium dropped from 140 to 131 mg/dL, and his muscles became stiff and painful. He was put back on steroids and salt intake was raised to 15 g. His ultimate replacement therapy was 12.5 mg of oral cortisone twice daily, 1 mg of fludrocortisone (Florinef), and at least 6 g of salt daily. This patient lived for another 20 years, maintaining a good quality of life, during which removal of a large pituitary chromophobe adenoma corrected severe narrowing of the visual fields. He died at the age of 80 from pulmonary emphysema.

PARATHYROID DISEASE

Hyperparathyroidism

Hyperparathyroidism raises the level of serum parathyroid hormone, which elevates serum calcium. Myopathy may occur with the more severe elevations and is usually manifested by muscle weakness. Myofascial pain is uncommon.[6] The diagnosis is now frequently made in asymptomatic patients because of routine measurement of serum calcium in chemical profiles. Fibromyalgia may occur and usually clears with correction of the hypercalcemia. The treatment of choice is usually surgical removal. Mild, asymptomatic disease may be kept under observation; especially in poor-risk patients.

Hypoparathyroidism

Hypoparathyroidism usually occurs as a result of removal, or damage to the parathyroid glands during thyroid surgery, but may occur spontaneously. It results in low serum calcium which, when severe, causes acute muscle spasms and tetany. Acute spasms may be relieved by elevation of the serum calcium with IV injection of 10% calcium gluconate as a bolus or slow drip. Protracted hypocalcemia responds to ingestion of large doses of vitamin D_2, or calciferol, about 50,000 units/day, or calcitriol in a dose of 0.25 μg orally twice daily. Patients on sustained therapy must have periodic evaluations to ascertain that the serum calcium level is not overcorrected.

SUMMARY

Virtually all metabolic disorders affect skeletal muscle and may cause pain, spasm and trigger points. This report considers a number of endocrine disorders in which myofascial pain may occur. Case reports of myopathy in a patient with thyrotoxicosis, and in a patient with a pituitary tumor and secondary adrenal insufficiency are presented. More detailed discussions are presented for the two endocrine disorders most commonly encountered by practitioners who diagnose and treat endocrine-related myofascial pain and trigger points, thyroidal deficiency, and the female monopause.

Menopausal patients commonly complain of myofascial pain. Recognition of this clinical relationship is essential since conventional physical therapy and injections of trigger points may be ineffective, or subject to relapse if the patient is not treated with steroids.

Thyroidal deficiency states are commonly associated with myopathy. The data presented reveal an increasing awareness of syndromes of peripheral resistance to thyroid hormones. The Refetoff syndrome of GRTH, considered a rarity since 1967, has in the past year been called the "tip of an iceberg."

Data on therapeutic trials with thyroid hormones in chemically euthyroid patients with symptoms of hypothyroidism, relatively low-oxidative metabolism, and symptomatic low metabolism are presented. Myofascial pain is the second most common complaint. Many patients have had clinical improvement confirmed by improvement in oxidative metabolism, and a decrease in serum cholesterol—a marker of metabolic response to thyroid hormone. The condition differs from the Refetoff syndrome in that it does not produce the feedback signals, inappropriate secretion of T_4 and TSH. Absence of a feedback signal makes detection difficult. Clinical acuity is an essential first step in making the diagnosis. The resistance would occur at a site different from that of the Refetoff syndrome, possibly in the postreceptor cascade of biological reactions that translate the receptor signal into the biological action of the cell.

Hypometabolism, the first proposed form of peripheral resistance, was rejected 30 years ago.

Measurement of oxidative basal metabolism by the BMR is an essential test in the diagnosis and study of peripheral resistance to thyroid. The test was obsoleted a number of years ago by formal agreement between Blue Cross/Blue Shield, and a number of medical organizations, although it continues to be used in research laboratories dealing with peripheral resistance to thyroid hormones. Unfortunately, most practitioners no longer have access to this important diagnostic measurement. The practitioner dealing with myofascial pain syndromes in which peripheral resistance to thyroid is considered a factor, will have to do what many practitioners have done for many years, administer therapeutic trials in doses of about 0.15 mg T_4, or its equivalent without direct objective confirmation other than the serial measurement of serum cholesterol, and rely on clinical judgement to adjust, or discontinue treatment. Hopefully computerized analytic systems now available will again be used in routine metabolic evaluation.

REFERENCES

1. Bessman SP, Geiger PJ: Transport of energy in muscle: The phosphoryl creatine shuttle, *Science* 211:448, 1981.
2. Blandford RL, Samanta AC, Burden AC, et al: Muscle contractures associated with glucocorticoid deficiency, *Br Med J* 291:127, 1985.
3. Cohen E, Personal communication, 1959.
4. Craig FA, Crispin Smith J: Serum creatine phosphokinase activity in altered thyroid states, *J Clin Endocrinol* 25:723, 1965.
5. Debre R, Semelaigne G: Syndrome of diffuse muscular hypertrophy in infants causing athletic appearance and its connection with congenital myxedema, *Am J Dis Child* 50:1351, 1935.
6. De Meirleir K, Golstein J, Jonckheer MH, et al: Hypothyroidism with normal thyroid hormone levels as a consequence of autoimmune thyroiditis and peripheral resistance to thyroid hormone, *Acta Clin Belg* 35:107, 1980.
7. Frame B, Heinze EG, Block MA, et al: Myopathy in primary hyperparathyroidism, *Ann Intern Med* 66:1022, 1968.
8. Gergely J: Biochemical aspects of muscle structure and function. In Walton JN, editor: *Disorders of voluntary muscle*, ed 2, London, 1981, Churchill Livingstone, p 102.
9. Keating R: Metabolic insufficiency (editorial), *J Clin Endocrinol Metab* 18:531, 1958.
10. Kraus H, Personal communication, 1992.
11. Kurland GS, Hamolsky MW, Stone Freedberg A: Metabolic insufficiency, *J Clin Endocrinol Metab* 18:531, 1957.
12. Levin ME: "Metabolic Insufficiency," a double blind study using triiodothyronine, thyroxine, and placebo, *J Clin Endocrinol Metab* 20:106, 1960.
13. Mc Ardle B: Metabolic, and endocrine myopathies. In Walton, JN, editor: *Disorders of voluntary muscle*, Edinburgh, 1974, Churchill Livingstone, p 735.
14. Mixon AJ, Parrilla R, Ransom SC, et al: Correlation of language abnormalities with localization of mutations in the B-thyroid hormone receptor in 13 kindreds with generalized resistance to thyroid hormone: Identification of four new mutations, *J Clin Endocrinol Metab* 75:1039, 1992.
15. Ramsey I: Thyroid disease and muscle dysfunction, St Louis, 1974, Mosby–Year Book.

16. Refetoff S: Thyroid hormone resistance syndromes. In Braverman LE and Utiger RD, editors: *Werner and Ingbar's the Thyroid,* Philadelphia, 1991, JB Lippincott, p 735.

17. Refetoff S, De Wind LT, De Groot LJ: Familial syndrome combining deaf mutism, stippled pract, goiter, and abnormally high PBI: Possible target organ refractoriness to thyroid hormone, *J Clin Endocrinol Metab* 27:279, 1967.

18. Richardson HB, Shorr E: Creatin metabolism in atypical Graves disease, *Trans Assoc Am Physicians* 50:156, 1935.

19. Rives KL, Furth ED, Becker DV: Limitations of the ankle jerk test, *Ann Intern Med* 62:1139, 1965.

20. Shapiro MS, Trebich C, Shilo L, et al: Myalgias and muscle contracture as the presenting signs of Addison's disease, *Postgrad Med J* 64:222, 1988.

21. Shorr E: An evaluation of the clinical applications of the vaginal smear method, *J Mt Sinai Hosp* 12:667.

22. Shorr E, Richardson HB, Mansfield JS: Influence of thyroid administration on creatine metabolism in myxedema of adults, *Proc Soc Exp Biol Med* 32:1340, 1935.

23. Sonkin LS: Paired BMR and serum cholesterol measurements in therapeutic trials with thyroid hormones in patients with normal levels of TSH and/or T_4, or PBI and symptoms suggesting thyroid deficiency (abstract 678), Endocrine Society 60th Annual Meeting, 1978.

24. Sonkin LS: Endocrine disorders and muscle dysfunction. In Gelb H, editor: *Clinical management of head, neck, and TMJ pain and dysfunction,* Philadelphia, 1985, JB Lippincott, p 137.

25. Sonkin LS: Myofascial pain in metabolic disorders. In Kraus H: *Diagnosis, and treatment of muscle pain,* Chicago, 1988, Quintessence.

26. Thorn GW: Creatine studies in thyroid disorders, *Endocrinology;* 20:628, 1936.

27. Thorn GW, Eder HA: Creatine studies in chronic thyrotoxic myopathy, *Am J Med* 1:538, 1946.

28. Thyroid hormone resistance syndrome may affect thousands of unsuspecting americans, *NIH Observer* 1 (winter): 1991.

29. Williams R: Hypometabolism (metabolic insufficiency). In Williams R, editor: *Textbook of endocrinology,* ed 3. Philadelphia, 1962, WB Saunders.

Chapter 4

Psychological Considerations in Myofascial Pain, Fibromyalgia, and Related Musculoskeletal Pain

Roy C. Grzesiak, Ph.D.

Clarification of the possible roles of psychological factors in myofascial pain and other musculoskeletal pain problems is a complex undertaking. First, there is a psychology of pain that is complex and multifactorial in nature suggesting that the role of psychological factors in the etiology of myofascial pain ranges from none at all to considerable, if not exclusive. The clinician must be attuned to signs that point to possible complicating psychological factors in the patient's presenting behavior. Second, a biopsychosocial perspective on fibromyalgia and myofascial pain indicates that proper treatment and management approaches will vary considerably from patient to patient and that progress, or the lack of it, in physical rehabilitation may be the only indication of whether the prescribed treatment program is correct. The focus of this chapter is on offering a comprehensive but practical clinical approach to the psychological evaluation and management of patients with musculoskeletal pain syndromes. After a brief theoretical introduction to concepts such as chronic pain and its attendant psychological features, attention is on *what to look for* in the clinical screening of patients with myofascial and related musculoskeletal pain as well as *what to do* in terms of patient management when psychological or psychosocial factors appear to be complicating the picture. Additionally, an overview of common psychological assessment and treatment approaches is provided. However, to reiterate, the focus is primarily on clinical management.

CHRONIC PAIN AND THE PAIN-PRONE PATIENT

Physicians and other health care professionals who work exclusively with pain patients often develop a skewed and distorted view of chronic pain. Not only do they often end up sounding like psychiatrists,[22] but they frequently fall victim to some form of stereotyping with respect to a favored cause of chronic pain. The relationship between pain and depression affords an excellent example. The majority position on the relationship between pain and depression is that the depression seen in chronic pain patients is a consequence of living with the pain; there is only equivocal experimental, empirical, or clinical support for such a notion. Depression can be either cause, concomitant, or consequence of pain.[24, 47] Perhaps the attitude reflects an implicit apology for the need to include psychological care in the management of people who are "in pain." One of the facts that is often lost in chronic pain work is that there are many persons with persistent pain who do not become "chronic pain patients." In other words, they continue to cope, work, love, and embrace life, even with pain. In fact, even within any given sample of chronic pain patients, Turk and Rudy[95, 96] have identified factors that suggest that patients seen in specialty pain clinics and programs are not representative of chronic pain patients as a whole. Recent studies examining the role of biopsychosocial factors in the development of chronic pain suggest that it is the psychological component of the matrix that leads to chronicity, not the biological component.[79, 94] In fact, a recent prospective investigation indicated that anxiety was the psychosocial antecedent that predicted chronicity in herpes zoster (postherpetic neuralgia).[27]

Before considering chronic pain in more detail, it is informative to review the various components of pain. A frequently used schema has been proposed by Loeser[60, 61] (Fig 4–1). In this schema, *nociception* refers to the potentially tissue-damaging mechanical, thermal, or chemical energy impinging on specialized nerve endings that can initiate the transmission of a signal into the nervous system. *Pain* is the perception of that signal in the central nervous system. While pain perception can occur as a consequence of nociception, pain can also be perceived when no tissue-damaging energy has impinged, or continues to impinge, on the nervous system. Pain syndromes reflecting this latter concept would be the various central pain syndromes. *Suffering* is where psychological factors enter the picture. Suffering refers to the negative emotional reactions that can complicate the clinical presentation. *Pain behavior* refers to those observable behaviors that suggest to the observer that the individual is experiencing pain. The concept of pain behavior was proposed first by Fordyce and associates.[35, 36] Considering these multifaceted components of overall pain experience, it is no wonder that patients often present us with complicated and confusing clinical pictures.

What is *chronic* pain? Why is it important to recognize when a continuing pain problem represents a chronic as opposed to an acute condition? While definitions of chronic pain vary, the consensus among pain professionals holds that

FIG 4–1. Concepts of pain. (From Loeser JD: Concepts of pain. In Stanton-Hicks M, Boas RA, editors: *Chronic low back pain,* New York, 1982, Raven Press, pp 145–148. Used by permission.)

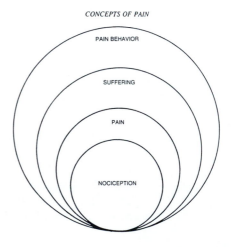

CONCEPTS OF PAIN

PAIN BEHAVIOR

SUFFERING

PAIN

NOCICEPTION

pain that continues for more than 3 months is the "most convenient point of division between acute and chronic pain."[68] Briefly, chronic pain is pain that continues over time, unresponsive to appropriate medical, surgical, or pharmacologic treatment, lacks biological utility, is frequently associated with depression, and should not be managed with narcotic analgesics[90] (Table 4–1). In fact, Chapman and Bonica[15] have warned that the two major dangers in failing to recognize a pain as chronic are unnecessary surgery and risk of addiction.

While there is no singular pain-prone personality, there are certainly pain-prone *personalities*. The concept of pain-prone personality originated in the work of Engel[29, 30] who noticed that his patients who lacked definitive physical findings to account for their pain shared a number of common denominators in terms of their early psychosocial and developmental experiences. These early experiences included physically or verbally abusive parents; harsh or punitive parents who then overcompensated with rare displays of affection; cold or distant parents who were only warm and solicitous of the child when the latter was ill; a parent who suffered from chronic illness or pain; and various other parent-child interactions involving guilt, aggression, or pain. Engel proposed that these early developmental events predisposed a person to pain-proneness. Further, he stated that these pain-prone persons superimposed an individual psychic signature on their somatically or psychogenically based pain sensation. This individual psychic signature usually complicates symptom presentation. In fact, Engel offered that the more complex the symptom picture, the greater the likelihood that psychological factors were at play. It is important to note that pain-proneness does not reflect a singular personality type but rather is found in a variety of personality and characterologic organizations.

Empirical support for the concept of pain-proneness can be found in three recent studies. Adler and associates[1] compared psychogenic pain patients with three other pain and illness-related control groups and found that the former recalled significantly more early psychosocial and developmental trauma. In a recent study investigating the correlation of traumatic psychosocial-developmental events on the outcome of spinal surgery it was found that these traumatic events had the capacity to severely compromise postsurgical outcomes.[86] Finally, extensive investigations of back pain by Blumer and

TABLE 4–1.

Distinctions Between Acute and Chronic Pain*

Acute	Chronic
Symptomatic	A disease in itself
Biologically useful	Less diagnostic utility
Induces anxiety	Induces depression
Narcotics indicated; undertreatment is a concern	Narcotics contraindicated
Little potential for addiction	Potential addiction
Pathologic origin recognized	Pathologic origin unclear, often complex interaction
Cure likely	Cure may be impossible

*From Tait RC: *Curr Concepts Pain* 1:10–15, 1983. Used by permission.

Heilbronn[6, 7] have demonstrated a similar configuration of early experiences that they believe predispose to depression and subsequently to pain. They have termed this the *dysthymic pain disorder*.[6, 7] These early traumas are frequently not remembered by pain patients and reflect unconscious processes that have been either repressed, dissociated, or otherwise foreclosed from consciousness. It is only when illness, trauma, or pain trigger these early psychodynamic factors that the patient's clinical presentation, course of treatment, and ultimate rehabilitation are affected.[45]

The above thesis should not be taken as suggesting that *all* chronic pain patients have dysfunctional early psychosocial-developmental histories, for that certainly is not the case. But some do. Pain experience reflects the multifactorial interaction of biopsychosocial processes. For example, chronic pain may reflect simple learning, failure to cope, dysfunctional coping capacities, irrational beliefs about pain and suffering, chronic postural problems, musculoskeletal hyperreactivity, as well as more hidden psychological difficulties such as pain-prone tendencies.

MYOFASCIAL PAIN, FIBROMYALGIA, AND RELATED MUSCULOSKELETAL PAIN

Turning specifically to myofascial pain syndrome, fibromyalgia, and related musculoskeletal pain, a brief review of the literature is in order. While a comprehensive review is beyond the scope of this chapter, a number of comprehensive surveys are available.[8, 9, 39, 56, 62] As a whole, while these reviews are thorough and comprehensive, their conclusions are disappointing. For example, they point out that concepts such as primary fibromyalgia, secondary fibromyalgia, fibrositis, myofascial pain syndrome, and psychogenic rheumatism all have considerable overlap and many of the early studies failed to provide clear-cut operational definitions for the syndromes being investigated. Consequently, there is much confusion as to exactly which syndrome is being studied in many of the reports. Similarly, attempts to define psychological and psychiatric variables have been less than clear on methodology, sample characteristics, and illness parameters. Consequently, a more pragmatic approach to presenting this information is to deconstruct it into its component features and present them as summary modules. Accordingly, the following concepts will be summarized: the fibromyalgic personality; depression, in its premorbid, current, and lifetime occurrences; somatization; stress, anxiety, and muscle tension; nonrestorative sleep disturbance; and phenomenology.

The Fibromyalgic Personality

Historically, persistent pain problems that have ill-defined causes have been subjected to personality stereotyping. For example, common terms in the older psychosomatic literature include migraine personality, rheumatic personality, temporomandibular joint (TMJ) personality, and so on. So too has a "fibromyalgic personality" been characterized. Smythe has been an adamant proponent of this concept: "These patients set high standards and are as demanding of themselves as they are of others. They are caring, honest, tidy, committed, moral, industrious—virtuous to a fault."[89] While empirical support for this personality configuration has not been forthcoming, such discrepancy between the empirical and the clinical literature is not unusual. Research efforts to validate personality types as they relate to pain-related and other psychosomatic problems have been plagued by problems of depth of assessment. It may well be that this highly moral, hard-working, perfectionistic type of person can be found in any subset of pain patients and that the final symptomatic outcome will reflect the interaction of personality type with physical predisposition or diathesis and disease or injury.

Clinicians have found this "workaholic" personality style in many chronic pain sufferers. Sarno[80-85] has stressed chronic character style, avoidance of conflict, and unawareness of anxiety as contributory to neck and back muscular pain. He has noted that many of his patients are conscientious, compulsive, responsible, and hard-working; they are self-motivated and critical of themselves and others. In a recent paper, Coen and Sarno[21] have explained that one of the primary tension generators in this type of personality is not the psychic conflict proper but rather avoidance of awareness of the conflict so that conscious effort is turned toward external activities, productivity, success, etc., rather than toward one's inner emotional life.

This kind of personality style is also well documented in the research of Blumer and Heilbronn[6, 7] who have labeled it "ergomanic." Not unlike Engel's pain-prone personalities,[30] ergomanic persons work hard to maintain their image as "solid citizens." They have a history of excessive work performance, often hold more than one job, are uncomfortable with time off or vacations, do little to relax, and are pathologically self-reliant. They have maintained this pace from early in life, often having been forced to do so by a dysfunctional family constellation and when they finally suffer a painful trauma, they have extreme difficulty in allowing themselves to be ill, but finally succumb to their dependency needs to such an extent that treatment efforts are foiled. A study by Van Houdenhove[97] surveying a large sample of chronic pain patients for premorbid hyperactivity found a significant number (70%) fit the criteria described by Blumer and Heilbronn.[6, 7] A preliminary study by Ciccone and Grzesiak[19] reviewed work history and early psychosocial trauma in a sample of chronic neck and back patients. They found significance for the ergomanic traits as well.[19]

It may well be that the so-called fibromyalgic personality is not causal of fibromyalgia or fibrositis but that it is a significant contributor to the overall disablement when a patient does have soft tissue pathology. As such, it is not unique to fibromyalgia or myofascial pain dysfunction but reflects the interaction of a pain-prone premorbid personality with other biological variables or diatheses for this condition. As Blumer and Heilbronn have suggested,[7] it is clinically most useful to look at the pain problem and the mood as synchronous expressions of the patient's overall state of being.[7]

Depression: Cause, Consequence, or Concomitant

In psychological and psychiatric studies of fibromyalgia and myofascial pain syndrome, depression has been the most extensively studied, although a tally of results leaves us with more questions than answers. Again, definitional problems plague the literature. Myofascial pain syndrome, fibrositis, and fibromyalgia are mixed together in some of the studies. Furthermore, definitions of depression vary in terms of criteria, as do the psychometric and clinical investigative methods used to arrive at results. All that can be done at this point in time in terms of understanding the role of depression in these syndromes is to present the trends that seem apparent in the literature.

It has become a commonplace to expect chronic pain patients to be depressed. Many of the studies of depression in fibromyalgia, e.g., have used the MMPI (Minnesota Multiphasic Personality Inventory) as the primary psychometric index (the MMPI in psychodiagnostic evaluation is presented later) and, because it was designed for use with psychiatric, not medical, patients, its value is somewhat compromised. Nevertheless, MMPI results constitute a major part of the literature on the psychological aspects of fibromyalgia.

Payne and associates[76] compared patients with fibromyalgia, mixed arthritis, and rheumatoid arthritis on the MMPI and found that the MMPI profiles of the fibromyalgia group showed greater elevations and more variability. However, only the Hy scale (hypochondriasis) and the Hs scale (hysteria) were of clinically significant elevation; the D scale (depression) was not differentially elevated in the fibromyalgia group.[76] Similarly, Ahles and associates[2] compared patients with fibromyalgia with patients having rheumatoid arthritis as well as with normal controls and found the fibromyalgia group to have higher elevations on Hy, D, and Hs, but not to a pathologic degree. Another MMPI study conducted by Wolfe and associates[100] found Hy and Hs highest in the fibromyalgia group. So it seems clear that at least part of the so-called neurotic triad of hypochondriasis, depression, and hysteria is more significantly elevated in fibromyalgia patients. However, all three of these MMPI scales load heavily on somatic factors and patients with active, painful medical conditions are likely to score higher than either patient controls with painless medical conditions or normal controls. Based on the research presented thus far, it appears that psychological concerns such as somatic preoccupation, symptom endorsement, and denial of psychological difficulties figure more prominently in the clinical picture than does depression.

Targeting the relationship between depression and fibromyalgia for study, and using more standardized and structured clinical interview criteria, Hudson and associates[52] found that current as well as past episodes of depression were more common in the fibromyalgia group compared with rheumatoid arthritis patients and controls. Additionally, 64% of the fibromyalgia group recalled experiencing symptoms of depression prior to the onset of their muscle pain.[52] In another study, Kirmayer and associates[58] found that fibromyalgia patients had a somewhat greater incidence of lifetime depressive episodes than did patients with rheumatoid arthritis, although the difference did not reach significance. The psychiatric histories of first-degree relatives for both fibromyalgia and rheumatoid arthritis patients were also reviewed and it was found that family histories of those with fibromyalgia had more depression, although not significantly more.[58] Goldenberg[39] proposed that the above results suggest some form of psychobiological link between depression and fibromyalgia. Another study[2] used the Zung Depression Scale to compare patients with primary fibromyalgia, rheumatoid arthritis, and healthy controls, attempting to determine if fibromyalgia is a variant of depression. No differences were found for the two clinical groups although both groups had a subset of patients that appeared to have significant depression.[2]

Although the empirical evidence is meager, it does suggest a trend in that many of the studies suggest a somewhat greater incidence of premorbid, family, and lifetime occurrence of depression in persons who develop fibromyalgia. The evidence at this time is not sufficient to posit a causal psychosomatic relationship.

Somatization

Closely aligned to the concept of depression is the process of somatization. According to Kellner,[56] somatization disorder is one of the somatoform disorders in the current psychiatric nomenclature. Patients with somatization disorder have multiple somatic complaints (at least 13) beginning before the age of 30 years. Somatization refers to a subconscious process in which emotional distress is translated into bodily complaints. While Kellner prefers to restrict the use of either term to those patients who display *no* evidence of organic illness, the actual DSM-III-R (*Diagnostic and Statistical Manual of the American Psychiatric Association*, revised third edition) definition is not so stringent and patients can be labeled with one of the somatization processes or disorders in the presence of organic pathologic findings if the complaints and resulting social or occupational impairments are grossly in excess of what would be expected given the physical findings.

Hudson and associates[52] investigated the presence of somatization disorder in a sample of fibromyalgia patients and found it present in only 6% of cases. Similarly, Kirmayer and associates[58] studied the presence and coexistence of depression and somatization in fibromyalgia patients. They found only 5% of their sample met the criteria for somatization disorder. Although only a small percentage of fibromyalgia patients actually meet the criteria for somatization *disorder*, the authors argue that the fibromyalgia population does have many of the characteristics of somatization disorder, including frequent and varied somatic complaints in multiple organ systems, excessive health care utilization, and many surgeries in systems other than the musculoskeletal. Kirmayer and associates argue that it is important to look at somatization not as a disorder but as a process—one of the processes involved in illness behavior—and from that perspective gain a richer understanding of how the patient can impose idiosyncratic meaning on his or her symptoms.[58]

Stress, Anxiety, and Muscle Tension

Stress has been implicated as a major factor in the development of many painful conditions and it has been examined in relationship to fibromyalgia and myofascial pain syndrome. In a major review of orofacial pain syndromes, including myofascial pain dysfunction, Grzesiak[44] found that the literature supported stress as one of the major psychological factors leading to symptom formation or intensification.

Stress leads to muscle tension and there is ample evidence that prolonged muscle tension leads to pain. Is this a significant factor in fibromyalgia and other myofascial pain syndromes? One of the earliest studies investigating the role of life situations, emotions, and backache was reported by Holmes and Wolff.[51] They studied back pain patients that had no obvious physical findings to account for their pain and found that both life situations and strong emotions facilitated back pain. They used both amobarbital (Amytal) interviews and surface electromyographic (EMG) recordings to monitor levels of muscle tension across a variety of muscle groups. Because their subjects were not specifically defined as suffering from myofascial pain syndrome or fibromyalgia, the results may not be directly applicable. However, their findings are important and worth noting because of the implications for virtually all soft tissue pain problems. Most noteworthy is the fact that they found the majority of their patients to engage in hyperfunctioning of all the skeletal musculature. The subjects tended to be locked in a vigilant "on guard" pattern of sustained muscle contraction. These findings fit nicely with Sarno's observations described above in which personality style and psychic conflict generate tension which leads to back pain.[80-85]

In a study comparing patients with fibromyalgia with both a rheumatoid arthritis group and a normal control group, Ahles and associates[3] found that the fibromyalgia group reported a greater number of stressful life events. Importantly, using the MMPI as a major psychometric index, they found the fibromyalgia group could be subcategorized and that 31% of the sample showed significant psychological disturbance. In the presence of major stressors, this subgroup was more reactive in terms of symptom pattern. The authors point out that further studies looking at both major stressful life events and minor daily hassles may add another dimension to our understanding of the interaction of stress and muscle pain.[3] Unfortunately, there is not a major literature on stress and fibromyalgia. There is a significant literature on the relationship between stress, muscle tension, and myofascial pain dysfunction of the muscles of mastication and upper quarter.

Nonrestorative Sleep and Symptom Formation

The importance of sleep pattern dysfunction in fibrositis or fibromyalgia was first observed by Moldofsky and associates.[72, 73] Patients with fibromyalgia frequently have a nonrestorative sleep pattern so that they do not awaken feeling refreshed even after what seemed to be a good night's sleep. Additionally, they awaken with generalized musculoskeletal pain and stiffness, fatigue, and localized tender points. Sleep electroencephalographic (EEG) studies have shown that patients with fibromyalgia have an alpha intrusion into their delta or stage IV sleep.[72] This alpha intrusion is correlated with an increase in muscle tenderness. Furthermore, a study of normal volunteers in which delta sleep was experimentally disrupted showed the development of fibrositic trigger points.[73] Comparisons of fibromyalgia patients, chronic insomniacs, dysthymics and normals for EEG sleep patterns reveals that the *alpha EEG, non-rapid eye movement (NREM) sleep anomaly* is characteristic of fibromyalgia. Whereas normals, insomniacs, and dysthymics average approximately 25% duration in NREM sleep of alpha EEG sleep, those with fibromyalgia average 60% duration of NREM sleep occupied by the alpha EEG sleep anomaly.[48, 85] According to Moldofsky,[70] alpha EEG sleep may be a sensitive indicator of fibrositis but it is not specific to the disorder. The sleep anomaly has been found in healthy people who are asymptomatic.

Studies that pharmacologically manipulated sleep EEG frequencies using chlorpromazine or L-tryptophan have demonstrated that the alpha and delta frequencies are related to pain, energy, and mood.[71] In a review paper,[70] Moldofsky noted that psychological, environmental, and biological influences can disrupt sleep and, consequently, a wide range of factors can affect the fibrositis syndrome. Most notable are areas where minor trauma can lead to major changes in musculoskeletal complaints. Stressful life events, e.g., motor vehicle accidents, even minor ones, can lead to sleep disturbance, and musculoskeletal and mood symptoms. In addition to trauma, viral illness, immunocompromise, and painful articular disease may affect sleep, lead to alpha intrusion, and subsequent neuromuscular pain.[70] If one attempts to tie the above areas together, one gets a sense of the futility clinicians often experience when they try to differentiate biological variables from psychological ones. Conditions such as fibromyalgia, myofascial pain syndrome, and related musculoskeletal pain do truly reflect the multifactorial interaction of complex biopsychosocial processes.

Phenomenology

In a recent major review paper, Boissevain and McCain,[9] in addition to reviewing the psychological and psychiatric literature, focused on the phenomenology of fibromyalgia. Phenomenology refers to experience and many investigators believe that patients with fibromyalgia experience their symptoms as more painful, global, and debilitating than the pains suffered in other chronic conditions. Pain and physical discomfort are the main symptoms of fibromyalgia. A large number of studies comparing patients with fibromyalgia with those having other chronic pain conditions have documented higher pain and disability ratings for the fibromyalgia group,[101] lower threshold for pain over both tender and nontender points[13, 88] and more spontaneous and pervasive clinical pain.[32, 40, 100, 101] Boissevain and McCain[9] conclude that the pain of fibromyalgia is more severe and debilitating than the pain of other chronic pain syndromes, but that the relative psychopathologic and pathophysiologic contributions remain to be clarified.

IDENTIFYING THE POTENTIALLY CHRONIC PAIN PATIENT

The majority of primary pain practitioners do not have the luxury of a multidisciplinary team of specialists to evaluate the patient with myofascial pain, fibromyalgia, or other musculoskeletal pain complaints. Therefore, it is important for the clinician to be aware of early signs, symptoms, and behaviors that auger poorly for successful rehabilitation. All persons with persistent pain problems do not become chronic pain patients in terms of having virtually all areas of psychosocial existence affected by their pain. As noted earlier, it appears that psychosocial factors are the forces that drive any given persistent pain sufferer toward chronic pain syndrome. What are some of the early signs suggesting potential chronicity?

In an earlier paper, I attempted to identify some of the clinical signs that should alert the practitioner to the potential chronicity of his or her patient.[43] The patient who fails to respond to what should be appropriate treatment may be on the road to chronic pain syndrome. Typically, when the patient fails to respond to our ministrations, we question our diagnosis and treatment plan. That is good health care. However, it is also important to consider what the complicating factors may be that prevent improvement. Both excessive anxiety and clinical depression can confound treatment effects. Anxiety is a person's response to a real or imagined threat to either self or physical integrity. As such, anxiety is shaped by premorbid personality. Some patients are by nature or character more hysterical or hypochondriacal. Their symptoms are presented with flair, exaggeration, and drama. Although it does not make their symptoms less real, this anxious presentation is likely to confound the clinical picture and result in a clinical picture that is bigger than the sum of its parts. Depression, e.g., may inhibit the effectiveness of any given treatment.

When the patient appears depressed, it is appropriate for the primary practitioner to inquire about aspects of psychosocial functioning, e.g., recent stresses, job changes, mood, marriage, personal losses, and so on. Earlier in this chapter the psychosocial-developmental risk factors for chronicity were reviewed and, particularly when a psychologist or psychiatrist is not a member of the treatment team, the clinician may have to inquire into areas of family history, upbringing, the presence of physical, sexual, or emotional abuse, and so on. Was the patient exposed to significant others early in life who had chronic painful illness? Was the patient seriously ill as a child? If so, that patient as a child had the opportunity to learn or take in a repertoire of sick role and illness behaviors that may have laid dormant for many years until recent illness or injury triggered their release from memory and reenactment in the present painful illness. The patient who is drug-seeking may be a potentially chronic patient. When the patient presents with clear physical signs and symptoms but appears more concerned with what prescriptions the physician will write, there may be a hidden drug abuse problem. Patients who are eager to have releases from work or assignment to light duty may or may not be playing out the chronic syndrome. As recent studies have shown, the role of compensation factors such as litigation for work-related injuries and workers' compensation income often have little or no effect on motivation to return to work, and the evaluation of such potential disincentives must be individualized.[26, 64]

The above-mentioned aspects of the patient's clinical presentation are meant to alert the primary practitioner to the possibility of a persistent pain problem on its way to chronic pain syndrome. None of these factors, in and of themselves, are pathognomonic of incipient chronicity, but should serve as warning signs to the practitioner that a more comprehensive team approach may be necessary.

PSYCHOLOGICAL SCREENING AND EVALUATION

Many pain patients show an initial reluctance to undergo psychological screening or evaluation. This resistance is usually a function of beliefs such as the following: "They think the pain is all in my head," "The psychologist is trying to prove that my problems are mental," and the misinformed notion that a psychologist or psychiatrist can somehow divine just what portion of the patient's problem is mental as opposed to medical. The psychologist on meeting any pain patient for the first time must dispel these myths. At the initial meeting I try to deal with this resistance by explaining that there is no scientific way I can determine what, if any, portion of the pain problem is psychological. Instead, I explain that we have learned over the years that when persons live with pain for extended periods of time and treatments do not alleviate pain, it is not unusual for patients to find themselves upset over this state of affairs. I usually go on to explain that some patients become depressed, others irritable, some rely on medications, others fight with their spouses, and so on. I reassure them that these are all normal responses to an apparently insoluble situation and that in the interest of helping them as best we can, we need to have a picture of the entire person. Usually, this introduction is sufficient to enable the patient to talk about the pain and its impact on his or her life. Quite often, I am not able to get through this introduction before the patient begins talking about the pain's emotional impact on his or her life. Patients vary in their degree of psychological sophistication and it is important to tailor the introduction to the verbal and nonverbal responses coming from the patient.

Clinical psychologists screen and evaluate pain patients using three broad categories of data: (1) interview and observation; (2) psychological and psychometric tests; and (3) psychophysiologic data.[44] Psychologists vary in their preference for one type of datum over another; the majority of psychologists use the interview as well as clinical observation, while a smaller percentage will include psychological tests as well. A much smaller group will collect psychophysiologic information as part of their assessment.

Clinical Interview and Observation

Psychologists vary in interview style. Some prefer broad, open-ended inquiry, whereas others prefer highly structured and standardized interview formats. As Waldinger[98] has stated, we want our patients to tell us what is wrong. The clinical interview provides the psychologist with basic information on mental status, thought processes, emotions, perceptual functioning, intelligence, and motivation. The psychologist may also glean some information on the presence or absence of more formal psychiatric or psychological dysfunction. However, all of the above is routine and the focus will now turn to areas of investigation that are germane to assessment of the patient with pain. Elsewhere, Ciccone and Grzesiak[20] have provided a set of evaluative questions the physician can use to screen for psychological dysfunction in pain patients. These questions break down into three domains: (1) inappropriate illness behavior; (2) emotional disorder; and (3) premorbid risk factors.[20]

Inappropriate Illness Behavior

1. Is there persistent pain extending beyond the bounds of normal healing time?
2. Is there an identified physical cause for the patient's pain?
3. Does the patient's report of pain appear proportionate to the suspected or identified pathologic condition?
4. Is the distribution of pain, sensory loss, or motor weakness consistent with a dermatomal or myotomal distribution?
5. Is the complaint of pain or tenderness specific and limited to a single skeletal or neuromuscular structure? (This question may be inappropriate for myofascial and fibrositis patients because the syndrome is diffusely spread across the musculature.)
6. What behaviors does the patient perform to communicate pain and suffering to family members and health care providers?
7. What specific behaviors are performed by the patient's spouse, friends, and family in response to the patient's pain behavior?
8. What is the patient's current income and from what sources is it derived?
9. Is the patient using, abusing, or dependent on an addictive drug (narcotic analgesics or tranquilizers)?
10. Does the patient use alcohol as a means of controlling pain?
11. Who performs routine household chores such as grocery shopping, cooking, cleaning, and laundry?

12. How much of the patient's waking day is spent resting or reclining because of pain?

Emotional Disorder

13. Does the patient report or exhibit signs of excessive worry, nervousness, or anxiety?
14. If the pain is of traumatic origin, does the patient dwell on or ruminate about the traumatic incident; experience flashbacks, sleep disturbance, or nightmares; avoid situations that are reminiscent of the original trauma?
15. Does the patient report discrete periods of heightened anxiety or panic accompanied by such symptoms as shortness of breath, palpitations, feeling faint, or trembling, and associated with an intense fear of dying, losing control, or going insane?
16. Does the patient report more frequent loss of temper or feelings of hostility following the onset of pain?
17. When pain prevents the patient from engaging in a favorite activity or performing a routine chore, is there a tendency to feel angry or aggravated as opposed to frustrated?
18. Is the patient aware of any correlation between the onset of anger and an increase in pain symptoms?
19. Does the patient exhibit symptoms of depression such as prolonged periods of depressed mood, loss of interest or pleasure in most or all activities, disturbance of sleep or appetite, psychomotor agitation or retardation, frequent fatigue or loss of energy, diminished concentration, recurrent thoughts of death or suicidal ideation, and feelings of hopelessness or worthlessness?
20. If the patient admits to suicidal ideation, has he or she formulated a plan and does he or she express serious suicidal intent?
21. When the patient fails to meet social or work-related obligations, does the patient tend to blame himself or herself or feel guilty?
22. Does the patient frequently perform burdensome or otherwise unpleasant chores with the intent of helping others or winning social approval?

Premorbid risk factors

23. Does the patient have a premorbid history of hard-driving, work-oriented behavior?
24. Does the patient have a history of depression or other psychiatric disturbance?
25. Does the patient have a history of substance abuse or dependency?
26. Does the patient have a history of chronic pain or other stress-related medical illness?
27. Was the patient exposed to chronic illness during childhood?
28. Did the patient sustain the loss of a loved one early in life?
29. Was the patient a victim of physical or sexual abuse?

By asking the patient questions of this sort, the physician or other health care practitioner will develop some understanding for what the patient may be bringing to the clinical situation to make the overall presentation more problematic than it might be. The rationale underlying the above questions can be found in Ciccone and Grzesiak.[20]

Personality traits and states must be assessed to understand the individual with pain. Each patient brings to the pain situation his or her unique premorbid personality. Personality style has implications of emotional expression, cognitive style, behavioral response, and psychophysiologic reactivity. Many of these factors can maintain or exacerbate the pain experience. As has been pointed out above, many patients with fibromyalgia, myofascial pain syndrome, or ill-defined musculoskeletal pain will present with personality styles that are primarily obsessional and depressive in nature. They are perfectionistic, hypernormal, precociously responsible, aggressive, ambitious, and critical of self and others. They often present with an ergomanic orientation to work and life. The importance of determining developmental events suggestive of pain-proneness is extremely important and is dealt with below. Suffice it to say here that the focus of the interview should be on determining the idiosyncratic or unique meaning that the patient superimposes on the pain sensation.

Premorbid and reactive psychopathologic disorders must be evaluated. Both psychological dysfunction and psychiatric illness can play a role in causing or complicating a musculoskeletal pain problem. Earlier it was noted that depression is by far the most common emotional symptom or syndrome presenting along with persistent pain. Such depression may reflect premorbid functioning, be comorbid with the pain, or be a function of attempting to live with a persisting pain problem. In patients with chronic pain, it may be impossible to separate out pain from depression and, as Blumer and Heilbronn have stated,[7] pain and depression may become synchronous expressions of mood.

For purposes of this presentation, stress responses will be considered as part of a reactive psychopathologic disorder. Major and minor life events can be stressful depending on their appraisal by the individual. Major life events, including upheavals such as death of a parent, spouse, or child; serious illness; divorce; marriage; loss of job; and so on are often associated with the development of medical problems, including pain. Similarly, we have learned that the psychophysiologic and autonomic correlates of stress can build on the basis of repetitive daily hassles leading to stress-related illnesses, including pain. Finally, because so many musculoskeletal pain problems begin with either major or minor trauma, the clinician must be alert to signs of posttraumatic stress disorder (PTSD). PTSD can complicate the patient's clinical presentation and serve as a perpetuator of pain complaints.

A very small number of patients have pain as part of a more serious psychiatric illness. In addition to depression, pain can be a symptom in the anxiety disorders, bipolar illness, hysterical conversions, hypochondriasis, and schizophrenia.[37, 66]

The impact of pain on physical and personal functioning needs to be evaluated as well. In the presence of persistent pain, some persons continue to live their lives as best they can while others fall victim to a variety of dysfunctions such as unemployment, physical inactivity, reliance on medication, etc. In other words, they develop a "disability lifestyle." What appears critical to how dysfunctional any given individual becomes is coping capacity, or the lack of it. As I have said elsewhere, nowhere is the interaction of pain and function more apparent than in the area of inactivity. Pain may spread from one focal area to more generalized and pervasive sites on the basis of disuse and inactivity. This often leads to inappropriate postural adaptations which ultimately lead to more muscular pain and stiffness. Decreased physical functioning because of pain does not lead to less pain in the long run but to more pain.[44]

Psychological Testing

Psychological or psychometric testing adds a more formal and structured dimension to the clinical evaluation. Few psychological tests were developed specifically for the clinical assessment of the patient with pain. Because some psychologists specialize in measurement techniques, they have contributed to the design of procedures for evaluation of pain.

The Visual Analog Scale is one of the most popular methods for estimating clinical pain. The Pain Visual Analog Scale (PVAS) is a 10-cm line anchored at one end as "no pain" and at the other end by "unbearable pain."[67] Patients are told to indicate the intensity of their pain by a marking on the line between the two extremes. The examiner, if he or she wishes to quantify the results, can convert the mark into a numeric scale, using 0 to 100 mm as the range. Over the years there have been many variations on the PVAS such as using numbers or words rather than the simple line. However, Huskisson[53] has argued that by leaving the line simple with only the two anchor phrases at the extremes the evaluator is left with a sensitive scale possessing a virtually infinite number of data points. The PVAS can serve as a useful measure of pain as well as a repeated measure to document therapeutic change.

The McGill Pain Questionnaire (MPQ) was developed in the mid-1970s by Melzack.[65] Based in part on the components of the gate control theory of pain, the MPQ uses classes of words (verbal descriptors) that have been factorially derived to represent the sensory, affective, and cognitive components of pain experience. The verbal descriptor section of the MPQ provides the evaluator with three kinds of information on the patient's pain: (1) present pain intensity; (2) number of words chosen; and (3) pain rating index. When the MPQ is completed in its entirety it can also serve as a comprehensive, quasi-structured pain interview.

The Psychosocial Pain Inventory is one example of a number of relatively new structured evaluations designed specifically for pain patients.[50] This particular inventory was designed to assess the psychosocial aspects of the pain and, as such, it provides information on pain, psychosocial factors, pain-related treatments, secondary gain, interpersonal factors, and premorbid occupational satisfaction. Because its focus is predominantly psychosocial, it can be used to complement other psychometric procedures that assess personality, such as the MMPI.

The West Haven–Yale Multidimensional Pain Inventory was designed to supplement behavioral and psychophysiologic observations.[57] Initially labelled the WHYMPI, it is now better known as the MPI. The MPI provides three broad categories of information on the pain patient: (1) pain dimensions, including pain's interference with various areas of function, the role of significant others, pain severity, and mood; (2) specific responses of significant others; and (3) functional activities. The MPI is frequently used in both clinical practice and in research investigations.

The Minnesota Multiphasic Personality Inventory is one of the most thoroughly researched and frequently used personality questionnaires with both psychiatric and medical patients. Developed in the 1940s, the MMPI has been a matter of controversy in pain management for years. Critics maintain that its primary focus on personality and psychopathology makes it an inappropriate instrument for the evaluation of chronic pain patients. Rather than discard it from the evaluation process, I think a more practical approach is to understand that interpretation of the MMPI is a sophisticated process that must be accomplished by a skilled clinical psychologist who understands that using the MMPI with medical and pain patients requires some adjustment in interpretation. It is important to know that certain scales, e.g., those for hypochondriasis, depression, and hysteria, are somewhat elevated by virtue of the number of somatic items in them. Interpretation of the MMPI should combine information on the personality and psychopathologic dimensions as well as integration of the behaviors and defenses inherent in both high and low elevations on each of the clinical scales. In so doing, the clinician will bring to the diagnostic and treatment planning process useful information on some of the more idiosyncratic aspects of the pain patient's functioning.

Early interest in the MMPI with pain patients began with the publication of a study by Hanvik[49] comparing back pain patients with and without definitive physical findings to account for their pain. Hanvik found that the group of back pain patients with no organic findings produced a composite MMPI profile with elevations on Hy (hypochondriasis) and hysteria (Hs) with a D (depression) score within normal limits. These three scores are called the neurotic triad and the above-noted elevations for a V configuration that has been called the "conversion V" or "psychosomatic V." So for some time it was believed that the MMPI could differentiate between "real" pain and so-called psychogenic pain. However, extensive research that will not be detailed here has failed to consistently replicate a capacity to use the MMPI for diagnosis of psychogenic pain.

In 1978 Bradley and associates[10] published the first of several major studies on the MMPI with chronic back pain patients in which multivariate analysis was used to identify consistently recurring clusters of MMPI profile types. Studies such as Hanvik's used measures of central tendency and, as such, compared the mean scores of one group with those of the other. An unfortunate consequence of such an undertaking is a washing-out of individual differences within each group. The studies of Bradley and associates[10] found recurring profile types, one of which was the so-called conversion V. To my mind, this remains the prototypal approach to research using psychometric tests with pain patients and it has two important implications for the clinician. First, these studies demonstrate that persons with pain bring to the clinical situation their own unique premorbid personalities; some of these personality types are more frequently recurring, suggesting that some personality configurations may be more pain-prone than others. Second, the fact that several personality types have been identified in patients with chronic back pain suggests that this population is not psychologically homogeneous and, further, that psychological evaluation findings should be used to tailor a treatment program unique to the needs of the individual patient.

Other psychological tests have been used with pain patients as well but they will not be detailed here. Suffice it to say that the conclusions based on interview, observation, and psychometric evaluation must be accomplished by a psychologist trained in the clinical assessment of patients with pain. Routine application of psychological tests with pain patients may lead to gross misinterpretations of the results if the extenuating and distorting effects of living with pain are not taken into consideration.

Psychophysiologic Monitoring

As noted above, a small number of psychologists also gather information on psychophysiologic functioning as well. In the evaluation of patients with musculoskeletal pain syndromes the primary method of data collection is surface electrode monitoring of muscle activity. The reader may recall the study by Holmes and Wolff[51] mentioned earlier that used surface EMG recording as one of the measures. In many respects that study is a forerunner of the biofeedback explosion in the late 1960s and early 1970s when EMG biofeedback was applied to problems such as muscle tension headache. Psychophysiologic assessment has come a long way since those early days. Middaugh and Kee[69] have provided a thorough guide for the psychophysiologic assessment of neck, shoulder, and low back pain. They make the important point that static assessment of the EMG is often misleading, and proper evaluation of muscle function must involve muscles in function. Accordingly, the Middaugh and Kee program uses a muscle-by-muscle EMG evaluation[69] (Fig 4–2).

Assessment of neck and shoulder girdle musculoskeletal pain involves a three-component assessment. During the Quiet Sitting Test the patient sits in an armless straight-backed chair with hands on lap for 2 minutes; this position should allow the muscles being evaluated to become completely relaxed and EMG recordings will be at or very near the inherent noise level of the recording equipment. One is searching for elevated sitting baselines in the muscles being monitored. Second, the patient does the Shrug/Return Test in which he or she is asked to shrug both shoulders up, hold this position for 3 seconds, and then let the shoulders back down. The muscles are then monitored for 1 minute to assess recovery to baseline. This procedure is repeated three times. This component of the evaluation is the muscle's capacity to recover in a timely fashion. According to Middaugh and Kee, "the significant finding is a failure on the part of the individual patient to recover his own sitting baseline level within 30 seconds on two of three trials."[69, p. 150] Such findings are indicative of muscle hyperactivity and irritability. The third area of assessment involves the Abduct/Return Test in which the sitting patient is asked to raise (abduct) the arms

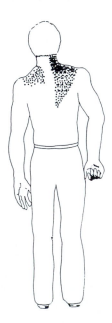

FIG 4–2. Common areas of reported pain in patients with chronic cervical and shoulder girdle pain. (From Middaugh SJ, Kee WG: Advances in electromyographic monitoring and biofeedback in the treatment of chronic cervical and low back pain. In Eisenberg MG, Grzesiak RC, editors: *Advances in clinical rehabilitation*, vol 1, New York, 1987, Springer, pp 137–172. Used by permission.)

straight out to the side to the horizontal position, hold that position for 3 seconds, and then lower the arms to the lap to resume baseline. Muscle activity is again observed for 1 minute and this procedure is repeated three times. Failure to recover to baseline after this test is another indication of muscle irritability in the muscles being monitored. The example in Figure 4–3 from Ciccone and Grzesiak[18] illustrates three different parameters of muscle abnormality. Comparing right and left shoulder shrugs and recovery to baseline suggests marked differences; the right shoulder is more active (hypertonic), is reactive when the muscles are at work (hyperactive), and fails to return to baseline in a timely manner (persistence).

Dynamic psychophysiologic assessment of the low back is similar to that of the shoulder girdle. Two or four muscle sites are evaluated on each patient; right and left lumbar paraspinous muscles and right and left lower thoracic paraspinous muscles with electrode placements being parallel to the spine and approximately 1 in. from midline (L4 and T8–12, respectively). Each patient undergoes a standing baseline in which he or she is asked to stand still, as straight as possible, with weight equally distributed between the two legs. The test is positive for muscle hyperactivity if one or both sides show sustained muscle activity. Trunk rotation is used to establish the absence or presence of inappropriate reciprocal activity between left and right as the trunk rotates in either direction. Trunk flexion is used to assess poor relaxation (muscle irritability), asymmetry, continued contraction, and failure to recover baseline. Middaugh and Kee point out that while shoulder muscle irritability is common (65%), only 26% of low back pain patients show similar irritability. Overall, the authors point out that these simple tests often identify problems of inappropriate and inefficient use of low back muscles for posture and movement. Both overuse and underuse of appropriate musculature are common.[69]

Other psychophysiologic parameters are occasionally used in assessment of the patient with musculoskeletal pain, perhaps the most frequent being temperature, on the premise that the persistent pain is tied into autonomic disregu-

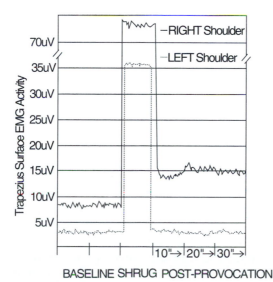

FIG 4–3. Dynamic electromyographic (EMG) assessment of upper trapezius muscle activity before, during, and after shoulder shrug provocation. (From Ciccone DS, Grzesiak RC: Chronic musculoskeletal pain: A cognitive approach to psychophysiologic assessment and intervention. In Eisenberg MG, Grzesiak RC, editors: *Advances in clinical rehabilitation*, vol 3, New York, 1990, Springer, pp 197–215. Used by permission.)

lation. However, that assessment tactic is not frequently used and will not be elaborated on here.

Taken as a complete package, the results of the clinical interview and observations, the psychological test findings, and the psychophysiologic assessment, the psychologist can make a substantial contribution to understanding the cognitive, behavioral, affective, and psychophysiologic dimensions of any given pain patient's problem. We now turn to how to use this information in the psychological treatment of patients with musculoskeletal pain.

APPROACHES TO PSYCHOLOGICAL TREATMENT

One of the major failings in behavioral medicine so far has been its inability to use psychological findings to do differential treatment planning. Turk has argued for customizing treatment plans and he states many pain programs fall victim to what he calls the "patient uniformity myth" and the "treatment uniformity myth."[92] It should be clear by now that all persistent musculoskeletal pain patients, whether they have myofascial pain syndrome or fibrositis, do not present with similar psychological and physiologic findings. People are different, yet few reports in the pain treatment literature address those differences in any significant way.

All patients with persistent pain do not require psychological treatment although, in an ideal program, all should have a psychological evaluation. We must customize treatment. An early example of defining treatment on the basis of affirmative and negative physical and psychological findings was offered by Brena and Koch[11] when they subdivided their patients on the basis of behavioral and tissue pathologic findings into four groups: (1) pain amplifiers (high pain behavior, low tissue pathologic changes), (2) pain verbalizers (low pain behavior, low tissue pathologic changes), (3) chronic sufferers (high pain behavior, high tissue pathologic changes), and (4) pain reducers (low pain behavior, high tissue pathologic changes). Clearly, each of these groups requires a treatment plan that weighs differently on medical and psychological interventions.

Psychological treatment approaches are diverse. Exactly how to divide them into reasonably discrete packages is no mean feat. For our purposes, the following section is divided into three components: (1) psychotherapy (including the small but meaningful empirical information on psychoactive medication), (2) self-regulatory approaches (relaxation, biofeedback, and hypnosis), and (3) multidisciplinary pain management.

Psychotherapy

In this section, behavioral management, cognitive therapy, and integrative psychodynamic psychotherapy are presented as well as some information on the use of psychoactive medication. Psychoactive medication does not fall within the purview of the psychologist. Yet, frequently, the medical team will seek out information on possible psychopharmacologic interventions from the psychologist. Ideally, a psychiatrist with psychopharmacologic expertise and an interest in pain management should be a member or a consultant to the treating physician or team, but such specialists are few and far between.

Behavioral management of the patient with musculoskeletal pain is an important component of any psychological treatment. Years ago, Fordyce[34] stated that pain behavior became chronic because it was rewarded while efforts the person might make to engage in well or healthy behavior went unnoticed or were actually discouraged. Therefore, the rewards or contingencies for displaying pain behavior were greater than those for healthy behavior. It is not my intention to present a behavioral management program here. However, key patient behaviors that are most appropriately managed with behavioral methods are activity levels, exercise performance, and medication intake. Chronic musculoskeletal pain patients often have had months, if not years, of inactivity and muscle disuse. Exercise is incompatible with pain behavior. The psychologist can assist the physician and the physical therapist in designing an exercise program in which the patient is unlikely to experience failure; a major impediment to rehabilitative progress is attempting to advance the patient in his or her activities too quickly. With both reconditioning and individualized therapeutic exercises it is important to determine the patient's baseline level of performance. After identifying that level of performance, a systematic schedule of slowly increasing activity goals can be established enabling the patient to improve his or her performance without experiencing failure.

When medication use is a problem, it is important to determine just how much pain medication is needed to cover the patient's discomfort so that he or she does not have breakthrough pain during participation in the rehabilitation program. As activity and exercise levels increase, pain medications are slowly decreased. One area where I take issue with an orthodox behavioral approach is in the attribution of responsibility. It is generally believed that instrumental learning can take place without thinking being involved. Therefore, the manipulation of behavior change can be viewed as a thoughtless process in which environmental contingencies are the sole shapers of behavior. Such an attitude takes away from the patient responsibility for his or her behavior. I believe it is better for patient motivation to educate the patient that, even though these environmental contingencies have an impact on behavior, it is the patient's own responsibility to determine the course of the rehabilitation program; responsibility for change can then become an internalized process.

Cognitive or cognitive-behavior therapy is by far the most commonly used of the psychotherapies in the management of patients with chronic pain. Turk and associates[93] have been the foremost proponents of the cognitive-behavioral position. Cognitive-behavioral therapy is not so much a theory as it is a pragmatic integration of a variety of psychological techniques borrowed from such diverse areas of psychology as behaviorism, social learning, rational-emotive therapy, and cognitive psychology. A focal concept in the cognitive-behavioral position is the idea that what people think about their illness and pain is actually more important than the illness or pain itself. Turk and associates have stated that "affect and behavior are largely determined by the way in which the individual construes the world."[93] Patients often maintain an inner dialogue with themselves, have automatic thoughts, self-statements, and private conceptualizations that add to their symptomatic distress. While affect, behavior, and cognition are given equal weight in the cognitive-behavioral position, a focus on behavior change is still believed to be the most efficient way to alter emotion and thought as well.

A major focus of cognitive-behavior therapy is coping; people often believe they have little or no control over what is happening to them. Cognitive-behavior therapy is active, educative, and interactive. The components of cognitive-behavioral therapy as applied to pain are as follows. First, there is developed a shared conceptualization of the patient's problems so that a psychologically based treatment is feasible. The scientific validity of this conceptualization is less important than its plausibility to the patient. Until both patient and therapist have a consensual understanding of how the treatment will work and what it aims to accomplish, treatment efforts are likely to work at cross-purposes. After reaching this shared conceptualization, therapy proceeds to the acquisition of necessary cognitive coping skills and behavioral strategies for managing pain-related dysfunction. Skill deficiencies are identified, new or improved cognitive skills are defined, rehearsed in the clinical setting, applied to mutually agreed-upon goals, and plans for implementing generalization and maintenance are developed. Although this sounds relatively simple, it is not in the actual clinical situation.

A somewhat similar cognitive approach to treatment of the chronic pain patient has been put forth by Eimers.[28] He uses the acronym PADDS to define his approach to pain management. PADDS refers to five components of his cognitive therapy approach. The first letter, *P*, stands for *p*acing. The importance of setting appropriate therapeutic goals and moving toward them in an orderly and nonexhaustive manner has been mentioned above. Too often, patients fail in their physical rehabilitation because they attempt to do too much, too fast. Pacing is an important component of any physical restoration program. *A* stands for *a*nxiety management; many of the techniques for anxiety management are spelled out below in the section on self-regulatory techniques. At this point it is sufficient to state that anxiety can negatively affect both pain experience and treatment participation. The first *D* stands for *d*istraction. The patient in pain can easily become focused and enmeshed in the overall pain experience, adding anxiety and augmenting the pain sensation. Distraction techniques change the gate on pain sensation; e.g., selective inattention, attention diversion, reinterpretation of sensation, and so forth can be used to modify the interactive effects of anxiety and pain sensation. The next D stands for the *d*isputation of negative thoughts. This procedure, similar if not identical to what is discussed in the next section on rational-emotive cognitive therapy, involves identifying underlying automatic thoughts and irrational beliefs and then challenging their validity. Finally, *S* stands for *s*topping negative thoughts and images through a cognitive technique called thought stopping.

A cognitive therapy based on rational-emotive psychotherapy has been presented by Ciccone and Grzesiak.[16-18] This approach does not set behavior, affect, and cognition on an equal footing but rather proposes that central to all affective, behavioral, and psychophysiologic dysfunctions are cognitively driven irrational beliefs and distorted interpretations of the meaning of pain. Using an ABC model of how irrational beliefs influence behavior and emotion, these authors spell out how to do cognitive analysis and treatment. Among the more common cognitive errors that lead to coping failure and inability to adapt to pain are "awfulizing," demandingness, low frustration tolerance, conditional self-worth, and attributing responsibility to external sources. By changing how one thinks about pain, one can modify adaptation to it as well as dampen the negative impact of pain on virtually all functional activities (Fig 4–4). In addition to its utilization as a cognitive psychotherapy, Ciccone and Grzesiak have also demonstrated how cognitive therapy and dynamic EMG assessment and treatment can be integrated.[18]

Integrative psychodynamic psychotherapy for patients with chronic pain has been proposed by Dworkin and Grzesiak.[25] Their integrative approach combines self-regulatory approaches and behavioral prescription with psychotherapy. The

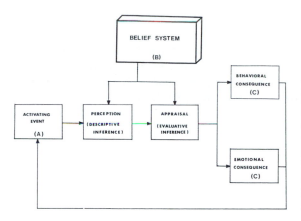

FIG 4-4. A cognitive model of human behavior and emotion. (From Ciccone DS, Grzesiak RC: Chronic musculoskeletal pain: A cognitive approach to psychophysiologic assessment and intervention. In Eisenberg MG, Grzesiak RC, editors: *Advances in clinical rehabilitation,* vol 3, New York, 1990, Springer, pp 197–215. Used by permission.)

psychotherapeutic interventions vary on a continuum from supportive to insight-interpretive depending on patient needs. According to the authors, if psychological involvement in chronic pain is conceptualized as varying from minimal to maximal, as potentially involving cognitive, behavioral, affective, psychophysiologic, and intrapsychic (unconscious) components, and as playing a role as cause, consequence, or concomitant, then the value of being able to bring an integrative psychotherapy to bear on the chronic pain patient's pain and suffering becomes clear. The authors stress the usefulness of this form of psychotherapy for working with pain patients who have psychopathology and/or personality disorder; they also stress the value of using adjunctive psychoactive medications when indicated.[25]

There are only two major studies evaluating the usefulness of psychotherapy with musculoskeletal pain problems. Both demonstrate significant success. Draspa[23] studied patients with muscular pain, many of them apparently having fibrositis or "psychogenic rheumatism" who underwent extensive psychological evaluation and then psychological treatment combining active and passive relaxation, education (reassurance that the pain was muscular and not medically dangerous), and insight-oriented psychotherapy. The insight-oriented focus was on demonstrating how their stress and inner psychological world were contributing to musculoskeletal strain and consequently pain. Two groups with muscle pain were used: one group received psychological treatment plus physical therapy, while the other received physical therapy only. Almost twice as many patients in the treatment group became pain-free compared with the pain controls.[23]

The other study was completed by Pomp[78] who did not use a control group but selected myofascial pain patients who failed to respond to conventional treatment. Symptom remission occurred during brief psychotherapy in 15 out of 23 patients, with an additional 2 patients becoming pain-free after psychotherapy was completed. According to the author, the aspects of psychotherapeutic process that led to symptom remission included relief from strong negative emotion, recognition of an invalid and unrealistic self-concept, development of a greater sense of self-competence or efficacy, and changes in the stress-creating aspects of the patient's environment.[78] Both of the above studies suggest that in selected musculoskeletal pain patients, one must deal with the interaction of personality, defense, coping style, and environment to attain pain relief.

Two recent clinical reports using psychotherapy with chronic pain patients have made similar points. Not unlike cognitive therapy, Shutty and Sheras[87] have used clinical examples to demonstrate the value of brief strategic psychotherapy to reframe problems faced by chronic pain patients in such a way as to provide them with new coping options. From a more psychoanalytic perspective Whale[99] reported on the successful use of brief psychoanalytic psychotherapy with chronic pain patients. Each of her cases revealed underlying blocked anger and an inability to mourn important losses. However, even when evaluation findings suggest psychologic dysfunction or psychiatric disturbance, psychotherapy may not prove to be an appropriate treatment. Tunks and Merskey[91] have stressed the importance of differentiating between the need for supportive or insight-oriented individual psychotherapy, group psychotherapy, and family therapy.

Psychopharmacologic intervention has achieved a prominent place in the pain management armamentarium. The tricyclic antidepressants, in particular, are now used routinely in the management of chronic pain. Turning specifically to the use of psychoactive medications in fibromyalgia and fibrositis there is only a meager literature supporting efficacy. In a controlled comparison of chlorpromazine and L-tryptophan for pain and mood symptoms in a sample of fibrositis patients, Moldofsky and Lue[71] found chlorpromazine to be more effective. In a double-blind study comparing amitriptylene and placebo, the group receiving the former showed improvements in morning stiffness, pain, sleep, and global functioning.[14] Goldenberg and associates[40] conducted a double-blind study of amitriptylene, naproxen, a combination of amitriptylene and naproxen, and placebo on fibromyalgic symptoms. They found the amitriptylene groups showed significant improvement on all measures. The combination of amitriptylene and naproxen was not better than amitriptylene alone.[40] In the final study to be reviewed here, Bennett and associates[4] studied cyclobenzaprine (cyclobenzaprine is structurally related to the tricyclic antidepressants) with placebo in a study comparing therapeutic response between a group with fibromyalgia and a control group. The fibromyalgia group showed significant improvement in pain intensity as well as a nonsignificant improvement in fatigue, tender point pain, and muscle tightness.[4]

In terms of psychopharmacologic intervention in fibromyalgia and myofascial pain syndrome, results are not promising, with the exception of using amitriptylene in low doses. The mechanisms by which this tricyclic antidepressant are effective remain unclear but appear to involve improvement in sleep pattern and serotonin uptake.

Self-Regulatory Approaches: Relaxation, Biofeedback, and Hypnosis

Relaxation and biofeedback are commonly used with chronic pain patients. It is appropriate to consider relaxation and biofeedback together as both allow the patient to experience a modicum of control over pain sensations. Hypnosis, on the other hand, is often viewed by patients as a surrendering of control, and hypnotic techniques often meet greater resistance than the other self-regulatory approaches.

Relaxation training is perhaps the most benign of the behavioral interventions. The rationale for relaxation training with musculoskeletal pain patients involves the notion that it is impossible to be relaxed and augment one's pain at the same time. Relaxation training is so widespread in behavioral medicine that it has been called the "aspirin of behavioral medicine." It is unfortunate that relaxation training is often viewed as a simple, rather straightforward technique. One should not look to the pain literature to understand the varieties of relaxation but to the stress management literature. In contemporary practice, relaxation training is usually one component of a much more comprehensive treatment package.

The origins of contemporary relaxation training lie in the work of Jacobson,[55] but few practitioners actually use a jacobsonian protocol because it is time-consuming and not fitted to the rather short-term treatment focus seen in most pain management settings. Nevertheless, relaxation approaches have proved useful in the overall management of diverse chronic pain problems, including musculoskeletal pain. Using a jacobsonian protocol, McGuigan[63] has pointed out that one must relax all the complexly interacting systems of the body. By directly relaxing the skeletal musculature, one also "relaxes" the central nervous system as well as the various components of the autonomic nervous system.[63] A key to relaxation training is not attempting to relax but in "turning off the power" to various muscle groups. In the Jacobson method, one works with only one muscle group at a time and, consequently, the process is quite extended over time.

More popular with psychologists working in pain management are the abbreviated forms of relaxation training. One of the more popular versions is that of Bernstein and Borkovec[5] who have divided the muscles into 16 major groups. Using a tense-relax strategy, the patient is taught to relax each of these groups. When the patient is proficient with relaxation at this level, a briefer version is introduced that combines some of the interrelated groups. When the patient is proficient with the combined muscle groups, instructions focus on relaxation by recall, therefore eliminating the need to go through the tense-relax paradigm. The final step is to induce a relaxed state by counting.

Another version of relaxation, a simple relaxation method, was introduced by French and Tupin[38] who added a meditation-like imagery component. This approach involves deep breathing, abbreviated tense-relax training for major muscles, and relaxing imagery. Grzesiak[41] applied this approach to chronic pain secondary to spinal injury and, in a clinical case follow-up study, found it successful in the majority of cases. One of the major values of relaxation training is that it enables the patient to develop a better sense of body functioning or somatic awareness. However, as the patient becomes more attuned to internal cues, the clinician must be aware of the possibility of untoward side effects. Jacobsen and Edinger[54] have reported on two patients who developed anxiety symptoms apparently related to underlying psychodynamic conflicts that were released by the relaxation paradigm. Relaxation approaches have been quite effective in the management of headache and back pain.[46]

Biofeedback is a form of psychophysiologic treatment that has developed a nearly overwhelming literature over the last two decades. The section of psychophysiologic assessment provided a brief introduction into how surface electrode EMG monitoring could be used to assess muscle functions. Before considering specific applications of biofeedback to problems of myofascial pain and fibromyalgia, some introductory comments are in order. In a brief review article,[42] Grzesiak pointed out that the use of biofeedback in pain management can be conceptualized as involving two targets. The first involves using biofeedback as a generalized relaxation or quieting procedure; the second involves using biofeedback to target specific areas of dysfunction believed to be related to the pathophysiology of the pain problem itself.[42] There is a relatively extensive literature on using biofeedback for tension headache, low back pain, and myofascial pain, but only one study on the biofeedback treatment of fibromyalgia. The extensive research on biofeedback applications to headache will not be included here.

Biofeedback involves monitoring a physiologic system of which we are not ordinarily aware, converting it electronically into signals (usually visual or auditory), and feeding back that information to the subject so that he or she can become aware of it and develop internal strategies for its modification. The use of static EMG biofeedback in the management of back pain has not had a particularly good record. Using as a rationale for the application of biofeedback the idea of muscle spasm, tension, and pain, Nouwen and Solinger[75] reported a controlled study of lumbar paraspinal EMG feedback. After a 20-session feedback period, they found that the treatment group had lowered EMG levels as well as lowered pain reports. However, on 3-month follow-up they found that although the treatment group continued to report improved pain, the resting paraspinal muscles had returned to baseline levels of activity.[75] This suggests that factors, possibly nonspecific therapeutic ones, were responsible for the pain improvement, not lowered levels of paraspinal muscle tension. A somewhat more sophisticated study was conducted by Large and Lamb[59] who used a counterbalanced design to treat chronic musculoskeletal pain patients (neck, low back, and fibrositis) with actual EMG biofeedback, EMG control, and a waiting list control. For patients with focal pain complaints, site-specific EMG was used, and for those with more generalized complaints, frontalis EMG was used. Interestingly, only those patients who began treatment with actual EMG feedback were able to achieve linear levels of improvement. The EMG control (a bogus feedback) actually had the lowest pain levels.[59] Both of these studies suggest the need for more research on the relationship between pain and muscle tension.

Because of equivocal findings such as the above, Nouwen and Bush[74] conducted a major review of the relationship between EMG levels and pain. They broke the data down on the basis of seven hypotheses. The hypothesis that resting levels of paraspinal EMG will be higher in low back pain patients has minimal support. The hypothesis that paraspinal EMG levels will be higher in low back pain patients during various movements and postures has some support. The hypothesis that low back pain patients have more reactive paraspinal musculature under stress has not been supported. The hypothesis that lowered paraspinal EMG levels are associated with lower pain levels has not received consistent support. The hypothesis that low back pain patients will have higher levels of paraspinal EMG while other muscle groups remain normal has not been supported. The hypothesis that low back pain patients will have greater general muscular and autonomic reactivity has not been supported. Finally, the hypothesis that low back pain patients will respond better to biofeedback-enhanced relaxation training than to simple relaxation training has not been supported. So one of the only areas where paraspinal muscle tension may play a role in back pain involves the differential patterning of paraspinal EMG. Return, if you will, to the data presented earlier on psychophysiologic assessment using dynamic EMG assessment. Middaugh and Kee,[69] e.g., provide a comprehensive EMG treatment program for cervical and low back pain based on their dynamic assessment.

Biofeedback treatment of myofascial pain and muscle tension has an equivocal track record. There appear to be more successful studies involving myofascial syndromes of the upper quarter. For example, Peck and Kraft[77] compared the outcomes of EMG treatment for a small group of tension headache, and back, shoulder, and jaw pain; while treatment outcomes were satisfactory for the tension headache group, the results were far less promising for the other pain problems. Another study[12] compared relaxation training with biofeedback in the treatment of myofascial pain dysfunction syndrome. Relaxation treatment appeared effective in reducing pain. Adding biofeedback to the relaxation program did not enhance effectiveness.[12] Overall, it appears that either relaxation training or EMG biofeedback is a promising treatment for myofascial pain of the upper quarter.

There is only one biofeedback study on fibromyalgia. Ferraccioli and associates[33] used EMG biofeedback to treat the pain associated with fibromyalgia. They found that 56% of their treatment group achieved long-lasting clinical benefit. Looking at those who failed to benefit from treatment, they found the subgroup that failed to benefit were clinically depressed. This study calls attention to the need to deal with both mind and muscle.[33] Many appropriate and potentially effective treatments will fail if psychopathology is not taken into consideration.

Hypnosis is probably one of the oldest nonmedicinal treatments known to man and, despite such an extended history, controversy continues over just what hypnosis is and how it works. One of the more common definitions of hypnosis is that it is a state of focused attention or heightened concentration.[102] Some refer to the hypnotic state as a dissociation phenomenon, while others equate it more to a relaxation response. Neither position is likely to be correct. Because the capacity to be hypnotized varies widely, it is most probable that a small percentage of the population can be put in a deeply dissociated state of mind in which they are amenable to suggestion, while at the other extreme, there are a small number of people who simply cannot surrender any personal control whatsoever. In the middle range are those persons for whom hypnosis is the equivalent of a relaxation response. Hypnotic applications to clinical pain are extensively documented but, for the most part, involve clinical case reports and anecdotal tales.

Four common hypnotic suggestions for modifying clinical pain have been reviewed by Wolskee.[102] The first involves direct suggestion of analgesia. In the hypnotic trance, suggestions are given of pain relief as well as imaginative transfer of sensation from pain to some other sensation such as numbness. The second group of suggestions involves filtering of pain. These suggestions often combine imagery with sensation to provide the patient with a sense of the pain being filtered through or out of the body. The third group of suggestions involves dissociation of the pain from the body. Again, with this approach, use of imagery is helpful and the patient is encouraged to stand aside or away from his or her pain. The fourth set of suggestions involves displacement of the pain sensation to another part of the body. These suggestions can be very effective in pain management. Evans [31] has counseled care in assessment of the patient who is a candidate for hypnotic pain relief. He is particularly concerned about the pain masking depression. If such is the case, too rapid or complete a removal of pain can lead to increased overt depression and suicidal ideation.[31]

Hypnotic techniques can be combined with other forms of psychological intervention as well. Techniques such as hypnotherapy and hypnoanalysis are often used to determine the deeper meanings and idiosyncratic aspects of how the patient's psychology interacts with pain sensation.

Patients can be taught self-hypnosis. Again, this is similar to training in the relaxation response and it enables the patient to have yet another positive coping skill for dealing with the more intense pain sensations. Both relaxation and self-hypnosis need to be learned and practiced at times when the pain is less intense. Intense pain is disruptive of concentration and the patient may be unable to engage in the induction.

All of the self-regulatory techniques require intensive training. One of the failures often seen in pain management is too limited a trial of any one of the above methods. One cannot teach relaxation, biofeedback, or self-hypnosis in one or two sessions. Yet, in my experience, many patients report that is exactly what happened to them.

Multidisciplinary pain management is often the only reasonable approach to managing the intractable pain patient. Specialty centers frequently use the services of physicians, psychologists, and physical therapists in addition to an array of consultants that are called on an as-needed basis. As persistent pain continues it may take on more psychological features. The nonpsychiatric physician rarely has the time, training, or inclination to listen to the patient in the same way that the psychiatrist or psychologist does. A team approach to evaluation, treatment planning, and implementation of that plan provides the patient with the most comprehensive care available. In the absence of a multidisciplinary setting, the physician managing these complicated cases of fibromyalgia, myofascial syndrome, and other related musculoskeletal pain should attempt to have access to both skilled physical therapy services and a psychologist or psychiatrist with an interest in pain problems.

SUMMARY

The role of psychological factors in fibromyalgia, myofascial pain syndrome, and related musculoskeletal pain is extremely variable. While there is some evidence that depression is more prevalent in the personal and family histories of patients with fibromyalgia, empirical and experimental support are neither consistent nor strong. Patients should also be assessed with attention to anxiety, stress, somatization, and nonrestorative sleep disorder. It is important to remember that all patients with persistent pain do not develop chronic pain syndromes in which virtually all areas of psychosocial activity are compromised. Those patients that do develop chronic pain syndromes are more likely to have a history that includes developmental and psychosocial risk factors. Careful screening of the patient may provide clues as to which patients may require more comprehensive management, including psychological services. Both biofeedback and psychotherapy have shown promise in the comprehensive management of the patient with musculoskeletal pain.

REFERENCES

1. Adler RH, Zlot S, Hurny C, et al: Engel's "psychogenic" pain and the pain-prone patient: A retrospective, controlled clinical study, *Psychosomatics* 51:87–101, 1989.
2. Ahles TA, Yunus MB, Masi AT: Is chronic pain a variant of depressive disease? The case of primary fibromyalgia syndrome, *Pain* 29:105–111, 1987.
3. Ahles TA, Yunus MB, Riley SD, et al: Psychological factors associated with primary fibromyalgia syndrome, *Arthritis Rheum* 27:1101–1106, 1984.

4. Bennett RM, Gatter RA, Campbell SM, et al: A comparison of cyclobenzaprine and placebo in the management of fibrositis, *Arthritis Rheum* 31:1535–1542, 1988.
5. Bernstein DA, Borkovec TD: *Progressive relaxation training*, Champaign, Ill, 1973, Research Press.
6. Blumer D, Heilbronn M: Chronic pain as a variant of depressive disease: The pain-prone disorder, *J Nerv Ment Dis* 170:381–405, 1982.
7. Blumer D, Heilbronn M: Dysthymic pain disorder: The treatment of chronic pain as a variant of depression. In Tollison CD, editor: *Handbook of chronic pain management*, Baltimore, 1989, Williams & Wilkins, pp 197–209.
8. Boissevain MD, McCain GA: Toward an integrated understanding of fibromyalgia syndrome. I. Medical and pathophysiological aspects, *Pain* 45:227–238, 1991.
9. Boissevain MD, McCain GA: Toward an integrated understanding of fibromyalgia syndrome. II. Psychological and phenomenological aspects, *Pain* 45:239–248, 1991.
10. Bradley LA, Prokop CK, Margolis R, et al: Multivariate analysis of the MMPI profiles of low back pain patients, *J Behav Med* 1:253–272, 1978.
11. Brena SF, Koch DL: "Pain estimate" model for quantification and classification of chronic pain states, *Anesthesiol Rev* 2:8–13, 1975.
12. Brooke RI, Stenn PG: Myofascial pain dysfunction syndrome: How effective is biofeedback-assisted relaxation training? In Bonica JJ, Lindblom U, Iggo A, editors: *Advances in pain research and therapy*, vol 5, New York, 1983, Raven Press, pp 809–812.
13. Campbell SM, Clark S, Tindall EA, et al: Clinical characteristics of fibrositis: A "blinded" controlled study of symptoms and tender points, *Arthritis Rheum* 26:817–824, 1983.
14. Carette S, McCain GA, Bell DA, et al: Evaluation of amitriptylene in primary fibrositis: A double-blind, placebo-controlled study, *Arthritis Rheum* 29:655–659, 1986.
15. Chapman CR, Bonica JJ: *Chronic pain*. Kalamazoo, Mich, 1985, Upjohn.
16. Ciccone DS, Grzesiak RC: Cognitive dimensions of chronic pain, *Soc Sci Med* 19:1339–1345, 1984.
17. Ciccone DS, Grzesiak RC: Cognitive therapy: An overview of theory and practice. In Lynch NT, Vasudevan S, editors: *Persistent pain: Psychosocial assessment and intervention*, Boston, 1988, Kluwer, pp 133–161.
18. Ciccone DS, Grzesiak RC: Chronic musculoskeletal pain: A cognitive approach to psychophysiologic assessment and intervention. In Eisenberg MG, Grzesiak RC, editors: *Advances in clinical rehabilitation*, vol 3, New York, 1990, Springer, pp 197–215.
19. Ciccone DS, Grzesiak RC: Psychological vulnerability to chronic pain: A preliminary study, Annual Meeting of the American Pain Society, St Louis, October 1990.
20. Ciccone DS, Grzesiak RC: Psychological dysfunction in chronic cervical pain: An introduction to clinical assessment. In Tollison CD, Satterthwaite JR, editors: *Painful cervical trauma: Diagnosis and rehabilitative treatment of neuromusculoskeletal injuries*, Baltimore, 1992, Williams & Wilkins, pp 79–92.
21. Coen SJ, Sarno JE: Psychosomatic avoidance of conflict in back pain, *J Am Acad Psychoanal* 17:359–376, 1989.
22. Crue BL Jr: Evaluation of chronic pain syndromes tape T 155, New York, 1978, BioMonitoring Applications.
23. Draspa LJ: Psychological factors in muscular pain, *Br J Med Psychol* 32:106–116, 1959.
24. Dworkin RH, Gitlin MJ: Clinical aspects of depression in chronic pain patients, *Clin J Pain* 7:79–94, 1991.
25. Dworkin RH, Grzesiak RC: Chronic pain: On the integration of psyche and soma. In Stricker G, Gold JR, editors: *Comprehensive handbook of psychotherapy integration*, New York, 1993, Plenum, pp. 365–384.
26. Dworkin RH, Handlin DS, Richlin DM, et al: Unraveling the effects of compensation, litigation, and employment on treatment response in chronic pain, *Pain* 23:49–59, 1985.
27. Dworkin RH, Hartstein G, Rosner HL, et al: A high-risk method of studying psychosocial antecedents of chronic pain: The prospective investigation of herpes zoster, *J Abnorm Psychol* 101:200–205, 1992.

28. Eimers BN: Psychotherapy for chronic pain: A cognitive approach. In Freeman A, Simon KM, Beutler LE, et al, editors: *Comprehensive handbook of cognitive therapy*, New York, 1989, Plenum, pp 440–465.
29. Engel GL: Primary atypical facial neuralgia: An hysterical conversion symptom, *Psychosom Med* 13:375–396, 1951.
30. Engel GL: "Psychogenic" pain and the pain-prone patient, *Am J Med* 26:899–918, 1959.
31. Evans FJ: Hypnosis and chronic pain management. In Burrows G, Elton D, Stanley G, editors: *Handbook of chronic pain management*, Amsterdam, 1987, Elsevier.
32. Felson DT, Goldenberg DL: The natural history of fibromyalgia, *Arthritis Rheum* 29:1522–1526, 1986.
33. Ferraccioli G, Ghirelli L, Scita F, et al: EMG-biofeedback training in fibromyalgia syndrome, *J Rheumatol* 144:820–825, 1987.
34. Fordyce WE: *Behavioral methods for chronic pain and illness*, St Louis, 1976, Mosby–Year Book.
35. Fordyce WE, Fowler RS, deLateur BJ: Application of behavior modification technique to problems of chronic pain, *Behav Res Ther* 6:105–107, 1968.
36. Fordyce WE, Fowler RS, Lehmann J, et al: Some applications of learning to problems of chronic pain, *J Chron Dis* 21:179–190, 1968.
37. France RD, Krishnan KRR: Pain in psychiatric disorders. In France RD, Krishnan KRR, editors: *Chronic pain*, Washington, DC, 1988, American Psychiatric Press, pp 117–141.
38. French AP, Tupin JP: Therapeutic application of a simple relaxation method, *Am J Psychother* 28:282–287, 1974.
39. Goldenberg DL: Psychiatric and psychologic aspects of fibromyalgia syndrome, *Rheum Dis Clin* 15:105–114, 1989.
40. Goldenberg DL, Felson DT, Dinnerman HA: A randomized controlled trial of amitriptyline and naproxen in the treatment of patients with fibromyalgia, *Arthritis Rheum* 29:1371–1377, 1986.
41. Grzesiak RC: Relaxation techniques in treatment of chronic pain, *Arch Phys Med Rehabil* 58:270–272, 1977.
42. Grzesiak RC: Biofeedback in the treatment of chronic pain, *Curr Concepts Pain* 2:3–8, 1984.
43. Grzesiak RC: Strategies for multidisciplinary pain management, *Compendium Continuing Educ Dent* 10:444–448, 1989.
44. Grzesiak RC: Psychological aspects of chronic orofacial pain: Theory, assessment and management, *Pain Digest* 1:100–119, 1991.
45. Grzesiak RC: Unconscious processes and chronic pain: On the foundations of pain-proneness, Annual Meeting of the American Psychological Association, Washington, DC, August 1992.
46. Grzesiak RC, Ciccone DS: Relaxation, biofeedback and hypnosis in the management of pain. In Lynch NT, Vasudevan S, editors: *Persistent pain: Psychosocial assessment and intervention*, Boston, 1988, Kluwer, pp 163–188.
47. Grzesiak RC, Perrine KR: Psychological aspects of chronic pain. In Wu W, editor: *Pain management: Assessment and treatment of chronic and acute syndromes*, New York, 1986, Human Sciences Press, pp 44–69.
48. Gupta M, Moldofsky H: Dysthymic disorder and rheumatic pain modulation disorder (fibrositis syndrome): A comparison of symptoms and sleep physiology, *Can J Psychiatry* 31:608–616, 1986.
49. Hanvik LJ: MMPI profiles in patients with low back pain, *J Consult Psychol* 15:350–353, 1951.
50. Heaton RK, Lehman RAW, Getto CJ: *Psychosocial Pain Inventory*, Odessa, Fla, 1980, Psychological Assessment Resources.
51. Holmes TH, Wolff HG: Life situations, emotions, and backache, *Psychosom Med* 14:18–33, 1952.
52. Hudson JI, Hudson MS, Pliner LF, et al: Fibromyalgia and major affective disorder: A controlled phenomenology and family history study, *Am J Psychiatry* 142:441–446, 1985.
53. Huskisson EC: Measurement of pain, *Lancet* 2:1127–1131, 1974.
54. Jacobsen R, Edinger JD: Side effects of relaxation treatment, *Am J Psychiatry* 139:952–953.

55. Jacobson E: *Modern treatment of tense patients,* Springfield, Ill, 1964, Charles C Thomas.
56. Kellner R: *Psychosomatic syndromes and somatic symptoms,* Washington, DC, 1991, American Psychiatric Press.
57. Kerns RD, Turk DC, Rudy TE: The West Haven–Yale Multidimensional Pain Inventory (WHYMPI), *Pain* 23:345–356, 1985.
58. Kirmayer LJ, Robbins JM, Kapusta MA: Somatization and depression in fibromyalgia syndrome, *Am J Psychiatry* 145:950–954, 1988.
59. Large RG, Lamb AM: Electromyographic (EMG) feedback in chronic musculoskeletal pain: A controlled trial, *Pain* 17:167–177, 1983.
60. Loeser JD: Concepts of pain. In Stanton-Hicks M, Boas RA, editors: *Chronic low back pain,* New York, 1982, Raven Press, pp 145–148.
61. Loeser JD, Black RG: A taxonomy of pain, *Pain* 1:81–90. 1975.
62. McCain FA, Scudds RA: The concept of primary fibromyalgia (fibrositis): Clinical value, relation and significance to other musculoskeletal pain syndromes, *Pain* 33:273–287, 1988.
63. McGuigan FJ: Progressive relaxation: Origins, principles, and clinical applications. In Woolfolk RL, Lehrer PM, editors: *Principles and practice of stress management,* New York, 1984, Guilford.
64. Mendelson G: Compensation, pain complaints, and psychological disturbance, *Pain* 20:169–177, 1984.
65. Melzack R: The McGill Pain Questionnaire: Major properties and scoring methods, *Pain* 1:277–299, 1975.
66. Merskey H: Psychiatric patients with persistent pain, *J Psychosom Res* 9:299–309, 1965.
67. Merskey H: The perception and measurement of pain, *J Psychosom Res* 17:251–255, 1973.
68. Merskey H, editor: Classification of chronic pain: Descriptions of chronic pain syndromes and definitions of pain terms, *Pain* 3(suppl):1986.
69. Middaugh SJ, Kee WG: Advances in electromyographic monitoring and biofeedback in the treatment of chronic cervical and low back pain. In Eisenberg MG, Grzesiak RC, editors: *Advances in clinical rehabilitation,* vol 1, New York, 1987, Springer-Verlag, pp 137–172.
70. Moldofsky H: Sleep and fibrositis syndrome, *Rheum Dis Clin* 15:91–103, 1989.
71. Moldofsky H, Lue FA: The relationship of alpha delta EEG frequencies to pain and mood in "fibrositis" patients with chlorpromazine and L-tryptophan, *Electroencephalogr Clin Neurophysiol* 50:71–80, 1980.
72. Moldofsky H, Scarisbrick P: Induction of neurasthenic musculoskeletal pain syndrome by selective sleep stage deprivation, *Psychosom Med* 38:35–44, 1976.
73. Moldofsky H, Scarisbrick P, England R, et al: Musculoskeletal symptoms and nonREM sleep disturbance in patients with "fibrositis" syndrome and healthy subjects, *Psychosom Med* 37:341–351, 1975.
74. Nouwen A, Bush C: The relationship between paraspinal EMG and chronic low back pain, *Pain* 20:109–123, 1984.
75. Nouwen A, Solinger JW: The effectiveness of EMG biofeedback training in low back pain, *Biofeedback Self Regul* 4:8–12, 1979.
76. Payne TC, Leavit F, Garron DC, et al: Fibrositis and psychologic disturbances, *Arthritis Rheum* 25:213–217, 1982.
77. Peck CL, Kraft GH: Electromyographic biofeedback for pain related to muscle tension: A study of tension headache, back and jaw pain, *Arch Surg* 112:889–895, 1977.
78. Pomp AM: Psychotherapy for the myofascial pain-dysfunction syndrome: A study of factors coinciding with symptom remission, *J Am Dent Assoc* 89:629–632, 1974.
79. Rudy TE, Turk DC, Zaki HS, et al: An empirical taxometric alternative to traditional classification of temporomandibular disorders, *Pain* 36:311–320, 1989.
80. Sarno JE: Psychogenic backache: The missing dimension, *J Fam Pract* 1:8–12, 1974.
81. Sarno JE: Chronic back pain and psychic conflict, *Scand J Rehabil Med* 8:143–153, 1976.
82. Sarno JE: Psychosomatic backache, *J Fam Pract* 5:353–357, 1977.

83. Sarno JE: Etiology of neck and back pain: An autonomic myoneuralgia, *J Nerv Ment Dis* 169:55–59, 1981.

84. Sarno JE: *Mind over back pain*, New York, 1984, Berkeley Books.

85. Saskin P, Moldofsky H, Lue FA: Sleep and posttraumatic pain modulation disorder (fibrositis syndrome), *Psychosom Med* 48:319–323, 1986.

86. Schofferman J, Anderson D, Hines R, et al: Childhood psychological trauma correlates with unsuccessful lumbar spine surgery, *Spine* 17:138–144, 1992.

87. Shutty MS, Sheras P: Brief strategic psychotherapy with chronic pain patients: Reframing and problem resolution, *Psychother* 28:636–642, 1991.

88. Simms RW, Goldenberg DL, Felson DT, et al: Tenderness in 75 anatomic sites: Distinguishing fibromyalgia patients from controls, *Arthritis Rheum* 31:182–187, 1988.

89. Smythe HA: Non-articular rheumatism and psychogenic musculoskeletal syndromes. In McCarty DJ, editor: *Arthritis and allied conditions,* ed 11, Philadelphia, 1988, Lea & Febiger, pp 1241–1254.

90. Tait RC: Psychological factors in chronic benign pain, *Curr Concepts Pain* 1:10–15, 1983.

91. Tunks ER, Merskey H: Psychotherapy in the management of chronic pain. In Bonica JJ, editor: *The management of pain,* vol 2, ed 2, Philadelphia, 1990, Lea & Febiger, pp 1751–1756.

92. Turk DC: Customizing treatment for chronic pain patients: Who, what, and why?, *Clin J Pain* 6:255–270, 1990.

93. Turk, DC, Meichenbaum D, Genest M: *Pain and behavioral medicine: A cognitive-behavioral perspective,* New York, 1983, Guilford.

94. Turk DC, Rudy TE: Toward an empirically derived taxonomy of chronic pain patients: Integration of psychological assessment data, *J Consult Clin Psychol* 56:233–238, 1988.

95. Turk DC, Rudy TE: Neglected factors in chronic pain treatment outcome studies—referral patterns, failure to enter treatment, and attrition, *Pain* 43:7–25, 1990.

96. Turk DC, Rudy TE: Neglected topics in the treatment of chronic pain patients—relapse, noncompliance, and adherence enhancement, *Pain* 44:5–28, 1991.

97. Van Houdenhove B: Prevalence and psychodynamic interpretation of premorbid hyperactivity in patients with chronic pain, *Psychother Psychosom* 45:195–200, 1986.

98. Waldinger RJ: *Psychiatry for medical students,* Washington, DC, 1984, American Psychiatric Press.

99. Whale J: The use of brief focal psychotherapy in the treatment of chronic pain. *Psychoanal Psychother* 6:61–72, 1992.

100. Wolfe F, Cathey MA, Kleinheksel SM, et al: Psychological status in primary fibrositis and fibrositis associated with rheumatoid arthritis, *J Rheumatol* 11:500–506.

101. Wolfe F, Smythe HA, Yunus MB, et al: The American College of Rheumatology 1990 criteria for the classification of fibromyalgia, *Arthritis Rheum* 33:160–172.

102. Wolskee PJ: Psychological therapy for chronic pain. In Wu W, editor: *Pain management: Assessment and treatment of chronic and acute syndromes,* New York, 1987, Human Sciences Press, pp 201–215.

Chapter 5

Disability Evaluation and Management of Myofascial Pain

Matthew Monsein, M.D.

Unfortunately, not all patients with myofascial pain syndromes respond successfully to treatment. There exist a small but significant number of patients who despite undergoing extensive treatment continue to complain of severe and often disabling pain. Often subsumed under the rubric of the chronic pain syndrome, these patients can be characterized by their clinical unresponsiveness to standard medical care, the presence of numerous psychosocial contributing factors, and the frustration confounding their physicians, themselves, and the medicolegal systems they are frequently involved with. In spite of treatment, they continue to complain of pain, often greater than one would expect based on the clinical findings alone. Associated with their complaints of pain are often a number of other dysfunctional behaviors. These may include excessive alcohol use or overdependence on narcotics, and even on over-the-counter medications; histrionic behavior, i.e., grimacing, groaning, bizzare posturing, or touch-me-not reactions in response to even the lightest palpation; and depression, anxiety, and other psychological distress. These patients have often developed extremely sedentary lifestyles secondary to their experience of pain, and are physically deconditioned. Most important, from the patients' and society's perspective, they have, owing to their experience of pain, become socially isolated, given up a number of recreational activities, and claimed disability from work.

The reasons for this pattern are unclear. Simons suggests that these patients have developed a post traumatic hyperirritability of their nervous system and of their trigger points. Each patient has suffered trauma usually from an automobile accident or fall severe enough to damage the sensory pathways of the central nervous system. The damage apparently acts as an endogenous perpetuating factor suspectible to augmentation by severe pain, additional trauma, vibration, loud noises, prolonged physical activity, and emotional stress. From the date of the trauma, coping with pain typically becomes the focus of life for these patients who previously paid little attention to pain. They are unable to increase their activity substantially without increasing their pain level.[30]

Others suggest that it is the psychosocial factors which are the dominant feature in the evolution of this pattern of behavior, and furthermore it is addressing these factors that is at the heart of successful rehabilitation of these patients.[17, 25] Assessing the clinical status of this group of patients, providing appropriate guidance toward rehabilitation, and interfacing with the various disability systems that they may be involved with remains for the physician an extremely challenging task.

Physicians often feel inadequate in addressing issues that society has demanded of them with the establishment of the various disability systems. Disability assessment is not a standard part of medical school or residency training. Physicians often resent the requirements of filling out lengthy forms and the involvement of attorneys. Finally, they may have concerns about their own ability based on their training and knowledge to delineate for society issues such as disability, percentage of bodily impairment, functional limitations, and the patient's ability or inability to work, particularly when this assessment is based on an understanding of the patient's subjective experience of pain.

In 1955, congressional hearings were held to establish whether physicians were able to determine disability by standard medical examinations. Physicians from almost every state and medical society were interviewed. A substantial majority of physicians felt that they were unable to determine disability purely on a medical basis. Moreover, most felt that intervening in the disability process would be in conflict with their therapeutic relationship with the patient.

> "Disability certification for purpose of cash benefits required the physician to mediate between the patient and the government's interest. In such gatekeeping rules, physicians would be "caught in a squeeze" and forced to "serve two masters." Patients could and would simply shop around for a doctor willing to provide evidence of their impairments, and friends and family, as well as patients, would put unbearable pressure on physicians reducing their ability to make good clinical judgments. Introducing such extensions into the doctor patient relationship would undermine its therapeutic effectiveness."[20]

Nevertheless, in spite of these objections, most disability systems do place considerable, if not total, dependence upon the treating physician's evaluation.

In the area of pain, particularly myofascial pain, this issue is even more problematic. By definition, pain is simply a personal and subjective experience known only to the patient. As clinicians, we can only observe the outer manifestations of this experience or the patient's pain behaviors. We are dependent on the patient's subjective complaints in assessing the severity of the problem.

In myofascial pain disorders, there are no agreed-on objective standards for assessing the anatomic severity of the condition. Specifically, while there are data to support the reliability and validity of pressure algometry, questions remain as to its sensitivity and it is still reliant on the patient's subjective response.[24] Furthermore, neither pressure algometry nor the more controversial thermography[5] has been accepted as a reliable standard by medical organizations such as the American Medical Association (AMA) or the American Academy of Orthopaedic Surgeons, or by the various disability systems such as Social Security disability or workers' compensation.

While Simons[30] believes that a palpable hardening of taut bands of muscle fibers passing through the tender spot in a shortened muscle and a local twitch response of the taut band are objective indications of myofascial pain, assessment of these findings depends on the sensitivity and clinical acumen of the examiner. Thus, at the present time, assessing a patient's level of pain and dysfunction, as well as determining how to help this select group of patients with myofascial pain syndromes who claim disability, remains a challenge.

The purpose of this chapter is threefold: first, to discuss various disability systems in the context of myofascial pain; second, to describe in more detail the psychosocial characteristics of patients who present with disability secondary to myofascial pain syndromes; and finally, to present a model for rehabilitation to assist these patients in returning to a more normal and functional lifestyle.

DISABILITY SYSTEMS

Most patients with myofascial pain are covered under one of four systems: Social Security Disability Insurance (SSDI), workers' compensation (WC), personal injury (PI), or long-term disability (LTD). Each system has its own characteristics established either through legislation, in the case of SSDI and WC, or in PI and LTD cases through a combination of legislation and individual policy formulation. In order to understand the implication of myofascial pain to each specific system, it is important to review the concepts of impairment and its relationship to pain and disability.

DEFINITIONS

Impairment

Impairment is defined as any loss or abnormality of psychological, physiologic, or anatomic structure or function that can be defined in terms of objective medical evidence such as radiographs or laboratory tests, standardized psychological tests, and objective clinical findings such as range of motion, muscle atrophy, sensory changes, and so forth.[4] It should be noted that trigger points are generally not included in the various systems that define medical impairment. Furthermore, the patient's subjective complaints, while critically important in defining disability and functional capacity, may or may not be considered in the establishment of a medical impairment, depending on the system (Table 5–1). At times, physicians are asked only to assess whether the patient has a physical or psychological condition and at other times are asked to actually give a percentage of impairment. The rationale for this concept dates back to models used in determining casualty and property damage where an insurance adjuster, for example, was capable of estimating the percentage of fire dam-

TABLE 5–1.

Comparison of Impairment (Disability)*†

System	Symptoms	ROM	Diagnosis	Other Physiologic	Functional Evaluation
Social Security	X	X		X	
California (WC)	X	X	X	X	X
Minnesota (WC)	X		X		
American Medical Association			X	X	
American Academy of Orthopaedic Surgeons	X		X	X	

*Modified from Mayer TG, Mooney V, Gatchel RJ, et al: *Contemporary conservative care for painful spinal disorders: Impairment evaluation issues and the disability system*, Philadelphia, 1991, Lea & Febiger, p 533. Used by permission.
†ROM = range of motion; WC = workers' compensation.

age to a building. The premise is that a physician has the same capability in terms of defining a percentage of damage to the body of an individual. While one may argue the reasonableness of this metaphor, as long as the current legal system remains, physicians will continue to be held responsible to define impairment as a percentage of the whole person or of an individual extremity.

In an attempt to gain some uniformity, several systems of impairment or disability determination have emerged. The factors utilized in determining impairment vary based on each individual system. For example, the AMA *Guides to the Evaluation of Permanent Impairment*,[4] which was first published in 1958 and is now in its fourth edition, is based primarily on anatomic features but does include diagnosis as well. This is also true of the American Academy of Orthopaedic Surgeons system, which was a modification of the AMA model.[15] The latter does, however, incorporate a scale for pain in patients with documented organic disorders. In Minnesota, WC impairment is defined in the state regulations and is based primarily on range of motion and radiographic findings, although clinical symptoms are also included.[36]

With specific regard to the issue of myofascial pain, let us take an example of someone with a cervical strain or whiplash injury. Using the AMA guidelines, two specific areas would be utilized in determining the percentage of impairment. First, as defined in Figure 5–1,A, assuming that the patient does not have any degenerative radiographic changes, he or she would receive a 4% permanent partial impairment of the whole person for the diagnosis of a cervical strain. This is based on the observation that not only does the patient have pain but there is clinical evidence of recurrent muscle spasm or rigidity. Assuming that there is loss of motion, there would be an additional percentage of impairment based on the findings as indicated in Figure 5–1,B, C, and D. Adding these together and using what the AMA calls a Combined Values Chart, one would be able to determine the actual percentage of physical impairment.

Pain in and of itself is not considered to be ratable in this example. In fact, pain is only considered to be ratable in the area of neuromuscular problems when it is associated with specific damage to a peripheral nerve. In this case, the pain needs to be associated with a sensory loss and is determined by multiplying the severity of pain and sensory deficits by the percentage of impairment associated with the particular nerve root or peripheral nerve involved.[4]

Pain associated with the soft tissue injury in our example is not ratable but is recognized as a factor that will contribute to decreased range of motion. In fact, pain, fear of injury, and neuromuscular inhibition are considered to be factors that may diminish range of motion due to either diminished effort or guarding, and in order for range of motion to be considered accurate, reproducibility is required. Specifically "the examiner must take at least three consecutive mobility measurements which fall within + or −10 percent or 5 percent (whichever is greater to be considered consistent)."[4]

In Minnesota, a person with the same type of injury would receive only a 3.5% permanent partial impairment, assuming that there were no abnormalities on their radiographs and that there was documented muscle spasm or rigidity associated with loss of motion (Fig 5–2). While one can certainly argue about the fairness of these various systems, they do point out the inconsistencies and ambiguities associated with the evaluation of impairment with myofascial pain.

In persons involved with personal injury cases, defining impairment may or may not be required depending on the legislative statutes and the whims of the attorneys. Often, in persons with soft tissue injuries where pain is a major

A

Disorder	% Impairment of Whole Person		
	Cerv	Thor	Lumb
I. Fractures			
A. Compression of one vertebral body			
0%-25%	4	2	5
26%-50%	6	3	7
>50%	10	5	12
B. Fracture of posterior elements (pedicles, laminae, articular processes, or transverse processes)	4	2	5
Note: Impairments due to compression of the vertebral body and to fractures of the posterior elements are combined using the Combined Values Chart.			
Note: When two or more vertebrae are compressed or fractured, combine all impairment values.			
C. Reduced dislocation of one vertebra	5	3	6
Note: If two or more vertebrae are dislocated and reduced, combine the impairment values using the Combined Values Chart.			
Note: An unreduced dislocation causes temporary impairment until it is reduced: then the physician should evaluate permanent impairment on the basis of the subjects' condition with the reduced dislocation. If no reduction is possible, then the physician should evaluate impairment on the basis of restricted motion and concomitant neurological findings in the spinal region involved, according to the criteria in this Chapter and in Chapter 4.			
II. Intervertebral disc or other soft tissue lesions			
A. Unoperated, with no residuals	0	0	0
B. Unoperated with medically documented injury and a minimum of six months of medically documented pain, recurrent muscle spasm or rigidity associated with none-to-minimal degenerative changes on structural tests	4	2	5
C. Unoperated, with medically documented injury and a minimum of six months of medically documented pain, recurrent muscle spasm, or rigidity associated with moderate to severe degenerative changes on structural tests, including unoperated herniated nucleus pulposus, with or without radiculopathy	6	3	7
D. Surgically treated disc lesion, with no residuals	7	4	8
E. Surgically treated disc lesion, with residual symptoms	9	5	10
F. Multiple operative levels, with or without residual symptomatology	Add 1%/level		
G. Multiple operations ("failed back surgery") with or without residual symptoms:			
1. Second operation	Add 2%		
2. Third or subsequent surgery	Add 1%/operation		
III. Spondylolysis and spondylolisthesis, unoperated			
A. Spondylolysis or Grade I (1%-25% slippage) or Grade II (26%-50% slippage) spondylolisthesis, accompanied by medically documented injury and a minimum of six months of medically documented pain, recurrent muscle spasm, or rigidity	7	4	8
B. Grade III (51%-75% slippage) or Grade IV (76%-100% slippage) spondylolisthesis, accompanied by medically documented injury and a minimum of six months of medically documented pain, recurrent muscle spasm, or rigidity	9	5	10
IV. Spinal stenosis, segmental instability, or spondylolisthesis, operated			
A. Single level operation, with no residuals	8	4	9
B. Single level operation, with residual symptoms	10	5	12
C. Multiple levels operated, with residual symptoms	Add 1%/level		
D. Multiple operations ("failed back surgery") with residual symptoms:			
1. Second operation	Add 2%		
2. Third or subsequent surgery	Add 1%/operation		

Note: List impairments separately for cervical, thoracic, and lumbar regions (Figures 83 a-c).

Note: All impairment ratings above should be combined with the appropriate values of residuals, such as:

1. Ankylosis (fusion) in the spinal area or extremities

2. Abnormal motion in the spinal area (i.e., objectively measured rigidity) or extremities

3. Spinal cord and spinal nerve root injuries, with neurologic impairment (see Upper Extremity and Lower Extremity sections of Chapter 3 and Peripheral Nervous System section of Chapter 4)

4. Any combination of the above using the Combined Values Chart.

FIG 5–1. A–D, determining the percentage of impairment due to specific disorders of the spine. (From Engelberg AL, editor: *Guides to the evaluation of permanent impairment,* ed 3, Chicago, 1988, American Medical Association. Used by permission.)

B

Abnormal Motion
Average range of *Flexion-Extension* is 135°.
Value to total range of cervical motion is 40%.

Flexion from neutral position (0°) to:	Degrees of Cervical Motion		% Impairment of Whole Person
	Lost	Retained	
0°	60°	0°	6
20°	40°	20°	4
40°	20°	40°	2
60°	0°	60°+	0

Extension from neutral position (0°) to:			
0°	75°	0°	6
25°	50°	25°	4
50°	25°	50°	2
75°	0°	75°+	0

Ankylosis

Region ankylosed at:	% Impairment of Whole Person
0° (neutral position)	12
20°	20
40°	30
60° (full flexion)	40

Region ankylosed at:	
0° (neutral position)	12
25°	20
50°	30
75° (full extension)	40

C

Abnormal Motion
Average range of *Lateral Flexion* is 90°.
Value to total range of cervical motion is 25%.

Right lateral flexion from neutral position (0°) to:	Degrees of Cervical Motion		% Impairment of Whole Person
	Lost	Retained	
0°	45°	0°	4
15°	30°	15°	2
30°	15°	30°	1
45°	0°	45°+	0

Left lateral flexion from neutral position (0°) to:			
0°	45°	0°	4
15°	30°	15°	2
30°	15°	30°	1
45°	0°	45°+	0

Ankylosis

Region ankylosed at:	% Impairment of Whole Person
0° (neutral position)	8
15°	20
30°	30
45° (full right/left lateral flexion)	40

FIG 5-1 (cont.).   For legend see previous page.

D

Abnormal Motion
Average range of Rotation is 160°.
Value to total range of cervical motion is 35%.

Right rotation from neutral position (0°) to:	Degrees of Cervical Motion		% Impairment of Whole Person
	Lost	Retained	
0°	80°	0°	6
20°	60°	20°	4
40°	40°	40°	2
60°	20°	60°	1
80°	0°	80°+	0

Left rotation from neutral position (0°) to:			
0°	80°	0°	6
20°	60°	20°	4
40°	40°	40°	2
60°	20°	60°	1
80°	0°	80°+	0

Ankylosis

Region ankylosed at:	% Impairment of Whole Person
0° (neutral position)	12
20°	20
40°	30
60°	40
80° (full right/left rotation)	50

FIG 5-1 (cont.).   For legend see page 95.

component of disability, a physician is only asked to give his medical opinion regarding whether the injury is permanent. In the case of long-term disability, impairment only needs to be established in order to confirm the veracity of the claimant. A much more critical issue has to do with the patients' functional capacities and their ability to return to their previous task vs. returning back to any type of further gainful employment. This is also the critical issue in determination of Social Security disability.

Thus, in conclusion, impairment is a definable loss of structure or function. It is not synonymous with disability and while there are certainly some persons with significant impairments who will be able to function with relatively normal activities of daily living and work full-time, others with a minimal medical impairment will find themselves extremely disabled owing to a combination of psychological, social, and behavior factors, in addition to their impairment and experience of pain.

Disability

Disability is defined as the limiting loss or absence of a person's capacity to meet personal, social, or occupational demands, or to meet statutory or regulatory requirements.[25] Disability reflects loss of function and is usually defined operationally in terms of inability to participate in social or recreational activities, other activities of daily living, and most important, in the individual's ability to perform work, based on a limitation of functional capabilities. Disability is a reflection of the patient's psychological and physical perception of his or

Subp. 2. Cervical spine. The spine rating is inclusive of arm symptoms except for gross motor weakness; sensory loss; and bladder, bowel, or sexual dysfunction. Bladder, bowel, or sexual dysfunction must be rated as provided in part 5223.0060, subpart 7. Permanent partial disability of the cervical spine is a disability of the whole body as follows:

A. Healed sprain, strain, or contusion:

(1) Subjective symptoms of pain not substantiated by objective clinical findings or demonstrable degenerative changes, 0 percent.

(2) Pain associated with rigidity (loss of motion or postural abnormality) or chronic muscle spasm. The chronic muscle spasm or rigidity is substantiated by objective clinical findings but without associated demonstrable degenerative changes, 3.5 percent.

(3) Pain associated with rigidity (loss of motion or postural abnormality) or chronic muscle spasm. The chronic muscle spasm or rigidity is substantiated by objective clinical findings and is associated with demonstrable degenerative changes.

(a) Single vertebral level, 7 percent; or

(b) Multiple vertebral levels, 10.5 percent.

B. Herniated intervertebral disc, single vertebral level:

(1) Condition not surgically treated:

(a) X-ray or computerized axial tomography or myelogram specifically positive for herniated disc; excellent results, with resolution of objective neurologic findings, 9 percent.

(b) Neck and specific radicular pain present with objective neurologic findings; and X-ray or computerized axial tomography or myelogram specifically positive for herniated disc; and no surgery is performed for treatment, 14 percent.

(2) Condition treated by surgery:

(a) Surgery with excellent results such as mild neck pain, no arm pain, and no neurologic deficit, 9 percent.

(b) Surgery with average results such as mild increase in symptoms with neck motion or lifting, and mild to moderate restriction of activities related to neck and arm pain, 11 percent.

(c) Surgery with poor surgical results such as persistent or increased symptoms with neck motion or lifting, and major restriction of activities because of neck and arm pain, 13 percent.

FIG 5–2. Determining the percentage of impairment in cervical spine injury: the Minnesota system. (From *Minnesota statutes annotated,* Minneapolis, 1989, West Publishing. Used by permission.)

her underlying condition or illness. Disability may result from a medical impairment, but the degree of disability does not necessarily conform to the level of impairment. In terms of work, for example, a professional piano player who loses a little finger would have the same impairment as a truck driver with a similar injury. The former, however, would be totally disabled with respect to employability, whereas the latter would not experience any disability with regard to employment. Moreover, in understanding disability, psychological and social factors need to be evaluated and integrated into the disability assessment.

In patients with myofascial pain syndromes, their psychological status, i.e., whether they are depressed or anxious; their personality style, i.e., whether they have a dependent personality, histrionic personality, or a tendency to somatize; the meaning of pain to that person, i.e., the fear of reinjury, concerns about having a more serious underlying medical condition; motivational factors, i.e., desire to return to work; relationship with their employer; litigation; other potential secondary gain factors; cultural issues; and family modeling, i.e., other family members with a history of disability—all can have a significant impact on the way patients perceive and express their condition. In terms of determining work-related disability, the patient's age, education, intelligence, the economic status of the community, work experience, and job availability are critical. The fact that the patient's symptoms of pain and subsequent disability are greater than what one would expect based on the clinical findings alone does not mean that the patient is malingering or consciously exaggerating his or her symptoms.[25] Obviously then, the determination of disability is an extremely complex and multifaceted process. Yet again, physicians are often asked to determine the patient's level of disability and in particular the capacity to work. Whereas impairment is a medical decision, disability is a legal one.

In the case of myofascial pain and disability, a patient's functional capacities are by definition a self-limited phenomenon secondary to the patient's perception of pain and his or her interpretation of that perception. This is ultimately what defines the patient's ability to perform activities of daily living, including work. In order for the physician to evaluate the patient's level of disability, obviously the accuracy of the patient's self-report is critical. Confirmation of the patient's reported limitations by family members can be helpful in defining functional limitations.

Another useful source of information regarding the patient's functional abilities is through the use of a standardized self-assessment questionnaire. While currently there does not exist a specific instrument that has been established as the gold standard in the assessment of disability and pain, there are a number of instruments, i.e., the SIP, WIMPY, and IMPATH that are currently in use.[18] Moreover, the Social Security Administration is in the process of attempting to develop standardized instruments for the evaluation of disability under their guidelines.

Another useful method for assessing disability is the functional capacity evaluation. This is performed by either a physical therapist or an occupational therapist and consists of a minimum of a 2- to 3-hour assessment up to a week-long assessment of the patient's physical and functional capabilities. Patients are asked to perform a number of activities on a repetitive basis. Repetitive testing is performed to maintain consistency and test for reliability. A skilled therapist is able to distinguish limitations due to physiologic capacities, i.e., muscle fatigue vs. pain-limited functions. While testing may be capable of measuring consistency of effort, the observation that inconsistencies are present does not distinguish between conscious input on the part of the patient vs. unconscious input. The former obviously implies malingering, whereas the latter may reflect the fear of increased pain, anxiety, or other psychological factors.

A well-performed functional capacity evaluation can certainly provide important data as to a person's functional capacities, and identify work restrictions. On completion of a functional capacity evaluation, information is provided as to the patient's capacities regarding sitting, walking, standing, lifting, ability to perform repetitive motions, and range of motion, as well as lifting and carrying capacities. Moreover, a well-performed functional capacity evaluation can also provide important data as to which patients, owing to physiologic limitations or pain behaviors, may be candidates for more intensive work-hardening programs, intensive pain rehabilitation, or other types of functional restoration programs.[12, 13] Information gathered by the physical therapist (Fig 5–3) allows the physician to generate restrictions required for a return-to-work plan (Fig 5–4).

Social Security Administration

Before leaving the issue of disability, it is important to discuss the Social Security Administration and its evaluation of myofascial pain, since in the United States, the largest disability system is that of the Social Security Admin-

						Client	
						Date	

Item	Percent of 8-hour Day					Restrictions	Recommendations
	0	1-5	6-33	34-66	67-100		
WEIGHT CAPACITY IN LBS.							
Floor to waist lift							
Waist to overhead lift							
Horizontal lift							
Push							
Pull							
Right carry							
Left carry							
Front carry							
Right hand grip							
Left hand grip							
FLEXIBILITY/POSITIONAL							
Elevated work							
Forward bending/sitting							
Forward bending/standing							
Rotation sitting							
Rotation standing							
Crawl							
Kneel							
Crouch-deep static							
Repetitive Squat							
STATIC WORK							
Sitting tolerance							
Standing tolerance							
AMBULATION							
Walking							
Stair climbing							
Step ladder climbing							
Balance							
COORDINATION							
R. upper extremity							
L. upper extremity							

Evaluator   Date

FIG 5–3.   A functional capacity evaluation in subacute spinal disorders. (From Mayer TG, Mooney V, Gatchell RJ, et al: *Contemporary conservative care for painful spinal disorders: Impairment evaluation issues and the disability system,* Philadelphia, 1991, Lea & Febiger, p 533. Used by permission.)

PATIENT: _____

I estimate this person is able to:

	Never	Occasionally (1-33%)	Frequently (34-66%)	Continuously (67-100%)
1. LIFT:				
a. up to 10 lb.	_____	_____	_____	_____
b. 11-25 lb.	_____	_____	_____	_____
c. 26-35 lb.	_____	_____	_____	_____
d. 36-50 lb.	_____	_____	_____	_____
e. 51-75 lb.	_____	_____	_____	_____
f. 76-100 lb.	_____	_____	_____	_____
2. CARRY:				
a. up to 10 lb.	_____	_____	_____	_____
b. 11-25 lb.	_____	_____	_____	_____
c. 26-34 lb.	_____	_____	_____	_____
d. 36-50 lb.	_____	_____	_____	_____
e. 51-75 lb.	_____	_____	_____	_____
f. 76-100 lb.	_____	_____	_____	_____
3. CAN THE PERSON PERFORM THE FOLLOWING TASKS:				
Push/Pull—Seated	_____	_____	_____	_____
Push/Pull—Standing	_____	_____	_____	_____
Bend	_____	_____	_____	_____
Squat	_____	_____	_____	_____
Crawl	_____	_____	_____	_____
Climb	_____	_____	_____	_____
Reach above shoulder level	_____	_____	_____	_____

4. CIRCLE THE NUMBER OF HOURS FOR EACH ACTIVITY:
Note: Does not have to total 8 hours.

									Continuously	With Rest
Sit	1	2	3	4	5	6	7	8 (hrs)	_____	_____
Stand	1	2	3	4	5	6	7	8 (hrs)	_____	_____
Walk	1	2	3	4	5	6	7	8 (hrs)	_____	_____
Sit/Stand	1	2	3	4	5	6	7	8 (hrs)	_____	_____

5. CAN PERSON USE HANDS FOR REPETITIVE ACTION SUCH AS:

	Simple Grasping	Firm Grasp	Fine Manipulating
Right	Yes _____ No _____	Yes _____ No _____	Yes _____ No _____
Left	Yes _____ No _____	Yes _____ No _____	Yes _____ No _____

6. CAN PERSON USE FEET FOR REPETITIVE MOVEMENTS, AS IN OPERATING FOOT CONTROLS?

Right	Left	Both
Yes _____ No _____	Yes _____ No _____	Yes _____ No _____

7. ANY RESTRICTIONS OF ACTIVITIES INVOLVED?

8. CAN PERSON NOW RETURN TO FORMER JOB?

Yes _____ No _____

CAN PERSON RETURN TO OTHER WORK ACCORDING TO RESTRICTIONS DEFINED ABOVE?

Yes _____ No _____

IF NOT, GIVE ESTIMATED DATE FOR RETURN TO WORK _____

Work part time? _____ hrs/day   Work full-time?   Yes _____ No _____
Disability rating _____% (if applicable)

9. COMMENTS: _____

_____

_____

_____

_____

_____

_____

_____

Physician	Date

FIG 5–4. Workers' compensation functional capacity form. (From Mayer TG, Mooney V, Gatchell RJ, et al: *Contemporary conservative care for painful spinal disorders: Impairment evaluation issues and the disability system,* Philadelphia, 1991, Lea & Febiger, pp 330–331. Used by permission.)

istration. Over 1.5 million people apply each year for Social Security disability. Of these, approximately 10% are considered to have a chronic pain syndrome. This implies that they have pain as their primary complaint without clinical findings to fully substantiate it.

In order to qualify for Social Security disability, a claimant has to prove that he or she is unable "to engage in any substantial gainful activity by reason of a medically determinable, physical, or mental impairment which can be expected to result in death or can be expected to last for a continuous period of not less than 12 months."[20] Furthermore, a physical or mental impairment is further defined as that which "would result from anatomic, physiologic, or psychological abnormalities that can be shown by medically acceptable clinical and laboratory techniques,"[20] and by regulation must be established by medical evidence consisting of symptoms, signs, and laboratory findings.

The Social Security regulations go on to define *symptoms* as the patient's own perception of his or her physical or mental impairment, *signs* as being anatomic, physiologic, or psychological abnormalities that can be observed with medically acceptable clinical techniques. *Laboratory findings* are manifestations of anatomic, physiologic, or psychological phenomena demonstrable by replacing or extending the perceptiveness of the observer's senses. They include chemical, electrophysiologic, roentgenologic, and psychological tests.[20]

In order to qualify for Social Security disability benefits, the claimant must go through a standardized procedure. First, he or she files a claim with one of the more than 1,300 Federal, district, and branch offices of the Social Security Administration. The claim is then referred to a state agency—the Disability Determination Service (DDS). Each claim is reviewed by a two-member team composed of a physician and disability examiner who make the initial decision regarding qualification for disability, the physician evaluating for medical impairment, and the disability evaluator being responsible for legal and administrative requirements. The team is required to assess the claimant based on a method established by regulation and known as the five-step sequential evaluation process (Fig 5–5,A). In order to qualify for Social Security disability, an individual must meet all five of the criteria.

Step 1 asks whether the patient is engaging "in sustainable gainful activities." This has been defined as earnings greater than $300 per month. Those persons not involved in substantial gainful activity progress to the second step. This asks whether the patient has a severe impairment. Impairment is defined as being severe when it is "judged to have a significant effect on the individual's capacity to perform work activities." By this definition, myofascial pain falls somewhere in between the lines. Specifically, there currently are no medically acceptable laboratory techniques by which the diagnosis can be made, and clinically both myofascial pain and fibromyalgia are considered, at least in the context of pain and disability, to be controversial diagnoses.

In 1984, Congress mandated the Secretary of the Department of Health and Human Services to appoint a commission for the evaluation of pain with the primary task of studying current pain policy and to recommend appropriate changes.[25] In addition, the commission was mandated to work in consultation with the National Academy of Sciences, and through the Institute of Medicine a more detailed study was commissioned. There was discussion and debate on the issue of myofascial pain. There was no consensus. According to the report, the discussion on this topic was "very heated," although all the clinicians acknowledged the existence of muscular involvement in back pain; some expressed strong doubts about the existence of myofascial trigger points. Similarly, others expressed strong doubts that the orthopedic view of the pathogenesis of back pain (disc rupture, nerve compression, etc.) is correct. Although advocates of the view that trigger points in referred pain are primary elements in the pathogenesis of many common pain symptoms acknowledged the absence of controlled clinical trials for this, they pointed to a rapidly growing literature reporting that the diagnosis is useful and common and asserted that efficacious treatment approaches have been developed. The committee did not reach agreement on this. Because of the debate, and in light of the increasing prominence of myofascial pain syndrome in clinical reports, the committee be-

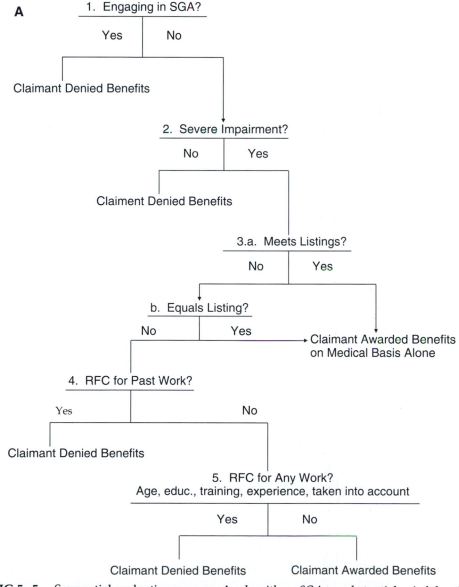

FIG 5–5. Sequential evaluation process. **A,** algorithm. *SGA* = substantial gainful activity; *RFC* = residual functional capacity. **B,** listings for musculoskeletal impairments. (From Osterweis M, Kleinman A, Mechanic D, editors: *Pain and disability: Clinical, behavioral, and public perspectives,* Washington, DC, 1987, National Academy Press.)

B

Disorders of the Spine

A. Arthritis manifested by ankylosis or fixation of the cervical or dorsolumbar spine at 30° or more of flexion measured from the neutral position, with X-ray evidence of:
1. Calcification of the anterior and lateral ligaments; OR
2. Bilateral ankylosis of the sacroiliac joints with abnormal apophyseal articulations; OR

B. Osteoporosis, generalized (established by X-ray) manifested by pain and limitation of back motion and paravertebral muscle spasm, with X-ray evidence of either:
1. Compression fracture of a vertebral body with loss of at least 50 percent of the estimated height of the vertebral body prior to the compression fracture, with no intervening direct traumatic episode; OR
2. Multiple fractures of vertebrae with no intervening direct traumatic episode: OR

C. Other vertebrogenic disorders (e.g., herniated nucleus pulposus, spinal stenosis) with the following persisting for at least 3 months despite prescribed therapy and expected to last 12 months. With both 1 and 2:
1. Pain, muscle spasm, and significant limitation of motion in the spine; AND
2. Appropriate radicular distribution of significant motor loss with muscle weakness and sensory and reflex loss.

Active rheumatoid arthritis and other inflammatory arthritis. With both A and B.

A. Persistent joint pain, swelling, and tenderness involving multiple joints with signs of joint inflammation (heat, swelling, tenderness) despite therapy for at least 3 months, and activity expected to last over 12 months; AND

B. Corroboration of diagnosis at some point in time by either:
1. Positive serologic test for rheumatoid factor; OR
2. Antinuclear antibodies; OR
3. Elevated sedimentation rate.

FIG 5-5 (cont.). For legend see previous page.

lieved that the topic and the controversy should be "brought to the attention of clinician and researchers."[25] Ultimately, the institute's publication on pain and disability included a discussion of myofascial pain syndromes by Simons,[30] but the issue of myofascial pain as an entity or as a cause of an impairment, in the context of Social Security disability, remains controversial.

The third step of the sequential evaluation process deals with whether the individual's impairment meets or equals the listings. In the case of musculoskeletal impairments, this generally includes findings associated with significant arthritis, ankylosis of joints, disc herniation, spinal stenosis, or osteoporosis. Thus, by definition, persons with myofascial pain would not meet the listings (Fig 5–5,B). However, if an individual does qualify based on this category, this does not mean that he or she does not qualify for Social Security disability. Rather, the claimant moves to the next step in the sequential evaluation process which has to do with residual functional capacity, i.e., does the patient's residual functional capacity allow him or her the ability to perform past relevant work? Essentially, a functional residual capacity is determined by the program physician on the basis of the limitations caused by the patient's impairment and symptoms. This determination is made by review of the medical records alone, no direct contact having been made with the patient at this point. If it is determined that the patient is unable to return to past relevant work, the final question is whether the patient is able to perform "any work that exists in the national economy." At this point, in addition to the functional impairment, age, education, training, and past work experience are also taken into account.

It is in the area of the fourth and fifth steps where pain becomes a factor. Case law has determined that the adjudicator may not disregard the claimant's subjective complaints solely because objective medical evidence does not fully support them. Adjudicators must give full consideration to all of the evidence presented relating to subjective complaints. This includes the patient's prior work record and observations by third parties and treating and examining physicians relating to such matters as the claimant's daily activities; the duration of frequency and intensity of pain; precipitating and aggravating factors; doses, effectiveness, and side effects of medication; and functional restrictions. These recommendations have to a large degree been incorporated in the Social Security Administration's current assessment of pain and disability.[20]

Thus, the determination of disability due to pain remains a challenge. Since pain is subjective, there always exists the possibility of conscious fabrication or exaggeration of symptoms by the claimant. More common, and of a deeper complexity, is the role of the various psychosocial variables and how they influence the claimant's perception of pain and ultimate disability. More specifically, does the granting of Social Security benefits for these individuals truly provide a safety net for the disabled, or does it merely represent a mechanism that fosters dependency on a governmental system and only serves further to disable potentially rehabilitatable individuals by legally authenticating their position? The answer remains unknown. Until further research is done, one can only surmise that a large part of the so-called chronic pain syndrome population does in fact fall into the category of myofascial pain patients.

MYOFASCIAL PAIN VS. THE CHRONIC PAIN SYNDROME

Patients with myofascial pain who despite appropriate medical treatment fail to respond and who continue to demonstrate significant pain behaviors, whose clinical presentation appears to be exaggerated, and whose time for healing is prolonged fall into the category of chronic pain syndrome. In order to understand these patients and the clinical evolution of their syndrome, an extensive history with the focus on psychosocial contributing factors is essential. Identifying and addressing the psychosocial factors often serves as the key to successful rehabilitation.[3, 7, 8, 11, 21, 33] While an exhaustive discussion of the many psychosocial issues interfering with the treatment and rehabilitation of patients with chronic myofascial pain is beyond the scope of this chapter, there are several critical risk factors that can be identified as part of the history and which certainly can predispose a person to the development of a chronic pain syndrome (Fig 5–6). Furthermore, if these issues are not taken into account as part of the assessment process, then the likelihood of any type of intervention proving successful is decreased significantly. Certainly, if a patient with acute myofascial pain has not responded to treatment in a reasonable time period, then it is likely that a referral to either a psychologist with extensive experience in pain assessment or to an interdisciplinary pain clinic for an evaluation is appropriate.

The appropriate length of time for the use of passive treatment modalities in defining the end of normal tissue healing is difficult. Physicians often err on the safe side, which only leads to further physical deconditioning and dysfunctional pain behaviors on the part of the patient. In Minnesota, a task force of

Chronic pain risk factors

Instructions: Place a checkmark next to each risk factor that is present.

1 Medical history	☐ Pain that persists despite appropriate treatment ☐ Physical deconditioning or prolonged inactivity ☐ Unrealistic expectations from treatment ☐ History of conflicting medical opinion ☐ Anger or dissatisfaction with medical care ☐ Life-long history of health problems
2 Pain behavior	☐ Dramatic description or display of pain ☐ Dependency on paraphernalia (canes, collars, etc.) ☐ "Doctor shopping"
3 Chemical dependency	☐ Overuse or preoccupation with medications ☐ Use of alcohol for pain ☐ History of alcohol or drug abuse and/or CD treatment
4 Emotional reactions	☐ Depression, social withdrawal ☐ Anxiety, worry, fear ☐ Anger, resentment, blaming, "power struggles" ☐ Overreaction to stress ☐ Complacency, too comfortable with disability
5 Vocational	☐ Job dissatisfaction or anger at employer ☐ Injured near retirement age ☐ Loss or threatened loss of job ☐ Unstable work history ☐ Limited education
6 Secondary benefits	☐ Avoidance of stressful situations ☐ Increased attention from family, including overprotection ☐ Financial compensation for disability ☐ Prospect of gain through litigation
7 Stress factors (Prior to or developing after the onset of pain)	☐ Role changes (retirement, "empty nest") ☐ Financial problems ☐ Marital discord, separation, divorce ☐ Illness or death in family ☐ Chemical dependency in family
8 Personality factors	☐ Passive or dependent ☐ Hypochondriacal or hysteroid ☐ Perfectionist or "workaholic"
9 Childhood trauma (Between birth and 16 years)	☐ Death, disability, or serious illness in family ☐ Chemical dependency in family ☐ Verbal or physical abuse in home

© Pilling Pain Clinic/Fairview Southdale Hospital.

FIG 5–6.   Checklist for chronic pain risk factors. *CD* = combination drug. (From Pilling LF, Clift RB: Instructions for use of the chronic pain risk factors checklist, *Modern Medicine* 54:83–84, 1986. Used by permission.)

the Department of Labor and Industry charged with defining this issue for workers' compensation cases has suggested that no passive therapy, i.e., passive physical therapy (PT), chiropractic care, massage, and such, should continue for more than 90 days following the date of the acute injury.

Clinically, the majority of patients with myofascial pain syndromes, when the problem becomes chronic, manifest findings associated with depression,[6, 26] i.e., sleep disturbance, irritability, fatigue, and anhedonia. In fact, Blumer and Heilbronn[1] believe that chronic pain may be simply a variant of a depressive disorder. Frequently, in obtaining a history on these patients, one finds a pattern of significant social disruption predating the injury. Often, there is a history of chemical dependency in the family system, a history of physical or sexual abuse, loss of a parent at an early age, or some event that places the patient in the role of a victim. Patients who are injured and become involved with disability systems often respond to this process either with a sense of hopelessness or anger. With time, they often develop a hostile dependent relationship with their physician, and the various disability systems. They express their frustration and anger at their lack of improvement and their dependency on the system, yet they continue to seek relief of their symptoms through further diagnostic tests, medications, or the use of passive PT modalities, i.e., trigger point injections, massage, heat, etc., which produce at best temporary improvement without any long-lasting benefit, and thus they remain stuck in the disability process. Recognition of the role of family dynamics in the patient's social environment often provides critical information regarding the clinical expression of a painful condition. This is illustrated by the following vignettes:

Case 1: A 47-year-old woman with a 12-month history of back pain diagnosed as a strain was referred to a multidisciplinary pain clinic because of her lack of response to PT. Physical examination revealed trigger point tenderness over the right gluteal muscle. Radiographs, including a computed tomography (CT) scan, were negative. *Her history revealed a longstanding pattern of physical abuse by her husband.* After she was injured, her husband stopped beating her.

Case 2: A 57-year-old laborer, father of five, with an eighth-grade education, suffered a cervical strain. Spinal films demonstrated multilevel degenerative disc disease. During the history, the patient's college-educated wife answered most of the questions directed toward the patient. She described him as being severely disabled and indicated that it was her opinion that there was no way that he would ever return to work. She said that her husband "couldn't even do anything" around the house and that she and her children had taken over essentially all of his former activities such as lawn care, car care, and driving. On physical examination, palpation of the cervical muscles elicited grimacing and groaning on the part of the patient's wife. When asked what was the matter, her response was, "You're hurting him."

Case 3: A 37-year-old factory worker with a 9-month history of back pain was evaluated. The physical examination showed trigger point tenderness over the quadratus and gluteal muscles with some decreased range of motion. His neurologic examination was normal and spinal films showed no degenerative changes. In spite of appropriate, conservative care, the patient remained disabled. During the history, he began a long diatribe regarding his work environment. His company had been sold to a large conglomerate and his boss of 15 years had been replaced "by a punk kid." He had told his new supervisor about a potential hazard associated with an oil spill on the floor, but was ignored. Then one day while carrying a box of parts, he slipped on that oil spill injuring his back.

In each of the above cases, psychosocial factors clearly influence the meaning of the painful experience to the patient and by inference the clinical expression of that condition. No amount or type of somatically oriented treatment will affect these factors. Even, when these issues are identified, however, this does not guarantee that they can be successfully addressed. Asking patients to confront and modify longstanding behavior patterns or identify repressed emotions can be extremely challenging. Thus, for many of these patients, ongoing counseling and appropriate follow-up are essential to maintain any gains made in an intensive rehabilitation center and to ensure long-term success.

Fear is a major component in the clinical presentation. Patients are often frightened that since they have not improved, they can only get worse. They are afraid that, despite undergoing multiple diagnostic tests, there must be some underlying condition that no one has been able to diagnose. They doubt their ability to return to gainful employment, fear that they may be "spied upon" by investigators working for the insurance carrier, and are petrified about losing their benefits, which serve as the barrier against poverty.

For many people involved with disability systems, their pain and resultant pain behaviors represent their only leverage in dealing with the complex medicolegal system in which they have become disempowered, being now fully dependent on the insurance carrier for their paycheck, on their physician for relief of their symptoms, and on their attorney for their future security. With time, the majority of these patients become extremely deconditioned. In our patient population, we have found that from an aerobic or cardiovascular standpoint, our pain patients are more deconditioned than persons undergoing cardiac rehabilitation following a myocardial infarction. As patients continue with their extremely sedentary lifestyles, limiting themselves in terms of activities of daily living, weight gain is common and often extensive, muscle mass and strength decrease, and endurance lessens. These patients require a holistic or biopsychosocial model of intervention. Because of the complexity of their clinical presentation, either a team approach utilizing active PT, i.e., exercise and reconditioning, psychological support, and appropriate medical supervision, or involvement in a more intensive pain management or functional restoration program integrating the above is mandatory.[16]

PAIN MANAGEMENT VS. PAIN TREATMENT

While some would argue, the primary role of a chronic pain rehabilitation program is not pain amelioration but rather functional restoration. Eliminating the patient's dependency on the physician, passive PT modalities, and the use of ineffective medications are primary goals. Empowering patients to regain functional activities, return to work, release their anger, and address their sense of indignation and victimization are critical. Shifting the focus from pain relief to normalization of living is the challenge.

As part of our assessment, patients are told that they are the ones responsible for getting well. If their pain actually lessens or goes away, we jokingly tell them that there won't be any extra charge and they should consider it a bonus. Deflecting the issue of pain relief and shifting the responsibility for eliminating pain from the clinician to the patient is empowering. The dynamic of searching for the magic bullet, which has not proved effective up to this point, is now diffused.

Pain management is not block therapy, spray and stretch, or acupuncture. Although many pain rehabilitation programs have used biofeedback, injections, PT, and so forth without success in eliminating or reducing pain, if these modalities can be presented from the perspective that they will help the patient better manage stress, improve his or her level of physical conditioning, and assist in a return to a functional lifestyle, rather than reduce or eliminate the pain, they may be helpful.[28] This approach needs to be viewed in opposition to the traditional acute model where the patient is treated like an infant and the responsibility for success or failure lies with the clinician in terms of making a proper diagnosis and treatment (Figs 5–7,A and B).

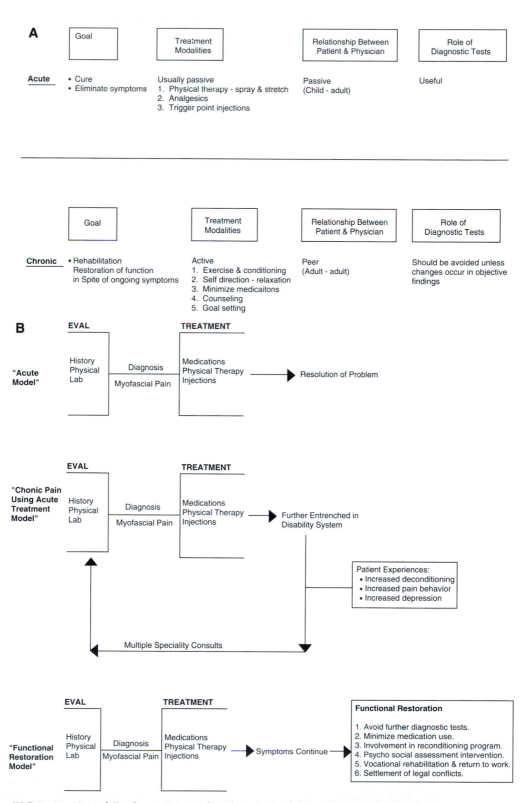

A

| Goal | Treatment Modalities | Relationship Between Patient & Physician | Role of Diagnostic Tests |

Acute
- Cure
- Eliminate symptoms

Usually passive
1. Physical therapy - spray & stretch
2. Analgesics
3. Trigger point injections

Passive
(Child - adult)

Useful

| Goal | Treatment Modalities | Relationship Between Patient & Physician | Role of Diagnostic Tests |

Chronic
- Rehabilitation
  Restoration of function
  in Spite of ongoing symptoms

Active
1. Exercise & conditioning
2. Self direction - relaxation
3. Minimize medicaitons
4. Counseling
5. Goal setting

Peer
(Adult - adult)

Should be avoided unless changes occur in objective findings

B

EVAL   TREATMENT

"Acute Model"

History
Physical
Lab

Diagnosis

Myofascial Pain

Medications
Physical Therapy
Injections

→ Resolution of Problem

EVAL   TREATMENT

"Chonic Pain Using Acute Treatment Model"

History
Physical
Lab

Diagnosis

Myofascial Pain

Medications
Physical Therapy
Injections

→ Further Entrenched in Disability System

Patient Experiences:
- Increased deconditioning
- Increased pain behavior
- Increased depression

Multiple Speciality Consults

EVAL   TREATMENT

"Functional Restoration Model"

History
Physical
Lab

Diagnosis

Myofascial Pain

Medications
Physical Therapy
Injections

→ Symptoms Continue

Functional Restoration
1. Avoid further diagnostic tests.
2. Minimize medication use.
3. Involvement in reconditioning program.
4. Psycho social assessment intervention.
5. Vocational rehabilitation & return to work.
6. Settlement of legal conflicts.

FIG 5–7.   **A** and **B**, the acute vs. the chronic model in pain management.

In order for patients to benefit from a pain rehabilitation program, proper screening is required. This should consist of a review of relevant medical records; an extensive history, with emphasis on identifying psychosocial contributing factors described previously; physical examination; review of the appropriate laboratory findings; and development of a treatment plan that is agreed upon by all concerned parties. In addition, absolute contraindications, i.e., primary substance abuse and psychosis, need to be ruled out.

MEDICAL RECORDS

Unfortunately, patients with chronic pain are not the best historians. They have often seen numerous physicians and undergone multiple diagnostic studies. In addition, if medication dependency or compensation issues are involved, they may intentionally leave out significant details. Thus, obtaining previous medical records from treating physicians, or at least an adequate summary of medical data, is mandatory.

THE HISTORY

As discussed earlier, the history should include, with careful documentation, the onset of the patient's problems with special emphasis on causation, the previous treating physicians, previous treatments, and the patient's response. The issue of causation is extremely important, particularly in the determination of workers' compensation and PI cases. In addition to describing the patient's current symptoms, documentation of alterations in lifestyle and social and recreational activities, as well as current activities, is essential. Identification of various psychosocial stressors should be sought. These include job dissatisfaction; family discord; psychological status; drug and chemical usage, including caffeine and nicotine; family history; economic factors, i.e., litigation; and previous pain problems. All of these contributing factors can complicate and influence the clinical manifestations of the patient's condition.

A Minnesota Multiphasic Personality Inventory (MMPI) or other appropriate psychometric testing, as well as evaluation by a competent psychologist or psychiatrist, should be considered in assessing a patient as a potential candidate for a pain rehabilitation program. Usually, a careful history will reveal critical important psychosocial factors that provide the key elements in understanding the clinical presentation of the patient.

PHYSICAL EXAMINATION

In terms of the physical examination, two important determinants need to be kept in mind. First, one wants to make sure that the diagnosis of myofascial pain is correct. In general, by the time patients are referred to a pain rehabilitation program, they have undergone extensive diagnostic tests, including radiographs and electrophysiologic evaluations, to rule out entrapment syndromes. However, the possibility of sympathetic-mediated pain is frequently overlooked. Therefore, it is critical to look for signs of skin temperature change, asymmetry, discoloration, swelling, and other signs associated with reflex sympathetic dystrophy when evaluating a patient.[28]

The other important aspect of the physical examination is identifying non-physiologic responses which suggest psychological distress and somatization. Findings such as Waddell's signs[34] (Table 5–2), exaggerated grimacing, or bizarre posturing suggest either conscious or unconscious exaggeration of symptoms. While nonphysiologic findings on physical examination are important to observe, they do not mean that the patient is malingering. Malingering implies conscious premeditated exaggeration, or confabulation on the part of the patient. Most experts in the field of pain consider malingerers to represent a small minority of chronic pain patients. A much higher percentage of these patients truly have an exaggerated pain perception and pain behaviors, often due to psychological factors. They may well be histrionic personality types or for various reasons have extremely poor pain threshholds. Psychometric testing reveals elevations on scales measuring histrionic or hysterical behavior or hypochondriasis.[10]

RADIOLOGIC EXAMINATION

Obviously, in myofascial pain syndrome radiographic findings are within normal limits in establishing the diagnosis. The fact that a spinal film may show degenerative changes such as facet hypertrophy or a bulging disc does not exclude the diagnosis of myofascial pain. The development of sophisticated imaging methods, particularly magnetic resonance (MR), comes as a mixed blessing for many of these patients. While providing excellent imaging, particularly of the anatomy of the disc, MR and CT scans often demonstrate abnormalities which are not clinically significant.[35] While physicians recognize the importance of correlating symptoms with the physical examination and radiologic findings, this is not necessarily true of plaintiff attorneys, unsophisticated patients, or administrative judges who often have the final say as to the relative clinical importance of these findings from the standpoint of disability and impairment ratings.

TABLE 5–2.

Comparison of Symptoms and Signs of Physical Disease and Abnormal Illness Behavior in Chronic Low Back Pain*

	Physical Disease and Normal Illness Behavior	Magnified or Inappropriate Illness Behavior
Symptoms		
Pain	Localized	Whole leg pain, tailbone pain
Numbness	Dermatomal	Whole leg numbness
Weakness	Myotomal	Whole leg giving way
Time pattern	Varies with time	Never free of pain
Response to treatment	Variable benefit	Intolerance of treatment, emergency admissions to hospital
Signs		
Tenderness	Localized	Superficial, widespread, nonanatomic
Axial loading	No lumbar pain	Lumbar pain
Simulated rotation	No lumbar pain	Lumbar pain
Straight leg raising	Limited on distraction	Improves with distraction
Sensory	Dermatomal	Regional
Motor	Myotomal	Regional, jerky giving way
General response	Appropriate pain	Overreaction

*From Waddell G, Bircher M, Finlayson D, et al: *Br Med J* 289:740, 1984. Used by permission.

Moreover, patients who lack the sophistication to understand the significance of x-ray findings commonly become frightened when they find that there are some "structural changes on their x-rays." It is not uncommon to find a patient presenting not with a complaint of back or neck pain, but rather with a complaint of a "bulging disc or stenosis." Once the patient has been told that there is an abnormality on the x-ray film, it is often difficult to reassure the patient that even with these findings, he or she can return to a functional lifestyle.

DEVELOPING A REHABILITATION PLAN

Once the patient has been evaluated, a specific rehabilitation plan needs to be established. While specific modalities vary among pain rehabilitation programs, all have certain features in common. The primary goal is returning the patient to a functional lifestyle, including work. It is important that at the end of treatment that a functional capacity evaluation be obtained and that appropriate functional restrictions be imposed. The patient needs to be told this and that he or she will be supported in returning to work despite the continuing discomfort. The message that is communicated is simply that chronic pain may indeed cause hurt and discomfort, but that this is not necessarily harmful.

Working closely with the employer, as well as with other members involved in the rehabilitation process, such as the rehabilitation counselor, is required. In our program, we have two full-time workers whose primary function is to interface with patients, employers, and insurers in helping to establish a return-to-work plan.

While pain management programs make various claims about how they are helping chronic pain patients deal with their pain, from the insurer's perspective, the only true measure of success is whether that patient returns to work. In this regard, there will always be a subgroup of pain patients who clearly have no intention of going back to work. Either they wish to retire or they have developed an extremely adversarial relationship with their employer. In these cases, like a marriage in trouble, counseling may save the relationship. At others times the best solution for both parties is a divorce. Likewise, in the vocational realm, at times the relationship between the employer and employee can be saved, differences can be worked out, and the patient can be successfully returned to work. In other instances, however, the degree of anger, resentment, and mutual enmity is so great that any attempt at resolution will be met with failure and it may be in everyone's best interest to resolve their differences through an administrative settlement. Particularly in the area of workers' compensation in which adversarial relationships exist between employer and employee, each side will attempt to exert whatever leverage is available to gain an advantage. In the case of the employer and the insurer, they are the ones that pay the bills and often direct medical care. The employer can certainly attempt to provide a job position within the restrictions of the individual.

The patient has fewer options in terms of leverage. In fact, the primary one is pain behavior. If a situation exists that the patient does not like, e.g., being placed in a monotonous light-duty position, the patient's only option is to hurt more. Since pain by definition is subjective, it is impossible to either substantiate or disprove this position. Again, this does not imply malingering, but merely represents a mechanism for survival from the patient's perspective. Acknowledging the patient's feelings, yet not necessarily acquiescing to the patient's position, is a difficult act of diplomacy.

In addition to helping the patient return to work, modalities that foster a sense of independence and self-sufficiency on the part of the patient are helpful. An exercise program that emphasizes flexibility, strength, and cardiovascular conditioning is critical to a reconditioning program. Again, the focus of exercise is not on the resolution of pain but rather on restoration of function.[29] Patients need to be reassured that during the early part of any type of physical reactivation program, they can expect to experience increased soreness. This does not mean that their condition is worse. On completion of an intensive 3- or 4-week pain rehabilitation program, continued involvement in a comprehensive conditioning program is critical. It may be another 3 to 6 months, if ever, before the patient actually notes diminution in his or her pain.

MEDICATIONS

Narcotics, benzodiazepines, and other potentially addictive drugs should be avoided in the long-term management of patients with myofascial pain.[19] While the use of narcotics is controversial in the management of nonmalignant pain syndromes,[22, 32] it is my experience that patients, particularly those with myofascial pain, do not need chronic narcotic or benzodiazepine use for pain management (Table 5–3). The chronic use of these medications can and often does enhance depression, lethargy, and effect motivation to return to work. In addition, the patient's ability to concentrate may be affected by the long-term use of these medications. Attempts should also be made to reduce the use of other medications, including nonsteroidal anti-inflammatory drugs (NSAIDs) and over-the-counter analgesics. While these medications may be useful in acute flare-ups, they have potential adverse side effects. It is my experience that many patients with myofascial pain can be weaned from NSAIDs and that they do not notice any major increase in their pain.

Antidepressants have been demonstrated to be useful in the treatment of myofascial pain syndromes. In patients with sleep disturbance, without major depressive symptoms, response has been favorable to very low doses of tricyclics. Amitryptyline (Elavil), doxepin (Sinequan), or nortriptyline (Pamelor) 5 to 10 mg or trazodone (Desyrel) 25 mg slowly titrated up to a level that allows the patient to sleep without undue side effects can prove quite effective. A more normal sleep pattern often has a positive effect on the patient's general functional ability as well as pain management. After 2 to 3 months, assuming the patient is back to a more functional lifestyle, is exercising, and utilizing other stress management strategies, an attempt can be made to decrease the antidepressant. Some patients, however, may require small amounts of antidepressant medication on a long-term basis.

PATIENT EXPECTATIONS

Before recommending a comprehensive pain rehabilitation program, it is important to negotiate with the patient and clearly define expectations. If the patient is looking for a quick fix or miracle cure, a functional restoration approach is not appropriate. The patient needs to find out for himself or herself whether

TABLE 5–3.

Indications for Long-Term Narcotic Use

Factors Indicating Poor Candidates for Long-Term Narcotic Use	Factors Indicating Possibly Appropriate Candidates for Long-Term Narcotic Use
1. No or minimal indications of structural pathologic changes, inflammation, or active disease process to substantiate pain complaints	1. Clear clinical, anatomic, and laboratory data to substantiate the diagnosis of a painful condition
2. History of previous alcoholism, substance abuse, or family history of substance abuse or involvement in chemical dependency treatment	2. No history either of chemical dependency on the part of the patient or on the part of the family.
3. Inappropriate or dramatic pain behaviors, or inappropriate use of canes, braces or other supportive devices	3. Pain behaviors appear to be appropriate to the clinical condition
4. History of previous psychological problems, especially depression or hysteria	4. No premorbid psychological dysfunction
5. Evidence of dependent personality style, e.g., heavy caffeine or nicotine use or compulsive overeating	5. The patient is not a heavy smoker, heavy caffeine user, nor does he or she demonstrate other signs of a compulsive lifestyle or dependent behavior pattern
6. No evidence that using narcotic medications allows the patient to improve function with respect to activities of daily living and vocational pursuits	6. The patient does function reasonably in spite of pain, but using narcotic medications appears to improve significantly the level of functioning
7. Unstable work history	7. Previous stable work history
8. History of physical, sexual, or emotional abuse	8. No history of physical, sexual, or emotional abuse
9. Poor family support system or a history of a dysfunctional family system	9. Good family support system
10. Noncompliance with treatment recommendations	10. All other reasonable attempts at pain control have failed, and the patient has demonstrated compliance

acupuncture, chiropractic, myofascial therapy, or some other type of passive modality will actually eliminate the symptoms. Attempting to force a reluctant or unwilling patient into a pain rehabilitation program often leads to increased mistrust and anger on the part of the patient and all attempts to support this person's rehabilitation will be met with resistance. Typically, our patients are asked to sign an agreement that outlines what can and cannot be offered. Thus, even before admission, the message is made clear that the patient is the one responsible for success. The job of the staff is not to "fix" the patient but to support him or her in making the necessary behavioral and perceptual changes required to deal with pain in a more functional manner and to return to a normal lifestyle (Fig 5–8). By setting appropriate boundaries from the start, there is far less of a chance of getting caught up in the patient's dependent and manipulative behaviors.

THE ROLE OF SELF-REGULATION TECHNIQUES

Self-regulation techniques, such as self-hypnosis, relaxation training, and biofeedback, can be helpful adjuncts in the treatment of myofascial pain syndromes. Stress, anxiety, and tension all increase levels of muscle tension and can certainly aggravate if not precipitate a myofascial pain problem.[2, 27] Patients are taught basic relaxation and particularly breathing techniques, emphasizing that these techniques be used throughout the day, rather than on an occasional basis.

**ABBOTT NORTHWESTERN HOSPITAL/SISTER KENNY INSTITUTE
CHRONIC PAIN REHABILITATION PROGRAM**

PATIENT/STAFF PARTNERSHIP

The purpose of the Chronic Pain Rehabilitation Program is to create an opportunity for individuals experiencing chronic or long-term pain to significantly improve the quality and enjoyment of their lives, to gain control over their pain, and to return to a more productive lifestyle.

The responsibility for the success or failure of the Program depends on the willingness of the participants to accept responsibility for their situation, to be open to the concepts being taught in the Chronic Pain Rehabilitation Program and, most importantly, to actually apply these concepts to their everyday life.

In order to achieve this purpose, I understand and am willing to comply with the following guidelines:

1. To participate fully and be on time for all required activities that are scheduled in the Chronic Pain Rehabilitation Program. This includes all scheduled activities, including evening sessions (for inpatients), staying to the end of each day, and arriving on time Sunday night prior to the beginning of each week.

2. Total abstinence from alcohol, marijuana, or other mood altering substances for the three-week period of time, including weekends, in order to allow my system to properly respond to pain management techniques.

3. To review all medication whether prescribed by a physician or over-the-counter items such as Aspirin, Tylenol, etc., at a private meeting with a staff nurse. The use of any medication during the three weeks must be approved by the Program's medical staff.

4. To wean completely from narcotic and other potentially harmful, addicting, and habit forming medications, understanding that periodic urine screening may be requested to monitor levels of addictive substances.

5. To attend the "Smoking Awareness" class if a smoker and sincerely attempt to reduce nicotine consumption.

6. To be willing to improve physical strength and endurance through an exercise program and to recognize that proper exercise needs to become integrated into my lifestyle.

7. To be willing to learn and put into practice pain management techniques such as acupressure, relaxation, imagery, breathing techniques, biofeedback, and/or self-hypnosis to control stress, pain, and anxiety.

8. To be willing to communicate any negative thoughts or feelings about the Chronic Pain Rehabilitation Program to appropriate staff members.

FIG 5–8.　The physician-patient agreement. (Courtesy of Abbott Northwestern Hospital/Sister Kenny Institute, St. Paul, Minn.)　　　　　　　　　　　　　　*(Continued.)*

9. To understand that Family Day is an important aspect of the Chronic Pain Rehabilitation Program. At least one family member or significant friend will participate fully by being present for the activities on Family Day.

10. To remain on the campus of Abbott Northwestern Hospital except on weekends, unless I have received permission to do so from a staff member.

11. To be careful to not interfere with the progress of fellow patients.

12. To make myself physically and psychologically fit, in order to return to work, normal activities, and a more productive lifestyle.

13. To cooperate with Aftercare follow-up, maintaining contact with staff by telephone or attending optional weekly/monthly sessions.

14. To make every attempt to attend the Final Aftercare session scheduled six months after the three-week program.

These issues are critical to the success of pain management and rehabilitation. Signature implies a self-responsibility commitment.

PATIENT/STAFF PARTNERSHIP

I, _____ HAVE READ, UNDERSTAND FULLY, AND AGREE TO COMPLY WITH THE STATEMENTS LISTED ABOVE.

ADDITIONAL AGREEMENTS:

_____   _____
PATIENT SIGNATURE   DATE

_____   _____
STAFF MEMBER WHO PROVIDED THESE   DATE
GUIDELINES TO PATIENT

FIG 5-8 (cont.).   For legend see previous page.

Teaching patients how to breathe in a controlled and rhythmic manner using their diaphragm often provides immediate reduction of stress and anxiety. Breathing is after all both an autonomic and a voluntary function. Persons under stress often demonstrate shallow breathing patterns, breathing from the chest as opposed to the diaphragm. This is not only inefficient, in that there is poorer oxygenation, but is also associated with fear and anxiety. Diaphragmatic breathing, on the other hand, is a more natural and efficient way of breathing. It is almost impossible to breathe diaphragmatically in a slow and rhythmic manner and experience tension and anxiety.[23]

COGNITIVE PSYCHOTHERAPY

The subject of psychological intervention with chronic pain patients needs to be approached carefully. As mentioned, patients with chronic pain are often resistant to looking at psychological factors. Recognition of psychological factors implies that the pain is not in their bodies, but "in their heads." They have a difficult time understanding how their feelings and emotions can affect their current situation. They are often extremely defensive about seeing a clinical psychologist, psychiatrist, or taking an MMPI. However, unless the issues associated with anger, family problems, job dissatisfaction, fear, mistrust, and other self-defeating behaviors are addressed, it is difficult to help the patient move forward. I have found that our most effective therapists are not necessarily Ph.D.'s or M.D.'s, but peer counselors who themselves have chronic pain and have successfully completed a pain program. Patients do need to work through their anger and depression. Following an injury, there is a loss. Patients have a right to be angry, but the challenge is how to help them refocus their anger in a positive and constructive way and to assume responsibility for their underlying condition rather than blaming an external force, i.e., their employer, physician, insurer, etc., or themselves.

A metaphor applicable to chronic pain is similar to that expressed by Kübler-Ross[14] in dealing with dying patients. Initially, following an injury, there is a loss. Patients often deal with this loss with a sense of denial, a belief that their symptoms will go away, and that they will get better. As time goes on, and the condition does not improve, they are often left with a sense of anger and depression. By helping patients move through this position to a point of acceptance, they are able to deal with their injury in a more healthy manner.

CONCLUSION

Myofascial pain is a common, perhaps the most common, cause of chronic musculoskeletal pain and disability. In one study, 85% of 283 patients presenting to a chronic pain clinic were diagnosed as having myofascial pain syndromes.[6] In another study of 296 patients presenting with head and neck pain, 55.4% had a primary diagnosis of myofascial pain.[9]

The cost to society is enormous. While no specific estimates regarding myofascial pain exist, it has been estimated that the total annual cost of low back care, including vocational retraining, medical care, compensation, and legal fees, approaches 40 to 50 billion dollars. The cost of medical care alone is $16 billion, half of that going to surgical treatment.[28] Combining the prevalence data with the economic costs certainly implies a tremendously high social and economic cost to society for myofascial pain syndromes. By the time the condition becomes chronic, psychosocial factors and physical deconditioning have played a critical role in the manifestation of the condition and subsequent disability. Identification of psychosocial risk factors, supporting the patient in developing healthy coping skills, and focusing on functional restoration rather than symptomatic relief are often the key to successful pain management.

Approaches to management should include limiting passive modalities to the acute stages or aggravations of a condition; avoiding long-term use of narcotics, benzodiazepines, NSAIDs, and over-the-counter drugs; reinforcing physical reactivation through a home exercise and conditioning program; and teaching appropriate stress management. Educating the patient on the interrelationships between stress, fear, depression, and deconditioning in terms of overall function is critical. When evaluating patients with a chronic pain syndrome, only by assessing the patients from a biopsychosocial perspective, addressing the individual biological, psychological, and social contributing factors, can one truly empower these persons to cope more effectively with their pain, and maximize their potential for rehabilitation.

REFERENCES

1. Blumer D, Heilbronn M: Chronic pain as a variant of depressive disease: The pain-prone disorder, *J Nerv Ment Dis* 170:381–406, 1982.
2. Cailliet R: *Soft tissue pain and disability*, Philadelphia, 1977, FA Davis.
3. Engel G: "Psychogenic" pain and the pain-prone patient, *Am J Med* 26:899–915, 1959.
4. Engelberg AL, editor: *Guides to the evaluation of permanent impairment*, ed 3, Chicago, 1988, American Medical Association, pp 37, 71, 236.
5. Fischer AA: Documentation of myofascial trigger points, *Arch Phys Med Rehabil* 69:286–291, 1988.
6. Fishbain DA, Goldberg M, Meagher R, et al: Male and female chronic pain patients categorized by DSM-III psychiatric diagnostic criteria, *Pain* 26:181–197, 1986.
7. Flor H, Turk DC, Scholz OB: Impact of chronic pain on the spouse: Marital, emotional, and physical consequences, *J Psychosom Res* 31:63–71, 1987.
8. Fordyce WE: Pain and suffering, *Am Psych* 43:276–283, 1988.
9. Fricton JR, Kroening R, Haley D, et al: Myofascial pain syndrome of the head and neck: A review of clinical characteristics of 164 patients, *Oral Surg Oral Med Oral Pathol* 60:615–623, 1985.
10. Frymoyer JW: Back pain and sciatica, *N Engl J Med* 318:291–298, 1988.
11. Frymoyer JW, Rosen JC, Clements J, et al: Psychologic factors in low-back-pain disability, *Clin Orthop* 195:178–184, 1985.
12. Isernhagen SJ: Functional capacity evaluation and work hardening perspectives. In Mayer TG, Mooney V, Gatchel RJ, editors: *Contemporary conservative care for painful spinal disorders*, Philadelphia, 1991, Lea & Febiger.
13. Keeley J: Quantification of function. In Mayer TG, Mooney V, Gatchel RJ, editors: *Contemporary conservative care for painful spinal disorders*, Philadelphia, 1991, Lea & Febiger, pp 290–307.
14. Kübler-Ross E: *On death and dying*, New York, 1969, Macmillan.
15. *Manual for orthopaedic surgeons in evaluating permanent impairment*, Chicago, 1966, American Academy of Orthopaedic Surgeons.
16. Mayer TG, Gatchel RJ: *Functional restoration for spinal disorders: The sports medicine approach*, Philadelphia, 1988, Lea & Febiger.
17. Merskey H: Psychosocial factors and muscular pain. In Fricton JR, Awad EA, editors: *Advances in pain research and therapy*. Vol 17: *Myofascial pain and fibromyalgia*, New York, 1990, Raven Press.
18. Monsein M: Soft tissue pain and disability. In Fricton JR, Awad EA, editors: *Ad-*

vances in pain research and therapy. Vol 17: *Myofascial pain and fibromyalgia,* New York, 1990, Raven Press.

19. Nies KM: Treatment of the fibromyalgia syndrome, *J Musculoskeletal Med* 9:20–26, 1992.
20. Osterweis M, Kleinman A, Mechanic D, editors: *Pain and disability: Clinical, behavioral, and public policy perspectives,* Washington, DC, 1987, National Academy Press, pp 6, 25, 35, 38–41, 198, 280.
21. Pope MH, Rosen JC, Wilder DG, et al: The relation between biomechanical and psychological factors in patients with low-back pain, *Spine* 5:173–178, 1980.
22. Portenoy RK: Opioid therapy for chronic noncancer pain: The issue revisited, *Am Pain Soc Bull* 1:4–7, 1991.
23. Rama S, Ballentine R, Hymes A: *Science of breath: A practical guide,* Honesdale, Pa, 1979, The Himalayan International Institute of Yoga Science and Philosophy.
24. Reeves JL, Jaegen G, Graff-Radford SB: Reliability of the pressure algometer as a measure of myofascial trigger point sensitivity, *Pain* 24:313–321, 1986.
25. *Report of the commission on the evaluation of pain,* Washington, DC, 1987, Government Printing Office, Social Security Administration Publication No. 64-031.
26. Romano JM, Turner JA: Chronic pain and depression: Does the evidence support a relationship?, *Psychol Bull* 97:18–34, 1985.
27. Sarno JE: Etiology of neck and back pain: An autonomic myoneuralgia?, *J Nerve Ment Dis* 169:55–59, 1981.
28. Schwartzman RJ: Reflex sympathetic dystrophy, *Arch Neurol* 44:555–561, 1987.
29. Sherman C: Managing fibromyalgia with exercise, the physician and sports, *Medicine,* 20:166–172, 1992.
30. Simons DG: Myofascial pain syndromes due to trigger points. In Osterweis M, Kleinman A, Mechanic D, editors: *Pain and disability: Clinical, behavioral, and public policy perspectives,* Washington, DC, 1987, National Academy Press, pp 285–292.
31. Stone D: *The disabled state,* Philadelphia, 1984, Temple University Press.
32. Turk DC, Brody MC: Chronic opioid therapy for persistent noncancer pain: Panacea or oxymoron?, *Am Pain Soc Bull* 1:4–7, 1991.
33. Turk DC, Rudy TE: Assessment of cognitive factors in chronic pain: a worthwhile enterprise?, *J Consult Clin Psychol* 54:760–768, 1986.
34. Waddell G: Clinical assessment of lumbar impairment, *Clin Orthop* 221:110–120, 1987.
35. Wiesel SW, Tsourmas M, Feffer HL, et al: A study of computer-assisted tomography: 1. The incidence of positive CAT scans in an asymptomatic group of patients, *Spine* 9:549–551, 1984.
36. *Worker's compensation permanent partial disability schedule,* Minneapolis, 1984, Minnesota Medical Association.

Chapter 6

Pressure Algometry (Dolorimetry) in the Differential Diagnosis of Muscle Pain

Andrew A. Fischer, M.D., Ph.D.

Point tenderness is a very frequent finding in patients with pain. Rosomoff et al.[43] found tender points or trigger points in 100% of patients with chronic non-malignant neck pain and in 97% of patients with low back pain. It is obvious that when tenderness is present the number one diagnostic task is to establish whether the degree of pressure pain sensitivity reached abnormal levels. This difficult decision can be made best by measurement of the pressure pain threshold using a dolorimeter.

Pressure threshold measurement quantifies tenderness, i.e., pressure pain sensitivity of tender spots and trigger points. *Pressure threshold* is the minimum pressure (force) that causes pain. Threshold is measured over hypersensitive spots (tender points or trigger points) in order to diagnose their location and to quantify the degree of pressure sensitivity that expresses their level of *activity*.[11, 16, 17, 23, 45, 48]

Pressure tolerance measurement assesses pain sensitivity. *Pressure tolerance* is the highest pressure one can endure under clinical conditions and expresses the patient's sensitivity to pain. Unlike pressure threshold, which quantifies sensitivity over tender spots, pressure tolerance is assessed on standard locations over the deltoid muscle and shin bone, focusing on nonsensitive tissue, i.e., avoiding pressure-sensitive points.[11, 16, 17, 39] The measurements over the two different tissues allows comparison of pressure pain sensitivity of muscles and bones.[16, 17]

SENSITIZATION OF NERVES—THE CAUSE OF TENDERNESS AND PAIN

Tenderness, i.e., increased *pressure pain sensitivity*, is quantified by a decrease in the pressure threshold. *Pressure pain threshold*, defined as the minimum pressure that induces pain, is the point at which the patient reports that the feeling of pressure changes into a painful sensation. Tenderness is the leading diagnostic sign of inflammation. Normal tissues do not generate real pain on pressure. The change of reactivity of the nerve fibers making the mechanical pressure painful is caused by a process called *sensitization*.[36] It is known that cell damage causes release of substances that induce inflammation, resulting in pain and sensitivity to pressure.[36] The main products of tissue damage include bradykinin, 5-hydroxytryptamine, prostaglandins, and a high concentration of potassium. The action of this group is then potentiated further by prostaglandins of the E type and bradykinin itself.[36] Increased sympathetic activity can release prostaglandins that further potentiate the effect of other inflammatory substances.[36] It is obvious that spontaneously occurring pain in the injured tissue, as well as its tenderness on pressure, is caused by the identical process of sensitization, which can be measured by decreased pressure pain threshold. Pressure threshold measurement thus reflects the activity of the inflammation. Dolorimetry makes it possible to quantify in clinical practice the increase of nerve sensitivity, which is the most frequent cause of pain.

Definitions

Tender spots is a general term expressing focal pressure pain sensitivity, i.e., tenderness limited to a point usually not larger than about 1 cm^2. Tender spots are not defined by any additional specific attributes or condition in which they occur.

Trigger points are small exquisitely sensitive areas of soft tissue, that sometimes shoot pain into a remote "reference pain zone" that is specific for each trigger point.[19, 52, 53] Leading authorities in pain management agree that the diagnostic criterion of trigger points is point tenderness. Kraus[28] defines trigger point as a "tender node" with possible hardening. Bonica[2] uses a similar definition.

Steindler,[51] who introduced the term, defined trigger point as a circumscribed area in which pressure produces a sudden sharp pain. This is the most valuable sign for locating the origin of the pain and for identifying the painful structures.

Myofascial trigger points are located in muscles and extend also to their fascial covers. In addition to point tenderness, myofascial trigger points are characterized by a palpable taut band of tender and contracted muscle fibers extending on both sides of the trigger point proper.[53] Snapping the taut band produces a twitch indicating the hyperexcitability of the involved muscle fibers. In addition, a trigger point can give rise to characteristic pain in a reference pain zone that is specific for each trigger point.[52, 53] Clinical observations, however, showed that the tender spots with taut bands frequently cause pain in the area of the maximum point tenderness, not in the reference zones.

CLINICAL APPLICATIONS OF PRESSURE THRESHOLD MEASUREMENT

Numerous physicians, physical therapists, and dentists during several years of use found that pressure threshold measurement is useful in clinical practice for evaluation of tender spots, trigger points, tender points of fibromyalgia, and inflammation. The clinical applications of pressure threshold measurement are:

I. Diagnosis of tenderness and its documentation.
   A. Quantification of pressure pain sensitivity (tenderness).
   B. Location of tender spots.

C. Long-term follow-up of a change in pain and its relation to local tenderness.

D. Evaluation of activity in inflamed joints.[20, 35]

II. For evaluation of treatment results.

A. The immediate results of trigger point injection or blocks by local anesthetics.

B. The immediate effect of pain-relieving measures such as heat, coolants, mobilization, physiotherapy, manipulation, traction, acupuncture, biofeedback, etc.

C. Effect of pain-relieving or anti-inflammatory medications.

D. Long-term effects of treatment.

Essentially, pressure threshold measurement is used to locate tender spots, and for quantification of their sensitivity.[2, 7, 11, 13, 15, 16] This information is useful not only for clinical diagnosis but also for documenting the presence of trigger points to the patient. Kraus[27] found pressure threshold measurements useful for clinical diagnosis of trigger points. If measurements are done before and immediately after treatment, as after injection,[11] stretch,[21] physical therapy[5, 15, 16] or manipulation,[55, 56] laser treatment,[41] acupuncture, transcutaneous electrical nerve stimulation (TENS), etc., the effects of intervention, improvement,[11] or the opposite[5] will be demonstrated. The findings can guide plans for further treatment and remove causes of failure.[5] Long-term follow-up, usually at 2-week to 2-month intervals, will demonstrate the patient's progress or lack of changes.[5, 11] The activity of an inflammatory process, including arthritis[35] and fibrositis-fibromyalgia,[45–49, 54] can be assessed easily by pressure threshold measurement. Somatic tenderness secondary to visceral pain can be quantified.[59] Healing of an amputation stump can be monitored.[14] The pressure threshold meter has been useful in the differentiation of tension-type migraine and cervicogenic headaches[4] and in follow-up of clinical improvement of back pain.[25]

Description of Pressure Threshold Meter

The pressure threshold meter (Fig 6–1) (distributed by Pain Diagnostics & Thermography Inc., Great Neck, N.Y.) consists of a rubber disc attached to the pole of a pressure (force) gauge. The gauge is calibrated in kilograms and pounds. The kilogram scale is used for clinical purposes. Since the surface of the rubber tip is exactly 1 cm^2, the readings are expressed in kilograms per square centimeter (kg/cm^2). A maximum hold feature maintains the indicator on the highest pressure achieved. Pressing the zeroing knob returns the indicator to the original resting position, which is not necessarily 0. Deviations of resting position do not affect the precision of measurements. The range of the meter is 0 to 10 kg with 0.1-kg divisions.

Technique of Pressure Threshold Measurement

The technique consists of three steps:

1. *Explain the procedure and position the patient properly.* Explain to the patient: "I am going to measure the pressure threshold, i.e., how much pressure induces discomfort. This method will allow us to assess your progress." Show the pressure threshold meter to the patient and explain, "I am going to increase pressure with this device slowly. It won't hurt you" (Fig 6–2). The patient lies

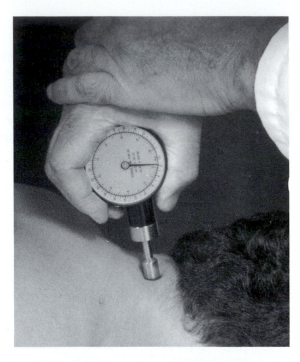

FIG 6–1.   Pressure threshold meter for quantification of tenderness.

with the side to be measured facing upward and is supported by pillows to allow complete relaxation. It is essential for accuracy that the muscles covering tender spots are relaxed. Careful palpation is used in order to detect spasm in areas to be measured. The patient is asked to relax. The patient can also be seated on an examination table for measurement in the extremities.

2. *Identify the maximum tender spot and mark it.* Have the patient pinpoint the maximum pain area with one finger (Fig 6–3). Palpate the painful area with

FIG 6–2.   The pressure threshold meter is shown to the patient and increasing pressure is applied over a visible area. The purpose of the test and the procedure are explained.

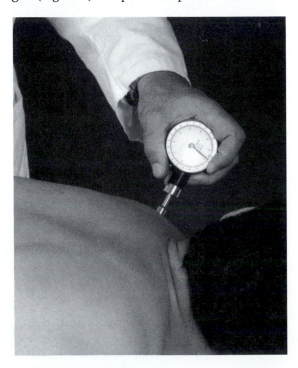

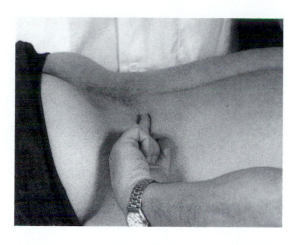

FIG 6–3. The patient is asked to point to the area of maximum pain using one finger.

the fingertip to identify the point of maximum sensitivity (Fig 6–4). Mark the maximum sensitive spot, preferably with a felt pen (Fig 6–5). (*Note:* Sometimes a patient will point to a reference zone into which the pain is radiating from a trigger point. Trigger points and referred pain patterns are described in Part II; see also the Appendix and Travell and Simons.[52, 53] The trigger points can be identified from the reference pain charts and their pressure threshold assessed. Treatment should be concentrated on the trigger point from which the pain originates.)

3. *Measure the pressure threshold* over the tender spot and a nontender control point. Apply the pressure gauge to the point of maximum sensitivity, placing the gauge at a 90-degree vertical angle to the skin (Fig 6–6). Instruct the patient, "Please say 'Yes' when you start to feel discomfort."

Increase the pressure continuously exactly at a rate of 1 kg/sec.[11, 57] by counting 1,001, 1,002, etc. while increasing the pressure so that the dial corresponds to your count, i.e., shows 1 kg when you say 1,001, etc. (Fig 6–7). The rate of pressure increments is thus guided by counting. Stop applying pressure and remove the gauge for reading immediately when the patient says *yes* indicating his or her pressure threshold. (*Note:* In some patients pain is demonstrated by pulling away or grimacing. In these cases we request again that the patient indicate the starting point of pain orally. Pulling away and grimacing is considered a later sign of pain than the verbal response.)

Mark a control reference point exactly on the corresponding opposite side,

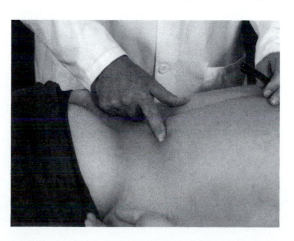

FIG 6–4. The examiner palpates with the index finger or thumb for the point of maximum tenderness.

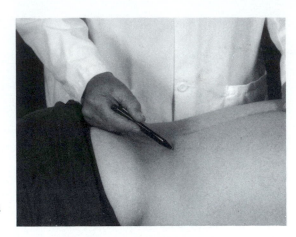

FIG 6–5. The point of maximum tenderness is marked.

Measure by tape or fingerbreadths the distance between the tender spot (trigger point) and the midline. Mark the corresponding distance from the midline on the opposite side (Fig 6–8). Palpate for tenderness or taut bands. If tenderness is present over the opposite side corresponding to the trigger point, bilateral involvement is considered. In this case a nontender spot in the same muscle that harbors the trigger point is employed as a reference. Measure the pressure threshold over the control point. Absolute values of pressure threshold for muscles frequently afflicted by trigger points[8] can be used as controls in case of bilateral tenderness. Slipping of the plunger caused by the rounded contour of the measured muscle (masseter, sternocleidomastoid, etc.) can be prevented by guarding the tip of the gauge between the thumb and index finger.[10]

Measuring and Circumventing Skin Tenderness When Muscle Sensitivity Is Recorded

Sometimes pressure pain sensitivity is present in the skin, and may interfere with measurement of deep tenderness in the muscles. Skin tenderness, however, does not prevent measurement of deep muscle pressure sensitivity, and can be circumvented in two different ways. When the patient indicates the pressure threshold at a relatively low level, it is suspected that the skin is abnormally sensitive. The increase of pressure is then continued further until a second threshold is achieved, which expresses the pressure sensitivity in deeper layers of the muscle. The presence of skin tenderness can be diagnosed and

FIG 6–6. The dolorimeter is applied over the marked tender spot, perpendicular to the surface of the muscle. Instruct the patient to say "Yes" when he or she starts to feel pain or discomfort.

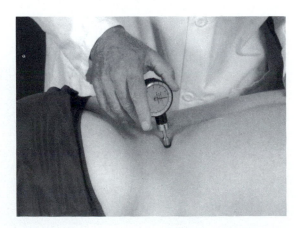

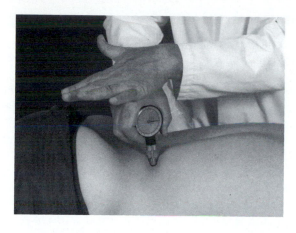

FIG 6–7. While one hand holds and stabilizes the gauge, the other hand applies the pressure. The examiner leans over the meter in order to increase the pressure mainly by body weight. It is important to increase the pressure at a rate of exactly 1 kg/sec.

quantified by pinching the skin. Normal skin is not painful on pinching or rolling. Skin pressure sensitivity can be quantified by measuring the pressure threshold over skin folded between the index finger and thumb or between the index finger and middle finger.

Recording the Pressure Threshold

1. Indicate the location of the measurement, including the right and left sides. We always record the right side first to prevent confusion.

2. Record the pressure threshold reading (kg/cm^2).

3. Record special circumstances under which the measurement was performed such as before or after therapy, after injection; recheck (compare with previous measurements), etc.

4. Spontaneous pain, not induced by pressure, can be rated on a scale of 0 to 10. The usual 0 to 5 scale is not sufficiently sensitive to express changes after therapy.

> *Example:* Before physical therapy, 10:05 A.M.: Gluteus medius m. Rt. 1.5 kg (spontaneous pain 5/10); Lt., 4.5 kg (no pain). After physical therapy, 11:01 A.M.: Rt. 3.5 kg (pain 3/10), Lt. 4.5 (pain 0).
>
> *Conclusion:* There was a decrease of tenderness and pain in the treated trigger point after therapy.

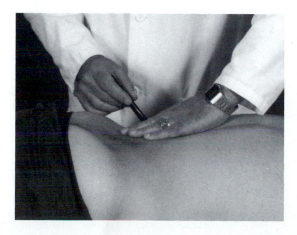

FIG 6–8. The distance of the maximum tender point from the midline is measured in centimeters, or fingerbreadths. A corresponding nonsensitive reference point on the opposite side is marked for a control measurement. In case of bilateral tenderness, a point that is not hypersensitive to pressure is used as a control.

Evaluation of Pressure Threshold

The following criteria can be used to assess abnormally low pressure thresholds indicating pathologic tenderness.

1. Side-to-side differences exceeding 2 kg are considered abnormal and clinically significant.[7, 11, 13, 16] This criterion is based on clinical experience. The difference of 2 kg expresses quantitatively the degree of tenderness that is considered pathologic on palpation by physicians experienced in using this procedure. Fischer found that hot spots on thermograms are markers of pressure-sensitive points.[16, 18] A 2-kg difference between the most tender point in the area of the hot spot and the contralateral normal tissue detected 87% of abnormalities.[16] This experimental data confirmed the clinical impression that a 2-kg difference is abnormal, and is useful for practical application of pressure algometry.

2. Normal values of pressure threshold were established for males and females in 50 control subjects without pain.[8] The averages and cutoff values are indicated in Table 6–1. The side-to-side difference is a more sensitive and individualized criterion. The normal values are to be used as a guideline because pain sensitivity varies considerably among individuals.

3. The patient's pain sensitivity can be assessed easily by pressure tolerance measurement.[6, 16, 17, 39, 45] The pressure tolerance test offers an additional reference in pain evaluation. Decreased pressure threshold over trigger points can be related to the patient's own general pain sensitivity. If pressure tolerance measured over normal tissues of deltoid muscle and shin bone is very high (see Table 6–2), even a relatively higher threshold over painful areas may indicate the presence of trigger points. (See discussion on evaluation of pressure tolerance below.)

4. A pressure threshold lower than 3 kg is usually abnormal.

Limitations of Pressure Threshold Management

Great caution should be exercised in clinical use of the method and employment of criteria owing to the very complicated problem of pain perception in different persons as well as in the same person under various conditions and

TABLE 6–1.

Summary of Abnormal Pressure Thresholds*

Muscle	Females		Males	
	Lowest	Average	Lowest	Average
Upper trapezius	2.0	4.0	2.9	4.7
Pectoralis			3.3	5.1
Levator scapulae	2.7	4.2	3.6	5.2
Supraspinatus	2.8	4.2	3.9	6.03
Teres major	2.7	4.0	4.1	6.0
Infraspinatus	3.0	4.8	4.6	6.9
Deltoid	3.1	4.8	5.1	7.3
Lumbar paraspinals	3.8	5.7	5.6	8.0
Gluteus medius	3.7	6.0	4.3	6.4

*Minimal pressure inducing pain: side-to-side differences higher than 2 kg/cm^2; absolute values generally lower than 3 kg/cm^2; lowest normal pressure threshold (84% security) and average values rounded up to 0.1 kg.

psychological states. On evaluation of results one should be aware of the fact that psychological tension, a change in the weather, the use of muscles harboring trigger points, and daily repetitive stresses increase tenderness and this in turn may be correctly reflected in lower pressure threshold readings.

Tender areas can be compared with nontender normal areas only if the tissues compared are of similar structure (muscle, tendon, ligament, etc.) and in areas which are normally equally sensitive to pressure: the lower part of the body is usually less sensitive to pressure than the upper back and neck. (Compare pressure thresholds in respective muscles in Table 6–1.)

The reproducibility of results collected by persons trained in pressure threshold measurement is sufficient for practical clinical use. Changes in pressure threshold obtained under standard conditions can be therefore regarded as reliable data (see Discussion).

Calibration of Pressure Threshold and Tolerance Gauges

A hook is provided, which can be screwed into the small opening located on the side of the gauge opposite the rubber tip and pole. A weight is attached to the hook while holding the gauge in hand so the reading in pounds or kilograms can be checked. (*Note:* The indicator may not return to zero. This difference does not affect the precision of the reading.)

PRESSURE TOLERANCE MEASUREMENT

Pressure tolerance is the highest pressure that the person can endure under the conditions of the examination. Pressure tolerance expresses the subject's sensitivity to pain. Unlike the pressure threshold measurement, which represents the minimum pressure inducing pain and which is used for quantification of tenderness in pressure-sensitive, abnormal areas, pressure tolerance is measured in two standard sites of normal tissues, avoiding tender spots; the deltoid muscles represent sensitivity to pain in muscles while the shin bone indicates the same over bony structures.[6, 39, 45]

Description of Pressure Tolerance Meter

The pressure tolerance meter consists of a rubber disc with a surface of exactly 1 cm^2 which is attached to a force (pressure) gauge. The rubber tip is identical with the one used in the pressure threshold meter. The gauge is calibrated in kilograms and pounds. For clinical purposes the metric (kg) scale is used.

The tolerance gauge has a similar construction as the pressure threshold meter with two important differences: The range of the tolerance gauge is extended to 20 kg, as compared to 10 kg with the threshold meter. Consequently the divisions on the tolerance gauge are also larger—0.2 kg vs. 0.1 kg on the threshold meter. The tolerance meter, gaining a higher range, loses somewhat in precision of measurement. The threshold meter, although more precise than the tolerance gauge, lacks sufficient range for high normal threshold[48] and tolerance measurements. Readings in 0.2-kg divisions for threshold are somewhat unusual and cumbersome. Therefore, for best results the use of both gauges— one for threshold (10 kg) and one for high threshold and for tolerance (20 kg), is recommended. The tolerance meter looks like the threshold meter and has

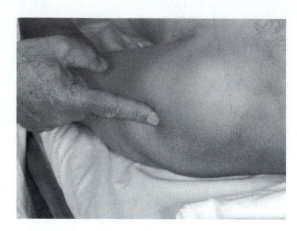

FIG 6–9. Pressure tolerance measurement. The deltoid muscles are palpated for tenderness. Only *non*tender areas are measured.

identical features: it also holds automatically the maximum pressure achieved. A zeroing button is located at the index finger when the gauge is held in the right palm, with the dial facing the eyes (see Fig 6–1).

Technique of Pressure Tolerance Measurement

1. *Explain the procedure to the patient:* "I am going to increase the pressure with this instrument. Say 'Stop' when you want me to stop the pressure. Results will help in assessing the cause of your pain and in prescription of the most effective treatment. The procedure is not painful."

2. *Positioning of patient:* Pressure tolerance is measured with the patient supine and relaxed. The clothing over the deltoid muscle and shin bone is removed.

Measurements are taken on both sides and repeated once in order to assure reproducibility and to increase the reliability of the measurements. Average values of both deltoid and tibia measurements are calculated.

3. *Procedure of measurement, Deltoid:* The bulk of the middeltoid muscle, the part of the deltoid on the side of the humerus, is palpated. Pressure is exerted by a finger over the height of the bulk and around it in order to rule out local tenderness or palpable abnormal consistency (edema, fibrositis, etc.) (Fig 6–9). The measurement of tolerance should avoid hypersensitive areas.

If there is tenderness over the deltoid or its parts, then several additional, presumably normal muscles are palpated in order to rule out or confirm generalized muscle tenderness. Biceps, triceps, shoulder blade muscles, thoracic paraspinals, the quadriceps femoris, and hamstrings are palpated in order to rule out tenderness. In case of generalized tenderness, both deltoids are measured with the addition of some of the other muscles, listed above, to demonstrate their involvement.

The rubber tip of the pressure tolerance meter (20-kg range) is applied to the bulkiest part of the deltoid muscle, selecting a spot which is not more tender than the surrounding area (Fig 6–10).

Pressure tolerance measurement can be combined with readings of threshold in the same procedure. Using the combined procedure, the patient is instructed as follows: "Say 'Yes' when you start feeling discomfort." The pressure over the deltoid or tibia is increased continuously at a speed of 1 kg/sec. When the patient says "yes," the increase of pressure is stopped, the threshold

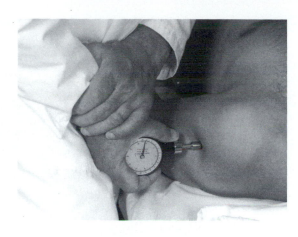

FIG 6–10. The examiner applies pressure mainly by leaning with the thigh and body against the meter.

value is read and memorized, but the meter is not removed from the skin. The second instruction follows immediately: "Say when to stop." When the patient says "Stop," the gauge is removed and the maximum value held expressing tolerance is read.

Isolated tolerance measurement, not combined with threshold readings in the same location, requires the command, "I am going to increase the pressure slowly. Say 'Stop' when you want me to stop."

Tibia: The site of measurement is selected by palpation over the inner anterior aspect of the leg about 5 cm distal to the upper end of the tibia (Fig 6–11). Tender areas are avoided. If tenderness is experienced over the area below the knee, palpation is extended further distally. Usually the anterior crest of the tibia is not tender and serves well as a reference (Fig 6–12). The nontender area to be measured is marked. The same procedure of measurement as described for the deltoid is utilized. If the tibial crest is measured, the tip of the meter needs to be guided between the index finger and thumb in order to prevent it from sliding off the bone (Fig 6–13).

Since considerable force may be required for pressure tolerance measurement, it is useful to use the examiner's body weight to provide the necessary pressure. When the shin bone is measured the examiner leans over the meter using his or her body weight, while watching the meter for the rate of increase. Deltoid pressure tolerance can be measured by pushing the meter by the examiner's body (thigh or hip) while stabilizing and guiding the instrument with both hands to prevent the tip from slipping (see Fig 6–13).

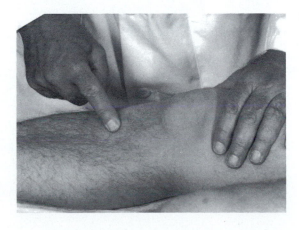

FIG 6–11. Pressure pain tolerance measurement over the tibia. The first step is to palpate for nontender areas over the medial tibial flare.

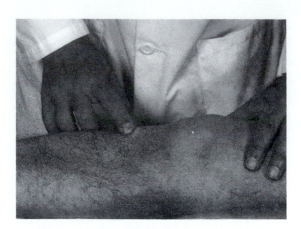

FIG 6–12. If the tibial flare is tender, then the anterior edge of the tibia is palpated since this region is usually nontender.

Evaluation of Pressure Tolerance

Normal values and cutoff points for pressure tolerance are indicated in Table 6–2. The numbers in the table are to be used as a guideline since tolerance in different cultural groups, mood, and psychological status vary substantially.[37] Males have higher pressure tolerance than females. Athletes' rates are usually higher than those of inactive people. The lower body has higher threshold and tolerance values than the upper body (see Table 6–1).

Significance of Relations Between Muscle and Bone Pressure Tolerance

1. *Both muscle and bone tolerance are decreased:* This condition indicates generalized decreased pain tolerance (hypersensitivity to stimuli). Physical therapy and other measures usually aggravate the pain. Antidepressant and biofeedback with counseling to develop coping mechanisms in order to increase pain tolerance should be considered.

2. *Both muscle and bone tolerance are increased:* This indicates good pain tolerance, which is seen frequently in athletes. If trigger points are detected by decreased threshold, the prognosis with local treatment is good. In view of general high pain tolerance, trigger points may be diagnosed even when the pressure threshold over the suspected area is relatively high (Table 6–3).

FIG 6–13. The *non*tender area is measured. Pressure is increased at a rate of 1 kg/sec. The pressure is applied by the examiner leaning his body over the meter using his or her weight as a source of force.

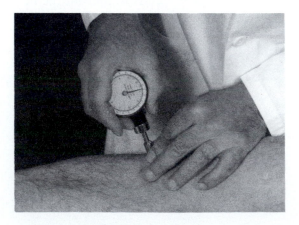

TABLE 6–2.

Maximum Tolerated Pressure (kg/cm^2)

Muscle	Lowest X̄−SD	Highest X̄+SD	Average SD	Lowest X̄−SD	Highest X̄±SD	Average SD
Deltoid	7.0	13.4	10.2 ±3.2	8.5	14.4	11.8 ±2.6
Midtibia	5.5	12.3	8.9 ±3.4	8.2	12.6	10.4 ±2.2

3. *Only muscle tolerance is decreased.* Bone tolerance may be normal or also decreased, but muscle tolerance is still lower than that of bone. Normally, tolerance is higher over the deltoid (soft tissue) than over the shin bone. If hypersensitive areas (spots) are avoided, as described above, the measurement reflects the sensitivity of muscle tissue not afflicted by local abnormality. Decreased tolerance over both deltoid muscles therefore indicates diffuse muscle tissue tenderness.[13, 16] This condition is completely different from point tenderness, which is limited to a small area, while the rest of the muscle tissue demonstrates normal pressure pain sensitivity.

If diffuse, i.e., nonpoint tenderness is present, the next question is whether the diffuse muscle tenderness diagnosed over the deltoids is present in other muscles, indicating generalized diffuse muscle tenderness. The back, lower back, pectoral, and extremity muscles are palpated by exerting pressure with the thumb or with the pressure tolerance meter, in order to establish the general spread of diffuse muscle tenderness. Generalized diffuse tenderness evidently indicates a condition that afflicts all muscles or most of them, and is usually caused by endocrine deficiency, particularly low thyroid or estrogen production.[50] In contrast, myofascial trigger points are localized, the tenderness is focal, i.e., limited to spots, while the rest of the muscle demonstrates normal pressure sensitivity. The concept of diffuse muscle tenderness means that in addition to decreased pressure thresholds over certain points, the entire rest of the muscle is also tender.

If pressure tolerance over the deltoid is lower than over the shin bone, local tenderness, i.e., tenderness limited to the deltoids, has to be ruled out by a measurement over other nontender muscles. If tolerance is decreased over all muscles, generalized muscle disorder should be considered.[16] Hypothyroidism should be ruled out by triiodothyronine (T_3), thyroxine (T_4), and thyroid-stimulating hormone (TSH) levels and ovarial dysfunction by vaginal smear with a cell maturation study and determination of blood estrogen levels.[50]

4. A narrowed span between threshold and tolerance over normal muscles indicates hysterical personality.[37]

TABLE 6–3.

Diagnostic Significance of Relation Between Pressure Tolerance Over Muscles and Bones

Muscle Tolerance	Bone Tolerance	Diagnosis
Decreased	Decreased	Low pain tolerance
Increased	Increased	High pain tolerance
Decreased	Normal	Muscle tenderness
Normal	Decreased	Osteoporosis?
Narrowed difference between pressure threshold and tolerance		Hysterical personality

DISCUSSION

Several clinicians and investigators confirmed usefulness of quantitative measurement of local tenderness, which is the hallmark for diagnosis of trigger points and tender points in fibromyalgia.*

Force gauges attached to a rubber disc were used for measurement of pain sensitivity. Head called the device an "algometer," meaning "measurement of pain," and employed it to study the thalamic syndrome.[26] Keele[26] called a similar device a "pressure algometer" and established normal values over the forehead. A flat circular end of 0.5 cm was used and the calibration ranged to 7.7 kg. Clinical experience with patients suffering from trigger points and deep tenderness showed that for measurement of *deep tissue tenderness* in muscles, a disc with a 1-cm^2 surface was more suitable.[16] This conclusion has been confirmed by Smythe et al.[48]

A force gauge with a flat disc plunger of 1-cm^2 surface has been introduced attached to a force gauge ranging up to 10 kg. The device is suitable for measuring the minimal pressure that induces pain (threshold) over tender areas located in deep tissues (tender spots, trigger or tender points) and is called the *pressure threshold meter*.[16] While pressure algometers were employed for assessment of general sensitivity to pain in normal tissues, the pressure threshold meter is primarily used for quantification of tenderness in hypersensitive spots.

Reliability of Pressure Threshold and Tolerance Measurements

The reliability of pressure algometer readings between different observers was assessed in schizophrenics by Merskey et al.[37] and in normal subjects by Merskey and Spear.[38] The pressure was increased smoothly at a consistent rate of 1 kg/sec, as recommended by Keele.[26] The forehead and tibia were investigated. A total of 69 subjects were examined, of which 10 were females. The subjects indicated when the pressure began to hurt. The mean values for the forehead were 3.75 ±0.82 for males and 2.74 ±0.91 for females. The lower pain tolerance of females is consistent with previous reports. The pressure ("It hurt a lot") over the shin for 20 males was 5.98 +1.49.

The conclusion of the study was that the pressure at which a subject first describes awareness of pain (threshold) correlates well between different observers, occasions, and sites.[38] The authors indicated that the pain threshold depends a great deal upon such factors as attitude, sex, and cultural role. The conclusion was made that the pressure pain has a degree of reliability which makes possible its quantitative use for investigation of emotional states, anesthesia, and analgesia.[38] This is particularly so where each individual serves as his own control, since the scale of readings taken in each person tends to be less than that of readings taken on several people.[38]

Pressure Threshold in Evaluation of Tender Spots

The interobserver correlation coefficients for pressure pain measurements have ranged from .67 to .88. Intraobserver correlations were even better, ranging from .71 to .92.[35, 39, 42] Mikkelson et al.[39] showed in a group of 18 fibromyalgic patients high intraobserver reliability of .85; interobserver reliability was .90. Jensen and co-workers,[23, 24] Orbach and Gale,[40] Lautenschlager et al.,[33, 34]

*References 2, 11, 13, 16, 17, 21, 23–25, 28–30, 32–35, 37, 40, 44–49, 55–57, 59.

and Shiffmann et al.[44] showed good reliability and validity of pressure pain measurements. Jensen[23] provides a good review of the topic.

There was no difference on repeated measurements or at five separate sessions.[40] Smythe et al.[49] found a standard deviation among the observers of 0.9 kg and an intraobserver variation of about 0.7 kg. Smythe[48] also emphasized that a larger scale, as in the pressure tolerance meter (20-kg range), is necessary for normal values. Scudds[45] reported an interrater reliability of .95 using the pressure threshold meter at four points in healthy subjects. Such levels can be achieved only by careful standardization of the procedure[45] and sufficient training.[42]

Reeves et al.[42] and Jaeger et al.[22] investigated the reliability of the pressure meter as an objective measure of myofascial trigger point pain sensitivity. Two experimenters independently applied a pressure meter to five trigger point locations in a sample of 13 patients with myofascial headaches. Correlations showed significant interexperimenter reliability of pressure meter readings for trigger point pain threshold ranging from $r = .68$ to $r = .86$. Only one trigger point failed to reach significance. The authors of this valuable study concluded: "The pressure meter is shown to be a reliable measure of trigger point pain threshold."[42] In another study the same authors found r values for intertester correlations for five trigger points higher than .67. Findings indicate that "reliable readings can be obtained by testers when they are required to locate and measure the same unmarked trigger point locations."[42] A third study on the validity of trigger point measurement included eight patients.[42] In addition to five trigger point locations, an adjacent muscular area was measured. The results conclusively showed that the measurements differentiated sensitive points from the entire muscle group. The conclusion of the group of Reeves and Jaeger was the following: "Our studies indicate that the algometer is a valid and reliable measure of trigger points in the head and neck region, making it a valuable tool for clinician and experimenter."[42]

Fischer and Chang[18] demonstrated in 14 patients with low back pain statistically significant lower thresholds over trigger points, which were corroborated by hot spots on thermograms. Pressure threshold on the normal side was 6.2 kg/cm^2 as compared with 4.85 over the trigger points. The difference was significant at a $P < .001$ level. The temperature difference, 1.15° C, was also significant at $P < .05$. In a follow-up study Fischer[16] measured pressure thresholds in tender spots occurring in the areas of focal increased heat emission (hot spots) on thermograms. Hot spots were documented to be related to hypersensitive points. Pressure threshold was significantly lower in tender spots found in the area of hot spots observed on the thermogram averaging 4.85 ±2.36 kg/cm^2 vs. 8.69 ±3.07 kg/cm^2 over the opposite normal area ($P < .0001$). Hot spots were therefore considered an objective marker of tender spots on the thermogram. Using hot spots as markers of focal tenderness, Fischer investigated how much pressure difference vs. the normosensitive tissue should be considered abnormal. Evidently this is a crucial question for clinical use of algometry for diagnosis of abnormal tenderness. A side-to-side difference of 1.5 kg/cm^2 detected 97.8% of tenderness in areas of hot spots. A difference of 2 kg/cm^2 vs. the opposite normal side indicated 87.0% of hot spots. For clinical purposes the 2-kg/cm^2 side-to-side difference is therefore reliable and recommended as a criterion of abnormal pressure pain threshold. Significantly lower pressure thresholds in tender points and trigger points and hot spots described by Fischer[11, 16, 18] have been confirmed by Kruse and Christiansen.[30] They found pressure thresholds of 1.54 ±0.24 over trigger points as compared to 4.73 ±1.01 ($P < .001$) over control areas. Jimenez[25] reported pressure measurement to be useful in evaluation of patients in a pain clinic. The clinical improvement correlated well with increases in pressure measurements.[25]

Normal values of pressure threshold were established in muscles of 50 healthy persons (24 males and 26 females). The side-to-side difference was significant in only one muscle (infraspinatus) in females. Again, the identical findings over corresponding sites of measurement proved the high reproducibility and validity of threshold measurement. Muscle tenderness is an important sign of endocrine insufficiency, and pressure measurement is helpful in the diagnosis of the condition as well as in documentation of improvement with treatment. Airaksinen et al.[1] found the pressure threshold meter to be reliable for detection of latent trigger points. Kraus[27] found pressure threshold measurements useful in clinical practice for documentation of trigger points and their reaction to treatment.

Algometry in Diagnosis of Fibromyalgia and Evaluation of Treatment Results

The name *fibromyalgia*, meaning "muscle fiber pain," was coined by Yunus[60, 61] (see also Chapter 1), to replace fibromyositis since the condition is not an inflammatory disorder. Fibromyalgia is characterized by tender spots called *tender points*. Algometry has been used extensively for quantification of tender points in fibromyalgia. When using dolorimetry for differential diagnosis of muscle pain, the main notion to be kept in mind is that trigger points occur in isolated muscles or muscle groups and their spread is usually limited to regions such as the neck, shoulder, upper back, lower back, and extremities. Only trigger points caused by systemic disorders, such as endocrine dysfunction, particularly hypothyroidism and estrogen deficiency, are generalized, i.e., spreading to the upper and lower body, bilateral, with usually symmetric sensitivity. In endocrine disorders, however, as mentioned above, in addition to widespread point tenderness, there is also diffuse abnormal pressure pain sensitivity over the rest of the muscle.[16, 17] The tenderness is therefore not confined to a point, but affects diffusely the entire muscle tissue, albeit to a lesser degree than tender spots.

In contrast to the local or regional distribution of myofascial trigger points, fibromyalgia is a systemic disorder that affects not only muscles but extends to other tissues as well. The location of tender points considered by different authors to be diagnostic of fibromyalgia, as well as the number necessary to achieve diagnostic conclusions, varies. Yunus derived such criteria (see Chapter 1). The latest criteria were published in the American College of Rheumatology multicenter study organized by Wolfe.[58]

The presently recognized criteria for abnormal pressure pain sensitivity diagnostic of fibromyalgic tender points is about 4-kg pressure provided by the thumb. This pressure can, of course, be quantified easily by dolorimetry using the proper head with a surface of 1 cm². Smythe et al.[47] showed that the 1-cm² surface is most effective in detection of tender points.

The location of myofascial trigger points is limited to muscles. In myofascial trigger points the pressure sensitivity usually extends from the maximum tender spot to the origin and insertion of the muscle in the form of a taut band.[28, 29, 52, 53] One major difference between myofascial trigger points and tender points diagnostic of fibromyalgia is their location. Tender points in fibromyalgia are confined to nine typical sites. Fischer[17] pointed out the contradiction that only three out of the nine pairs (each being bilateral) of points diagnostic for fibromyalgia (muscle fiber pain) are located over the muscle. These include the trapezius at the midpoint of the upper border, the supraspinatus at regions above the scapular spine near the medial border, and the gluteal upper outer quadrant of the buttocks in the anterior fold of the muscle. The rest of the tender points—the occiput, anterior cervical at intertransverse spaces C5–7, the second rib at the costochondral junction, the lateral humeral epicondyle at a point 2 cm distal to the epicondyle, the greater trochanter posterior to the trochanteric prominence, and the knee at the medial fat pad proximal to the joint line—are evidently not muscular points.

In addition to tenderness over 11 of the 18 diagnostic points (nine pairs) the diagnosis of fibromyalgia requires widespread pain defined as axial plus upper and lower segment plus left- and right-sided pain.[58]

Lautenschlager et al.[33, 34] have proved the usefulness of algometry in the diagnosis of fibromyalgia. They used a hard small plunger. This specific head, for which normal values and the sensitivity and the specificity of pressure threshold measurement for diagnosis of fibromyalgia were established, is available as an alternate tip to the pressure threshold and pressure tolerance meters (Pain Diagnostics & Thermography Inc.). Smythe et al.[47, 48] evaluated two different types of dolorimeters, the traditional Chatillon with a foot plate of 1.54 cm^2 and the pressure threshold meter with 1-cm^2 surface, introduced by Fischer. The authors concluded that the Fischer instrument gave lower readings at tender sites (10th percentile to 2.4 vs. 2.9 kg and higher values at nontender sites. . . . The small dolorimeter was more sensitive to the differences among sites. It was similarly more sensitive to the variations among subjects.[47]

The 1-cm^2 plunger is evidently the method of choice since a larger surface includes more normal tissue, decreasing the sensitivity and specificity of measurement. In addition, the authors found no significant order effects. Interobservers' standard deviation was 0.858 kg for all data, 0.748 for the large meter, and 0.944 for the smaller head.[47] The authors concluded that "the Fischer dolorimeter showed advantages in this study, with more tender points, less control points and fewer observations off the scale".[47] Smythe et al.[48] found a strong relation between control and fibrositic site tenderness, with control thresholds twice as high. They were able to differentiate well between fibrositic and control points but findings also revealed that fibrositic patients have a generally lower pressure pain sensitivity. This conclusion corresponds to that of other authors' findings.[39, 45, 53] Scudds et al.,[45] using the pressure threshold meter, were able to differentiate myofascial pain syndrome from fibrositis. The discriminating power of the four main study variables between the two groups led to a highly significant discriminant function which had a correct classification to groups of almost 80%. The middle deltoid and anterior tibia were used as control points to measure pain tolerance. The trapezius, costal cartilage, elbow, and medial fat pad of the knee were investigated as fibrositic tender points. A "total pain threshold index" was derived from the four points over the deltoids and shin bones and a total myalgic index from the eight fibrositic tender points. Simms et al.[46] also found algometry useful in the diagnosis of fibromyalgia.

It can be concluded that the pressure threshold and tolerance meters cover the range of normal to tender points and assist in quantification of tender spots and in differentiating them from normal control sites.

Normal values for pressure tolerance over the tibia and deltoid muscles were established in males and females.[6] Side-to-side differences were statistically not significant. Mikkelson et al.[39] found lower pressure tolerance over the tibia and deltoid in a Finnish population compared with the American study.[6] Pressure tolerance measurement showed lower values in fibromyalgia patients than in controls, showing the clinical efficacy of the method.[39]

Pressure Threshold in Evaluation of Inflammation (Arthritis)

Pressure threshold was used successfully for evaluation of inflammation in animals.[3] Hyperalgesia showed a high negative correlation with the logarithm of anti-inflammatory medication ($r = .983$).[3] McCarthy et al.[35] were able to determine more quantitatively the initial degree of involvement in arthritis as well as the subsequent spread of disease activity. Hollander and Young[20] and Lansbury[32] also found algometry useful in the evaluation of arthritis.

Pressure Threshold in Evaluation of Visceral Pain and Related Paraspinal Somatic Tenderness

Measurement of deep visceral tenderness was used successfully in patients with abdominal pain due to pancreatitis, cholecystopathy, and duodenal ulcer.[59] The range of gauges was up to 3.6 kg. The diseased side showed a 1.0-kg lower threshold which improved to a 0.2-kg difference compared with the sound side when pain was controlled by paraspinal anesthesia. Similarly, paravertebral tender points showed a difference vs. the healthy side of 0.2 kg when pain was present. The difference was reduced when the patient felt no pain at the time of the examination.

Tissue Compliance and Thermography

Fischer used thermography to demonstrate the presence of trigger points.[13, 16, 18] A *tissue compliance meter* is a hand-held mechanical instrument which serves as an extension of the physical examination (Pain Diagnostics & Thermography Inc.). Changes in muscle tone (spasm, spasticity) or consistency that are diagnosed by palpation can be documented quantitatively and objectively by tissue compliance measurement.[11, 13] Increased resistance (decreased softness or compliance) in the form of a taut band is recognized as diagnostic of myofascial trigger points.[52, 53] The presence of a harder consistency[28, 29, 31] in trigger points identified by pressure threshold measurement can be corroborated objectively using tissue compliance measurement.[9, 13, 16, 29]

SUMMARY

1. *The pressure threshold meter* is a pocket-sized force gauge fitted with a rubber disc tip of 1 cm^2. Documentation of trigger points by quantifying local tenderness is useful for diagnostic purposes and evaluating the effect of therapy. The effect of therapy or spontaneous improvement, as well as impairment of the condition, can be documented quantitatively.

2. *Pressure tolerance*, the maximum force tolerated, expresses sensitivity to pain. Lower tolerance readings over both muscle and bone indicate generalized

lower pain tolerance requiring specific treatment. Lower tolerance over muscles as compared to bone represents a reversal of the normal ratio and indicates a generalized muscle disorder. A narrowed range between threshold and tolerance occurs in the hysterical personality. High tolerance is seen frequently in athletes and allows diagnosis of the presence of trigger points even when the threshold is relatively high over the painful area. The reliability and validity of pressure threshold and tolerance measurements have been proved statistically (see Discussion).

3. The *tissue compliance meter* is a new hand-held instrument. Spasm, spasticity, edema, hematomas, taut and fibrotic bands, fibrositic nodules, taut bands of trigger points, and other soft tissue pathologic conditions can be documented.[9, 12] Normal values have been established for pressure threshold, tolerance, and tissue compliance.

REFERENCES

1. Airaksinen O, Pontinen OJ: The reliability of the pain threshold algometry on latent myofascial trigger points in healthy Finnish students, First International Symposium on Myofascial Pain and Fibromyalgia, Minneapolis, 1989.
2. Bonica JJ: *The management of pain,* Philadelphia, 1990, Lea & Febiger.
3. Bonnet J, et al: Platelet-activating factor acether (PAF-acether) involvement in acute inflammatory and pain processes, *Agents Actions* 11:559–562, 1981.
4. Bovim G: Cervicogenic headache, migraine, and tension-type headache. Pressure-pain threshold measurements, *Pain* 51:169–173, 1992.
5. Fischer AA: Diagnosis and management of chronic pain in physical medicine and rehabilitation. In Ruskin AP, editor: *Current therapy in physiatry,* Philadelphia, 1984, WB Saunders, pp 123–145.
6. Fischer AA: Pressure tolerance over muscles and bones in normal subjects, *Arch Phys Med Rehabil* 67:406–409, 1986.
7. Fischer AA: Pressure threshold meter: Its use for quantification of tender spots, *Arch Phys Med Rehabil* 67:836–838, 1986.
8. Fischer AA: Pressure algometry over normal muscles. Standard values, validity and reproducibility of pressure threshold, *Pain* 30:115–126, 1987.
9. Fischer AA: Clinical use of tissue compliance meter for documentation of soft tissue pathology, *Clin J Pain* 3:23–30, 1987.
10. Fischer AA: Letter to the editor, *Pain* 28:411–414, 1987.
11. Fischer AA: Pressure threshold measurement for diagnosis of myofascial pain and evaluation of treatment results, *Clin J Pain* 2:207–214, 1987.
12. Fischer AA: Documentation of muscle pain and soft tissue pathology. In Kraus H, editor: *Diagnosis and treatment of muscle pain,* Chicago, 1988, Quintessence, pp 55–65.
13. Fischer AA: Documentation of myofascial trigger points, *Arch Phys Med Rehabil* 69:286–291, 1988.
14. Fischer AA: Pressure threshold: a valuable method in evaluation of stump problems and healing, *Arch Phys Med Rehabil* 69:732, 1988.
15. Fischer AA: Pain and spasm alleviation by physiotherapy, *Arch Phys Med Rehabil* 69:735, 1988.
16. Fischer AA: Application of pressure algometry in manual medicine, *J Manual Med* 5:145–150, 1990.
17. Fischer AA: Differential diagnosis of muscle tenderness and pain, *Pain Manage* (Jan/Feb) 30–36, 1991.
18. Fischer AA, Chang CH: Temperature and pressure threshold measurements in trigger points, *Thermology* 1:212–215, 1986.
19. Hackett GS: *Ligament and tendon relaxation treated by prolotherapy,* ed 3, Springfield, Ill, 1958, Thomas, pp 27–36, 70.
20. Hollander JL, Young DG: The palpameter: An instrument for quantitation of joint tenderness, *Arthritis Rheum* 6:277, 1963.

21. Jaeger B, Reeves JL: Quantification of changes in myofascial trigger point sensitivity with the pressure algometer following passive stretch, *Pain* 27:203–210, 1986.
22. Jaeger B, et al: Reliability of the pressure meter as an objective measure of myofascial trigger point pain sensitivity, *Pain* (suppl 2), 1984.
23. Jensen K: Quantification of tenderness by palpation and use of pressure algometers. In Fricton JR, Awad EA, editors: *Advances in pain research and therapy*, New York, 1990, Raven Press, pp 165–181.
24. Jensen K, et al: Pressure pain threshold in human temporal region. Evaluation of a new pressure algometer, *Pain* 25:313–323, 1986.
25. Jimenez AC: Serial determinations of pressure threshold tolerance in chronic pain patients, *Arch Phys Med Rehabil* 66:545–546, 1985.
26. Keele KD: Pain-sensitivity tests—the pressure algometer, *Lancet* 636–639, 1954.
27. Kraus H: Musculofascial pain. In *Pain control: Practical aspects of patient care*, 1981, Masson.
28. Kraus H: *Diagnosis and treatment of muscle pain*, Chicago, 1988, Quintessence.
29. Kraus H, Fischer AA: Diagnosis and treatment of myofascial pain, *Mt Sinai J Med* 58:235–239, 1991.
30. Kruse RA, Christiansen JA: Thermographic imaging of myofascial trigger points: A follow-up study, *Arch Phys Med Rehabil* 73:819–823, 1992.
31. Lange M: *Die Muskelhärten* (Myelgelosen), Munich, 1931, Lehmann.
32. Lansbury J: Methods for evaluating rheumatoid arthritis. In Hollander JL, editor: *Arthritis and allied conditions*, Philadelphia, 1967, Lea & Febiger, pp 269–291.
33. Lautenschlager J, et al: Lokalisierte Druckschmerzen in der Diagnose der generalisierten Tendomyopathie (Fibromyalgia), *Z Rheumatol* 48:132–138, 1988.
34. Lautenschlager J, et al: Die Messung von Druckschmerzen im Bereich von Sehnen und Muskeln bei gesunden und Patienten mit generalisierter Tendomyopathie (fibromyalgie-Syndrom), *Z Rheumatol* 47:397–404, 1988.
35. McCarthy DJ Jr, Gatter RA, Phelps P: A dolorimeter for quantification of articular tenderness, *Arthritis Rheum* 8:551–559, 1965.
36. Mense S: Peripheral mechanisms of muscle nociception and local muscle pain, *J Musculoskeletal Pain* 1:133–170, 1993.
37. Merskey H, Gillis A, Marszalek KS: A clinical investigation of reactions to pain, *J Ment Sci* 108:347–355, 1962.
38. Merskey H, Spear FG: The reliability of the pressure algometer, *Br J Soc Clin Psychol* 3:130–136, 1964.
39. Mikkelson M, et al: Muscle and bone pressure pain threshold and pain tolerance in fibromyalgia patients and controls, *Arch Phys Med Rehabil* 73:814–818, 1992.
40. Ohrbach R, Gale EN: Pressure pain threshold in normal muscles: Reliability, measurement effect and topographic differences, *Pain* 39:257–263, 1989.
41. Pontinen PJ, Airaksinen O: The effort of low power infra-red laser on latent myofascial trigger points, First International Symposium on Myofascial Pain and fibromyalgia, Minneapolis 1989, pp 8–10.
42. Reeves JL, Jaeger B, Graff-Radford SB: Reliability of the pressure algometer as a measure of myofascial trigger point sensitivity, *Pain* 24:313–321, 1986.
43. Rosomoff HL, et al: Physical findings in patients with chronic intractable benign pain of the neck and/or back, *Pain* 37:279–287, 1989.
44. Schiffman E, et al: A pressure algometer for myofascial pain syndrome: reliability and validity testing. In Dubner R, Gebhart GF, Bond MR, editors: *Proceedings of the Fifth World Congress on Pain*, Amsterdam, 1988, Elsevier.
45. Scudds RA, et al: A comparative study of pain, sleep quality and pain responsiveness in fibrositis and myofascial pain syndrome, *J Rheumatol* 16(suppl 19):120–126, 1989.
46. Simms RW, et al: Tenderness in 75 anatomic sites, *Arthritis Rheum* 31:182–187, 1988.
47. Smythe HA, et al: Relation between fibrositic and control tenderness: Effects of dolorimeter scale length and footplate size, *J Rheumatol* 19:284–289, 1992.
48. Smythe HA, et al: Control and fibrositic tenderness. Comparison of two dolorimeters, *J Rheumatol* 19:768–771, 1992.
49. Smythe HA, et al: Tender shins and steroid therapy, *J Rheumatol* 18:1568–1572, 1991.
50. Sonkin LS: Endocrine disorders and muscle dysfunction. In Gelb H, editor: *Clinical*

management of head, neck and TMJ pain and dysfunction, Philadelphia, 1985, WB Saunders.

51. Steindler A: *Lectures on the interpretation of pain in orthopedic practice*, Springfield, Ill, 1959, C Thomas.
52. Travell JG, Simons DG: *Myofascial pain and dysfunction. The trigger point manual*, Baltimore, 1983, Williams & Wilkins.
53. Travell JG, Simons DG: *Myofascial pain dysfunction. The trigger point manual. The lower extremities*, vol 2, Baltimore, 1992, Williams & Wilkins.
54. Tunks E, et al: Tender points in fibromyalgia, *Pain* 34:11–19, 1988.
55. Vernon HT: Pressure pain threshold evaluation of the effect of spinal manipulation on chronic neck pain: A single case study, *J Can Chiropractic Assoc* 32:191–194, 1988.
56. Vernon HT, et al: Pressure pain threshold evaluation of the effect of spinal manipulation in the treatment of chronic neck pain: A pilot study, *J Manipulative Physiol Ther* 13:13–16, 1990.
57. White KP, McCain GA, Tunks E: The effects of changing the painful stimulus upon dolorimetry scores in patients with fibromyalgia, *J Musculoskeletal Pain* 1:43–58, 1993.
58. Wolfe F, et al: The American College of Rheumatology 1990 criteria for the classification of fibromyalgia. Report of the Multicenter Criteria Committee. *Arthritis Rheum* 33:160–172, 1990.
59. Yamagata S, et al: A diagnostic re-evaluation of electric skin resistance, skin temperature and deeper tenderness in patients with abdominal pain, *Tohoku J Exp Med* 118(suppl):183–189, 1976.
60. Yunus MB: Research in fibromyalgia and myofascial pain syndromes: Current status, problems and future directions, *J Musculoskeletal Pain* 1:23–41, 1993.
61. Yunus M, et al: Primary fibromyalgia, *Am Fam Physician* 25:115–121, 1982.

PART *II*

TRIGGER POINT MANAGEMENT

Chapter 7

Trigger Points

Edward S. Rachlin, M.D.

EPIDEMIOLOGY

Regional myofacial pain syndromes (defined as local and referred muscular pain arising from trigger points) are a major cause of disability and chronic pain, and play a factor in most workers' compensation cases involving pain.[8] Of 283 consecutive chronic pain patients who were examined independently by a neurosurgeon and physiatrist, 85% were found to have a diagnosis of primary myofacial pain.[6] Of 296 patients complaining of head and neck pain, 54.6% were diagnosed as having primary myofascial pain syndrome.[6] Schiffman and colleagues[30] found the prevalence of masticatory myalgia (pain with muscle tenderness) to be present in 50% of the population, though the majority of the people in this study did not feel their symptoms were severe enough to seek treatment. Smythe[39] found that approximately 30% of the patient population have at least one tender point. Sola et al.[43] surveyed 200 asymptomatic young adults to determine the presence of asymptomatic trigger points (latent trigger points) in the shoulder girdle muscles. Hypersensitive areas (trigger points) were found in 54% of the female subjects and 45% of the male subjects. Ninety-nine (49.5%) subjects had one or more trigger points. Referred pain was demonstrated in 12.5% of all subjects. Four muscles—the trapezius, levator scapulae, infraspinatus, and scalenus—accounted for 84.7% of the trigger points, the trapezius (34.7%) and the levator scapulae (19.7%) occurring most frequently. The incidence of myofascial pain syndromes appears to be higher in women than men, and though trigger points have been diagnosed in children and young adults they are most often seen in the age range of 31 to 50 years.[15, 43] More women than men appear to develop symptomatic myofascial pain and seek treatment[15] (Table 7–1).

Untreated myofascial pain syndromes can become chronic pain conditions. A study of 164 myofascial pain syndrome patients showed the mean duration of pain was 5.8 years for men and 6.9 years for women, with a mean of 4.5 clinicians seen in the past for the pain.[9] Chronic pain conditions not only cause disability due to pain but can also be responsible for related conditions, including depression, physical deconditioning due to lack of exercise, sleep disturbances, and other psychological and behavioral disturbances.[9, 22]

The persistent and chronic nature of untreated myofascial pain syndromes

TABLE 7–1.

Epidemiology of Trigger Points

Higher in women than men
Most common in 30- to 50-year age range
Most commonly found in the following muscles:
 trapezius, levator scapulae, axial postural
 muscles
Chronic pain clinics study reported incidence of
 85% of patients having myofascial pain
 syndrome
Asymptomatic shoulder girdle trigger points are
 found in 54% of females and 45% of males

explains the large numbers of myofascial pain patients seeking help at pain clinics. Understanding myofascial pain syndromes and fibromyalgia has become of major importance in pain management (see Chapter 5).

ETIOLOGY

Healthy muscles do not have active trigger points. Muscles become vulnerable when they are under acute or chronic stress.[17] Trigger points may occur in any skeletal muscle and arise from multiple causes (Fig 7–1). Trigger points may develop after prolonged periods of spasm, tension, stress, fatigue, and chill.[17] Stress and tension are among the most common causes of trigger points.[18] They occur most frequently in axial muscles used to maintain posture. This is due to the constant tension and microtrauma of poor postural habits, both in everyday living and in the workplace. Occupational or recreational activities which require repeated stress on a specific muscle or muscle group similarly cause

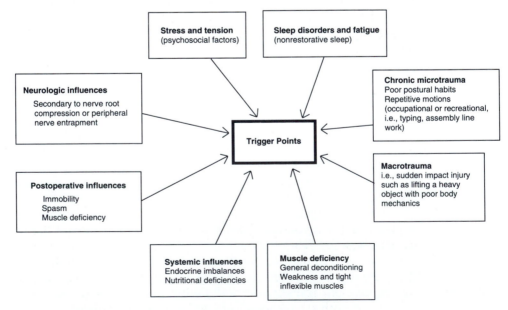

FIG 7–1. Trigger points—causes and contributing factors.

chronic stress leading to trigger points. Predisposing activities include holding a telephone receiver between the ear and shoulder to free the arms, prolonged bending over a table, sitting in chairs with poor back support and improper height of armrests or none at all, poor sitting posture when typing or working with computers for long periods, or loading heavy boxes using improper body mechanics (see Chapter 17).

Trigger points may develop in patients suffering from connective tissue disorders such as osteoarthritis, rheumatoid arthritis, and myositis.[28] Physical deconditioning secondary to chronic illness, or lack of exercise in general, may predispose patients to trigger points. Trigger points may develop in patients with fibromyalgia (see Chapter 1).

Nonrestorative sleep patterns (disturbance in stage 4 sleep) have been found by Moldofsky[24] to be a cause of muscular pain, and the development of tender points associated with fibromyalgia as well as myofascial pain syndromes.

Secondary trigger points may result in areas of pain due to nerve root compression from discogenic disease as well as peripheral nerve entrapment. Postlaminectomy pain may be due to trigger points which were present prior to surgery or developed afterward.[27, 29]

Although vitamin and nutritional deficiency may be found in patients with myofascial pain, the specific role of nutrition in the cause and treatment of myofascial pain syndrome requires further investigation and controlled studies. Vitamins are necessary for healthy neurologic functioning and oxygen metabolism. Adequate B vitamins such as thiamine, pyridoxine, niacin, and vitamin B_{12} are essential for healthy nerve function. Vitamin C is important for muscle and preventing capillary fragility. Nutritional deficiencies, including calcium, potassium, iron, and magnesium, may affect the irritability of myofascial trigger points.[50]

Multiple trigger points may result from endocrine imbalance, e.g., estrogen deficiency and hypothyroidism (see Chapter 3).

Acute and chronic trauma together with overuse syndromes commonly give rise to symptomatic trigger points. Trigger points are often overlooked in the treatment of athletic injuries. A common cause of failure in achieving therapeutic results in the management of tennis elbow is the lack of diagnosis and treatment of trigger points in the extensor and supinator muscles of the forearm.

Postoperative care of fractures and postoperative care after musculoskeletal surgery should include an examination for muscle tension, muscle deficiency, muscle spasm, and trigger points as a possible cause of persistent complaints. Soft tissue injury due to trauma or surgery, accompanied by inactivity, muscle tension, muscle spasm, and muscle deficiency, is a frequent cause of symptomatic trigger points.

Muscle Spasm

Muscle spasm is the painful involuntary contraction of muscle caused by chronic or acute trauma, excessive tension, or organic disorders. Aside from pain, muscle spasm creates shortening of muscles and limits motion. Untreated spasm and the "protective" immobility due to pain lead to decreased local blood flow in the muscles, causing more pain and contraction, resulting in a vicious cycle of muscle spasm and pain.

Muscle Tension

In our culture in which there is insufficient outlet to express the natural fight-or-flight response, we are all subject to tension.[17] Although the outlet for the release of tension is unavailable, the stimuli causing tension still exist. The result is prolonged contraction of muscles or muscle groups, ultimately causing pain. Tension may have postural, emotional, or situational causes. Postural tension occurs when a stressful position, such as holding the telephone between the shoulder and ear, or slouched sitting, is repeated frequently and for prolonged periods of time. Emotional tension can be triggered by pleasurable as well as unpleasurable emotional experiences, and causes muscular tension when it is constantly present. Situational tension arises when one is forced to adjust to unpleasant circumstances, such as an unpleasant work atmosphere.

Muscle Deficiency

Adequate muscular fitness is necessary to meet the daily requirements of walking, lifting, and stretching. When muscles are weak or stiff, they are considered deficient. When muscle deficiencies are present they make one prone to injury. Muscle deficiency itself can also be a source of pain. For example, weakening of abdominal muscles during pregnancy can bring on back pain. Premature ambulation after immobilization of the lower extremity can cause pain by overstretching and overloading tight, weak muscles.

The four types of muscle pain described by Hans Kraus, trigger points, muscle spasm, muscle tension, and muscle deficiency are interrelated and must be managed comprehensively (see Chapter 13 and Fig 8–1).

DEFINITION AND TYPES OF TRIGGER POINTS

Myofascial trigger points are small circumscribed hyperirritable foci in muscles and fascia, often found within a firm or taut band of skeletal muscle.[3, 17, 19, 49] Myofascial trigger points may also occur in ligaments, tendons, joint capsule, skin, and periosteum. They have been described as tender nodes of degenerated muscle tissue that can cause local and radiating pain. Historically, they have been referred to as *Muskelhärten* (muscle hardening) or *Myogelosen* (myogelosis) hardenings by Lang,[19] as myalgic spots by Gutstein,[12] and were later described as trigger points by Steindler.[45] Travel and Simons have published extensively on trigger points and referred pain patterns.[50] In regional myofascial pain syndromes trigger points may be limited to a single muscle or to several muscle groups.[19] Palpating the trigger point may elicit a local or referred pain pattern, or both, that are consistent and characteristic of the primary muscles involved.[3, 12, 17, 19, 38, 40, 49] The distant area of referred pain has been called the zone of reference.[40, 49] Referred pain patterns do not correspond to dermatomal, myotomal, or sclerotomal patterns. Kellgren[14] confirmed the specificity of muscular and ligamentous referred pain patterns by studying the effect of muscular injections using 0.1 to 0.3 mL of hypertonic saline. All referred pain patterns that have been reported have not been universally confirmed by clinical investigators.[25] Presenting symptoms may include pain; muscle weakness; decreased joint motion; paresthesia; autonomic symptoms, including sweating; lacrimation; localized vasoconstriction; coryza; and pilomo-

TABLE 7–2.

Myofascial Trigger Points: Symptoms and Physical Findings

Symptoms	Physical Findings
1. Local and referred pain patterns	1. Local tenderness
2. Pain with isometric/isotonic muscle contraction	2. Referred pain
	3. Single or multiple muscle involvement
3. Muscle stiffness and limited joint motion	4. Palpable nodules ("knots")
	5. Firm or taut bands in muscle
4. Muscle weakness	6. "Twitch response"
5. Paresthesia and numbness	7. Jump sign
6. Proprioceptive disturbances: loss of balance, dizziness, tinnitis	8. Muscle shortening
	9. Limited joint motion
7. Symptoms of autonomic dysfunction: lacrimation, coryza, pilomotor activity	10. Muscle weakness

tor activity. Trigger points that are located in the head and neck may cause proprioceptive disturbances such as problems with balance, dizziness, and tinnitus (Table 7–2). Trigger points may be classified as primary, secondary, satellite, active, or latent[50] (see Fig 7–2).

Primary trigger points develop independently and not as the result of trigger point activity elsewhere.

Secondary trigger points may develop in antagonistic muscles and neighboring protective muscles as the result of stress and muscle spasm. It is common for patients to experience the pain of a secondary trigger point after a primary trigger point is eliminated.

Satellite trigger points can develop in the area of referred pain as the result of persistent resting motor unit activity in the muscle.[50]

Patients may receive only partial or temporary relief from trigger point man-

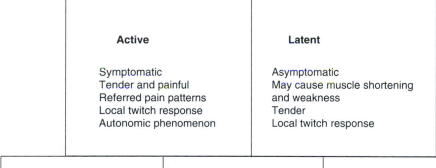

FIG 7–2. Types of trigger points.

agement if treatment is limited to secondary or satellite trigger points. Multiplication of trigger points results from the development of secondary and satellite trigger points. This chain reaction of trigger point multiplication may be initiated by several factors, including muscle weakness, postural abnormalities, and tension.[19] This combination of factors may sometimes explain the persistence of pain in the postlaminectomy patient, or "failed back syndrome."[27, 29]

Active trigger points are always tender, painful, and symptomatic. Pain may be present at rest and during motion. Palpation of the trigger point may cause a local or specific referred pain pattern, or both. Snapping palpation of a taut band of muscle fibers or needling of the trigger point may cause a visible "local twitch response" of the muscle or skin, or both. A more common reaction to trigger point palpation is the "jump response"[12]: the patient tends to jump or suddenly move away from the examiner's palpating hand. Movement to avoid pain is often accompanied by a vocal reaction. Referred pain patterns are specific for primary trigger points.[3, 11, 14, 17, 19, 41, 49] Specific knowledge and understanding of referred pain patterns are necessary to avoid the mistake of treating trigger points (satellite) in the referred pain areas and overlooking the primary trigger point. The most common trigger point locations are illustrated in Figure 8–4. Table 8–4 illustrates pain patterns frequently misdiagnosed as common orthopedic conditions.[27] See Appendix for diagrams of pain areas and common muscle trigger points that may be responsive for local or referred pain.

Latent trigger points are asymptomatic and do not require treatment unless they are activated. They are often found coincidentally on palpation. Latent trigger points are tender and may demonstrate a local twitch response. Although latent trigger points do not cause pain they may be a cause of muscle shortening and weakness. It is not uncommon to find latent trigger points on physical examination in patients who are asymptomatic. Latent trigger points are found most frequently in the shoulder girdle muscles, the trapezius and levator scapulae being the most common.[42, 43]

Uncertainty in diagnosis can exist when differentiating the tender points found in fibromyalgia[33, 39, 53] with the findings of trigger points in myofascial pain syndromes.[36, 37] Multiple, symmetric bilateral tender points occur in specific locations in fibromyalgia (see Chapters 1 and 2). Myofascial pain trigger points may occur in any skeletal muscle and may be singular or multiple. They may be found in the same locations as the tender points of fibromyalgia. When the findings of a palpable taut band, local twitch response, and referred pain pattern are present, the diagnosis of trigger point is obvious.[50] Confirmation of these findings by independent examiners, however, is not consistent enough to establish their presence as the sole criteria for the differential diagnosis between a tender point and trigger point.[25, 51] Taut muscle bands and muscle twitches were found commonly in subjects with no disease. A preliminary study of tender points and trigger points in persons with fibromyalgia, myofascial pain syndrome, and no disease found taut muscle bands and muscle twitches were common (50% and 30%, respectively) and noted equally in the three groups.[51]

At this stage of our knowledge of trigger point diagnosis and pathology, the significance of tender areas must be judged within the clinical context. It is not unusual for tender points and trigger points, as defined, to coexist in fibromyalgia, both requiring an appropriate therapeutic approach.

Small tender lipomas, which may represent fat herniations, may be found in the sacroiliac area. These tender nodules should not be mistaken for trigger points. Episacroiliac lipomas may refer pain to the groin and lateral aspect of the thigh.[26] Local anesthetic and steroid may be injected into the tender area with good therapeutic results. If symptoms return, surgery may be indicated. This is not a frequent surgical indication. Clinical correlation should strongly support this diagnosis before surgery is considered.

HISTOPATHOLOGY

Golgowsky and Wallraff[10] described biopsy findings in palpable hardenings of hip and back muscles. They found waxy degeneration of muscle fibers, destruction of fibrils, agglomeration of nuclei, and fatty infiltration. No control groups were included for comparisons. The findings were nonspecific.[52] Miehlke et al.[21] carried out biopsies of the upper trapezius, dividing them into four groups, groups 1 to 4 differing in symptomalogy and findings. Palpable hardenings were reported in groups 3 and 4. Biopsy of groups 3 and 4 demonstrated marked degeneration of the fibers as well as changes in the interstitial connective tissue. Yunus et al.[52] note that muscle fiber changes in groups 3 and 4 were similar to those reported by Golgowski and Wallraff,[10] but both studies were uncontrolled. Group 1 had generalized pain without palpable findings; biopsies in this group were normal. These studies indicate that trigger points may begin as a neuromuscular dysfunction and progress to a dystrophic pathologic state.

In a study conducted by Bengtsson et al.[1] 77 biopsies from 57 patients showed "motheaten" fibers in 35 of 57 patients and "ragged red fibers" in 15 of the 41 trapezius muscles biopsied.[8] Fassbender and Wegner[5] looked at biopsies of patients with probable myofascial pain syndromes of fibrositis. The majority of the biopsies were abnormal, initially showing swollen mitochondria and motheaten myofilaments, progressing to necrosis of myofilaments, progressing necrosis of myofilaments, irregularity of sarcomeres, and greatly reduced glycogen stores. The final stage examined demonstrated dissolution of contractile elements.[4] Other histologic studies of fibrositic tissue have confirmed the findings of Fassbender and Wegner, as well as changes in enzyme patterns and increased amounts of water, mucopolysaccharides, and ground substance.

Although abnormalities are reported they are nonspecific and inconsistent. The significance of these findings in relation to hormonal and abnormal clinical states remains unclear and requires further study[52] (Chapter 1).

The Pathophysiologic Development of a Trigger Point

The formation or activation of a trigger point may be due to an acute injury or chronic microtrauma to the muscle (e.g., sustained muscle contraction due to tension and poor posture). This stress creates a disruption of the sarcoplasmic reticulum which causes the release of free calcium ions. In the presence of adenosine triophosphate (ATP), the free calcium stimulates actin and myosin interaction and increased metabolic activity.[48] The increased metabolic activity activates an increase in the release of serotonin, histamine, kinins, and prostaglandins. These substances raise the sensitivity and firing of groups III and IV muscle nociceptors which converge with other visceral and somatic inputs, creating the perception of local and referred pain.[31, 34, 35] The pain, by way of the central nervous system, stimulates motor units, inducing muscle spasm and splinting. If the muscle spasm and secondary splinting go untreated a vicious muscle pain–spasm cycle is initiated, causing decreased local blood flow to the muscle, and therefore decreased ATP and calcium pump action. This results in

interaction of free calcium and ATP and increased contractile activity, perpetuating the pain-spasm cycle. Over time this cycle of events leads to sustained
noxious metabolites in the area which build up in the connective tissue, eventually creating localized fibrosis. The pain caused by the fibrotic tissue stimulates more motor unit firing, leading back to the muscle spasm cycle. The cycle
can be broken by restoring normal muscle length and addressing the cause and
contributing factors (Fig 7–3).

Mechanisms of Referred Pain

Selzer and Spencer[32] postulated five neurologic mechanisms to explain referred pain: (1) convergence-projection, (2) peripheral branching of primary af-

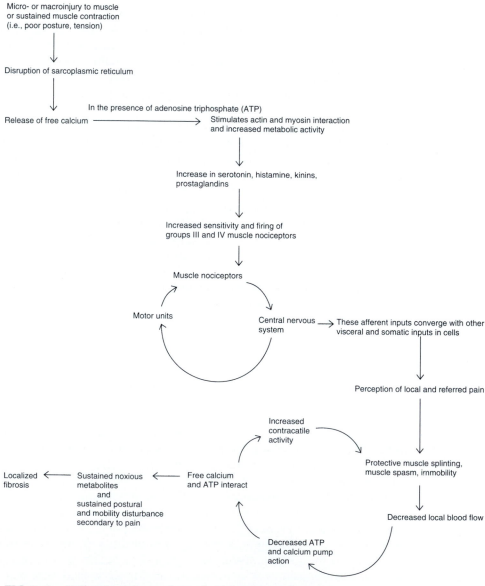

FIG 7–3. Pathophysiology of myofascial pain syndromes.

ferent nociceptors, (3) convergence-facilitation, (4) sympathetic nervous system activity, and (5) convergence or image projection at the supraspinal level.

Convergence-Projection. One nerve cell in the spinal cord may receive messages regarding pain from two different sources. The nerve may relay information about the internal organs and from nociceptors coming from the skin or muscles, or both. The brain has no mechanism for distinguishing whether the message comes from the skin, the muscles, or visceral organs. When the brain interprets messages it attributes the pain to the skin or muscles rather than internal visceral organs. Referred pain in trigger points may be pain which is "initiated by the muscle nociceptors but referred to the area served by other somatic receptors that converge on the spinothalamic tract cell."[37]

Peripheral Branching of Primary Afferent Nociceptors. A single neuron may serve several areas of the body by branching out. It is possible for the brain to interpret messages from one part of the body as coming from another. In the case of a nerve that serves both the leg and the lower back the message of pain in the back may be interpreted as coming from the leg.

Convergence-Facilitation. This hypothesis suggests that neural activity (somatic afferent impulses from the skin), which is generally below threshold, may be influenced in such a way by visceral impulses that they excite the spinothalamic tract fibers. This mechanism of pain production places the active myofascial trigger point in the position of acting as a peripheral pain generator.[32, 37]

Sympathetic Nervous System Activity. Stimulation of sympathetic nerves may cause pain in the referred pain area by two mechanisms: (1) by restricting blood flow to vessels that serve sensory nerve fibers and (2) releasing substances that sensitize primary afferent nerve endings in the area of referred pain.

Convergence or Image Projection at the Supraspinal Level. Pain pathways may converge at the thalamic or cortical level causing image projection of a referred pain pattern.

Mechanism of Pain Relief Following Stretch and Spray

Vapocoolant spray cools the skin by evaporating quickly. A sudden drop in skin temperature causes stimulation of skin afferent sensory fibers which affect polysynaptic reflexes in the spinal cord, closing the pain "gate" and preventing reflex hyperstimulation of muscle or the sensation of pain at higher centers. This temporary anesthesia then allows increased passive stretching of the muscle which has a direct therapeutic affect on the trigger point and restoration of normal muscle length[4] (Fig 7–4).

When cold, in the form of ice or vapocoolant spray, is applied to an area of the body, the metabolic rate and inflammation are decreased. Vasoconstriction causes a decreased blood flow in the area. The muscle can no longer contract once the metabolic rate drops. This cooling relieves muscle spasm. Nerve activity is also reduced. In the treatment of trigger points and muscle spasm, ice or vapocoolant spray is used to relieve pain and muscle spasm. Ethyl chloride spray is especially effective because it combines: (1) intense stimulation of a cold

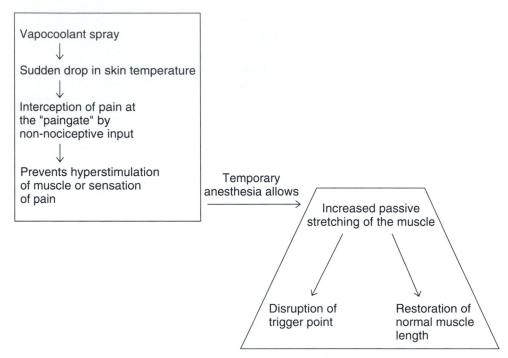

FIG 7–4.   Mechanism of pain relief following stretch and spray.

shock and rapid rate of change in skin temperature, (2) some degree of direct depression of cutaneous receptors by cooling, and (3) effects analogous to those produced by a light stroking massage[16, 46, 49] (see Chapter 9 for a discussion of fluorimethane and ethyl chloride vapocoolant spray).

MECHANISMS OF PAIN RELIEF FOLLOWING TRIGGER POINT INJECTION

Several mechanisms have been suggested, which, theoretically, may contribute to the inactivation of trigger points by injection.[50]

1. Mechanical disruption of the trigger point by disrupting muscle elements or nerve endings
2. Depolarization of nerve fibers due to the release of intracellular potassium which occurs with mechanical disruption of the muscle fibers
3. In contrast to dry needling, injected fluid, such as a local anesthetic or saline, diluting nerve-sensitizing substances
4. Local vasodilation effect of procaine increasing the energy supply and removal of metabolites in the area
5. Interruption of feedback mechanisms by local anesthetic
6. Focal necrosis depending on which local anesthetic is injected, as noted in animal experimentation[2]

In addition to the above, pain relief may occur due to an increase in endogenous opioids (i.e., neurohormonal β-endorphins or somatospecific dorsal horn enkephalins).[13]

ELECTROMYOGRAPHY

Electromyography (EMG) studies have shown that the trigger point and the associated taut band do not constitute a muscle spasm. A trigger point is electrically silent at rest and shows abnormal electrical activity when palpated.[4, 37] The muscle which harbors referred pain, however, is electrically active at rest.[47] It has been suggested that satellite trigger points develop as the result of this constant resting motor unit activity.[50] Simons[34] noted increased motor unit action potentials associated with the visible signs of a local twitch response following a snapping palpation of taut muscle bands. The motor unit electrical activity of the muscular bands with trigger points was found to be significantly higher than that of normal muscles tested.[7]

Sola and Williams[44] stimulated the area of the trigger point with negative galvanic current. This resulted in erythema over the trigger point area. They also used a neurodermanometer which indicated that there was decreased skin resistance in the area. They suggested that these findings indicate localized irritability around the trigger point due to an altered vascular motor activity.[44]

REFERENCES

1. Bengtsson A, Henriksson KG, Larsson J: Muscle biopsy in primary fibromyalgia: Light-microscopical and histochemical findings, *Scand J Rheumatol* 15:1–6, 1986.
2. Benoit PW: Effects of local anesthetics on skeletal muscle, *Anat Rec* 169:276–277, 1971.
3. Bonica JJ: Management of myofascial pain syndromes in general practice, *JAMA* : 732–738, June 1957.
4. Campbell SM, Bennett RM: *Fibrositis*, St Louis, 1986, Mosby–Year Book.
5. Fassbender HG, Wegner K: Morphologie und Pathogenese des Weichteilrheumatismus, *Z Rheumaforsch* 32:355–374, 1973.
6. Fishbain DA, Goldberg M, Steele R, et al: DSM-III diagnoses of patients with myofascial pain syndrome (fibrositis), *Arch Phys Med Rehabil* 70:433–438, 1989.
7. Fricton JR, Auvinen MD, Dykstra D, et al: Myofascial pain syndrome: Electromyographic changes associated with local twitch response, *Arch Phys Med Rehabil* 66:314–317, 1985.
8. Fricton JR, Awad EA, editors: *Advances in pain research and therapy*, vol 17, New York, 1990, Raven Press.
9. Fricton JR, Kroening R, Haley D, et al: Myofascial pain syndrome of the head and neck: A review of clinical characteristics of 164 patients, *Oral Surg* 60:615–623, 1985.
10. Glogowsky G, Wallraff J: Ein Beitrag zur Klinik und Histologie der Muskelhärten (Myogelosen), *Z Orthop* 80:237–268, 1951.
11. Good MG: Rheumatic myalgias, *Practitioner* 146:167–174, 1941.
12. Gutstein M: Diagnosis and treatment of muscular rheumatism, *Br J Phys Med* 1:302–321, 1938.
13. Hameroff SR, Crago BR, Blitt CD, et al: Comparison of bupivacaine, etidocaine, and saline for trigger-point therapy, *Anesth Analg* 60:752–755, 1981.
14. Kellgren JH: A preliminary account of referred pains arising from muscle, *Br Med J* 2:325–327, 1938.
15. Kraft GH, Johnson EW, LaBan MM: The fibrositis syndrome, *Arch Phys Med Rehabil* 49:155–162, 1968.
16. Kraus H: The use of surface anesthesia in the treatment of painful motion, *JAMA* 116:2582–2583, 1941.
17. Kraus H: *Clinical treatment of back and neck pain*, New York, 1970, McGraw-Hill.

18. Kraus H, editor: *Diagnosis and treatment of muscle pain*, Chicago, 1988, Quintessence.
19. Lang M: *Die Muskelhärten (Myogelosen)*, Munich, 1931, Lehmann.
20. Mense, In Fricton JR, Awad EA, editors: *Advances in pain research and therapy*, vol 17, New York, 1990, Raven Press.
21. Miehlke K, Schulze G, Eger W: Clinical and experimental studies on the fibrositis syndrome. *Z Rheumaforsch* 19:310–330, 1960.
22. Moldofsky H, Scarisbrick P, England R, et al: Musculoskeletal symptoms and non-REM sleep disturbance in patients with "fibrositis syndrome" and healthy subjects, *Psychosom Med* 37:1975.
23. Moldofsky H: Sleep and musculoskeletal pain, *Am J Med* 81(suppl 3A):85–89, 1986.
24. Moldofsky H, chairman: Workshop on sleep studies, *Am J Med* 81(suppl 3A):107–109, 1986.
25. Nice DA, Riddle DL, Lamb RL, et al: Intertester reliability of judgments of the presence of trigger points in patients with low back pain, *Arch Phys Med Rehabil* 73:893–898, 1992.
26. Pace JB: Commonly overlooked pain syndromes responsive to simple therapy, *Postgrad Med* 58:107–113, 1975.
27. Rachlin ES: Musculofascial pain syndromes, *Medical Times: The Journal of Family Medicine* January, 1984, pp 34–47.
28. Reynolds MD: Myofascial trigger point syndromes in the practice of rheumatology, *Arch Phys Med Rehabil* 62:111–114, 1981.
29. Rubin D: Myofascial trigger point syndromes: An approach to management, *Arch Phys Med Rehabil* 62:107–110, 1981.
30. Schiffman E, Fricton J, Daley D, et al: Prevalence and treatment needs of subjects with temporomandibular disorders, *J Am Dent Assoc* (in press).
31. Schwartz RG, Gall NG, Grant AE: Abdominal pain in quadriparesis: Myofascial syndrome as unsuspected cause, *Arch Phys Med Rehabil* 65:44–46, 1984.
32. Selzer M, Spencer WA: Convergence of visceral and cutaneous afferent pathways in the lumbar spinal chord, *Brain Res* 14:331–348, 1969.
33. Simms RW, Goldenberg DL, Felson DT, et al: Tenderness in 75 anatomic sites, *Arthritis Rheum* 31:182–187, 1988.
34. Simons DG: Electrogenic nature of palpable bands and "jump sign" associated with myofascial trigger points, *Adv Pain Res Ther* 1:913–918, 1976.
35. Simons DG: Myofascial trigger points, a possible explanation, *Pain* 10:106–109, 1981.
36. Simons DG: Fibrositis/fibromyalgia: A form of myofascial trigger points? *Am J Med* 8(suppl 3A):93–98, 1986.
37. Simons DG: In Fricton JR, Awad EA, editors: *Advances in pain research and therapy*, vol 17, New York, 1990, Raven Press.
38. Simons DG, Travell JG: Myofascial origins of low back pain: 1. Principles of diagnosis and treatment, *Postgrad Med* 73:99–108, 1983.
39. Smythe H: Referred pain and tender points, *Am J Med* 81(suppl 3A):90–92, 1986.
40. Sola AE: Treatment of myofascial pain syndromes. In Benedetti C, Chapman R, Moriocca R, editors: *Advances in pain research and therapy*, vol 7, New York, 1984, Raven Press, pp 467–485.
41. Sola AE: Trigger point therapy. In Robers JR, Hooges JR, editors: *Clinical procedures in emergency medicine*, Philadelphia, 1985, WB Saunders, 824–835.
42. Sola AE, Kuitert JH: Myofascial trigger point pain in the neck and shoulder girdle, *Northwest Med* 54:980–984, 1955.
43. Sola AE, Rodenberger MS, Gettys BB: Incidence of hypersensitive areas in posterior shoulder muscles: A survey of two hundred young adults, *Am J Phys Med* 34:585–590, 1955.
44. Sola AE, Williams RL: Myofascial pain syndromes, *Neurology* 6:91–95, 1956.
45. Steindler A: *Lectures on the interpretation of pain in orthopedic practice*, Springfield, Ill, 1959, Charles C Thomas.
46. Travell J: Ethyl chloride spray for painful muscle spasm, *Arch Phys Med* 33:291–298, 1952.
47. Travell J: Myofascial trigger points: Clinical view. In Bonica JJ, Albe-Fessard D, editors: *Advances in pain research and therapy*, vol 1, New York, 1976, Raven Press, 919–926.

48. Travell J: Identification of myofascial trigger point syndromes: A case of atypical facial neuralgia, *Arch Phys Med Rehabil* 62:100–106, 1981.
49. Travell J, Rinzler SH: The myofascial genesis of pain, *Postgrad Med* 11:425–434, 1952.
50. Travell JG, Simons DG: *Myofascial pain and dysfunction: The trigger point manual*, Baltimore, 1983, Williams & Wilkins.
51. Wolfe F, Simmons DG, Fricton J, et al: The fibromyalgia and myofacial pain syndromes: A preliminary study of tender points and trigger points in persons with fibromyalgia, myofascial pain syndrome and no disease, *J Rheumatol* 19:944–951, 1992.
52. Yunus MB, Masi AT, Aldag JC: A controlled study of primary fibromyalgia syndrome: Clinical features and association with other functional syndromes, *J Rheumatol* 16:62–71, 1989.
53. Yunus MB, Masi AT, Calabro JJ, et al: Primary fibromyalgia (fibrositis): Clinical study of 50 patients with matched normal controls, *Semin Arthritis Rheum* 11:151–171, 1981.

Chapter 8

History and Physical Examination for Regional Myofascial Pain Syndrome

Edward S. Rachlin, M.D.

Therapeutic results in the management of regional myofascial pain due to a trigger point pathologic condition depend on an accurate diagnosis and total assessment of all factors related to muscle pain. Myofascial trigger points should not be evaluated as a single entity, but as one component of interrelated causes of muscle pain (muscle spasm, muscle tension, muscle deficiency, and trigger points) (see Chapter 13 and Fig 8–1). The necessity for a thorough history and physical examination cannot be overemphasized (Table 8–1).

The physician who treats patients with myofascial pain must not only be knowledgable but interested in the patient as a human being. A proper history takes time and should not be rushed. All factors contributing to the pain must be investigated. A history of trauma and the findings of trigger points may not in themselves be sufficient to explain the occurrence of symptoms, the patient's progress, or the chronicity of symptoms. An attack of pain may be precipitated by emotional problems, tension, business strain, physical activities at work, or athletic activities to which the patient is unaccustomed. Endocrine problems (e.g., hypothyroidism) may contribute to the development and prolongation of myofascial pain. A complete medical and surgical history should be obtained to rule out other causes of pain, followed by a history focused on myofascial pain.

HISTORY

The myofascial pain history emphasizes the patient's current complaints, the history of onset, characteristics of pain, referred pain patterns, and the factors that precipitate and prolong symptoms. Information is obtained concerning previous episodes of pain, treatment, and response to treatment.

Current Complaints

Current complaints may include pain, stiffness, fatigue, deep tenderness, muscle weakness, restricted joint motion, a specific referred pain pattern, autonomic symptoms (e.g., lacrimation, coryza), and proprioceptive disturbances (e.g., dizziness, poor balance).

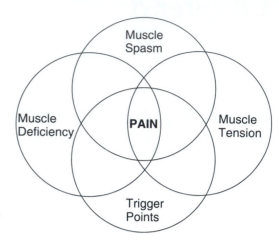

FIG 8–1.   The four interrelated types of muscle pain.

Characteristics of Pain

Location and Type of Pain

Patients are asked to point to the area of pain with one finger. They may be given a body diagram and asked to describe the location and type of pain they are experiencing by noting it on the diagram (Fig 8–2). If the patient complains of hip pain when referring to the back, or speaks of a generalized pain, a drawing will help him or her to be more specific. The drawing can be completed by

TABLE 8–1.

Patient Evaluation: History and Physical Examination for Myofascial Pain Syndrome*

A. History
  1. Medical and surgical history
    a. System review
    b. Trauma
    c. Previous medical conditions and treatment
    d. Surgical procedures
    e. Chronic debilitating disorders (e.g., arthritis)
    f. Endocrine disorders
    g. Dental problems
    h. Allergies
    i. Medications
  2. History related to myofascial pain
    a. Characteristics of pain
    b. History of onset: current and past episodes
    c. Occupational activities
    d. Athletic activities
    e. Sleep problems
    f. Psychological factors which contribute to tension
    g. Endocrine symptoms
    h. Temporomandibular joint symptoms

B. Physical examination
  1. Complete physical examination as indicated
  2. Observation of patient's posture and movement
  3. Postural examination
  4. Muscle evaluation
    a. Range of motion
    b. Flexibility of muscles
    c. Muscle strength
    d. Muscle spasm
    e. Muscle tension
    f. Trigger points
  5. Neurologic examination
C. Diagnostic studies (as indicated)
  1. Laboratory tests
    a. Blood chemistries, urinalysis
    b. CBC
    c. ESR
    d. T_3, T_4 RIA
  2. Radiologic studies
    a. CT scans
    b. MRI
    c. Myelogram
  3. Neurologic testing
    a. EMG and nerve conduction studies

*CBC = complete blood count; ESR = erythrocyte sedimentation rate; T_3 = triiodothyronine; T_4 = thyroxine; RIA = radioimmunoassay; CT = computed tomography; MRI = magnetic resonance imaging; EMG = electromyography.

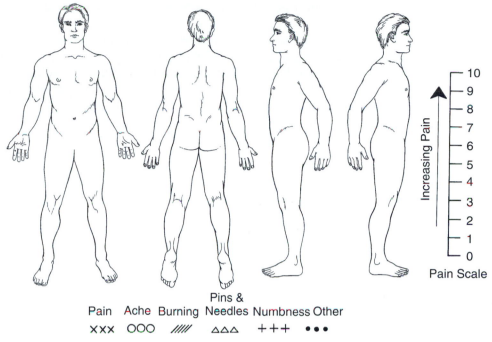

Pain	Ache	Burning	Pins & Needles	Numbness	Other
✕✕✕	○○○	/////	△△△	+++	●●

FIG 8–2.   Pain drawing.

the patient or the examiner. Areas are marked using different symbols representing different types of sensations (e.g., pain, ache, burning, numbness, pins and needles). Referred pain patterns can be visualized. On the drawing, the patient can indicate precisely where the pain is located, indicating which area is most or least frequently painful. The sequence of the history of the symptoms can be noted. The drawing not only serves as a useful way to identify the presenting problem but also becomes a record for comparison with pain on later visits so that recovery can be observed. A series of such drawings represent a pictorial description of the patient's clinical course.

Patient's Rating of Pain

The patient is asked to rate his or her pain on a scale of 0 to 10 (0 = no pain, 10 = extreme pain). This number is written down or marked on the scale and may be used as a future indicator of the patient's progress (see Fig 8–2). An additional body diagram can be used by the examiner to mark tender points and trigger points.

Description of Pain

Patients are asked to describe their pain. Is the pain constant or intermittent? What is the type of pain (i.e., deep, dull, burning, shooting, localized, diffuse, radiating)?[8, 9] If the patient describes a referred pain typical of cervical and lumbar radiculopathy, disc involvement should be ruled out. Active trigger points in the lumbar, gluteal, trapezius, and levator scapulae areas may cause symptoms resembling nerve root compression.[13] The referred pain may be felt close to the primary trigger point or may be a distance away. Specific referred pain patterns are characteristic of myofascial trigger points. Referred pain patterns do not follow dermatomal, myotomal, or sclerotomal patterns (see Table 8–2).

Effects of Rest and Activity

Is the pain relieved by rest or activity? Trigger points may cause pain at rest or can be aggravated by physical activity. Passive and active motion of shortened muscles harboring trigger points elicit pain. Pain after exertion may result from muscle weakness. Pain that occurs with the onset of movement following rest is typical of arthritis or muscle stiffness. Pain of sudden onset with lightning radiation and persistence may indicate nerve root involvement and must be differentiated from radiating pain due to trigger points. Pain may be caused by improper posture or tension. Pain of delayed onset after trauma is typical of muscle strain, and activation of trigger points (active or latent). Trigger point pain which occurs after inactivity can be relieved by short periods of joint movement. Trigger point pain which occurs after activity can be relieved with moist heat, slow gentle stretching, and short periods of rest.

Pain Relief

What have patients found to be effective in relieving their pain? Patients may have treated themselves for some time by taking hot baths or applying hot packs or ice. They may have been treated previously by other health practitioners. Ask about the positive and negative effects of prescription and over-the-counter drugs that they have been or are taking. Ask if they have received physical therapy (modalities and manual) and what the effects of physical therapy were. Were they given an exercise program with proper supervision and instruction on how to perform the exercises? (See Chapter 13.)

History of Onset

When was the patient first aware of the pain? Is there a history of physical or emotional trauma? Did the pain occur suddenly or increase over a prolonged period of time? Was there a specific incident or activity which preceded it? Knowledge of the activity can give clues to which trigger point may have been activated.

Patients with trigger points frequently have a history of pain in a specific muscle or muscle group which recurs following specific activities or situations. Symptoms may be of several years' duration. Patients may experience long periods of remissions during which time trigger points may be asymptomatic and which are referred to as latent trigger points. Latent trigger points are found most frequently in shoulder girdle muscles.[27, 28]

Review of Contributing Causes

Prolonged muscle tension or recurrent spasm. Patients with trigger points often describe muscle spasms and tension. Muscle spasm occurs in muscles which have been shortened owing to prolonged inactivity. Pain may be most intense upon awakening because of the shortened position of the muscle during sleep. Any activity which requires the patient to remain in a fixed position for a length of time may have this effect.

Pain Related to Occupational Activities

Inquire about the patient's job and how the work is performed. Repetitive movements, poor postural attitudes at work, and poor body mechanics may give rise to trigger points or aggravate latent trigger points. Permanent relief of symptoms will require instruction in proper posture and body mechanics. Emotional stress in the workplace should not be overlooked as a contributing factor in muscle tension.

Properly constructed chairs should be available for sedentary work. Does the patient sit in a chair of proper height, with a back support, and proper supportive armrests to prevent muscle tension and stress? Constant tightening and hunching of the shoulders is a common cause of cervical and trapezius pain in drivers and typists. Holding a telephone between the ear and shoulder to free both hands when talking for long periods is a frequent cause of neck pain. Muscle tension and strain during the workday owing to poor body mechanics or environmental conditions must be addressed if therapy is to succeed (see Chapter 17).

Athletic Activities. Does the patient exercise regularly? Do exercises include stretching and relaxation, warm-up, and cool-down? Most patients with regional myofascial pain syndrome and fibromyalgia will give a history of inactivity. Fibromyalgia patients will profit from an aerobic exercise program (see Chapter 2). Trigger points are frequent sequelae of athletic injuries resulting from micro- and macrotrauma. In taking an athletic history, details concerning the nature of the activity are necessary to determine the factors contributing to the onset and prolongation of symptoms. A knowledge of techniques unique to specific sports may be helpful in treating athletic injuries. Trigger points are a frequent cause of tennis elbow. This may result from faulty tennis equipment, poor stroke, or prolonged unaccustomed playing (overuse syndrome). Excessive repetitive movements such as practicing tennis serves or hitting a bucket of golf balls may produce or activate latent trigger points in the shoulder girdle muscles. Back pain in a tennis player may be caused by arching the back in performing an American twist serve. In this case treatment must be extended to correcting the serving technique.

Tension. Emotional stress and tension play a major role in muscle tension and trigger point formation.[23] It is essential to take a psychosocial history to find out if the patient is suffering from business, personal, family, or marital problems. Does the patient like his or her work? Is there constant stress in the workplace? Is the patient receiving psychotherapy? Does the patient appear tense? It is important to prescribe ways of decreasing stress as part of the treatment programs. Examples of ways to decrease stress are:

- Hobbies (e.g., music)
- Taking a walk
- Aerobic exercise
- Biofeedback
- Deep relaxation techniques, meditation
- Psychological counseling
- Couples/family counseling
- Altering occupational circumstances, e.g., workload, personal interrelationships
- Drug therapy (if necessary, prescribed by a physician)

Fishbain et al.[4, 5] found a high incidence of depression, anxiety, conversion (somatosensory disorders, alcohol and drug dependence, and personality disorders) among chronic pain patients. This does not imply that all people with pain suffer from these conditions, but does imply that there may be a link between muscle pain and mental, emotional, and personality disorders.[4, 5]

Stress and tension may be related to a past history of duodenal ulcer, ulcerative colitis, emotional depression, sleep disorder, or irritable colon.

Arthritis.   Does the patient have a history of joint pain and swelling? Pain, decreased joint mobility, and shortening of muscles predispose the surrounding muscles to the development of trigger points.[24] Muscles surrounding arthritic joints often harbor active trigger points which are overlooked as a source of pain and weakness in arthritic patients. During examination for signs of myofascial disorders Reynolds[24] found that the number of tender points and local twitch responses in women with rheumatoid arthritis was twice that found in women free of rheumatic illness. A study of 164 patients with head and neck myofascial pain syndromes showed that 42% of patients had a codiagnosis of joint problems. It is suspected that the reflex muscle splinting, which occurs as a means to protect a painful joint from aggravating movement, contributes to the development of trigger points.[7] A similar process develops in patients who suffer from chronic debilitating diseases.

Trauma and Surgery.   Is there a history of trauma or surgical procedures? Injuries and surgical procedures may lead to the formation of trigger points causing repeated episodes of pain. Patients who have had back surgery are more likely to have trigger points than those who have not. Active or latent trigger points may be present prior to, or may result from surgery. Preoperative and postoperative evaluation for trigger points is necessary to prevent unnecessary surgery and improve postoperative results.

Endocrine Disorders.   Myofascial pain and trigger points may be associated with hypothyroidism and estrogen imbalances.[26, 29] Signs of hypothyroidism include: brittle nails, dry skin, hair loss, constipation, depression, dry hair, difficulty losing weight, feeling cold, lethargy, and menstrual irregularity. Is the patient menopausal? Was menopause associated with hot flashes, vaginitis, or nervousness? Was estrogen given? Treatment of trigger points will not give lasting relief if endocrine problems contributing to muscle disorders are not treated. Endocrine problems should be treated prior to beginning trigger point injections (see Chapter 3 for discussion of the endocrine aspects of myofascial pain).

Dental Problems.   Grinding or clenching of the teeth may play a role in neck and upper back pain. This can be related to mechanical disturbances involving the teeth and temporomandibular region as well as to tension (see Chapter 11).

Dentists and orthodontists have noted that bite difficulties, regardless of their origin (teeth, temporomandibular joint, emotional problems), often result in tension, and later in spasm and trigger points of the masticatory muscles[14] (see Chapter 11).

Sleep Problems.   Sleep disturbance is frequently associated with both myofascial pain syndrome and fibromyalgia. Patients report insomnia, waking in the night with inability to return to sleep, or inability to fall asleep. The diagnosis of fibromyalgia syndrome includes multiple bilateral tender points found in specific locations together with a frequent history of unrestorative sleep (see Chapters 1 and 2). Does the patient wake up with pain or stiffness? Unrestorative sleep as a cause of myofascial trigger points has been described by Moldofsky.[18-20] Is there a cause of sleeplessness (e.g., pain, sleep apnea, psychological stress)?

Neurologic Symptoms.   Does the patient have symptoms of muscle weakness, sensory loss, or paresthesia? Symptoms related to proprioceptive disturbances include dizziness, tinnitis, and problems with balance (unsteady gait). Patients may complain of lacrimation or coryza due to autonomic dysfunction. Are there bladder or bowel irregularities? Trigger points may cause symptoms of nerve entrapment or referred pain patterns that may be mistaken for nerve root compression (e.g., disc herniation)[13, 22] (Table 8–2).

Routine Inquiries.   Before treating a patient with a trigger point injection one must make several routine inquiries: Is the patient diabetic? Is there a history of allergy? Is the patient allergic to procaine or lidocaine? Is the patient on medications, particularly anticoagulants? Does the patient have a bleeding disorder? Does the patient have a history of fainting? Is pain experienced in other parts of the body (e.g., other joints or muscles)? Multiple areas of pain may indicate a systemic disease. Is the patient pregnant? History of recent and past infections (e.g., hepatitis, human immunodeficiency virus (HIV)–positive). Does the patient have or has he or she recently had a local or systemic infection? The presence of infection is a contraindication to trigger point injection (see Chapter 9 for contraindications to trigger point injections).

PHYSICAL EXAMINATION

A complete physical examination is performed as indicated. The physical examination should include observation of the patient's movement and posture, testing of range of motion, muscle strength, and neurologic integrity, palpation of muscles, and algometry, if available (see Chapter 6).

A general physical examination with appropriate laboratory testing is important whenever the possibility of a systemic disease is present and to rule out other causes of muscle pain. Emphasis of the examination will differ according to the nature of the patient's complaints. The examination will elicit information to evaluate muscle abnormalities (spasm, tension, muscle deficiency, trigger points), skeletal and postural abnormalities, and neurologic dysfunction.

Observation

Observe the patient's movement during the history taking. A person suffering from myofascial trigger points learns how to move in ways that are least painful. The patient may hold the neck stiff or walk with a shortened gait in order to limit movement that causes muscle pain. The practitioner sensitive to this will carefully observe the way the patient enters the room, the way the patient walks, sits, and holds his or her head. Does the patient list to one side? This may be due to a disc lesion, but is more often caused by acute muscle spasm in the back due to muscle strain. It may also be a result of trigger points. Does

TABLE 8–2.

Pain Patterns Frequently Misdiagnosed as Common Orthopedic Conditions*

Locations of Muscular Trigger Points	Pain Pattern	Commonly Confused With Trigger Point Pain
Temporal, masseter, and occipital muscles	Radiation to head, headache, neck pain	Cervical arthritis, cervical syndrome
Sternocleidomastoid	Neck pain	Meniere's disease, intracranial abnormality
Scalenus muscles, posterior neck muscles	Dizziness, numbness in 4th and 5th fingers, headaches	Peripheral nerve entrapment, cervical syndrome
Trapezius (upper)	Neck and shoulder pain	Cervical arthritis
Supraspinatus	Arm pain	Cervical disc, bicipital tendinitis
Infraspinatus	Arm pain	Cervical disc, bursitis of shoulder, bicipital tendinitis
Rhomboid (upper and lower)	Interscapular, scapular, and dorsal pain	Arthritis of dorsal spine, glenohumeral arthritis, radiculopathy
Pectoral	Arm pain	Bursitis (shoulder), cardiac pain, cervical radiculopathy
Deltoid	Upper back, neck, and arm pain	Cervical radiculopathy, bursitis (shoulder)
Forearm muscle group	Forearm and elbow pain	Epicondylitis
Sacrospinalis	Pain radiating downward to buttock	Sciatica, herniated disc
Tensor fascia, gluteus medius	Pain radiating to lateral aspect of thigh and leg	Herniated disc, bursitis
Piriformis	Sciatic radiation	Herniated disc
Adductor longus	Groin pain	Arthritis of hip, adductor muscle strain
Gastrocnemius	Calf and leg pain	Tennis leg, plantaris tendon or gastrocnemius rupture
Soleus	Heel pain	Calcaneal bursitis, Achilles tendinitis
Adductor hallucis	Pain in metacarpophalangeal (MCP) joint area of big toe	Gout, arthritis of MCP joint of big toe
Tibialis anterior	Pain in front of leg and big toe	Herniated disc, anterior compartment syndrome
Vastus medialis semimembranosus, sartorius	Knee pain	Chondromalacia, arthritis of knee
Peroneus longus	Ankle pain	Arthritis of ankle
Interossei of foot	Foot pain, radiating to toes	Morton's neuroma, metatarsalgia

*From Rachlin ES: Musculofascial pain syndromes, *Medical Times, The Journal of Family Medicine*, January 1984, pp 34–47. Used by permission.

the patient show signs of tension by maintaining the shoulders in an elevated posture during the interview and not relaxing the upper extremities?[23]

Postural Examination

Evaluate key postural muscles when appropriate. Structural measurements for skeletal abnormalities such as scoliosis, leg length measurements, and chest expansion are done. Poor postural habits, including forward head position, rounded shoulders, slouched sitting, and knee hyperextension, are noted.

Muscle Evaluation

Joint Mobility

Trigger points may cause shortening of muscles, limited joint motion, and joint contractures. Pain may accompany any attempt to extend the joint. Some patients may not be aware of the restricted motion which may develop insidiously due to inactivity and lack of full use ("functional disuse"). Limited joint motion may also be a cause of trigger points (Fig 8–3).

Muscle Strength

A muscle evaluation comparing the left and right sides is performed. Joint stiffness and muscle weakness may be the presenting symptoms. If the patient has complaints referable to the back, perform the Kraus-Weber test to evaluate muscle deficiencies (see Chapter 13). The Kraus-Weber test is not performed if the patient is in acute pain.

Muscle Tension

Muscle tension may be the cause of the patient's pain. Does the patient let go or tighten up when asked to perform certain motions? Reflexes that are difficult to obtain without distraction may be a sign of tension. Tension can be evaluated in the Kraus-Weber test when patients are asked to slowly reach toward the floor with their knees straight. The tense patient may reach farther on the second attempt when instructed to "relax and let go." Does the patient maintain his or her shoulder in a hunched position?

Muscle Spasm

Muscles in spasm may be hard, rigid, and inflexible. Muscle spasm must be relieved before the examiner can palpate specific trigger points. Proper trigger point examination requires the muscles to be relaxed. The patient should be reevaluated after muscle spasm has been successfully treated (see Chapter 9 for discussion of postinjection physical therapy program).

Trigger Points

Trigger points can be diagnosed by palpation of muscle. The patient may be able to direct the physician to the trigger point and describe the area of local and referred pain. Generally, the examiner uses tips of the fingers with the hand relaxed and the fingers slightly bent. If the patient's muscles become tense it is necessary to wait until they are relaxed again. As noted above, trigger points cannot be diagnosed if the muscle is in spasm. If the patient has normally firm

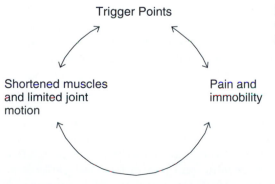

FIG 8–3. Muscle shortening and decreased joint motion secondary to trigger points.

muscles or excessive adipose tissue the examiner may place one hand on top of the other to increase the strength of the palpating hand. Trigger point tenderness must be differentiated from the tenderness typical of fibrositis. In fibrositis the subcutis is characterized by tenderness elicited by rolling and squeezing the skin.[14]

Trigger points may be identifiable to the examiner as tender, small hard knots or nodules, or a tender area in a firm taut band of muscle fibers surrounded by normal muscle tissues.[9] Trigger points may measure 2 to 5 mm in diameter.[6] The firm localized area may also be palpated when the muscle is gently stretched. The patient will report pain when the trigger point is touched and may jump away from the examiner's hand, wince, or cry out (a reaction known as the "jump response").[9] A local "twitch response" (muscle or skin twitch) may be visible as the trigger point is palpated or touched with a needle. A trigger point will often refer pain to a distant area. Patterns of referred pain are specific and constant for individual muscles. A knowledge of referred pain patterns is necessary to know where to look for the primary trigger point which requires treatment. Lasting results are only achieved when the primary trigger point is treated.[9, 15, 16, 30]

Trigger points occur most frequently in the muscles used to maintain posture (axial muscles) (Fig 8–4). They may occur as a single muscle trigger point or in multiple muscles. Examine neighboring muscles and the antagonists for secondary trigger points, which often become painful after the primary trigger point is eliminated. The gluteal muscles should be included when examining the lumbar area. A cervical examination should include the anterior cervical as well as the posterior muscles. The finding of local tenderness in a taut band of muscle fibers together with a local twitch response and referred pain has not been diagnosed with sufficient consistency by independent examiners in a controlled blind study to consider their presence as absolute requirements for the diagnosis of trigger point.[21, 32] In a recent study, taut muscle bands and muscle twitches were common and found equally in persons with fibromyalgia, myofascial pain, and no disease.[32] The clinical findings for the identification of trigger points, as described by Travell and Simons,[31] may not always be present in regional myofascial pain syndrome (MPS). The interpretation of the findings of tenderness depends on clinical correlation.

Tender Points

Tender points are subjective areas of tenderness, not accompanied by other signs of trigger points (Table 8–3). Multiple bilateral symmetric tender points in specific areas are found in fibromyalgia. Agreement is lacking in deciding the actual number of tender points required for diagnosis (see Chapter 1).[25, 33] Tender points and trigger points can occur simultaneously in fibromyalgia patients. The American College of Rheumatology has established criteria for the classification of fibromyalgia in addition to empirical criteria suggested for the diagnosis of MPS (see Chapter 1). Diffuse multiple tender areas or multiple trigger points may indicate an endocrine problem which requires investigation. The significance of the finding of tenderness must be judged within the clinical context. Tenderness may not represent the tender points of fibromyalgia or the trigger points of MPS. The patient who is "tender all over" may represent a case of psychogenic rheumatism. Psychological factors, factors related to secondary pain, individual pain perception, and pain behavioral patterns must all be considered in evaluating the subjective complaint of tenderness. Melzak et al.[17]

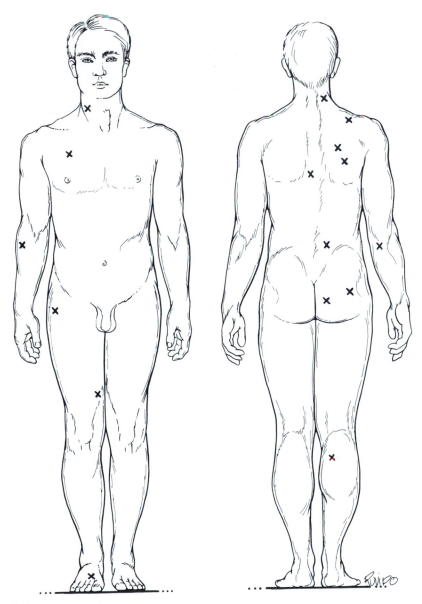

FIG 8–4.   Most frequent locations of myofascial trigger points.

noted a high degree of correspondence (71%) between the spatial distribution and associated pain patterns of trigger points and acupuncture points.

Neurologic Examination

A neurologic examination is performed for evidence of nerve root pressure, peripheral nerve entrapment, disc herniation, and neurologic disease. Trigger points may cause nerve entrapment. Examination includes testing for reflex loss, pathologic reflexes, sensory loss, and localized muscle weakness. Examination for referred pain patterns due to trigger points in the lumbar area include straight leg raising tests in addition to testing for hip joint abnormalities. The clinician will also examine for findings of autonomic dysfunction, i.e., sweat-

TABLE 8–3.

Trigger Points vs. Tender Points

Trigger Points	Tender Points
1. Local tenderness, taut band, local twitch response, jump sign	1. Local tenderness
2. Can be singular or multiple	2. Multiple
3. May occur in any skeletal muscle	3. Occur in specific locations and are symetrically located
4. Specific referred pain pattern	4. Do *not* cause referred pain
5. May have autonomic and proprioceptive symptoms	

ing, lacrimation, localized vasoconstriction, coryza, and pilomotor activity. Proprioceptive findings may include unsteadiness, poor balance, abnormal gait, or lack of dexterity.

Algometry

Algometry can be a valuable asset in the diagnosis of myofascial pain. Local tenderness can be assessed by using a pressure gauge devised by Fischer[3] (see Chapter 6). Tolerance to pressure is lower in areas where trigger points are present than in areas of normal muscle. The patient's sensitivity to pain is described by the pressure threshold, the minimum pressure or force that causes the patient discomfort, and by the pressure tolerance, the maximum pressure tolerated.[1, 2]

Tissue compliance is the consistency of the tissue with regard to its resistance to pressure.[3] The tissue compliance meter developed by Fischer enables a quantitative measurement of the softness or firmness of the muscle tissue. The meter is pressed against the skin and gauges the depth of penetration for a given amount of pressure (see Chapter 6).

Jaeger and Reeves[10] used the pressure algometer to quantify changes in myofascial trigger point sensitivity following passive stretching. They found that the trigger point sensitivity decreased in response to passive stretching and that intensity of referred pain is related to the sensitivity of the associated trigger point.[10]

Dermographia has been reported both in myofascial pain syndromes (T1) as well as in fibromyalgia. Yunus et al.[34] have found that if mechanical or chemical stimulation is applied in a uniform and standardized way, dermographia can be regarded as the most objective finding in primary fibromyalgia.

PAIN PATTERNS TYPICAL OF SPECIFIC MYOFASCIAL TRIGGER POINTS

Referred pain patterns are characteristic of individual muscle trigger points[9, 11, 12, 14, 16, 30] (see Chapter 10 and Appendix). The primary trigger point may be distant from the area of complaint. A knowledge of pain patterns enables the physician to locate the primary trigger point responsible for symptoms (see Table 8–2).

Trigger points may be found in any skeletal muscle. Figure 8–4 illustrates the most frequent locations of myofascial trigger points encountered in orthopedic practice (see Chapter 11 for common head and orofacial trigger points). Trigger points may represent more than a single muscle (see Fig 8–4). The areas illustrated are:

1. Posterior neck muscles
2. Sternocleidomastoid and scalenus muscles
3. Trapezius
4. Infraspinatus
5. Supraspinatus
6. Levator scapula, rhomboid, thoracic paraspinalis
7. Lumbar paraspinalis (sacrolumbar), quadratus lumborum
8. Gluteal muscles (maximus, medius, minimus), tensor fasciae latae, piriformis
9. Rectus femoris, vastus medialis
10. Flexor and extensor muscles of the forearm
11. Pectoral muscles (major, minor)
12. Foot muscles (interossei)

Trigger points causing referred pain patterns are often overlooked as the cause of symptoms and confused with common orthopedic diagnoses, e.g., cervical disc herniation, bicipital tendonitis, bursitis, arthritis, and lumbar disc herniation. Table 8–2 demonstrates referred pain patterns of trigger points which may be erroneously diagnosed as representing specific common orthopedic conditions. Preoperative muscle evaluation and treatment may avoid necessary surgery and will increase the success of surgery if it is necessary.

After completion of the history and physical examination, appropriate laboratory work may be indicated, depending on the findings and the area of the body to be treated. Basic laboratory work-up may include: blood chemistries, complete blood count (CBC), sedimentation rate, urinalysis, triiodothyronine (T_3) and thyroxine (T_4) radioimmunoassays, and serum levels of vitamins B_1, B_6, B_{12}, folic acid, and vitamin C if vitamin deficiency is suspected as a cause of trigger points.[31] Routine roentegenograms and further studies include computed tomography (CT) scans, magnetic resonance imaging, myelogram, or electrical diagnostic studies. Consultation may include neurologic, rheumatologic, psychological, orthopedic, and, less frequently, vascular when arterial disease must be ruled out (e.g., Leriche's syndrome as a cause of buttock and leg pain). There are no abnormal routine laboratory findings or radiographic studies diagnostic of regional MPS.

REFERENCES

1. Fischer AA: Advances in documentation of pain and soft tissue pathology, *Medical Times, The Journal of Family Medicine*, December 1983, pp 24–31.
2. Fischer AA: Diagnosis and managemnt of chronic pain in physical medicine and rehabilitation. In Ruskin AP, editor: *Current therapy in physiatry: Physical medicine and rehabilitation*, Philadelphia, 1984, WB Saunders.
3. Fischer AA: Tissue compliance meter for objective, quantitative documentation of soft tissue consistency and pathology, *Arch Phys Med Rehabil* 68:122–124, 1987.

4. Fishbain DA, Goldberg M, Meagher R, et al: Male and female chronic pain patients categorized by DSM-III psychiatric diagnostic criteria, *Pain* 26:181–197, 1986.
5. Fishbain DA, Goldberg M, Steele R, et al: DSM-III diagnoses of patients with myofascial pain syndrome (fibrositis), *Arch Phys Med Rehabil* 70:433–438, 1989.
6. Fricton JR: Clinical care for myofascial pain, *Dent Clin North Am* 35:1–26, 1991.
7. Fricton JR, Awad EA, editors: *Advances in pain research and therapy*, vol 17, New York, 1990, Raven Press.
8. Good MG: Rheumatic myalgias, *Practitioner* 146:167–174, 1941.
9. Gutstein M: Diagnosis and treatment of muscular rheumatism, *Br J Phys Med* 1:302–321, 1938.
10. Jaeger B, Reeves JL: Quantification of changes in myofascial trigger point sensitivity with the pressure algometer following passive stretch, *Pain* 27:203–210, 1986.
11. Kellgren JH: A preliminary account of referred pains arising from muscle, *Br Med J* 2:325–327, 1938.
12. Kellgren JH: Observations on referred pain arising from muscle, *Clin Sci* 3:175–190, 1938.
13. Kraus H: "Pseudo-disc," *South Med J* 60:416–418, 1967.
14. Kraus H: *Clinical treatment of back and neck pain*, New York, 1970, McGraw-Hill.
15. Kraus H, editor: *Diagnosis and treatment of muscle pain*, Chicago, 1988, Quintessence.
16. Lang M: *Die Muskelhärten (Myogelosen)*, Munich, 1931, Lehmann.
17. Melzack R, Stillwell DM, Fox EJ: Trigger points and acupuncture points for pain: Correlations and implications, *Pain* 3:3–23, 1977.
18. Moldofsky H, Scarisbrick P, England R, et al: Musculoskeletal symtoms and non-REM sleep disturbance in patients with "fibrositis syndrome" and healthy subjects, *Psychosom Med* 37:341–351, 1975.
19. Moldofsky H: Sleep and musculoskeletal pain, *Am J Med* 81(suppl 3A):85–89, 1986.
20. Moldofsky H, chairman: Workshop on sleep studies, *Am J Med* 81(suppl 3A):107–109, 1986.
21. Nice DA, Riddle DL, Lamb RL, et al: Intertester reliability of judgments of the presence of trigger points in patients with low back pain, *Arch Phys Med Rehabil* 73:893–898, 1992.
22. Rachlin ES: Musculofascial pain syndromes, *Medical Times, The Journal of Family Medicine* January 1984, pp 34–37.
23. Rachlin ES, Kraus H: Management of back pain, *Intern Med* 8:1987.
24. Reynolds MD: Myofascial trigger point syndromes in the practice of rheumatology, *Arch Phys Med Rehabil* 62:111–114, 1981.
25. Simons DG: Fibrositis/fibromyalgia: A form of myofascial trigger points? *Am J Med* 8(suppl 3A):93–98, 1986.
26. Sola AE: Trigger point therapy. In Robers JR, Hedges JR, editors: *Clinical procedures in emergency medicine*, Philadelphia, 1985, WB Saunders, pp 674–686.
27. Sola AE, Kuitert JH: Myofascial trigger point pain in the neck and shoulder girdle, *Northwest Med* 54:980–984, 1955.
28. Sola AE, Rodenberger MS, Gettys BB: Incidence of hypersensitive areas in posterior shoulder muscles: A survey of two hundred young adults, *Am J Phys Med* 34:585–590, 1955.
29. Sonkin LS: Myofascial pain in metabolic disorders. In Kraus H, editor: *Diagnosis and treatment of muscle pain*, Chicago, 1988, Quintessence, 91–95.
30. Travell J, Rinzler SH: The myofascial genesis of pain, *Postgrad Med* 11:425–434, 1952.
31. Travell JG, Simons DG: *Myofascial pain and dysfunction: The trigger point manual*, Baltimore, 1983, Williams & Wilkins.
32. Wolfe F, Simons DG, Fricton J, et al: The fibromyalgia and myofascial pain syndromes: A preliminary study of tender points and trigger points in persons with fibromyalgia, myofascial pain syndrome and no disease, *J Rheumatol* 19:944–951, 1992.
33. Yunus MB, Denko CW, Masi AT: Serum B (β)-endorphin in primary fibromyalgia syndrome: A controlled study, *J Rheumatol* 13:183–186, 1986.
34. Yunus MB, Masi AT, Aldag JC: A controlled study of primary fibromyalgia syndrome: Clinical features and association with other functional syndromes, *J Rheumatol* 16:62–71, 1989.

Chapter 9

Trigger Point Management

Edward S. Rachlin, M.D.

INDICATIONS FOR TRIGGER POINT INJECTION

Not all trigger points require needling. Many active trigger points may respond to a physical therapy program (see Chapters 13, 14, and 15). This is especially true in the early stages of trigger point formation (the neuromuscular dysfunctional stage) prior to the development of fibrotic pathologic changes (the dystrophic stage) (Fig 9–1). Trigger point injection and needling is the most effective and best treatment in cases of chronic trigger points with fibrotic scar formation. Trigger point injection is indicated in patients who have symptoms and findings consistent with active trigger points (trigger points causing symptoms). Latent trigger points are asymptomatic and do not require treatment. Latent trigger points may cause muscle stiffness and weakness which often is not noticed by the patient. They are often found on routine examination in asymptomatic persons as incidental findings.[14]

To be considered for injection, trigger points should be reasonably limited in number and suitable for injection therapy. Multiple tender points and trigger points found in patients suffering from fibromyalgia or endocrine disturbances are not suitable for initial trigger point injection therapy. Evaluation and treatment is indicated before considering trigger point injection (see Chapter 3). After several weeks of endocrine therapy the patient is reevaluated to determine which tender spots or trigger points remain. The finding of tenderness in itself is not an indication for trigger point injection. The significance of tenderness requires an understanding of the total clinical context (see Chapter 7 under Definition and Types of Trigger Points). Patients with fibromyalgia may also have myofascial pain trigger points. It is not unusual to find both conditions coexisting.

Active trigger points will usually require treatment before placing the patient on an exercise program. Exercise in the presence of trigger points may activate symptoms. A noninvasive therapeutic approach including physical therapy modalities (see Chapter 15), soft tissue mobilization techniques (see chapters 13 and 14), and an exercise program may be tried prior to injection therapy. The post–trigger point injection follow-up program described below is recommended as a conservative therapeutic treatment approach. Active exercise is a vital part of the treatment program to achieve therapeutic results and

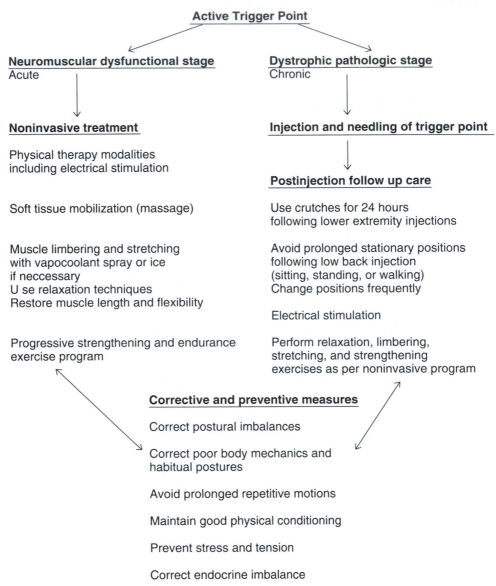

FIG 9–1.   Treatment of myofascial trigger point.

prevent recurrences. The patient may respond favorably to any or all of the physical therapy techniques. Injection and needling of trigger points is a beginning, not an end, to therapy. It enables the patient to begin a therapeutic exercise program, which must be incorporated in a comprehensive treatment plan for the management of myofascial pain (Fig 9–2).

Muscle tenderness must be correlated with other clinical factors. In treating pain due to trigger points it is not always necessary to require the finding of a taut band and local twitch response with a referred pain pattern on palpation to determine that injection is appropriate. A recent study of intertester reliability of judgments of the presence of trigger points in patients with low back pain in which 12 randomly paired therapists examined 50 patients for 197 trigger points using the criteria of Travell and Simons[16] disclosed that different therapists were unable to reliably determine when a trigger point is present in a patient with low back pain. This study was limited to low back pain patients and

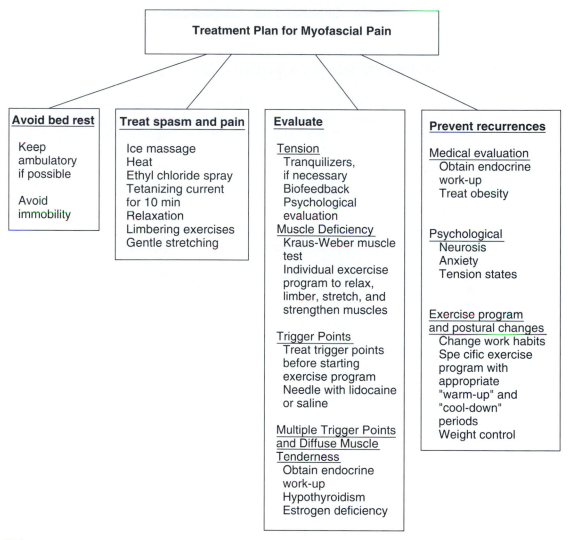

FIG 9–2. Treatment plan for myofascial pain.

cannot be generalized to patients with other diagnoses.[12] Further controlled studies of the reliability of referred pain patterns are indicated. Many of the reported referred pain patterns are common; others are rare.

Depending on the total clinical context, the finding of tender points in the classic areas of trigger point locations coinciding with the patient's complaints, together with a "jump sign," is sufficient to justify trigger point injection. In cases of referred pain it is not sufficient to inject only the trigger point in the referred pain area (zone of reference). The primary trigger point causing the pain must be found and treated to obtain a lasting result (see Fig 8–4 and Table 8–2).

CONTRAINDICATIONS TO TRIGGER POINT INJECTION

1. Do not inject in the presence of systemic or local infection.
2. Do not inject patients with bleeding disorders or patients on anticoagulants without proper medical evaluation and control.

3. Avoid injections in patients who are pregnant.

4. Avoid injections in patients who appear to be or feel ill.

REASONS FOR FAILURE IN TRIGGER POINT INJECTION

1. Success in trigger point injection depends on the ability of the patient to receive proper postinjection follow-up care (see below). Patients who are unable to receive follow-up care, as outlined later in this chapter, owing to occupational circumstances, lack of medical facilities, or problems related to traveling a long distance to the treatment facility, should not begin a program involving trigger point injections. Injection of ligamentous trigger points does not require the follow-up trigger point injection program because ligamentous trigger points do not cause the muscle spasm that is often seen after muscular trigger point injection.

2. Patients with multiple trigger points due to endocrine disturbance (e.g., hypothyroidism [see Chapter 3] or fibromyalgia [see Chapters 1 and 2]) should receive appropriate systemic care and be reevaluated before attempting any local injections to relieve symptoms.

3. Do not inject while muscles are in spasm. Muscular trigger points cannot be properly diagnosed in the presence of muscle spasm. Muscle spasm must first be treated (see below for follow-up management of trigger point injections, and Chapter 15 for the treatment of muscle spasm.) Palpation of trigger points becomes possible after muscle relaxation is achieved.

4. Emotionally unstable patients do not respond well to surgically invasive procedures[7] and also are unpredictable. Some patients receive no relief whereas others become addicted to all forms of treatment and request repeated injections, always receiving some relief but never enough to discontinue treatment. This type of treatment requires both professional judgment and integrity as to whether to start treatment and how long to continue it. Decisions may sometimes be clearer after a short period of treatment.

5. Patients with low pain thresholds will usually find the experience very tension-provoking and do not do well. Tranquilizers (diazepam [Valium]) may be tried prior to injection.

6. Do not inject more than one trigger point area at a time. For example, inject the gluteal and lumbar areas on separate visits. Multiple site injections covering many areas cause muscle spasm and irritation which interfere with muscle rehabilitation.

7. Tenderness in the referred pain area may represent secondary trigger points or satellite trigger points and not the primary trigger points causing the patient's symptoms. Limiting injections to trigger points in the referred pain area and omitting the primary trigger point will give only temporary relief.

8. Do not omit the injection of trigger points in neighboring muscle groups which contribute to symptoms.

9. Do not use procaine or lidocaine in patients who are allergic to these drugs. Avoid aspirin-like drugs 1 week prior to injections.

10. In adequate medical work-up, e.g. omitting radiographs or other tests necessary for proper diagnosis.

11. Complications of injection may include puncture of the lung, entering a major blood vessel, neurologic symptoms, infection, allergic reaction. Injections must be performed cautiously with a knowledge of the local anatomy and proper technique (see discussion of complications, below).

12. Avoid using needles that are too thin or too short to accomplish trigger point needling.

TRIGGER POINT INJECTION TECHNIQUE

Equipment

The basic equipment for trigger point injection includes the following (Fig 9–3):

- Povidone-iodine (Betadine).
- Sterile gauze pads, 4 × 4 in.
- Forceps.
- Clamp.
- Needles:
    16-gauge 1.5-in. for withdrawal of anesthetic solution.
    22- to 25-gauge 1.5-in. for scalenus and sternocleidomastoid muscles, and interrosei.
    25-gauge 1.5-in. for temporomandibular joint muscles.
    22-gauge 1.5-in. for cervical and suboccipital areas, upper extremities, and ankle and foot.
    21-gauge 2.0-in. for extremities.
    20- to 21-gauge 3-in. for lumbar and gluteal areas.
    25-gauge 2.0-in. for gastrocnemius (a thinner gauge is used because of muscle sensitivity).

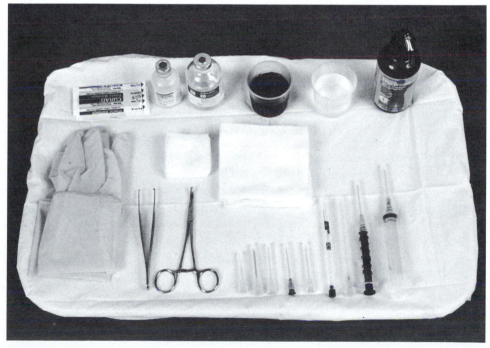

FIG 9–3. Basic equipment for trigger point injection includes sterile gloves, sterile gauze pads, forceps and clamp, povidone-iodine (alcohol may be used in addition), lidocaine, isotonic saline, vapocoolant spray, needles and syringes of various sizes, Band-Aids. See text for details.

If sterilization equipment is available, nondisposable needles and syringes may be used.

- A tray with sterile covering is used to hold syringes and needles of various sizes. These are determined depending on the muscle injected.
- Sterile gloves.
- Vapocoolant spray (ethyl chloride or fluorimethane).
- Plastic strip bandages (Band-Aids).
- Solutions for injections 0.5% procaine, 1% lidocaine, isotonic saline. Do not use epinephrine. Isotonic saline or dry needling may be used in patients who are allergic to local anesthetics. Steroids may be used for ligamentous trigger points.
- Procaine or lidocaine may be used for local anesthetic.

Procaine hydrochloride 0.5% (Novicain) exhibits the following characteristics:

1. Potent vasodilation.
2. Relatively high incidence of allergic reactions (typical of ester-type local anesthetics).
3. Short action.
4. Onset of action 6 to 10 minutes.
5. Lower systemic toxicity.

Lidocaine hydrochloride 1% (Xylocaine) exhibits the following characteristics:

1. Allergic reactions are virtually nonexistent (amide local anesthetic).
2. Rapid onset of action.
3. Longer duration than procaine.
4. Greater potency.
5. More profound anesthesia

Long-acting anesthetics (e.g., bupivacaine) have also been used.

Dry Needling

The elimination of trigger points by needling depends mainly on the mechanical disruption of the trigger point rather than the solution used during injection. A study by Jaeger and Skootsky[5] noted reduction in local trigger point tenderness to be only dependent on penetration of the trigger point with a needle. Reduction in the referred symptoms of myofascial pain was greater with injection of a solution but was independent of the kind used (saline and procaine were used).[5]

Dry needling is effective.[9] However, greater postinjection pain has been reported.[9, 10] The effectiveness of treatment has been found to be related to the intensity of pain produced at the trigger zone and the precision in needling the exact site of maximal tenderness. The immediate analgesia produced has been called the "needle effect."[9] Garvey et al.[2] found trigger point therapy to be a useful adjunct in the treatment of low back pain. They found the injected substance is apparently not the critical factor, since direct mechanical stimulus to the trigger point gave symptomatic relief equal to that of treatment with various types of injected medication.

Steps in Injection Technique

Communicate with the patient. Inform the patient that pain is to be expected when a trigger point is encountered and explain the importance of indicating when pain is felt. The use of local anesthetic provides a short period of pain relief following the injection. It is not used to avoid the feeling of pain when the trigger point is encountered. Although trigger points may sometimes be felt with the tip of the needle as hard nodules and fibrotic areas, we depend on the patient's reaction to confirm the contact with a trigger point. A needle inserted into normal tissue will not normally cause complaints of pain. Patients readily learn to distinguish between the sensation in normal muscle and the pain felt when a trigger point is encountered. Most of the time patients will tell their physician whether a trigger point has been encountered. Pain may be experienced locally in addition to referred pain.

1. The patient is positioned comfortably. The position will depend on the muscle to be injected. It is best to do injections with the patient lying down. Vasodepressor syncope (fainting) can occur during or after local anesthetic injection. Advising the patient to take deep breaths in and out, concentrating on breathing during the injection, will help in decreasing pain sensation and promote relaxation. Communicate with the patient during the injection. In unusual cases, relaxation techniques, self-hypnosis, or tranquilizers (diazepam) to relax the patient sufficiently for trigger point injection may be necessary.

2. Identify the primary trigger point and bony landmarks. It is important to know the anatomy of the area to perform the injections properly and avoid complications. Distinguish between primary trigger points and trigger points in referred pain areas. Frequently, multiple trigger points are found involving neighboring muscles. The most symptomatic trigger points are injected first. Trigger points in neighboring muscles may become symptomatic and require treatment after the primary trigger point has been eliminated. When injecting more than one trigger point or muscle group a second trigger point may be injected 2 days later while the patient is receiving follow-up care for the preceding trigger point injection.

3. Trigger point injection is performed under sterile conditions. Sterile gloves are worn after surgical washing of the hands. Sterile gloves permit identification of trigger points by palpation after surgical preparation of the skin and immediately prior to injection. The ability to palpate the trigger point avoids the necessity of scratching the skin with a needle to mark the trigger point area. A sterile covered tray is used to receive instruments (clamps, syringes, needles, and sponges). An assistant opens the packages of sterile and selected syringes and needles and places them on the tray. Fig 9–4 shows the equipment used

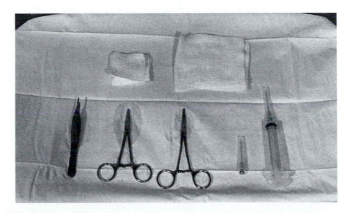

FIG 9–4. Instruments to be used are placed on a sterile tray.

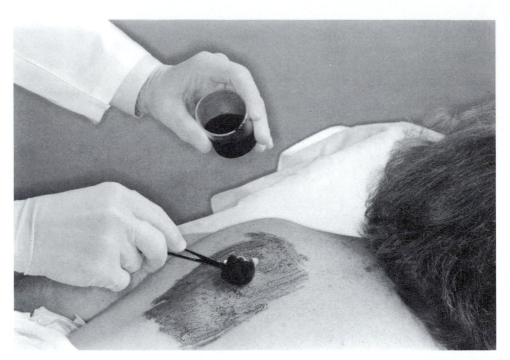

FIG 9–5.   Skin is prepared with povidone-iodine using sterile technique. Provide a generous area of sterility.

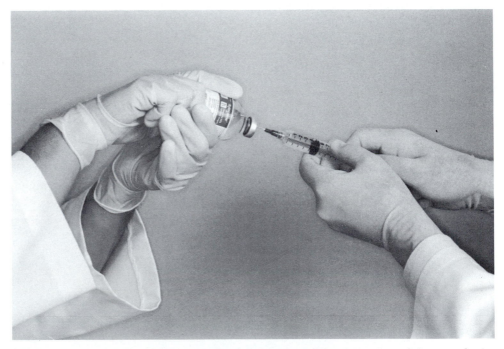

FIG 9–6.   Assistant holds the lidocaine bottle inverted for aspiration of the anesthetic.

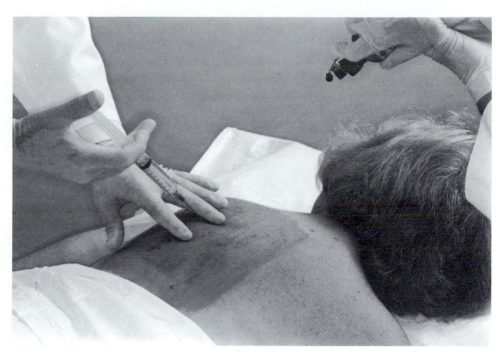

FIG 9–7. Application of a vapocoolant spray prior to injection decreases needle insertion pain.

for trigger point injection. When injection is performed the sterile tray will have only those needles and syringes which are to be used. It is best to keep syringes and needles out of the patient's sight.

4. The skin is prepared with povidone-iodine using 4- × 4-in. gauze pads. Drape the area of injection if necessary (Fig 9–5). Be aware of the sterile area which is demarcated by the povidone-iodine preparation. Do not violate sterility by touching the unsterile surroundings.

5. The assistant holds the lidocaine bottle inverted; usually 10 mL of lidocain is withdrawn (Fig 9–6). Do not use epinephrine.

6. Prior to injection, the assistant may spray a vapocoolant sparingly on the site chosen for injection. An anesthetic spray decreases needle insertion pain, thereby decreasing the patient's anxiety and muscle tension prior to injection (Fig 9–7). Avoid excessive use of vapocoolant spray which increases bleeding immediately following injection and may frost the skin. The use of sterile gloves permits palpation and the identification of trigger points immediately prior to injection and enables the physician to isolate the trigger points between two fingers (Fig 9–8) or between the fingers and thumb (Fig 9–9). A taut band may or may not be palpated. The patient is reminded to take slow deep breaths and to inform the physician when pain is felt.

7. When a trigger point is encountered, several milliliters of anesthetic is injected. Do not inject anesthetic prior to the patient noting that a trigger point has been encountered. The patient may experience local or referred pain, or both. A muscle twitch is often seen when the trigger point is struck. The trigger point may feel fibrotic. If the anesthetic is injected prematurely trigger points will not be recognized. Palpation must be performed for additional areas of tenderness before concluding that all trigger points were found and injected. After injection and needling the patient may quickly note relief of symptoms.

If a "no-touch" sterile technique (no hand-to-skin contact) is used, two

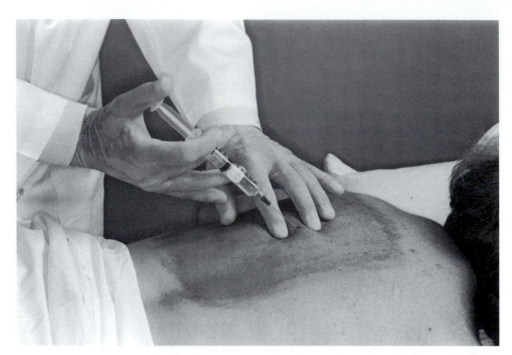

FIG 9–8.   Injection of trigger point in the left rhomboids. Using under sterile precautions the trigger point may be isolated between the index and middle fingers.

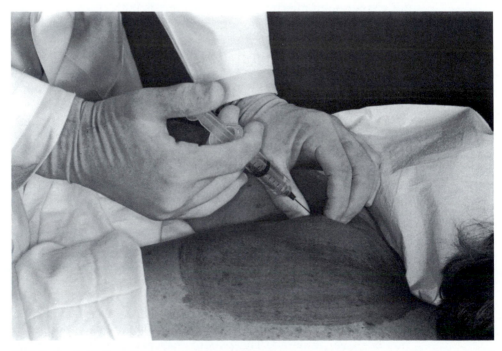

FIG 9–9.   Injection of trigger point isolating the trigger point between the fingers and thumb.

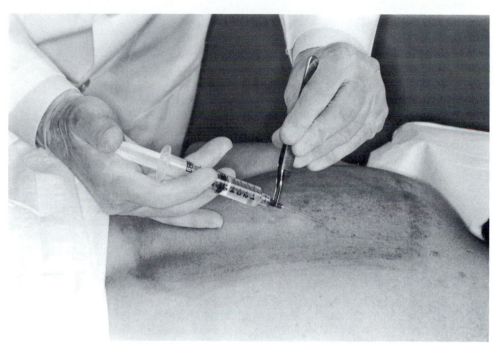

FIG 9–10. No-touch technique using forceps to control the stability and direction and depth of the syringe and needle.

hands are required for injection. The stability of the syringe and needle is accomplished by using forceps to hold the hub of the needle or syringe to control the depth and direction of needling. Sterility of the skin should not be violated (Fig 9–10). The trigger point is marked with a needle scratch for identification prior to injection.

8. Technique of injection may include multiple entries into a single muscle using different entry points, in addition to using a single entry and withdrawing but not bringing the needle out of the skin and changing directions in a circular fanlike covering of the trigger point area (Fig 9–11). The needle is used in a probing fashion in search of additional trigger points. Needling is performed without withdrawing the needle, which is moved in and out in different directions in a controlled fashion. A combination of techniques can be used. Trigger points are most often found in the areas of origin and insertion.

The multiple dry needling technique resembles that used by Gunn[3] in treating muscle shortening and muscle spasm based on his theory of the neuropathic cause of myofascial pain. Gunn uses an acupuncture technique using acupuncture needles. Although the techniques appear to overlap, the concept and the objective are quite different. Needling is referred to as intramuscular stimulation based on a neuropathic origin for musculoskeletal pain rather than a local phenomenon found in myofascial structures such as muscle fascia or ligaments.[3] Tenderness is found in the area of motor points.[4]

9. Aspirate prior to injection. This is extremely important when the possibility of entering arteries, large veins, and penetrating the chest cavity is present. The needle should be angled tangentially, and not vertically, when injecting in the area of the chest wall to avoid entering the intercostal space (Fig 9–12) (see discussion of complications, below). A needle 1.0 to 1.5 in. long should be used when injecting the region of the chest wall. Do not inject if blood or bubbles are aspirated when injecting in the chest area. The needle depth

FIG 9–11. **A,** single-entry injection using a circular fanlike covering of the trigger point area. **B,** multiple separate needle entries for needling and injection. **C,** combination of multiple needle entries and circular fan technique of individual trigger point area.

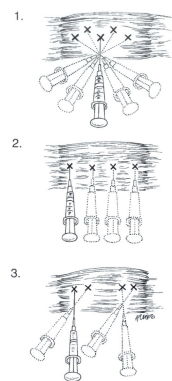

FIG 9–12. Injection of pectoralis muscles. Needle is directed tangentially in relationship to the chest cavity, avoiding the intercostal space. The syringe is stabilized with one hand to control the direction and depth of the needle once the trigger point is encountered. Aspirate prior to injection. Avoid pneumothorax.

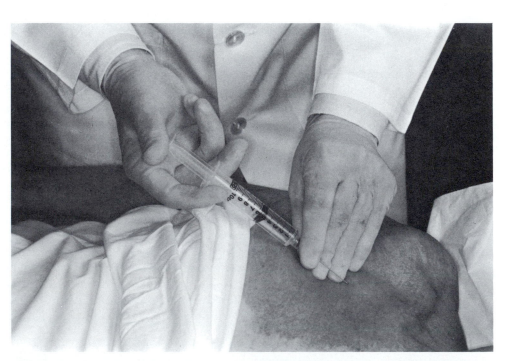

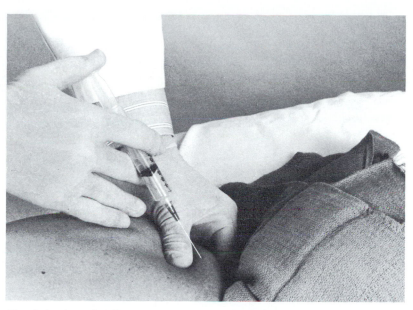

FIG 9–13.   Injection of right trapezius muscle. Grasp the trapezius between the thumb and index finger, elevating the trapezius muscle to avoid puncturing the chest cavity (see Chapter 10).

should be well controlled and the syringe stabilized when injecting in the chest wall area. Stabilize the syringe with the hand holding the syringe resting gently on the patient, holding the hub of the needle and syringe between the thumb and index finger while aspiration is performed. After aspiration with the syringe and needle still stabilized in the same position, injection is performed. To avoid entering the chest cavity when injecting the trapezius, elevate the trapezius muscle by grasping the muscle between the thumb, index, and middle fingers and gently lifting the muscle (see Fig 10–36). Aspirate prior to injections (Fig 9–13). The same technique is used for injection of the sternocleidomastoid muscle (Fig 9–14). The needle should be directed parallel to the frontal plane of the patient or tangential to the patient when injecting the quadratus lumborum and lumbosacral muscles (Fig 9–15 and Fig 10–1).

10. Do not inject if severe cramping pain is felt. Cramping pain is typical of radiculopathy and may represent a needle encountering a nerve.

11. If bleeding is encountered, remove the needle and apply pressure over the injected area to diminish hematoma formation.

12. Band-Aids are applied over each puncture area following the injection unless the patient is allergic to adhesives. Figure 9–16 shows a patient who has had trigger point injections for the rhomboids.

13. Inquire about unusual sensations, e.g., numbness, paresthesia, and muscle weakness, in the lower or upper extremities, depending on the injection given. The patient should remain on the treatment table for a few minutes following injection therapy.

14. For successful and lasting therapeutic results the trigger point injection is only the first step in relieving symptoms. The patient should be treated on 3 or 4 successive days following the trigger point injection and adhere to the trigger point follow-up program in its entirety (see below).

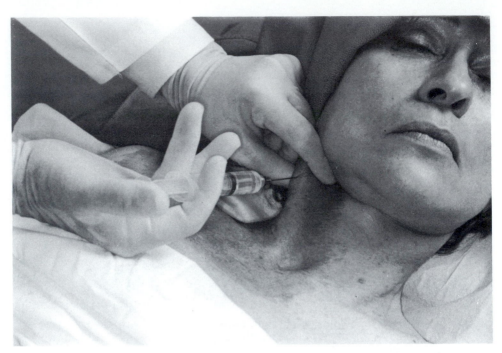

FIG 9–14. Injection of sternocleidomastoid muscle is performed by grasping the muscle between the thumb and index finger to localize the trigger point area and control localization of the needle. Aspirate prior to injection. Avoid the external jugular vein (see Chapter 10).

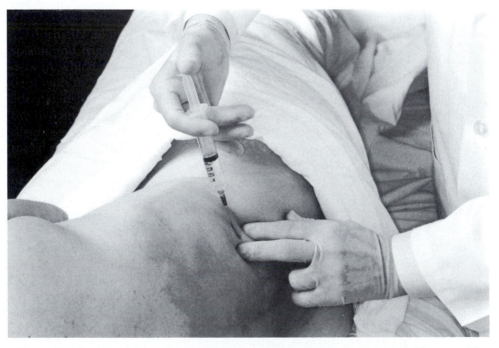

FIG 9–15. Positioning of the needle for injection of the quadratus lumborum. The needle is directed parallel or tangentially to the frontal plane of the patient.

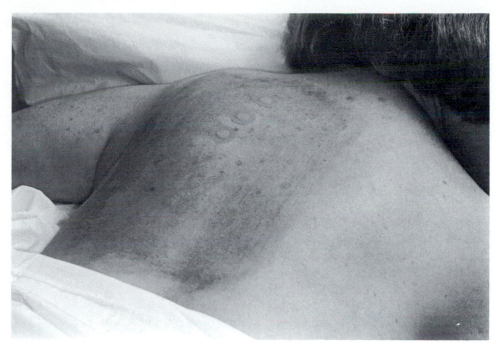

FIG 9–16. Band-Aids are applied over the injection sites of the left rhomboid muscles.

The injection of muscle groups, rather than individual muscles, is usually performed, e.g., injection and needling of the gluteal area includes the glutus maximus, minimus, and medius, the pectoralis major and minor, and the thoracolumbar paraspinal muscles.

Injection for Ligamentous Trigger Points

Ligamentous trigger point injections are given directly into the area of tenderness. Steroid is often used with a local anesthetic. The postinjection follow-up program is not necessary for ligamentous trigger point injection. Although it is not usual to require physical therapy for muscle spasm following a ligamentous trigger point injection, the conditioning of muscles and the use of physical therapy for both therapeutic purposes and prevention must not be overlooked.

Patient Advice

Patients should be advised of the possible complications of trigger point injection (see discussion of complications, below). The patient should be aware that although pain may be relieved almost immediately, more often pain and muscle soreness may persist for several days. Infection is a potential complication. The patient should be alerted to any signs of unusual swelling, progressive pain, and warmth and redness occurring in the area of the injection. These signs, together with temperature elevation, should alert the patient and physician to the possibility of infection. The patient should be reassured that areas of ecchymosis following injection are frequent and will be reabsorbed.

When injecting more than one muscle or muscle group the next trigger point may be injected 2 days later while the patient is receiving follow-up care for the preceding trigger point injection.

PHYSICAL THERAPY PROGRAM FOR FOLLOW-UP MANAGEMENT OF TRIGGER POINT INJECTIONS (NONINVASIVE THERAPY PROGRAM)

Therapeutic success following trigger point injection depends on the ability to provide proper follow-up care. The postinjection follow-up program and exercise regimen is based on the methodology of Dr. Hans Kraus.[7] The physical therapy program outlined below is performed after injection and must be followed in its entirety. The same therapeutic program is used as a noninvasive treatment approach when trigger point injection may not be necessary. Each injection should be followed by 3 to 4 successive days of physical therapy treatments to relax the muscle, avoid muscle spasm, and relieve postinjection pain. Therapy includes electrical stimulation, vapocoolant spray and gentle limbering motions, and stretching techniques (active and passive) followed by an exercise program. Active motion is an important part of the stretching as well as the exercise program. Relaxation must be achieved prior to stretching.

The prevention and treatment of muscle spasm is a vital part of the physical therapy program and is the first objective to be addressed. The following principles should be observed[7]:

1. Relief of pain.
2. Gentle movements to achieve relaxation, flexibility, and normal muscle length.
3. Do not pass the pain limit.
4. Do not cause pain with movement.

Postinjection Physical Therapy Program

Electrical Stimulation. Electrical stimulation is given to relieve and prevent the muscle spasm that often follows trigger point injection and needling. Electrical stimulation (sinusoidal current, surged, ramped) is administered for 15 minutes. If spasm is present in treating low back pain precede the sinusoidal current with 10 minutes of tetanizing current to fatigue the muscle. Electrical stimulation also aids in treating postinjection hematoma and edema. Tetanizing current can enhance the production of β-endorphins for mild anesthesia in addition to muscle relaxation (see Chapter 15). Some patients find electrical stimulation uncomfortable, promoting tension rather than relaxation. These patients are best treated with moist heat or infrared. (Heat should be used with caution immediately after multiple trigger point injections to prevent hematoma.) Electrical stimulation is used in preparation for exercise.

Relaxation and Limbering. Relaxing and gentle limbering movements including active and active-assistive exercise. Exercises are performed with or without the aid of vapocoolant spray or ice to restore flexibility and range of motion. A coolant is usually necessary in the initial stage of therapeutic exercise and stretching. Moist heat may be applied beforehand for comfort.

Stretching. Progressive passive and active stretching is performed with or without vapocoolant spray or ice to restore full muscle length and joint range of motion. Active and active-assistive stretching is an important part of the exercise program.

Spray and Stretch. Spray and stretch is an alternative noninvasive approach used in the treatment of trigger points and an excellent adjunct to follow-up care for trigger point injection.[6, 7, 15] A cold stimulus is used to provide hypoesthesia to a trigger point area and an area of shortened muscle, thus allowing increased stretch with less pain. The spray and stretch is repeated until normal muscle length is attained. (Do not permit the area to become excessively cold.) It is the stretching rather than the coolant itself which directly helps to inactivate the trigger point and obtain normal muscle length. Kraus[6] was the first to introduce the technique of vapocoolant spray using ethyl chloride in muscle rehabilitation. He stresses the importance of exercise during and following the vapocoolant spray treatment ("spray and limbering").[8] Although ethyl chloride is the most effective vapocoolant, it is not available in many institutions because of its flammable nature. The properties of the three most common coolants are summarized in Table 9–1. The procedure for the use of spray and stretch is as follows:

1. Assess the patient's movements and the direction of limited motion. Identify the shortened muscles and trigger points that are responsible for limitation in range of motion. Treat the primary trigger points and those in the referred pain area.

2. Position the patient so that he or she is comfortable with the body parts supported. The patient should be warm to avoid muscle spasm or tension due to chilling.

3. Stabilize one end of the muscle. One end of the muscle must be stabilized so that the other end can be both actively and passively stretched.

TABLE 9–1.

Common Coolants for Spray-and-Stretch Technique

Ethyl chloride
1. Acts as a general anesthetic
2. Colder than fluorimethane
3. Flammable
4. Potentially explosive when 4% to 15% of vapor is mixed with air
5. Toxic vapor

Fluorimethane
Not as cold as ethyl chloride
1. Nonflammable
2. Nonexplosive
3. Contributes to the depletion of the ozone layer

Ice
1. Nonflammable
2. Nonexplosive
3. Nontoxic
4. More difficult to use correctly; can cause undesirable wetness on the skin

4. Apply the cold stimulus. Vapocoolant spray or ice should be applied over the length of the muscle at an even pace covering the entire muscle and referred pain areas while the muscle is passively and actively stretched to its end range within the patient's pain limit. Two to three layers of coolant may be applied.

Continue steps 1 to 4 until normal muscle length has been reached, warming the area between applications. If ice is used, place plastic around the cube or "lollipop" to avoid dripping on the patient; wetness on the skin diffuses the cooling effect. Travell and Simons[16] provide specific instructions on how to apply vapocoolant or ice. While the muscle is passively stretched the coolant is administered in unidirectional parallel sweeps, applying it two to three times in the direction of the referred pain at a rate of 4 in./sec with the spray bottle held at a 30-degree angle 18 in. from the skin.[16] These exact details of application are not universally accepted. Most therapists will modify these guidelines.

Full range of motion is achieved by encouraging active motion with the help of vapocoolant spray beginning, with limbering movements[8] in addition to passive stretch. Muscles should be relaxed prior to stretching. Emphasis is placed on the patient's active movements.

5. Active motion and use of moist heat. Following the spray and stretch the patient should perform a few sets of five repetitions of active range-of-motion exercises with the treated part. The patient should also be instructed in stretching and active range-of-motion exercises to be done at home. At this stage some practitioners apply moist heat to increase muscle relaxation; others do not find this necessary.

6. The use of vapocoolant or ice is contraindicated in the case of allergy or hypersensitivity to cold.

Massage.   Massage and other manual physical therapy techniques are valuable modalities in the treatment of trigger points. These techniques are also used to facilitate muscle relaxation. Indications and techniques are described in Chapters 14 and 15.

Exercise Program.   The following instructions outline the principles discussed in Chapter 12. The exercise program should be tailored to the individual patient's requirements. Test the patient for specific muscle weaknesses, flexibility, and signs of tension (Kraus-Weber exercises; see Chapter 12). Begin all exercise programs with relaxation and limbering of muscles prior to stretching and strengthening. Exercises must be done in a relaxed and unhurried manner. It is better to do fewer exercises unhurried than rush through the full exercise program.

Relaxation.   Begin and end all therapy and exercise programs with relaxation. The patient should lie supine with pillows under the knees. Instruct the patient to close the eyes and take deep, slow breaths. The patient may rotate the head gently from side to side and then shrug the shoulders up while inhaling and let them drop while exhaling (see discussion of relaxation exercises in Chapter 12).

Exercises performed under tension will not promote the relaxation of muscles necessary for proper stretching. Each exercise is performed only three to four times. Too much repetition promotes muscle stiffening and should be avoided. Exercises are added progressively. Do not give too many exercises in one session. Reverse the sequence of exercises so that all exercises are done for a total of six to eight repetitions, ending the exercise session with relaxation. Exercises are taught to the patient by the therapist and are performed with the help and guidance of the therapist during the physical therapy sessions. These sessions are to be performed and continued in a home program. The patient is not to be presented with a sheet of exercises without proper instruction on how they are to be performed. After the patient completes the exercise program and is symptom-free he or she may progress to exercises promoting endurance and strength, which may include the use of free weights, and Universal or Nautalus equipment. The patient must be made aware that the ability to achieve relaxation and the performance of prescribed exercises are the most important aspect of the rehabilitation program. Exercises must be done regularly as described, beginning with warm-up exercises and ending with a cool-down. This is especially important prior to and after athletic activities to prevent injury and maintain the muscles in a relaxed, flexible, and normal length. Most athletic injuries occur as a result of muscle deficiency.

Corrective and Preventive Measures.   The patient's education prior to discharge should include factors that precipitate and may continue the patient's symptomatology. This may include adaptive changes in the workplace, changes in postural habits (see Chapter 16), and changes of a psychological and psychosocial nature that reduce tension. A corrective program must be instituted to achieve therapeutic results and prevent recurrences. Address endocrine disorders (see Fig 9–2).

Frequency of Treatment.   Trigger point injections may be given two times per week provided each injection can be followed by 3 to 4 successive days of physical therapy. Following the injection of all trigger points the exercise program is continued until the patient can complete the full exercise program properly. A level of flexibility, strength, and endurance should be achieved prior to returning the patient to his or her occupation. This depends on the individual's requirements.

Patient Instructions.   The patient is instructed as follows:

1. Following injection for the lumbar and gluteal areas, the patient is instructed to avoid prolonged walking, sitting, or lying down. Positioning should be changed frequently after injections of trigger points. In the lower extremities the patient should use crutches for 24 hours to avoid limping, pain, and muscle spasm. A sling may be used for the upper extremity.

2. The patient should be aware that the immediate relief of pain may be temporary. Soreness may be present for 24 to 48 hours.

3. The patient should be made aware of the possibility of infection following injection and is advised to report any unusual signs of infection such as pain, swelling, redness, or warmth.

4. After trigger point injection other trigger points in neighboring muscles may become symptomatic. This appears as a "shifting-type pain," and is a common phenomenon. Secondary trigger points that produce symptoms require treatment.

5. Patients should avoid traveling long distances to the treatment facility

for follow-up physical therapy. Prolonged travel promotes muscle spasms and jeopardizes therapeutic results.

6. The patient is to perform home exercises as directed (see Chapter 12)

COMPLICATIONS OF TRIGGER POINT INJECTIONS

Complications of trigger point injections may be due to the side effects and reactions to local anesthetics or to injection technique.

Allergic Reaction to Local Anesthetics

The patient may develop hives, dermatitis, pruritus, bronchospasm, or anaphylaxis following the injection of local anesthetics. Most allergies are due to the *p*-aminobenzoic acid groups and the preservative methylparaben. The use of an amide-type local anesthetic without preservative is recommended to avoid allergic reactions, e.g., lidocaine. Procaine is typical of an ester-type local anesthetic.[13]

Treatment.   Treatment of an allergic reaction is as follows:

1. Maintain ventilation and oxygenation.
2. Epinephrine 0.2 to 0.5 mL of 1:1,000 solution subcutaneously with repeat doses at 3-minute intervals as necessary.
3. Epinephrine by intravenous (IV) infusion of 1:50,000 solution to treat hypotension.
4. Antihistamine, e.g., diphenhydramine 50 to 80 mg intramuscularly (IM) or IV.
5. Steroids
6. Atropine.

Prevention.   The physician must take a history of any allergic condition. The history should include inquiries concerning allergy to local anesthetics and drugs, asthma, and food allergies. Perform a skin test if necessary. Use saline or dry needling technique if allergy is suspected.

Toxic Symptoms

Toxic symptoms are related to drug dose. Excessive local anesthetic cerebral blood levels may cause seizures. Toxic symptoms may include ringing in the ears, and a feeling of tingling around the mouth and facial muscles. It is important to aspirate before injecting to avoid injecting into a vein or artery. Intravascular injection may be responsible for producing a toxic level of local anesthetic. The amount used in trigger point injection should fall far below the maximum average dose for an adult. A maximum dose of lidocaine is 500 mg. The dose should not exceed 2 mg/lb.[11] The average dose used for trigger point injection is 5 to 10 mL).

Treatment.   Seizures are treated by (1) Maintaining ventilation and oxygenation, and (2) Performing cardiopulmonary resuscitation if hypotension occurs.

Anaphylaxis

A systemic reaction due to hypersensitivity to local anesthetics may occur during the injection or moments afterward. The *symptoms* are urticaria, angio-edema, wheezing, shortness of breath, hoarseness, tachycardia, and hypotension.

Treatment. Anaphylaxis is treated with:

1. Epinephrine 0.2 to 0.5 mL of 1:1,000 solution subcutaneously with repeat doses at 3-minute intervals as necessary.
2. Oxygen
3. IV fluids and volume expanders.
4. Epinephrine IV 1:50,000 solution to treat hypotension.
5. Aminophyline 0.25 to 0.5 g IV for bronchospasm.
6. Corticosteroid IV.

Prevention. Prevention mandates careful history taking with respect to allergies, skin testing if necessary, and the use of saline or dry needling if there is a question of allergy.

Neuropathy

Neuropathic injuries may be due to local mechanical trauma of the needle or to a toxic reaction to injected medications. The nerve may be traumatized when nerve fibers are penetrated by the needle or when local anesthetics are injected intraneurally.[1] The paresthesia that may be obtained with trigger point injection must be distinguished from the pattern of paresthesia of neural origin. Paresthesia due to trigger points is diffuse and nonspecific. In contrast, paresthesia or pain due to neural injury follows a specific nerve distribution; do not inject when these symptoms are present. A cramping pain may indicate injection into a nerve. If motor or sensory symptoms occur, obtain a baseline electromyography study which will aid in determining a preexisting nerve abnormality. This can be compared with a study done after several weeks, if necessary.

Prevention. A knowledge of anatomy will prevent injecting of peripheral nerves. The risk of nerve injury is reduced if a short beveled needle is used instead of a standard long beveled needle.[13]

Hematoma Formation

Always aspirate before injections and when performing dry needling. Aspiration will alert the physician to an arterial or venous puncture. Do not inject if blood is withdrawn. Withdraw the needle and apply pressure to avoid bleeding. If an artery is punctured apply only enough pressure to prevent bleeding without occluding the artery, so that the pulse can still be palpated. Maintain the pressure for 7 to 10 minutes. This will permit blood flow and enable the puncture wound to close. Complete occlusion of the artery will prevent blood flow which is necessary for closure of the arterial puncture wound. Venous puncture wounds will close with compression that occludes the vein.

If a hematoma appears to be developing or is present, apply pressure to stop the bleeding and follow with ice and compression. If a large hematoma forms in the thigh with persistent swelling, follow-up radiographs should be taken after several weeks to determine if calcification of the hematoma has occurred.

Prevention.   Needling should not be performed on patients who are on anticoagulants. A knowledge of anatomy is necessary to avoid arterial and venous structures.

Pneumothorax

Always aspirate prior to injection when injecting a trigger point in the area of the chest wall. Aspiration of air bubbles into the syringe indicates a puncture of the pleural cavity. The syringe used, however, must have a tight-fitting, airtight attachment between the needle and the syringe. If air bubbles are encountered injection is not performed.

Coughing or chest pain during the injection suggests that the pleura may have been punctured. An x-ray film should then be obtained. If a pneumothorax is present it must be treated appropriately. Only a small number of pneumothorax cases require chest tube drainage. A small pneumothorax involving 10% to 25% of the pleural space may be asymptomatic and may not need treatment. In the case of a modest pneumothorax the patient may develop tachycardia, restlessness, and diminished breath sounds on the affected side. Serial radiographs should be obtained to assess the progression of the pneumothorax. A tension pneumothorax may cause a collapsed lung and mediastinal shift. A tension pneumothorax may be life-threatening and requires emergency care including chest tube insertion.

Although small pleural puncture wounds most often heal without specific treatment, recognition and observation are necessary to prevent extension of the opening in the pleura. The patient should avoid any strenuous activity.

Prevention.   Always aspirate prior to injection. Observe if air bubbles are present in the syringe. Aspiration of blood will also indicate if the physician has entered the intercostal artery.

Angle the needle tangentially to the chest wall to avoid entering the intercostal space. Angle the needle in a caudal direction over the rib cage area to avoid injury to the intercostal artery as well as to the pleura. Do not direct the needle perpendicular to the chest wall (see Fig 9–12 and discussion of trigger point injection technique, above).

Control the depth of the needle by holding the needle stationary with one hand resting on the patient's body for stability and injecting with the other (see Fig 9–12). Debilitated patients are a risk. Patients who have thin chest walls are at high risk for pneumothorax; a small needle, e.g., a 22-gauge 1.5-in. short beveled needle, should be used in these patients.

Infection

Patients are instructed to report any signs of infection, including an increase in warmth, redness, swelling, and pain over the area of injection. Aspirate any collection of infected hematoma for culture and sensitivity prior to prescribing antibiotics. Incision and drainage of an abscess may be necessary.

Prevention.   Avoid trigger point injection in patients with systemic or local infections; use sterile technique; observe precautions in patients who are at high risk for infection, such as debilitated patients, patients on steroids, and diabetic patients.

Abdominal Puncture Wounds

Abdominal puncture wounds usually close without difficulties. Puncturing the rectosigmoid wall can cause infection.

Needle Breakage

Do not insert the full length of the needle into the muscle when injecting. When probing for trigger points using a circular fanning technique (Fig 9–11), withdraw the needle to a more superficial plane without exiting the skin and reinsert when changing direction.

REFERENCES

1. Carron H, Korbon GA, Rowlingson JC: *Regional anesthesia techniques and clinical applications,* Orlando, Fla, 1984, Grune & Stratton.
2. Garvey TA, Marks MR, Wiesel SW: A prospective, randomized, double-blind evaluation of trigger-point injection therapy for low-back pain, *Spine* 14:962–964, 1989.
3. Gunn CC: *Treating myofascial pain: Intramuscular stimulation (IMS) for myofascial pain syndromes of neuropathic origin,* Seattle, 1989, University of Washington.
4. Gunn CC, Milbrandt WE: Tenderness at motor points: An aid in the diagnosis of pain in the shoulder referred from the cervical spine, *J Am Osteopath Assoc* 77:196–212, 1977.
5. Jaeger B, Skootsky SA: Double blind, controlled study of different myofascial trigger point injection techniques (abstract), *Pain* 31:5292, 1987.
6. Kraus H: The use of surface anesthesia in the treatment of painful motion, *JAMA* 116:2582–2583, 1941.
7. Kraus H: *Clinical treatment of back and neck pain,* New York, 1970, McGraw-Hill.
8. Kraus H, Fischer AA: Diagnosis and treatment of myofascial pain, *Mt Sinai J Med* 58:235–239, 1991.
9. Lewit K: The needle effect in the relief of myofascial pain, *Pain* 6:83–90, 1979.
10. Malamed SF: *Handbook of local anesthesia,* ed 2, St Louis, 1986, Mosby–Year Book.
11. Mulroy MF: *Regional anesthesia,* Boston, 1989, Little Brown.
12. Nice DA, Riddle DL, Lamb RL, et al: Intertester reliability of judgments of the presence of trigger points in patients with low back pain, *Arch Phys Med Rehabil* 73:893–898, 1992.
13. Raj PP: *Handbook of regional anesthesia,* New York, 1985, Churchill Livingstone.
14. Sola AE, Rodenberger MS, Gettys BB: Incidence of hypersensitive areas in posterior shoulder muscles: A survey of two hundred young adults, *Am J Phys Med* 34:585–590, 1955.
15. Travell J, Rinzler SH: The myofascial genesis of pain, *Postgrad Med* 11:425–434, 1952.
16. Travell JG, Simons DG: *Myofascial pain and dysfunction: The trigger point manual,* Baltimore, 1983, Williams & Wilkins.

Chapter 10

Injection of Specific Trigger Points

Edward S. Rachlin, M.D.

Muscles of the Trunk

QUADRATUS LUMBORUM

Symptoms and Pain Pattern

- Low back pain present at rest as well as with motion of the lumbar areas.
- Limited range of motion of the lumbosacral spine due to pain and muscle stiffness. Patient may feel immobilized.
- Coughing and sneezing can cause pain in the low back without radiation.
- Pain may radiate to the lower extremity or anteriorly to the inguinal region including the scrotum and testicles.[18, 20]
- Referred pain may be limited to the sacroiliac region and buttocks[44] (Fig 10–1).
- Referred pain to the anterior abdominal wall.[36]

Findings on Examination

- Palpation of trigger points may cause local as well as referred pain. With the patient in the prone position, palpate trigger points lateral and deep to the iliocostalis lumborum. It is sometimes helpful in palpating beneath the iliocostalis lumborum to have the patient lying on the uninvolved side with slight forward rotation of the upper body.
- Muscle spasm.
- Muscle spasm will prevent an adequate examination for trigger points. Muscle spasm should be treated and relieved prior to trigger point evaluation. (See postinjection follow-up program in Chapter 9.)
- Functional scoliosis.
- Limited motion in the lumbar area.

Differential Diagnosis

- Kidney stone.
- Trochanteric bursitis.

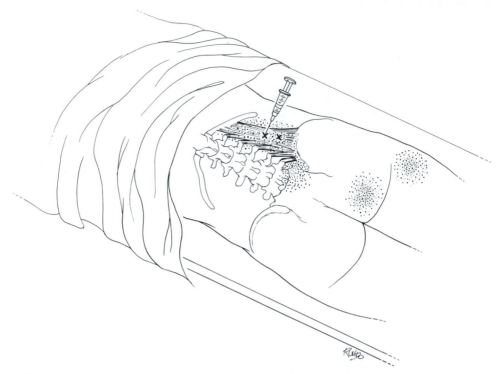

FIG 10–1.   Quadratus lumborum. Injection of trigger points *(X's)* in the right quadratus lumborum with the patient in the prone position. Injection may also be performed with the patient lying on the uninvolved side. Trigger point pain pattern is shown by *stippling.* Direct the needle tangentially or parallel to the frontal plane of the patient.

- Herniated lumbar disc.
- Lumbosacral sprain.

Anatomy

> *Origin:* the iliolumbar ligament and posterior iliac crest.
> *Insertion:* 12th rib and transverse processes of L1–4.
> *Action:* fixation of last two ribs; flexes the spine laterally.

Noninvasive Therapy

The post-trigger point injection follow-up program described in Chapter 9 is recommended as a conservative therapeutic treatment approach. Noninvasive therapy can include:

- Physical therapy modalities (e.g., electrical stimulation and warm packs; see Chapter 15).
- Manual physical therapy techniques (e.g., massage and the Trager Approach; see Chapters 13 and 14).
- Active and passive stretching and limbering of muscles with or without the use of vapocoolant spray or ice. Active exercise is part of the stretch-and-spray technique. Limbering and relaxation of muscles are necessary prior to stretching. Contract-relax techniques may be used.
- Stretch and spray for the quadratus muscle: The patient should lie on the uninvolved side. Stretching of the quadratus lumborum is achieved by

rotating the upper body forward and upward, opening the area between the 12th rib and pelvis. The right hip and pelvis are stabilized. Stretching is also achieved in the sitting position in the bend-rotation exercise by lateral rotation and flexion as described in back exercises in Chapter 12. Electrical stimulation, limbering of muscles, and warm packs should precede stretch and spray to relax muscles.

- Exercises and a home program for the low back are described in Chapter 12. Exercise programs include relaxation, limbering, stretching, and strengthening. When the patient is free of pain and full motion has been achieved, progress to strength and endurance programs.

Injection Technique

Position patient in the prone or side-lying position on the uninvolved side. Trigger points are palpated lateral and deep to the border of the iliocostalis lumborum muscle. Inject only the trigger points in the lower portion of the quadratus lumborum to avoid the diaphragm area. Direct the needle tangentially or parallel to the frontal plane of the patient (see Figs 10–1 and 9–15,J); the injection technique is described in Chapter 9).

Needle size: 1.5, 2.0, 3.0 in., 20 gauge.

Solution: Any one of the following solutions may be used: 0.5% procaine; 1.0% lidocaine; saline and dry needling in case of allergy. Do not use epinephrine.

Precautions

- Do not inject the upper portion of the quadratus lumborum to avoid causing a pneumothorax.
- Direct the needle tangentially or parallel to the frontal plane of the patient.

Postinjection Follow-Up Physical Therapy Program

The patient should receive 3 to 4 consecutive days of treatment. Physical therapy should include electrical stimulation, relaxation, limbering, and stretching of the involved muscle using vapocoolant spray or ice as needed combined with and followed by an exercise program. Active and active-assisted exercises are an integral part of the physical therapy program (see Chapter 9 for details).

Exercise and Home Program

Exercises for the quadratus lumborum and back muscles are prescribed. Exercises should at first be performed under the guidance of a therapist. When the patient is free of pain and full motion has been achieved, progress to strength and endurance programs. Begin and end exercise session with relaxation and stretching. (See Chapter 13 for exercise details.)

Corrective and Preventive Measures

- Failure to do warm-up exercises prior to athletic activities predisposes to the development of trigger points and the activation of latent trigger points. Continue the exercise program to avoid recurrence.
- Correct foot deformities, e.g., flatfoot. Prescribe orthoses as necessary.
- Correct leg length inequality with heel lifts.

- Recommend a buttock lift for small hemipelvis or scoliosis as indicated.[45]
- Proper chair design, e.g., backrest with lumbar support, armrests of proper height; feet should rest comfortably on the floor (see Chapter 16).
- Prescribe a lumbar roll if necessary.

LATISSIMUS DORSI AND TERES MAJOR

Symptoms and Pain Pattern

- Pain may be experienced over the midthoracic area, lower medial aspect of the scapula, anterior aspect of the shoulder, and in the posterior axillary region[22, 45] (Fig 10–2).
- Pain may radiate to the medial aspect of the arm to the fourth and fifth fingers.
- Working for long periods with the arms elevated and forward may cause trigger points, or aggravate latent trigger points.

Findings on Examination

- With the patient supine the arm is abducted and externally rotated. The latissimus dorsi is grasped between the thumb and index finger to palpate

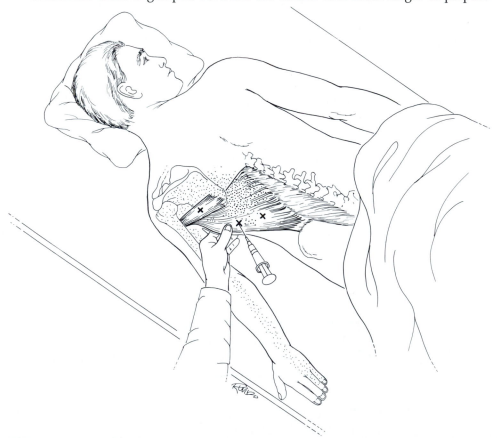

FIG 10–2.   Latissimus dorsi and teres major. Injection of trigger points *(X's)* in the latissimus dorsi and teres major with the patient prone. Injection may also be performed with the patient supine. Anatomic landmarks are noted. Pain pattern *(stippling)*. Area of trigger point is grasped between the thumb and fingers.

for trigger points. Palpation may also be performed with the patient prone.

- Local and referred pain may be elicited.
- Range-of-motion assessment may reveal limitation in elevation and external rotation.

Differential Diagnosis

- Cervical disc herniation.
- Thoracic outlet syndrome.
- Intrathoracic disease.
- Dorsal sprain.

Anatomy

Latissimus Dorsi

Origin: spinous processes and supraspinous ligaments of the lower thoracic vertebrae, lumbar fascia, posterior part of the crest of the ilium, all four ribs, and from the angle of the scapula.
Insertion: The floor of the bicipital groove.
Action: adduction, medial rotation, and extension of the arm.

Teres Major

Origin: back of the inferior angle and axillary border of the scapula.
Insertion: front of the humerus bicipital groove.
Action: medial rotator and adductor of arm.

The teres major is superior and adjacent to the latissimus dorsi. Anatomically it is an extension of the latissimus dorsi and both are treated together.

Noninvasive Therapy

The post–trigger point injection follow-up program described in Chapter 9 is recommended as a conservative therapeutic treatment approach. Noninvasive therapy can include:

- Physical therapy modalities (e.g., electrical stimulation and warm packs; see Chapter 15).
- Manual physical therapy techniques (e.g., massage and the Trager Approach; see Chapters 13 and 14).
- Active and passive stretching and limbering of muscles with or without the use of vapocoolant spray or ice. Active exercise is part of the stretch-and-spray technique. Limbering and relaxation are necessary prior to stretching. Contract-relax techniques may be used.
- Stretch and spray for the latissimus dorsi and teres major: Include the trigger point and referred pain area. Use vapocoolant or ice (see Chapter 9). Stretch in the direction of abduction, external rotation, and extension. Electrical stimulation, limbering of muscles, and warm packs should precede stretch and spray to relax muscles.
- Exercises and a home program for the shoulder are described in Chapter 12. Exercise programs include relaxation, limbering, stretching, and strengthening. When the patient is free of pain and full motion has been achieved, progress to strength and endurance programs.

Injection of Trigger Point

With the patient prone or supine the trigger point is located and may sometimes be able to be held between the thumb and index finger or isolated between the index and middle fingers. The needle is inserted into the raised tissue between the thumb and index finger. The needle should be directed tangentially or parallel to the thorax (see Fig 10–2 and Chapter 9 for injection technique).

Needle size: 1.5 in., 22 gauge.

Solution: Any one of the following solutions may be used: 0.5% procaine; 1.0% lidocaine; saline and dry needling in case of allergy. Do not use epinephrine.

The teres major may also be injected over its scapular origin in addition to the posterior axillary area.

Precautions

Control the depth of the needle. Direct the needle tangentially or parallel to the chest wall to avoid a pneumothorax (see Chapter 9 for complications). Maintain the trigger point area between two fingers or the finger and thumb when possible.

Postinjection Follow-Up Program

The patient should receive 3 to 4 consecutive days of treatment. Physical therapy should include electrical stimulation, relaxation, limbering, and stretching of the involved muscle using vapocoolant spray or ice as needed combined with and followed by an exercise program. Active and active-assisted exercises are an integral part of the physical therapy program (see Chapter 9 for details).

Exercise and Home Program

Exercises should at first be performed under the guidance of a therapist. When the patient is free of pain and full motion has been achieved, progress to strength and endurance programs. Begin and end the exercise session with relaxation and stretching (See Chapter 12 for exercise details.)

Corrective and Preventive Measures

- Avoid working with the arms elevated and forward for long periods.
- Do warm-up exercises for the back and upper extremities before athletic activities (see Chapter 12).
- Patients who have walked with crutches for a prolonged period of time develop shortness of the latissimus dorsi, e.g., paraplegic patients. Encourage stretching and range-of-motion exercises for the upper extremities.

THORACOLUMBAR PARASPINAL MUSCLES
Sacrospinalis, spinalis

Symptoms and Pain Pattern

- Thoracolumbar muscles, both superficial and deep, are treated as a group rather than individually.
- Injection is into the muscle group rather than to individual muscles. The sacrospinalis muscle or erector spinae consists of the iliocostalis, longissimus, and spinalis.
- These muscles may refer pain to the upper dorsal area, flank, and buttock[4, 11, 12, 16, 18, 44] (Fig 10–3).
- Trigger points in the dorsal musculature may cause radiating chest pain and pleurodynia.[4] The deep paraspinal muscles include the semispinalis thoracis, multifidi, and rotators.
- Trigger points found in the deep paraspinal muscle may give rise to thoracic pain and pain over the spinous processes, in addition to coccygodynia.[7, 44]
- Lumbar muscle trigger points may refer pain to the abdomen.[11, 12]

Findings

- Patients with thoracolumbar and low back pain demonstrate restricted spinal motion due to pain, muscle stiffness, muscle spasm, muscle shortening, and trigger points.
- Trigger point examination should be performed with the patient prone with a pillow under the abdomen as well as in the side-lying position.

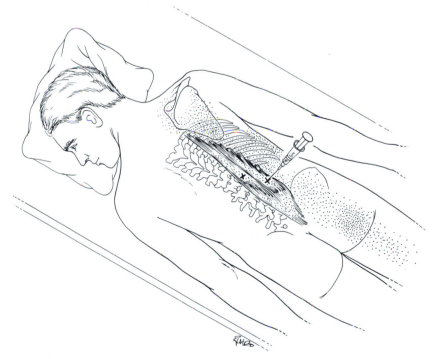

FIG 10–3. Thoracolumbar paraspinal muscle. Injection of trigger points *(X's)* in the right lumbar paraspinal muscles with the patient supine. Direct the needling tangentially in relation to the frontal plane of the patient. Anatomic landmarks are noted. Trigger point pain pattern is shown by *stippling*.

- Trigger points may be palpable both superficially and deep causing local and referred pain to the buttocks or chest area.
- Neighboring muscle groups often develop trigger points (e.g., gluteal, tensor fasciae latae).

Differential Diagnosis

- Herniated disc.
- Lumbosacral sprain.
- Dorsal lumbar sprain.
- Kidney stones.
- Spinal fractures.
- Metastatic disease.

Anatomy

The sacrospinalis (erector spinae) includes the iliocostalis, longissimus, and spinalis. The three muscle groups have an extensive common origin. Three columns arise from the common origin.

Origin: sacral spines and transverse processes, lumbar and lower thoracic spinous processes, posterior part of crest of the ilium.

The above muscles are arranged in three columns.

Outer Column
Iliocostalis Thoracis
Origin: upper border of angles of lower six ribs.
Insertion: upper borders of ribs 1–6, transverse process of C7.

Costalis
Origin: lower six ribs.
Insertion: upper six ribs.

Costocervicalis
Origin: upper three to six ribs.
Insertion: Transverse processes of C4–6.

Intermediate Column
Longissimus Thoracis
Origin: sacral spines and transverse processes, lumbar and lower thoracic spinous processes, posterior part of crest of the ilium;
Insertion: transverse process of all thoracic and lumbar vertebrae, lower ten ribs.

Longissimus Cervicis
Origin: transverse processes of T1–5.
Insertion: transverse processes of C2–6.

Longissimus Capitis
Origin: transverse processes of T1–7, articular processes of C5–7.
Insertion: posterior margin of mastoid process.

Medial Column
Spinalis
Origin: thoracic spines of T11 and L1–2.
Insertion: thoracic spines of T1–8.

Spinalis Cervicis
Origin: spinous processes of C7 and T1–2.
Insertion: spinous processes of C2–5.
Action: iliocostalis acts as extensor, lateral flexor, and rotator of the spine to the same side; longissimus thoracis and cervicis extend the spine and bend the spine to one side.

Noninvasive Therapy

The post–trigger point injection follow-up program described in Chapter 9 is recommended as a conservative therapeutic treatment approach. Noninvasive therapy can include:

- Physical therapy modalities (e.g., electrical stimulation and warm packs; see Chapter 15).
- Manual physical therapy techniques (e.g., massage and the Trager Approach; see Chapters 13 and 14).
- Active and passive stretching and limbering of muscles with or without the use of vapocoolant spray or ice. Active exercise is part of the stretch-and-spray technique. Limbering and relaxation are necessary prior to stretching. Contract-relax techniques may be used.
- Stretch and spray: Stretching is performed in flexion, rotation of the spine, and lateral bending to the opposite side. The back exercise program (see Chapter 12) also includes stretching in the sitting position. Electrical stimulation, limbering of muscles, and warm packs should precede stretch and spray to relax muscles.
- Exercises and home program for the paraspinal muscles (see Chapter 12 for back exercise and see Chapter 14 for massage techniques). Exercise programs include relaxation, limbering, stretching, and strengthening. When the patient is free of pain and full motion has been achieved, progress to strength and endurance programs.

Injection Technique

See diagram.
The patient is placed in the prone position with a pillow under the abdomen. Identify trigger points. Injection is performed under sterile precautions. Injection is performed in the thoracolumbar area without specific anatomic differentiation of individual muscles. *The muscles are treated as a group* (see Fig 10–3, and Chapter 9 for injection technique).
Needle sizes: 2.0, 3.0, 3.5 in. 20–22 gauge.
Solution: Any one of the following solutions may be used: 0.5% procaine; 1.0% lidocaine; saline and dry needling in case of allergy. Do not use epinephrine.
Multiple needle entries are required in addition to approaching the trigger point directly. Both superficial and deep trigger points are injected as a group.

Multiple entries usually encounter trigger points that are missed on palpation. Injections should be performed with the needle directed tangentially in the lower lumbar area. The direction of the needle should be angled parallel or tangential to the frontal plane of the patient to avoid penetrating too deeply in the upper lumbar area. Lidocaine 10 mL is usually sufficient. To avoid entering the intervertebral space when injecting the deep paraspinalis (e.g., the multifidi), angle the needle in a caudal direction in relation to the laminae which slant caudally guarding the intercostal space. This is the same principle used in injecting in the area of the rib cage to avoid entering the intercostal space.

Postinjection Follow-Up Physical Therapy Program

The patient should receive 3 to 4 consecutive days of treatment. Physical therapy should include electrical stimulation, relaxation, limbering, and stretching of the involved muscle using vapocoolant spray or ice as needed combined with and followed by an exercise program. Active and active-assisted exercises are an integral part of the physical therapy program (see Chapter 9 for details).

Exercise and Home Program

Exercises for the low back are prescribed. Exercises should at first be performed under the guidance of a therapist. When the patient is free of pain and full motion has been achieved, progress to strength and endurance programs. Begin and end exercise sessions with stretching and relaxation (see Chapter 12 for exercise details).

Corrective and Preventive Measures

- Correct postural foot deformities (e.g., use orthoses for flatfeet). Use an appropriate heel lift in case of leg length discrepancy.
- Correct lumbar-pelvic asymmetry (e.g., sitting with an appropriate cushion under one buttock in case of scoliosis or small hemipelvis).[44]
- Correct faulty postural habits (e.g., improper sitting and standing). Use correct method of lifting at work (see Chapter 16).
- Eliminate stress and tension as a cause of back pain.
- Instruct the patient in proper sleeping positions.
- Use a firm mattress and bed board.
- Use a properly designed chair and a lumbar roll (see Chapter 16).
- Use a lumbosacral support in acute pain for ambulation as a temporary measure.
- Continue exercise program to avoid recurrence.
- Eliminate metabolic causes of muscle pain.

SERRATUS POSTERIOR SUPERIOR

Symptoms and Pain Pattern

- Pain over the scapula, most pronounced over the upper medial border.
- Pain may radiate to the posterior aspect of the shoulder, upper arm, forearm, to the hand, and fifth finger.[44]

- Pain in the area of the medial scapula border may be difficult to distinguish from symptoms caused by the rhomboids or trapezius muscles.

Findings on Examination

- Palpation of trigger points may cause local and referred pain.
- The insertion of the serratus posterior superior muscle extends to the rib margins which are covered by the medial border of the scapula. Palpation of this area is best accomplished by abducting the scapula. To move the scapula laterally the arm can be brought around to the front of the chest or permitted to hang forward with the patient in the prone position. It is difficult to distinguish trigger points in the region of the origin and medial portion of the muscle because of the overlying rhomboids and trapezius muscles.

Differential Diagnosis

- Rhomboid and trapezius trigger points.
- Cervical radiculopathy.
- Subscapular bursitis.

Anatomy

Origin: spinous processes of C7, and T1–3.
Insertion: outer surfaces of ribs 2–5 lateral to the rib angles.
Action: elevator of the upper ribs.

Noninvasive Therapy

The post–trigger point injection follow-up program described in Chapter 9 is recommended as a conservative therapeutic treatment approach. Noninvasive therapy can include:

- Physical therapy modalities (e.g., electrical stimulation and warm packs; see Chapter 15).
- Manual physical therapy techniques (e.g., massage and the Trager Approach; see Chapters 13 and 14).
- Stretching is minimally effective in treating the serratus posterior superior. Stretch and spray of neighboring muscles which harbor trigger points, such as the rhomboids and trapezius, would be effective. Flexing the upper thoracic spine does not accomplish the type of stretch that is therapeutically effective. Emphasis should be placed on massage techniques which include ischemic compression, the use of electric modalities, and the treatment of neighboring muscles.

Injection of Trigger Point

The patient lies on the uninvolved side. The scapula is abducted and the trigger point is specifically localized and held between two fingers. The needle is directed to the rib to avoid the intercostal space. Aspirate prior to injection.

The needle is directed tangentially in relation to the chest wall to avoid causing a pneumothorax (Fig 10–4; see also Fig 9–5,G for injection technique when approaching the chest wall, e.g., the pectoralis muscle.)

Needle size: 1.5, 2.0 in., 21 gauge.

Solution: Any one of the following solutions may be used: 0.5% procaine; 1.0% lidocaine; saline and dry needling in case of allergy. Do not use epinephrine.

Precautions

- Aspirate prior to injection.
- Angle the needle tangentially in relation to the chest wall.
- Avoid the intercostal space.

Postinjection Follow-Up Physical Therapy Program

The patient should receive 3 to 4 consecutive days of treatment. Physical therapy should include electrical stimulation, relaxation, limbering, and stretching of the neighboring muscle using vapocoolant spray or ice as needed combined with and followed by an exercise program. Active and active-assisted exercises are an integral part of the physical therapy program (see Chapter 9 for details).

Exercise and Home Program

Exercises should at first be performed under the guidance of a therapist. When the patient is free of pain and full motion has been achieved, progress to

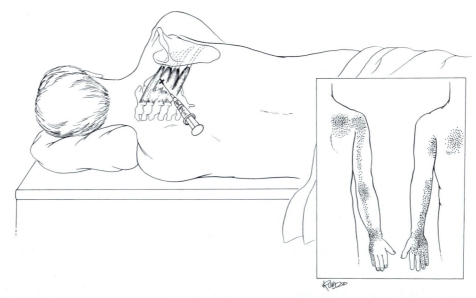

FIG 10–4. Serratus posterior superior. Injection of trigger point *(X)* in the right serratus posterior superior. Localize the trigger point by palpation and direct the needle in the direction of a rib and tangentially in relation to the chest wall to avoid entering the intercostal space. Aspirate prior to injection. Trigger points in the region of muscle insertion are more easily palpated with abduction of the right scapula. Observe precautions to prevent pneumothorax. *Inset,* trigger point pain pattern *(stippling).*

strength and endurance programs. Begin and end exercise sessions with stretching and relaxation (See Chapter 12 for exercise details.)

Corrective and Preventive Measures

- Correct sitting and standing postures for cervical, dorsal, and lumbosacral spine (e.g., avoid head-forward posture, round-shouldered posture, and use lumbar roll for sitting).

SERRATUS POSTERIOR INFERIOR

Symptoms and Referred Pain Pattern

- Patients report pain in the upper lumbar and lower dorsal area (Fig 10–5).
- Symptoms may be aggravated by activities requiring rotation of the torso.
- Patients can often put their finger on the tender spot.

Findings on Examination

- Local tenderness over trigger points.
- Trigger points are located over the rib area.
- Pain with rotation to the opposite side.

Differential Diagnosis

- Kidney stone.
- Nephritis.

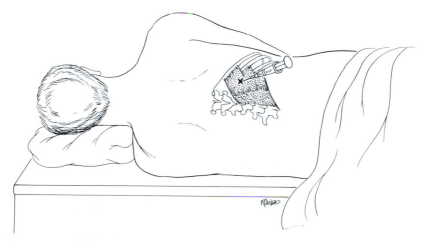

FIG 10–5. Serratus posterior inferior. Injection of trigger point in the serratus posterior inferior *(X)*. The trigger point should be well localized between the index and middle fingers or index finger and thumb. Avoid the intercostal space. The patient may be injected in the prone or side-lying position. Aspirate prior to injection. Direct the needle toward a rib pointing the needle in a caudal direction tangent to the chest wall. Pain pattern is shown by *stippling*.

- Lumbar-dorsal sprain.
- Fracture of the rib.

Anatomy

Origin: spinous processes of T11, T12, L1, and L2.

Insertion: ribs 9–12; muscle fibers are directed upward and laterally to insert on the surfaces of the lower four ribs.

Action: maintains stability of the lower ribs; depressor of the lower ribs.

Noninvasive Therapy

The post–trigger point injection follow-up program described in Chapter 9 is recommended as a conservative therapeutic treatment approach. Noninvasive therapy can include:

- Physical therapy modalities (e.g., electrical stimulation and warm packs; see Chapter 15).
- Manual physical therapy techniques (e.g., massage and the Trager Approach; see Chapters 13 and 14).
- Active and passive stretching and limbering of muscles with or without the use of vapocoolant spray or ice. Active exercise is part of the stretch-and-spray technique. Limbering and relaxation are necessary prior to stretching. Contract-relax techniques may be used.
- Stretch and spray for the serratus posterior inferior is performed with the patient in the sitting position. Flex the thoracolumbar area with rotation to the opposite side. This exercise and stretch are a part of the low back exercise program described in Chapter 12. Electrical stimulation, limbering of muscles, and warm packs should precede stretch and spray to relax muscles.
- Exercises and a home program for the low back are described in Chapter 12. Exercise is done progressively. Exercises for flexion and rotation in the thoracolumbar area are included. Exercises include sitting with forward bending in flexion as well as with rotation. Exercise programs include relaxation, limbering, stretching, and strengthening. When the patient is free of pain and full motion has been achieved, progress to strength and endurance programs. Begin and end exercise sessions with relaxation and stretching.

Injection of Trigger Point

Position patient in prone or side-lying position on the uninvolved side. Trigger points are palpated and isolated between the index and middle fingers over the rib area. The needle is directed over the rib tangentially to avoid entering the intercostal space (see Fig 10–5), and Chapter 9 for injection technique.

Needle size: 1.5 in., 20–22 gauge.

Solution: Any one of the following solutions may be used: 0.5% procaine; 1.0% lidocaine; saline and dry needling in case of allergy. Do not use epinephrine.

Precautions

- Avoid pneumothorax.
- Direct the needle tangentially over the rib.
- Avoid the intercostal space.
- Aspirate prior to injection.

Postinjection Follow-Up Physical Therapy Program

The patient should receive 3 to 4 consecutive days of treatment. Physical therapy should include electrical stimulation, relaxation, limbering, and stretching of the involved muscle using vapocoolant spray or ice as needed combined with and followed by an exercise program. Active and active-assisted exercises are an integral part of the physical therapy program (see Chapter 9 for details).

Exercise and Home Program

Exercises for the serratus posterior inferior include exercises for the back and thoracolumbar area (see Chapter 12 for back exercises). Exercises should at first be performed under the guidance of a therapist. When the patient is free of pain and full motion has been achieved, progress to strength and endurance programs. Begin and end exercise sessions with stretching and relaxation.

Corrective and Preventive Measures

- Avoid repetitive twisting of the torso or remaining in a rotated posture for prolonged periods. This may require correcting the working environment.
- Excessive repetitive hitting of golf balls (practice sessions) may cause or aggravate latent trigger points.
- Correct poor sitting posture, which may be due to pelvis asymmetry (e.g., use a cushion under one buttock as necessary).
- Correct leg length discrepancies (e.g., with a heel lift).

SERRATUS ANTERIOR

Symptoms and Referred Pain Pattern

- Pain over the anterior, lateral, and posterolateral chest wall[46] (Fig 10–6).
- Pain at rest and with movements of the rib cage.
- Referred pain may be noted over the inner border of the arm radiating to the fourth and fifth fingers.[43]
- Pain may be aggravated with deep breathing.

Findings on Examination

- Local trigger point tenderness is usually located in the midaxillary line between ribs 4–8.
- Referred pain pattern may be elicited with trigger point palpation.

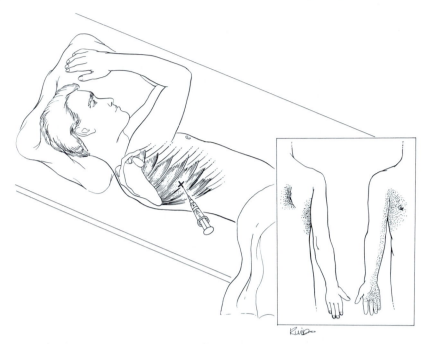

FIG 10–6. Serratus anterior. Injection of trigger point *(X)* in the right serratus anterior muscle in the midaxillary line. The patient is lying on the uninvolved side. Avoid entering the intercostal space. Aspirate prior to injection. *Inset,* pain pattern *(stippling).*

Differential Diagnosis

- Fracture of the rib.
- Cervical radiculopathy.
- Strain of serratus anterior muscle.

Anatomy

Origin: outer surfaces of the upper eight ribs.

Insertion: ventral aspect of the whole length of the vertebral body of the scapula.

Action: holds the medial border of the scapula against the thorax; abducts the scapula, rotating it so that the glenoid cavity faces upward to support the arm when it is raised above the shoulder; may also act in forced inspiration.

Noninvasive Therapy

The post–trigger point injection follow-up program described in Chapter 9 is recommended as a conservative therapeutic treatment approach. Noninvasive therapy can include:

- Physical therapy modalities (e.g., electrical stimulation and warm packs; see Chapter 15).
- Manual physical therapy techniques (e.g., massage and the Trager Approach; see Chapters 13 and 14).
- Active and passive stretching and limbering of muscles with or without

the use of vapocoolant spray or ice. Active exercise is part of the stretch-and-spray technique. Limbering and relaxation are necessary prior to stretching. Contract-relax technique may be used.

- Stretch and spray for the serratus anterior is accomplished with the patient in the side-lying position lying on the uninvolved side. Stretching of the serratus anterior is achieved by actively and passively bringing the patient's arm backward and downward using a vapocoolant spray or ice if needed. Electrical stimulation, limbering of muscles, and warm packs should precede stretch and spray to relax muscles.
- Exercises and a home program for the serratus anterior are described in Chapter 12 in the discussion of shoulder and upper extremity exercises. Exercise programs include relaxation, limbering, stretching, and strengthening. When the patient is free of pain and full motion has been achieved, progress to strength and endurance programs. Begin and end exercise programs with relaxation and stretching.

Injection of Trigger Point

Position the patient in the supine or side-lying position on the uninvolved side. Trigger points are palpated. The needle should be directed tangentially in relation to the chest wall, directing the needle over a rib to avoid the intercostal space (see Fig 10–6). Isolate the trigger point between the index and middle fingers. (See Chapter 9 for injection technique.)

Needle size: 1.5 in., 21 gauge

Solution: Any one of the following solutions may be used: 0.5% procaine; 1.0% lidocaine; saline and dry needling in case of allergy. Do not use epinephrine.

Precautions

- Aspirate prior to injection.
- Avoid causing a pneumothorax.
- Direct the needle toward the rib to avoid the intercostal space.
- To control the position and depth of the needle the needle and syringe may be stabilized with one hand while the other hand is used for injecting.
- Direct the needle tangentially in relation to the chest wall.

Postinjection Follow-Up Physical Therapy Program

The patient should receive 3 to 4 consecutive days of treatment. Physical therapy should include electrical stimulation, relaxation, limbering, and stretching of the involved muscle using vapocoolant spray or ice as needed combined with and followed by an exercise program. Active and active-assisted exercises are an integral part of the physical therapy program (see Chapter 9 for details).

Exercise and Home Program

Exercises should at first be performed under the guidance of a therapist. When the patient is free of pain and full motion has been achieved, progress to strength and endurance programs. Begin and end exercise sessions with stretching and relaxation. (See Chapter 12 for exercise details.)

Corrective and Preventive Measures

- Proper warm-up activities prior to performing exercises include pushups or overhead weightlifting.
- Relaxation and stretching exercises prior to and after exercise sessions.

RECTUS ABDOMINIS AND OBLIQUUS

Symptoms and Pain Pattern

Sola,[34, 35] Kelly,[13] Kellgren,[11, 12] Lang,[20] Travell and Simons,[45] Melnick,[23] and Slocumb,[33] have reported referred pain patterns involving the abdominal muscles. Both somatovisceral and viscerosomatic interactions have been reported.

- Trigger points may cause abdominal pain, vomiting, diarrhea, urinary bladder symptoms, and referred pain to the lower back. Trigger point patterns have been reported in the obliquus, transverse abdominis and rectus abdominis muscles. Trigger points in the rectus abdominis are a frequent result of muscle strains in athletic injuries (e.g., sit-ups). Often a history of a specific incident of trauma is lacking.
- Pain resulting from trigger points appears to persist long after an initial strain may have healed. Pain may be localized to the abdominal area (Fig 10–7). Different symptoms have been attributed to the upper, mid, and lower portions of the rectus abdominis.[44] The upper rectus abdominis re-

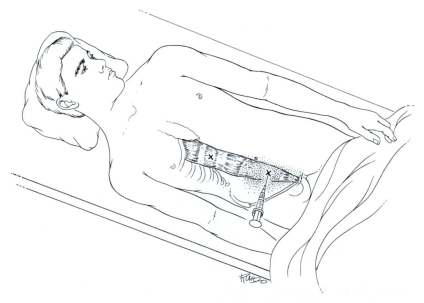

FIG 10–7.   Rectus abdominis. Injection of trigger points *(X's)* in the right rectus abdominis with the patient supine. Anatomic landmarks are noted. Pain pattern is shown by *stippling.* Direct the needle tangentially to the abdominal wall.

fers pain to the midback in addition to producing abdominal symptoms characteristic of indigestion. The periumbilical area causes a colic-like pain. The lower rectus abdominis refers pain to the low back area in addition to simulating the pain of appendicitis when the trigger point is on the right side.

- Melnick[23, 24] has described symptoms due to trigger points in the abdominal area: heartburn related to trigger points at the insertion of the abdominal muscles along the right costal margin from the xiphoid process to the angle of the ribs; abdominal fullness, nausea, and vomiting related to trigger points in the midline of the upper abdomen; and diarrhea resulting from trigger points in the left or right angle of the lower abdomen.

Findings on Examination

- Tenderness on palpation may cause local tenderness and referred pain patterns, in addition to abdominal symptoms.
- Placing the muscle under tension may produce characteristic pain (e.g., raising both legs, lifting both heels off the examining table, or performing sit-ups).

Differential Diagnosis

- Multiple causes of abdominal pain (e.g., appendicitis, gallbladder disease, diverticulitis).
- Abdominal muscle strain.

Anatomy

External Oblique
Origin: outer surfaces of the lower eight ribs.

Insertion: posterior fibers into the interior half of the iliac crest; the rest of the muscle inserts through the anterior superior iliac spine to the pubic tubercle and crest; the aponeurosis between these two points is thickened to form the inguinal ligament.

Internal Oblique
Origin: transverse processes of the lumbar vertebrae.

Insertion: lower borders of the lower six costal cartilages by an apneurotic sheet with the linea alba, to the pubic crest and illiopectineal line by the conjoined tendon.

Transversus Abdominis
Origin: lower six costal cartilages of the transverse processes of the lumbar vertebrae.

Insertion: by an aponeurotic sheet to the midline attached to the xiphisternun, to the pubic crest and iliopectineal line.

Rectus Abdominis
Origin: medial head in front of the body of the pubis and the lateral head from the top of the crest of the pubis.

Insertion: the anterior aspect of the fifth, sixth, and seventh costal cartilages, and the lower border of the seventh.

Action: flexion of the pelvis on the trunk or the trunk on the pelvis.

Action: external oblique, internal oblique, and transversus compress the abdominal viscera, flex the trunk, and act as muscles of expiration.

Pyrimadalis Muscle

Origin: a small triangular muscle inside the rectus sheath arising from the crest of the pubis.

Insertion, the linea alba.

Noninvasive Therapy

The post–trigger point injection follow-up program described in Chapter 9 is recommended as a conservative therapeutic treatment approach. Noninvasive therapy can include:

- Physical therapy modalities (e.g., electrical stimulation and warm packs; see Chapter 15).
- Manual physical therapy techniques (e.g., massage and the Trager Approach; see Chapters 13 and 14).
- Active and passive stretching and limbering of muscles with or without the use of vapocoolant spray or ice. Active exercise is part of the stretch-and-spray technique. Limbering and relaxation are necessary prior to stretching. Contract-relax techniques may be used.
- Stretch and spray for the rectus abdominis muscle is performed by arching the patient's back to achieve extension of the back. The legs may be supported by a stool off the examining table.[45] Spray is applied over the abdomen over the trigger point area and referred pain area. Electrical stimulation, limbering of muscles, and warm packs to relax muscles should precede stretch and spray.
- Exercises and a home program for the abdominal muscles are described in Chapter 12. Exercise program includes relaxation, limbering, stretching, and strengthening. When the patient is free of pain and full motion has been achieved, progress to strength and endurance programs.

Injection of Trigger Point

Needle size: 1.5 and 2.0 in., 21 gauge.

Solution: Any one of the following solutions may be used: 0.5% procaine; 1.0% lidocaine; saline and dry needling may be used in case of allergy. Do not use epinephrine. Injection is performed with the patient supine (see Fig 10–7).

Precautions

- Do not inject perpendicular to the patient.
- The needle should be directed tangentially to the abdominal wall.
- Trigger points should be isolated between two fingers or between the thumb and index finger. Localizing the trigger point and elevating it away from the abdominal cavity avoids puncturing the abdominal cavity.
- The needle should be well localized into the trigger point area.

Postinjection Follow-Up Physical Therapy Program

The patient should receive 3 to 4 consecutive days of treatment. Physical therapy should include electrical stimulation, relaxation, limbering, and stretching of the involved muscle using vapocoolant spray or ice as needed combined with and followed by an exercise program. Active and active-assisted exercises are an integral part of the physical therapy program (see Chapter 9 for details).

Exercise and Home Program

Exercises are performed to strengthen the abdominal muscles. Partial sit-ups are done progressing to full sit-up exercises. Exercises should at first be performed under the guidance of a therapist. When the patient is free of pain and full motion has been achieved, progress to strength and endurance programs. Begin and end exercise sessions with stretching and relaxation (see Chapter 12).

Corrective and Preventive Measures

- Correct abdominal weakness with a progressive exercise program.
- Avoid excessive stress caused by poor body mechanics during gymnastics, athletic activities, and postural attitudes at work.
- Eliminate intraabdominal pathologic conditions (visceral disease) which may be a cause of abdominal trigger points.
- Warm-up and cool-down exercises should be performed with all exercise and athletic activities.

PECTORAL MUSCLES
Pectoralis major, pectoralis minor

Symptoms and Pain Pattern

- A trigger point in the pectoral muscle is often found to be the cause of pain in the upper arm.[18, 20]
- Pain may be noted over the pectoral area in front of the chest.[7, 46]
- Referred pain is noted over the deltoid area and may radiate to the upper and lower forearm or may be localized to the upper and lower forearm (Fig 10–8).
- Radiation to the fourth and fifth fingers has been reported in addition to cardiac arrythmias due to trigger points between the fifth and sixth right ribs.[20, 43]
- Trigger points may develop in the chest wall from pain due to coronary artery disease.[43]
- Pectoral pain due to chest wall tenderness may resemble pain of cardiac origin.[2]

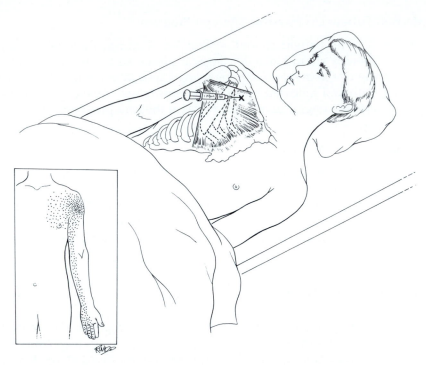

FIG 10–8.   Pectoralis major and minor. Injection of trigger points *(X's)* in the pectoral muscles. Direct the needle tangentially in relation to the chest wall to avoid puncturing the pleura. Aspirate prior to injection. Avoid the intercostal space. *Inset,* pain pattern *(stippling).*

Findings on Examination

- Tender trigger points over the pectoral area may cause referred pain to the deltoid, and upper and lower arm.
- Active trigger points in the pectoralis minor which cause muscle shortening have been reported to be responsible for a diminished radial pulse in addition to arterial compression when the shoulder is abducted.[44]

Differential Diagnosis

- Cardiac pain.
- Costochondritis (Tietze's syndrome).
- Cervical radiculopathy.
- Subdeltoid bursitis.

Anatomy

Pectoralis Major:

Origin: medial half of anterior surface of the clavicle, the whole length of the front of the sternum, front of the upper six costal cartilages, and external rectus sheath.

Insertion: lateral lip of the bicipital groove of the humerus.

Action: adducts the arm, medially rotates and flexes the arm.

Pectoralis Minor

The pectoralis minor lies under the cover of the pectoralis major.
Origin: third, fourth, and fifth ribs near the costochondral junctions.
Insertion: medial border of the coracoid process.
Action: pulls the scapula forward and depresses the shoulder.

Noninvasive Therapy

The post–trigger point injection follow-up program described in Chapter 9 is recommended as a conservative therapeutic treatment approach. Noninvasive therapy can include:

- Physical therapy modalities (e.g., electrical stimulation and warm packs; see Chapter 15).
- Manual physical therapy techniques (e.g., massage and the Trager Approach; see Chapters 13 and 14).
- Active and passive stretching and limbering of muscles with or without the use of vapocoolant spray or ice. Active exercise is part of the stretch-and-spray technique. Limbering and relaxation are necessary prior to stretching. Contract-relax techniques may be used.
- *Pectoralis major:* Stretch and spray should be performed with abduction, external rotation, and extension of the arm, with the aid of vapocoolant spray or ice. Electrical stimulation, limbering of muscles, and warm packs may precede stretch and spray to relax the muscles.
- *Pectoralis minor:* Stretch and spray is performed by abducting and elevating the arm to pull the scapula back and elevate the shoulder.
- Exercises and a home program for the upper extremities are described in Chapter 9. Exercise programs include relaxation, limbering, stretching, and strengthening. When the patient is free of pain and full motion has been achieved, progress to strength and endurance programs.

Injection of Trigger Points

The pectoralis minor is palpated through the pectoralis major. The pectoral muscles are most often treated together. With the patient in the supine position, trigger points are identified and local areas of tenderness are injected (see Figs 10–8 and 9–12,G). Localize the trigger points between the index finger and middle finger or thumb. Avoid the intercostal space. (See Chapter 9 for injection technique.)

Needle size: 1.5 in., 21 gauge.

Solution: Any one of the following solutions may be used: 0.5% procaine; 1.0% lidocaine; saline and dry needling in case of allergy.

Precautions

- Direct the needle tangentially in relation to the chest wall to avoid puncturing the pleura and causing a pneumothorax.
- Aspirate before injecting or needling.
- See Chapter 9 for complications.

Postinjection Follow-Up Physical Therapy Program

The patient should receive 3 to 4 consecutive days of treatment. Physical therapy should include electrical stimulation, relaxation, limbering, and stretching of the involved muscle using vapocoolant spray or ice as needed combined with and followed by an exercise program. Active and active-assisted exercises are an integral part of the physical therapy program (see Chapter 9 for details).

Exercise and Home Program

Exercises for the upper extremity and pectoral muscles are prescribed. Exercises should at first be performed under the guidance of a therapist. When the patient is free of pain and full motion has been achieved, progress to strength and endurance programs. Begin and end exercise sessions with relaxation and stretching. (See Chapter 12 for exercise details.)

Corrective and Preventive Measures

- Avoid activities which require holding the arms out in front of the body for long periods.
- Correct standing and sitting postures, e.g., use the proper height of chair armrests and a lumbar roll.

STERNALIS

Symptoms and Pain Pattern

- Pain due to trigger points in the parasternal muscles is most often felt under the sternum[13, 25] (Fig 10–9).
- Laterally located trigger points may refer pain to the scapula, upper extremities, and ulnar distribution of the forearm and hand.[20, 43]
- Symptoms may resemble angina or myocardial infarction.
- Chest pain resulting from myocardiac insufficiency may also be a cause of active trigger points involving the sternalis and pectoral muscles.[43]

Findings on Examination

- Local tender areas over the sternum refer pain to the arm, forearm, and hand. Look for trigger points in neighboring muscles (cervical and pectoral).

Differential Diagnosis

- Costochondrities (Tietze's syndrome).
- Angina.
- Myocardial infarction.
- Pectoral muscle trigger points.

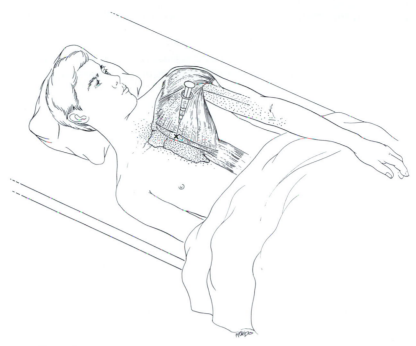

FIG 10–9. Sternalis. Injection of trigger point *(X)* in the sternalis with the patient supine. Observe precautions to avoid entering the chest cavity. Anatomic landmarks are noted. Pain pattern is shown by *stippling*.

Anatomy

Origin: deep aspect of the xiphoid and fifth, sixth, and seventh costal cartilages.

Insertion: posterior aspect of second to sixth costal cartilages.

Noninvavisive Therapy

The post–trigger point injection follow-up program described in Chapter 9 is recommended as a conservative therapeutic treatment approach. Noninvasive therapy can include:

- Physical therapy modalities (e.g., electrical stimulation and warm packs; see Chapter 15).
- Manual physical therapy techniques apply when the pectoral muscles are also involved (e.g., massage and the Trager Approach; see Chapters 13 and 14).
- Active and passive stretching and limbering of muscles when the pectoral muscles are involved, with or without the use of vapocoolant spray or ice. Active exercise is part of the stretch-and-spray technique. Limbering and relaxation are necessary prior to stretching. Contract-relax techniques may be used.

Injection of Trigger Point

Needle size: 1.5 in., 22–25 gauge.

Solution: Any one of the following solutions may be used: 0.5% procaine; 1.0% lidocaine; saline and dry needling in case of allergy. Do not use epinephrine.

Precautions

- Direct needle tangentially.
- Avoid the intercostal space.
- Aspirate prior to injection (see Chapter 9 for pneumothorax complications).

Postinjection Follow-Up Program

The patient should receive 3 to 4 consecutive days of treatment (see Chapter 9). Physical therapy should include electrical stimulation and massage techniques. If neighboring muscles (pectoralis major and minor) are involved, appropriate therapy including exercises are prescribed (see discussion of exercises for the upper extremity, Chapter 12).

Corrective and Preventive Measures

- Sternalis trigger points may develop secondary to trigger points in the pectoralis major or minor.
- Treat medical and physical conditions that cause chest pain.

Muscles of the Lower Extremities

GLUTEUS MAXIMUS

Symptoms and Pain Pattern

- Pain in the gluteal area is aggravated by walking or prolonged sitting and driving.
- Pain in the gluteal area at night.
- Pain usually remains localized in the gluteal area (Fig 10–10).
- Referred pain may felt be felt as coccygodynia.[45]
- Sciatic-type pain radiation has been described by several authors.[5, 7, 18, 20]
- The gluteus maximus is active in raising the trunk from a bent-forward position and can be activated with such activities as raising the trunk after leaning over a sink, or getting up from a chair with the trunk in a bent-forward position.

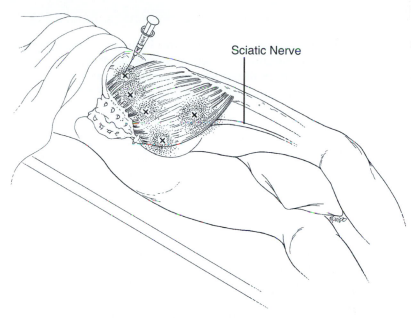

Sciatic Nerve

FIG 10–10. Gluteus maximus. Injection of trigger points *(X's)* in the gluteus maximus. Anatomic landmarks are noted. Avoid the sciatic nerve. Pain pattern is shown by *stippling*. Injection may be performed with the patient in the prone or side-lying position.

Findings on Examination

- Trigger point examination may be performed with the patient lying on the unaffected side with the knee flexed or with the patient prone.
- On palpation tender trigger points may be found next to the sacral attachments medially and distally as well as the region over the ischial tuberosity. Trigger points in the gluteal region can often be palpated as knots in the muscle, taut bands, or manifested only by the "jump sign." A jump sign is frequently elicited in this area (the patient quickly moves away when the painful trigger point is palpated).
- Gluteus maximus muscle strength may be tested by placing the patient in the prone position with the knee flexed to 90 degrees, hyperextending the thigh at the hip against resistance.
- Trigger points are often found laterally over the gluteus medius. Trigger points involving the gluteus maximus, medius, minimus, paraspinal area, and hamstrings, as well as tensor fasciae latae, often occur together in patients with low back pain.
- Antagonistic muscles, such as the rectus femoris and iliopsoas, may develop trigger points and also may require treatment.

Differential Diagnosis

- Ischial bursitis.
- Coccygodynia.
- Herniated disc.
- Arthritis of the hip presenting as posterior buttock pain.

Anatomy

Origin: area on ilium above and behind the posterior gluteal line, the lateral mass of the sacrum, the sacrotuberous ligament.

Insertion: back of the sacrotuberous ligament.

Action: extensor and lateral rotator of thigh.

Noninvasive Therapy

The post–trigger point injection follow-up program described in Chapter 9 is recommended as a conservative therapeutic treatment approach. Noninvasive therapy can include:

- Physical therapy modalities (e.g., electrical stimulation and warm packs; see Chapter 15).
- Manual physical therapy techniques (e.g., massage and the Trager Approach; see Chapters 13 and 14).
- Active and passive stretching and limbering of muscles with or without the use of vapocoolant spray or ice. Active exercise is part of the stretch-and-spray technique. Limbering and relaxation are necessary prior to stretching. Contract-relax techniques may be used.
- Stretch and spray for the gluteus maximus is performed with the patient lying on the uninvolved side. The hip is flexed bringing the knee to the abdomen. Use relaxation techniques to relax the gluteal muscles. Contract and relax the buttocks. When contracting the gluteal muscles in the supine position the patient should breathe in. Exhale with release or letting go of the contraction. This may be accompanied by the use of vapocoolant spray or ice if necessary. The therapist's hands should feel the contraction and relaxation of the muscle. The patient should be told that it is the relaxation ("letting go") of the muscle that is the most important part of the exercises. Electrical stimulation, limbering of muscles, and warm packs should precede stretch and spray to relax muscles.
- The exercise program for the hip and low back is described in Chapter 12. Include exercises which stretch the gluteus maximus area by bending forward in the sitting position. This should also be accompanied by appropriate relaxation and letting go. The patient should inhale when sitting up and exhale when bending forward. Movements should always be done slowly, smoothly, and with few repetitions (three to four).

Injection of Trigger Point

Trigger points may be palpated in the medial portion, lower midportion, and inferior portion of the gluteus maximus. A trigger point over the ischial bursa may be the cause of pain as well as trigger points below the crest of the ilium. Injection of trigger points should include multiple needle entries covering not only the area of the palpable tender trigger point but a search for additional trigger points throughout the muscle (see Fig 10–10). This would require injecting the four areas as noted in the figure. Trigger points over the area of the sciatic nerve should be well identified, isolated by palpation, and injected superficially, cautiously, and with avoidance of deep penetration. Injection may be performed with the patient prone with the pillow under the abdomen or in the side-lying position. (See Chapter 9 for injection technique.)

Needle size: Usually a 3-in., 21-gauge needle is necessary. For very thin persons a 1.5- to 2.0-in. needle may suffice.

Solution: Any one of the following solutions may be used: 0.5% procaine; 1.0% lidocaine; saline and dry needling in case of allergy. Do not use epinephrine.

Following injection apply pressure immediately. An ice compress may be used to prevent hematoma if excessive bleeding appears to be present or anticipated. The use of a moist heating pad or hot packs applied to the buttock for 5 to 10 minutes to reduce postinjection soreness should be done with caution. The use of hot packs after injection may encourage bleeding. Neither heat nor cold applications should be necessary following trigger point injection.

Precautions

- Avoid the sciatic nerve which lies at a midpoint between the ischial tuberosity and greater trochanter as illustrated in Figure 10–10).
- Tests for sciatic nerve involvement: Following injection the patient should not experience numbness, paresthesia in the lower extremity, or muscle weakness involving the foot.

Postinjection Follow-Up Physical Therapy Program

The patient should receive 3 to 4 consecutive days of treatment. Physical therapy should include electrical stimulation, relaxation, limbering, and stretching of the involved muscle using vapocoolant spray or ice as needed combined with and followed by an exercise program. Active and active-assisted exercises are an integral part of the physical therapy program (see Chapter 9 for details).

Exercise and Home Program

Exercises should at first be performed under the guidance of a therapist. Exercises include stretching of the gluteus maximus by flexing the hip and bringing the knee to the chest. This can be assisted and passively stretched by both the therapist and the patient at home. The patient must be given a home exercise program which includes active exercises as well as stretching. When the patient is free of pain and full motion has been achieved, progress to strength and endurance programs. Begin and end exercise sessions with stretching and relaxation. Exercise programs include relaxation, limbering, stretching, and strengthening. When the patient is free of pain and full motion has been achieved, progress to strength and endurance programs (see Chapter 12 for details).

Corrective and Preventive Measures

- An unbalanced sitting posture for prolonged periods may produce trigger points in the gluteal muscles. Trigger points that are symptomatic may require a doughnut-like pillow designed to take weight off specific trigger points. Poor sitting posture may aggravate latent trigger points.
- Avoid improperly constructed seat cushions. Cushions that have promi-

nences such as buttons may have an effect similar to carrying a wallet or other objects in the back pocket.
- Night pain may be helped by sleeping on the uninvolved side with a pillow between the thighs to avoid pressure on the gluteus maximus.
- Correct leg length discrepancies, e.g., with a heel lift.
- Correct foot abnormalities (flatfoot), e.g., with appropriate orthoses.

GLUTEUS MEDIUS

Symptoms and Pain Pattern

- Pain in the low back, buttock area, and lateral and posterior aspect of the thigh (Fig 10–11).
- Pain may be sciatic in nature involving the posterior aspect of the lower extremity.[17, 20, 33, 35]
- Symptoms are similar to those found with trigger points in the gluteus maximus and often occur together with active trigger points in the gluteus maximus as well as in the lumbar and tensor fasciae latae muscles.
- Prolonged sitting, walking, or lying directly on the trigger points will cause localized pain which may radiate to the lower extremity.

Findings on Examination

- Tender trigger points noted on palpation in the gluteus medius just below the iliac crest posteriorly and anteriorly.
- A nodule or taut band of muscle fibers may be palpable. A jump sign is a frequent finding.
- Posteriorly, the gluteus medius is covered by the gluteus maximus. Most

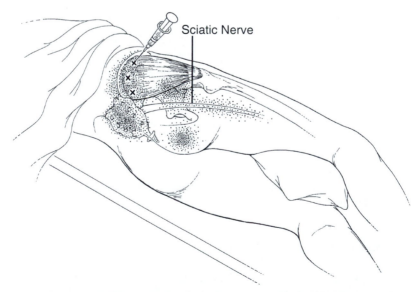

FIG 10–11.   Gluteus medius. Injection of trigger points in the right gluteus medius. Multiple trigger points (*X's*) are noted. Anatomic skeletal landmarks are shown together with the sciatic nerve. The patient is positioned lying on the uninvolved side. Injection may also be performed with the patient prone. Pain pattern is noted by *stippled area*.

often a neighboring muscle or muscles will also harbor trigger points. Trigger points in the sacrospinalis, quadratus lumborum, and tensor fasciae latae will be found together with involvement of all the gluteal muscles. This is often the combination of multiple trigger points found in patients with low back pain.

- Contracture of the muscle may be present.
- Test for muscle weakness by having the patient lie on the uninvolved side. Pressure is exerted on the abducted hyperextended leg with the knee in extension. Depending on the degree of weakness the patient may walk with a limp (gluteus medius limp). Slight weakness may cause postural changes such as scoliosis and pelvic tilt which can give rise to trigger points in the lumbar area.

Differential Diagnosis

- Herniated lumbar disc.
- Sciatica.
- Trochanteric bursitis.
- Leriche's syndrome.
- Sacroilaic joint dysfunction.
- Sciatic neuritis due to arthritis or diabetes.

Anatomy

Origin: outer surface of the ilium between the posterior and medial gluteal line.

Insertion. outer aspect of the greater trochanter.

Action. abducts thigh; prevents opposite side of pelvis from dropping when walking.

Noninvasive Therapy

The post–trigger point injection follow-up program described in Chapter 9 is recommended as a conservative therapeutic approach. Noninvasive therapy can include:

- Physical therapy modalities (e.g., electrical stimulation and warm packs; see Chapter 15).
- Manual physical therapy techniques (e.g., massage and the Trager Approach; see Chapters 13 and 14).
- Active and passive stretching and limbering of muscles with or without the use of vapocoolant spray or ice. Active exercise is part of the stretch-and-spray technique. Limbering and relaxation are necessary prior to stretching. Contract-relax techniques may be used.
- Stretch and spray for the gluteus medius is performed in the side-lying position. Positioning may be improved by placing a flat pillow under the uninvolved hip. Stretching of the gluteus is performed by adduction of the thigh bringing the leg both posteriorly as well as anteriorly to stretch both portions of the gluteus medius posteriorly and anteriorly. The patient may be moved back toward the edge of the table with the leg partly off the table in extension supported by the therapist. The thigh is ex-

tended posteriorly, adducted, and externally rotated. The leg is also brought forward to the opposite side of the table, the thigh extended, adducted, and internally rotated. Electrical stimulation, limbering of muscles, and warm packs may precede stretch and spray to relax the muscles. Stretching of muscle is also accomplished actively as well as with assistance during the exercise program. Active exercise is part of the stretch-and-spray technique. Use relaxation techniques (e.g., contract-relax). Electrical stimulation, limbering of muscles, and warm packs should precede stretch and spray to relax muscles.

- Exercise program: The exercise program for the gluteus medius is described in Chapter 12. Exercise programs include relaxation, limbering, stretching, and strengthening. When the patient is free of pain and full motion has been achieved, progress to strength and endurance programs.

Trigger Point Injection

Injection may be performed with the patient lying on the uninvolved side or prone (see Chapter 9 for technique). Tender trigger points are identified (see Fig 10–11).

Needle size: 3-in., 22 gauge, is usually used for needling the gluteal area. In the case of thin persons smaller needles of 1.5 to 2.0 in., 22 gauge, may be used.

Solution: Any one of the following solutions may be used: 0.5% procaine; 1.0% lidocaine; saline and dry needling in cases of allergy. Do not use epinephrine.

A small amount of vapocoolant spray over the needle entry area prior to injection decreases the pain of needle entry. Many patients report that avoiding needle entry pain decreases the discomfort of the procedure appreciably and avoids tensing. This effect varies with the individual patient. Look for additional trigger points in addition to the local tender area. The gluteus medius should be palpated and explored using multiple needle entries as noted in Figure 10–10. Multiple trigger points involving the gluteus maximus, gluteus minimus, quadratus lumborum, and tensor fasciae latae may be present. Each muscle group must be treated individually. The low back muscles, such as the sacrospinalis and quadratus lumborum trigger points, may be treated separately or together.

Precautions

- Following the injection the patient should not experience any paresthesia or muscle weakness in the lower extremity.
- Avoid injection in the area of the sciatic nerve, and avoid the greater sciatic notch area.
- Inject only one trigger point area or muscle group at a time. Postinjection spasm after multiple muscle group injections may prevent a proper rehabilitation program.

Postinjection Follow-Up Program

The patient should receive 3 to 4 consecutive days of treatment. Physical therapy should include electrical stimulation, relaxation, limbering, and stretching of the involved muscle using vapocoolant spray or ice as needed combined with and followed by an exercise program. Active-assisted and active exercises are an integral part of the physical therapy program (see Chapter 9 for details).

Exercise and Home Program

Exercises for the gluteus medius are prescribed. Exercises should at first be performed under the guidance of a therapist. When the patient is free of pain and full motion has been achieved, progress to strength and endurance programs. Begin and end the exercise sessions with stretching and relaxation. (See Chapter 12 for exercise details.)

Corrective and Preventive Measures

- Correct poor sitting and standing postures.
- Abnormalities of the pelvis such as a small hemipelvis may be corrected with a buttock lift.[44]
- Correct improper chair construction. Use a lumbar support to improve a car seat or chair.
- Remove objects from the back pocket, e.g., wallet.
- Correct leg length discrepancies, e.g., prescribe a heel lift.
- Correct foot abnormalities such as flatfoot or Morton's foot. Prescribe orthoses as necessary.

GLUTEUS MINIMUS

Symptoms and Pain Pattern

- The patient may experience pain over the buttock area in addition to sciatic referred-type pain radiating as far distally as the ankle (Fig 10–12).
- Anterior trigger points refer pain along the lateral thigh, lower buttock, and lateral aspect of the ankle.
- Posterior trigger points refer pain to the buttock area and posterior upper thigh in addition to the calf.[18, 20] Travell and Simons[45] make a distinction between radiating pain patterns due to anterior and posterior fibers. Other authors[4, 11, 12, 19] are not as specific when attributing sciatic pain from the gluteal muscle area.
- A similar pattern of pain is experienced by patients with trigger points in the gluteus maximus and gluteus medius.[13, 20]
- Pain is noted with sitting and walking.
- Night pain occurs when lying on the trigger point area.

Findings on Examination

- Trigger points may be found in the anterior and posterior portions of the muscle. Both may be palpated with the patient lying on the uninvolved side.
- Most often trigger points in the gluteus minimus are accompanied by trigger points in the surrounding muscles, e.g., the gluteus maximus, medius, piriformis, sacrospinalis, and latissimus dorsi.

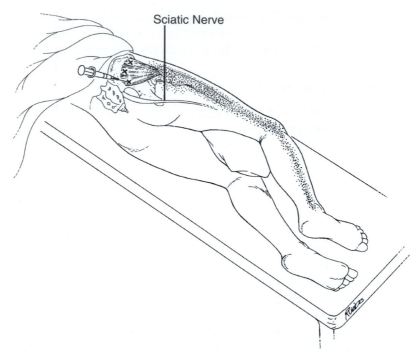

FIG 10–12. Gluteus minimus. Injection of trigger points *(X's)* in the gluteus minimus. Injection may be given with the patient in the prone or side-lying position. Anatomic landmarks and sciatic nerve are noted. Pain pattern *(stippling)* may extend to the ankle.

- Referred pain may cause the development of trigger points in the posterior aspect of the thigh.
- Examination of the gluteus minimus may reveal weakness of abduction and shortening of the muscle.

Differential Diagnosis

- Sciatic radiculopathy.
- Herniated lumbar disc.
- Trochanteric bursitis.
- Arthritis of the hip.
- Lumbar facet joint arthritis.
- Sacroiliac joint dysfunction.

Anatomy

Origin: outer surface of the ilium between the middle and inferior gluteal lines.
Insertion: the greater trochanter of the femur.
Action: abductor and medial rotator of the femur.

Noninvasive Therapy

The post–trigger point injection follow-up program described in Chapter 9 is recommended as a conservative therapeutic treatment approach. Noninvasive therapy can include:

- Physical therapy modalities (e.g., electrical stimulation and warm packs; see Chapter 15).
- Manual physical therapy techniques (e.g., massage and the Trager Approach; see Chapters 13 and 14).
- Active and passive stretching and limbering of muscles with or without the use of vapocoolant spray or ice. Active exercise is part of the stretch-and-spray technique. Limbering and relaxation are necessary prior to stretching. Contract-relax techniques may be used.
- Stretch and spray may be performed with the patient lying on the uninvolved side. Positioning may be improved by placing a flat pillow under the uninvolved hip. Stretching of the gluteus minimus is performed by adduction of the thigh bringing the leg both posteriorly as well as anteriorly to stretch both portions of the gluteus medius posteriorly and anteriorly. The patient may be moved back toward the edge of the table with the leg partly off the table in extension and supported by the therapist. The thigh is extended posteriorly, adducted, and externally rotated. The leg is also brought forward to the opposite side of the table, the thigh extended, adducted, and internally rotated. Electrical stimulation, limbering of muscles, and warm packs should precede stretch and spray to relax the muscles. Stretching of muscle is also accomplished actively as well as with assistance during the exercise program. Active exercise is part of the stretch-and-spray technique.
- Exercises and a home program for the gluteus minimus are described in Chapter 12. Exercise programs include relaxation, limbering, stretching, and strengthening. When the patient is free of pain and full motion has been achieved, progress to strength and endurance programs.

Injection of Trigger Points

Injection and needling may be performed with the patient lying on the uninvolved side (see Chapter 9 for technique). Tender trigger points are identified. In addition to local injection of the tender area, multiple needle entries may be necessary to probe for trigger points not felt on palpation. It is not unusual for the needle to penetrate the gluteus minimus and make contact with the ilium. Following injection, test for sciatic nerve symptoms and signs prior to permitting the patient to walk. The patient should remain on the table for a few minutes. Inquire about any abnormal sensation such as numbness or paresthesia in the lower extremity.

Needle size: 3 in., 22–20 gauge.

Solution: Any one of the following solutions may be used: 0.5% procaine; 1.0% lidocaine; saline and dry needling in case of allergy. Do not use epinephrine.

Postinjection Follow-Up Physical Therapy Program

The patient should receive 3 to 4 consecutive days of treatment. Physical therapy should include electrical stimulation, relaxation, limbering, and stretching of the involved muscle using vapocoolant spray or ice as needed combined with and followed by an exercise program. Active and active-assisted exercises are an integral part of the physical therapy program (see Chapter 9 for details).

Exercise and Home Program

Exercises include stretching for the gluteal and lumbar areas. Exercises should at first be performed under the guidance of a therapist. When the patient is free of pain and full motion has been achieved, progress to strength and endurance programs. Begin and end exercise sessions with stretching and relaxation. (See Chapter 12 for exercise details.)

Corrective and Preventive Measures

- Correct foot abnormalities (e.g., Morton's foot, flatfoot) and prescribe orthoses as indicated.
- Correct leg length discrepancy, e.g., prescribe an appropriate heel lift.
- Scoliosis due to small hemipelvis may be corrected by an ischial lift pad under the ischial area.[45]
- Correct postural stresses at work. Advise changing position frequently. Use a footstool when standing and working at a table or sink. (See Chapter 16).
- Avoid poor sitting and standing postures.
- Chairs should be properly constructed and adjusted for individual needs, e.g., the height of armrests, the need for lumbar support.
- Remove objects in the back pocket such as a wallet.[21]

PIRIFORMIS

Symptoms and Pain Pattern

- The patient may experience pain in the low back, buttock, and hip.
- Radiation of pain to the lower extremity involving the posterior thigh, calf, and foot (Fig 10–13). This pain pattern is referred to by Kraus[17] as "pseudo-disc".)
- Paresthesia may be experienced in the lower extremity.
- Pain may be noted after prolonged sitting or driving.[8]
- Pain occurs with prolonged stooping and squatting.[42]
- Sciatic pain may occur with symptoms of entrapment of the sciatic nerve.[15, 19, 28, 44]
- Pace and Nagle[26] have reported dyspareunia as a symptom of the piriformis syndrome.

Findings on Examination

- Piriformis syndrome[41] is seen more frequently in women than men in a 6:1 ratio.
- Palpation may reveal tenderness of the piriformis muscle and is often noted in the sciatic notch.
- To palpate the piriformis muscle, the patient should lie on the uninvolved side with the hip flexed and a pillow between the upper and lower legs.
- A taut band extending over the length of the piriformis (from the greater trochanter to the sacrum) may be found.
- Steiner et al.[40] found the most common trigger area to be located 3 cm

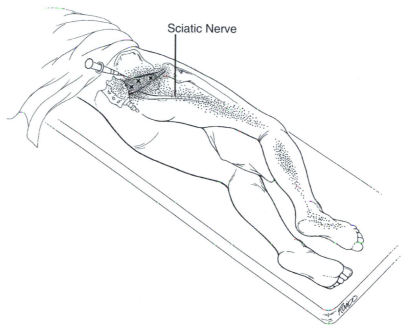

Sciatic Nerve

FIG 10–13. Piriformis. Injection of trigger points in the right piriformis muscle *(X's)*. The sciatic nerve is shown in addition to anatomic details. Injection is performed with the patient lying on the uninvolved side. A pillow is placed between the knees. The hip is flexed. Pain pattern is shown by *stippling*.

caudal and lateral to the midpoint of the lateral border of the sacrum. The second trigger point is located closer to its trochanteric insertion.[40]

- Piriformis tenderness with trigger points may also be palpated by rectal or intrapelvic examination.[1, 9, 26, 44] Coccygodynia is often caused by trigger points and spasm of the levator ani and coccygeus muscles.
- On palpation of a trigger point a referred pattern of pain may be elicited.
- Diminished sensation in the lower extremity or depressed or absent ankle jerk with mild footdrop may represent neurologic findings resulting from trigger points in the piriformis.
- Restriction in internal rotation on the involved side.
- A positive Trendelenburg's test.
- Pain and weakness on testing abduction strength in the seated position.
- Adduction may be limited and painful.
- The patient may maintain the leg in external rotation due to pain experienced with internal rotation.
- A leg length discrepancy may be noted in addition to asymmetry of the pelvis (e.g., hemipelvis).

Differential Diagnosis

The following conditions must be differentiated and are often mistaken for piriformis trigger points:

- Herniated intervertebral disc.
- Peripheral nerve entrapment can occur as a piriformis syndrome without trigger points.

- Sacroiliitis.
- Facet syndrome.

Anatomy

Origin: front of the middle three pieces of the sacrum.
Insertion: tip of greater trochanter.
Action: lateral rotation of the thigh, abduction of the thigh when the hip is flexed.

Noninvasive Therapy

The post–trigger point injection follow-up program described in Chapter 9 is recommended as a conservative therapeutic treatment approach. Noninvasive therapy can include:

- Physical therapy modalities (e.g., electrical stimulation and warm packs; see Chapter 15).
- Manual physical therapy techniques (e.g., massage and the Trager Approach; see Chapters 13 and 14).
- Active and passive stretching and limbering of muscles with or without the use of vapocoolant spray or ice. Active exercise is part of the stretch-and-spray technique. Limbering and relaxation are necessary prior to stretching. Contract-relax techniques may be used.
- Stretch and spray for the piriformis is performed with the patient lying on the uninvolved side with the hip flexed to 90 degrees. Stretch is done in the direction of adduction and internal rotation. Electrical stimulation, limbering of muscles, and warm packs should precede stretch and spray to relax the muscles. Stretching of muscle is also accomplished actively as well as with assistance during the exercise program. Active exercise is part of the stretch-and-spray technique.
- Exercise and home program. Exercises include hip abduction with the limb in moderate external rotation. Piriformis muscle stretching is accomplished by adducting the thigh with the hip flexed. See Chapter 12 for hip and low back exercises. Exercise programs include relaxation, limbering, stretching, and strengthening. When the patient is free of pain and full motion has been achieved, progress to strength and endurance programs.

Injection of Trigger Point

Injection is accomplished with the patient lying on the unaffected side with the thigh flexed to approximately 60 to 45 degrees (see Fig 10–13). The knee is dropped to the plinth. A pillow is placed between the knees. Identify the trigger point by palpation. Several authors have recommended that injection of trigger points in the medial region of the muscle be performed bimanually. One finger palpates the trigger point either by the rectal or vaginal approach and the other directs the needle externally in the direction of the intrapelvic palpating fingertip.[26, 45] (See Chapter 12 for injection technique.)
Needle size: 2, 3 in., 20 gauge

Solution: Any one of the following solutions may be used: 0.5% procaine; 1.0% lidocaine; saline and dry needling in case of allergy. Do not use epinephrine.

Precautions

- Postinjection complications: Test for sciatic nerve involvement following injection, including diminished sensation or muscle weakness. (See Chapter 9 for complications.)

Postinjection Follow-Up Program

After injection the patient is instructed not to sit, stand, or walk for prolonged periods. He or she is advised to change position often. The patient should receive 3 to 4 consecutive days of treatment. Therapy should include electrical stimulation, relaxation, limbering, and stretching of the involved muscle using vapocoolant spray or ice as needed combined with and followed by an exercise program (see Chapter 9 for details).

Exercise and Home Program

Exercises should at first be performed under the guidance of a therapist. When the patient is free of pain and full motion has been achieved, progress to strength and endurance programs. Begin and end exercise sessions with stretching and relaxation (see Chapter 12 for piriformis, hip, and low back exercise details). Advise the use of a pillow between the legs when sleeping on the side. Exercises should include stretching of the piriformis by adducting the thigh with the hip flexed and the pelvis stabilized (countertraction on the crest of the ilium).

Corrective and Preventive Measures

- Correct leg length inequality, e.g., with a heel lift.
- Postural corrections of small hemipelvis or scoliosis may require a buttock lift when sitting.[45]
- Correct foot deformities (e.g., flatfoot, Morton's foot) and prescribe orthoses.
- Patient must avoid prolonged unsupported lateral rotation of the leg on the accelerator when driving.
- Avoid sitting for long periods with the ankle crossed on the opposite knee.[43]

TENSOR FASCIAE LATAE

Symptoms and Pain Pattern

- Pain over the lateral aspect of the hip[7] (Fig 10–14).
- Referred pain may radiate to the greater trochanter area extending distally to the outer aspect of the thigh and below the knee. This pattern of referred pain may be mistaken for lumbar radiculopathy[11, 12, 17, 20] (see Fig 10–14).

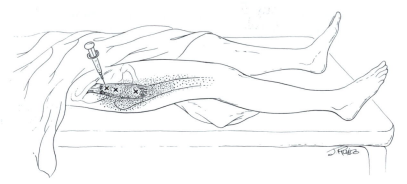

FIG 10–14.   Tensor fascia latae. Injection of trigger points in the right tensor fascia latae *(X's)*. Anatomic landmarks are noted including the origin and insertion of the muscle. The patient is supine with a small pillow under the knee. Pain pattern is shown by *stippling*.

- Pressure on the trigger point may cause pain when the patient lies on the involved side.
- Since trigger points in the gluteal muscles are frequently present together with those of the tensor fasciae latae, symptoms of gluteal muscle trigger points may also occur.
- Pain may be present with walking or running activities.

Findings on Examination

- Trigger points may be palpated along the tensor fasciae latae with the patient in the supine position or lying on the uninvolved side.
- The muscle extends laterally and inferiorly inserting into the iliotibial band.
- Tenderness may be found over the greater trochanter and in the area of referred pain.
- Contracture of the tensor fasciae latae causes contracture of the iliotibial band which can be demonstrated by a positive Ober's test. Ober's test for contraction of the iliotibial band is performed with the patient lying on the uninvolved side. The leg is abducted, the knee is flexed to 90 degrees, and the abducted leg is released. If the iliotibial tract is normal the thigh should drop to the adducted position. In the presence of contracture of the fasciae latae or iliotibial band the thigh remains abducted when the leg is released.[10] In less severe cases when a degree of tightness is present, limited adduction of the hip occurs.
- Palpation may cause a referred pain pattern to the outer aspect of the hip and lower extremity (see Fig 10–14).

Differential Diagnosis

- Herniated disc.
- Trochanteric bursitis.
- Neuralgia paresthetica.[15]

Anatomy

Origin: outer surface of ilium, between the tubercle of the crest and the anterior superior iliac spine.

Insertion: iliotibial tract below the greater trochanter of the femur.

Action: assists gluteus maximus in tightening the iliotibial band.

Noninvasive Therapy

The post–trigger point injection follow-up program described in Chapter 9 is recommended as a conservative therapeutic treatment approach. Noninvasive therapy can include:

- Physical therapy modalities (e.g., electrical stimulation and warm packs; see Chapter 15).
- Manual physical therapy techniques (e.g., massage and the Trager Approach; see Chapters 13 and 14).
- Active and passive stretching and limbering of muscles with or without the use of vapocoolant spray or ice. Active exercise is part of the stretch-and-spray technique. Limbering and relaxation are necessary prior to stretching. Contract-relax techniques may be used.
- Stretch and spray for the tensor fascia latae is performed with the patient side-lying on the uninvolved side. Electrical stimulation, limbering of muscles, and warm packs should precede stretch and spray to relax the muscles. Begin stretch and spray with the knee extended to promote adduction, increasing knee flexion as adduction increases. As with all stretch movements about the hip, the pelvis must be stabilized. Follow with active stretching.
- Exercises and a home program for the hip and knee are described in Chapter 12. Exercise programs include relaxation, limbering, stretching, and strengthening. When the patient is free of pain and full motion has been achieved, progress to strength and endurance programs.

Injection of Trigger Point

The tensor fasciae latae may be palpated in the supine position or with the patient lying on the uninvolved side. Trigger point injection may be performed in the supine or side-lying position (see Fig 10–14). A search for all trigger points is essential. Multiple entries and the use of a fanning, circular technique are necessary for proper trigger point treatment. Injection of lidocaine is performed after the trigger point is encountered. (See Chapter 9 for trigger point injection technique.)

Needle size: 1.5 or 3.0 in., 21 gauge.

Solution: Any one of the following solutions may be used: 0.5% procaine; 1.0% lidocaine; saline and dry needling in case of allergy. Do not use epinephrine.

Postinjection Follow-Up Physical Therapy Program

The patient should receive 3 to 4 consecutive days of treatment. Physical therapy should include electrical stimulation, relaxation, limbering, and stretching of the involved muscle using vapocoolant spray or ice as needed combined with and followed by an exercise program. Active and active-assisted exercises are an integral part of the physical therapy program (see Chapter 9 for details).

Exercise and Home Program

Exercises include stretching of the tensor fascia latae. Stretch and spray with the patient in the side-lying position. Hip abduction is followed by adduction permitting gravity to assist in the adduction maneuver. The stretch is first done with the leg extended, brought into the position of adduction. This progresses to performing the exercise with the knee flexed. The patient should be relaxed, permitting the flexed knee to fall assisted by gravity until it touches the plinth. The knee is then extended and the leg abducted. Exercises should at first be performed under the guidance of a therapist. When the patient is free of pain and full motion has been achieved, progress to strength and endurance programs. Begin and end exercise sessions with relaxation. (See Chapter 13 for exercise details.)

Corrective and Preventive Measures

- Correct leg length inequality, e.g., with a heel lift.
- Correct foot deformities: calcaneal valgus, flatfoot, Morton's foot. Prescribe orthoses as needed.

HAMSTRING MUSCLES
Semimembranosus, semitendinosus, biceps femoris

Symptoms and Pain Pattern

- Pain from the hamstrings is noted in the gluteal region, lower thigh, and upper portion of the leg[13] (Fig 10–15).
- Pain may be referred by the biceps femoris to the lateral aspect of the knee posteriorly.[4, 6, 44]
- The semitendinosus or semimembranosus may refer pain to the medial side of the back of the knee.[7, 32]
- Symptoms may occur with walking or sitting.[27]
- Compression of trigger points will give rise to symptoms.

Findings on Examination

- Tender trigger points over the hamstrings may cause local or referred pain extending approximately to the gluteal area, distally to the posterior aspect of the thigh and the back of the knee.
- In cases of hamstring tightness and trigger points, the gluteal and lumbar areas should also be examined for trigger points.
- Limited straight leg raising with pain in the low back.
- Pain in the posterior aspect of the thigh and the back of the knee may be

mistaken for a positive straight leg raising test owing to sciatic nerve irritation.

Differential Diagnosis

- Herniated lumbar disc.
- Peripheral neuritis.
- Knee disorders, e.g., osteoarthritis, torn posterior horn of meniscus.
- Ischial bursitis.

Anatomy

Biceps Femoris, Long Head
Origin: ischial tuberosity.
Insertion: head of fibula, lateral condyle of tibia.
Action: extends thigh, flexes leg.

Biceps Femoris Short Head
Origin: linea aspera, intermuscular septum.
Insertion: lateral condyle of tibia.
Action: flexes leg.

Semitendinosus
Origin: ischial tuberosity.
Insertion: medial body of the tibia behind the sartorius and inferior to the gracilis.
Action: extends thigh, flexes leg.

Semimembranosus
Origin: ischial tuberosity.
Insertion: posteromedial aspect of tibial condyle.
Action: extends thigh, flexes leg.

Noninvasive Therapy

The post–trigger point injection follow-up program described in Chapter 9 is recommended as a conservative therapeutic treatment approach. Noninvasive therapy can include:

- Physical therapy modalities (e.g., electrical stimulation and warm packs; see Chapter 15).
- Manual physical therapy techniques (e.g., massage and the Trager Approach; see Chapters 13 and 14).
- Active and passive stretching and limbering of muscles with or without the use of vapocoolant spray or ice. Active exercise is part of the stretch-and-spray technique. Limbering and relaxation are necessary prior to stretching. Contract-relax techniques may be used.
- Stretch and spray: Electrical stimulation, limbering of muscles, and warm packs should precede stretch and spray to relax the muscles. Use vapocoolant spray or ice to encourage flexion of the thigh and extension of the leg. Examine neighboring muscles for trigger points and muscle tightness.

Lengthening neighboring muscles such as the adductor magnus followed by release of the gluteal muscles may be necessary prior to stretching the hamstring muscles.[46]

- Exercise and a home program for the hip and knee are described in Chapter 12. Exercise programs include relaxation, limbering, stretching, and strengthening. When the patient is free of pain and full motion has been achieved, progress to strength and endurance programs.

Injection of Trigger Point

The patient may be supine with the legs slightly externally rotated with the hip and knee in slight flexion. Injection may also be performed with the patient in the side-lying position or prone (Fig 10–15). It is preferable to do either the medial or lateral hamstring during one session. If more than one muscle group is injected, postinjection soreness and spasm may interfere with proper rehabilitation. It is essential to explore the length of the muscle by multiple needling in addition to any single trigger point that is found on palpation. (See Chapter 9 for injection technique).

Needle size: 1.5, 2.0, 3.0 in., 22 gauge.

Solution: Any one of the following solutions may be used: 0.5% procaine; 1.0% lidocaine; saline and dry needling in case of allergy. Do not use epinephrine.

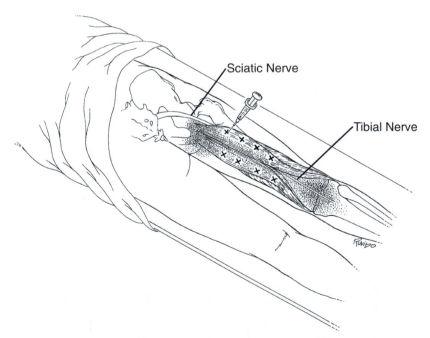

FIG 10–15. Hamstring muscles. Injection of trigger points in the right hamstring muscles with the patient prone. Injection of trigger points may be performed with the patient supine with the hip and knee in slight flexion and the leg externally rotated. It is preferable to do either the medial or lateral hamstring during one session. Injection of more than one muscle group promotes soreness and muscle spasm which may interfere with rehabilitation. Anatomic landmarks are noted including the sciatic nerve. Pain patterns are noted by *stippling*.

Postinjection Follow-Up Physical Therapy Program

The patient should receive 3 to 4 consecutive days of treatment. Physical therapy should include electrical stimulation, relaxation, limbering, and stretching of the involved muscle using vapocoolant spray or ice as needed combined with and followed by an exercise program. Active and active-assisted exercises are an integral part of the physical therapy program. Crutches are used for 24 hours following injection to prevent pain, spasm, and limping. (See Chapter 9 for program details.)

Exercise and Home Program

Exercises for the hamstrings are prescribed. Exercises should at first be performed under the guidance of a therapist. When the patient is free of pain and full motion has been achieved, progress to strength and endurance programs. Begin and end exercise sessions with stretching and relaxation. (See Chapter 12 for exercise details.)

Precautions

- Avoid the sciatic nerve (see Fig 10–14).

Corrective and Preventive Measures

- Avoid compression of the hamstrings by correcting poor sitting habits.
- Perform warm-up and cool-down exercises, which include hamstring stretches before and after athletic activity to prevent the development of trigger points and activation of latent trigger points.
- Continue home exercise program.

QUADRICEPS FEMORIS
Rectus femoris, vastus intermedius, vastus medialis, vastus lateralis
Single muscle trigger points in the muscles of the quadriceps femoris commonly cause trigger points in neighboring muscles.

RECTUS FEMORIS

Symptoms and Pain Pattern

- Trigger points in the rectus femoris refer pain to the lower thigh and anterior aspect of the knee.
- Pain at night occurring in front of the knee.[18, 20, 46]
- Feeling of weakness in the thigh.

Findings on Examination

- Tightness of the rectus femoris may be demonstrated in the side-lying position by extending the hip and flexing the knee. This can also be done with the patient lying in the supine position bringing the leg off the examination table and extending the hip and flexing the knee.

- Trigger points may be found on palpation along the entire length of the muscle. Most trigger points, however, are found in the regions of muscle origin and insertion. These areas are emphasized during examination for trigger points.[18]
- Quadriceps atrophy may be present due to disuse or symptomatic knee disorders.
- Chronic pain due to a knee abnormality may give rise to trigger points in the quadratus femoris muscles.

Differential Diagnosis

- Arthritis of the knee.
- Internal derangement of the knee.
- Chondromalacia.

Anatomy

Origin: the straight head from the anterior inferior iliac spine; the reflected head from the rim of the acetabulum.

Insertion: common tendon of quadriceps, upper border of patella, and through the patellar ligament to the tubercle of the tibia.

Action: extends leg, flexes thigh.

Noninvasive Therapy

The post–trigger point injection follow-up program described in Chapter 9 is recommended as a conservative therapeutic treatment approach. Noninvasive therapy can include:

- Physical therapy modalities (e.g., electrical stimulation and warm packs; see Chapter 15).
- Manual physical therapy techniques (e.g., massage and the Trager Approach; see Chapters 13 and 14).
- Active and passive stretching and limbering of muscles with or without the use of vapocoolant spray or ice. Active exercise is part of the stretch-and-spray technique. Limbering and relaxation are necessary prior to stretching. Contract-relax techniques may be used.
- Stretch and spray for the rectus femoris is performed in the side-lying position with the help of vapocoolant spray or ice. The hip is extended together with knee flexion. The trigger point area and reference areas are sprayed as necessary to give pain relief. A self-stretch can be performed in the same manner with the patient in the standing position flexing the knee and pulling the heel toward the buttock, the opposite hand holding the table or wall for balance. Hold the stretch for 10 seconds. Relax and repeat. Electrical stimulation, limbering of muscles, and warm packs may precede stretch and spray to relax the muscles. Stretching of muscle is

also accomplished actively as well as with assistance during the exercise program. Active exercise is part of the stretch-and-spray technique.

- Exercise and a home program for the rectus femoris are prescribed (see Chapter 12 for knee and hip exercises). Exercise programs include relaxation, limbering, stretching, and strengthening. When the patient is free of pain and full motion has been achieved, progress to strength and endurance programs.

Injection of Trigger Point

With the patient in the supine position, trigger points are identified and injected (see Chapter 9 for technique). Search for multiple trigger points emphasizing the area of origin and insertion (Fig 10–16).

Postinjection Follow-Up Physical Therapy Program

The patient should receive 3 to 4 consecutive days of treatment. Physical therapy should include electrical stimulation, relaxation, limbering, and stretching of the involved muscle using vapocoolant spray or ice as needed combined with and followed by an exercise program. Active and active-assisted exercises are an integral part of the physical therapy program.

Exercise and Home Program

Exercises for rectus femoris are prescribed. Exercises should at first be performed under the guidance of a therapist. When the patient is free of pain and full motion has been achieved, progress to strength and endurance programs.

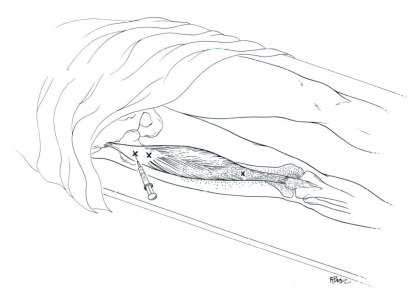

FIG 10–16.   Rectus femoris. Injection of trigger points *(X's)* in the right rectus femoris. Note trigger points in the area of origin and distally toward the area of insertion. The patient is supine. The trigger point pain pattern is shown by *stippling*. Anatomic landmarks are noted.

Begin and end exercise sessions with stretching and relaxation. (See Chapter 12 for exercise details.)

Corrective and Preventive Measures

- Avoid exercises that include deep squatting and knee bends greater than 90 degrees. Excessive squatting may damage a meniscus in addition to promotion of trigger points.
- Prolonged immobilization of the quadriceps can give rise to trigger points.

VASTUS MEDIALIS

Symptoms and Pain Pattern

- The vastus medialis may demonstrate atrophy in cases of knee abnormality and following surgery.
- Atrophy and trigger points may cause weakness giving rise to feelings of giving way of the knee or buckling.
- Pain is located in the knee joint area and lower thigh[19, 20, 44] (Fig 10–17).

Findings on Examination

- Tender trigger points in the vastus medialis.
- Atrophy of the vastus medialis.
- Weakness of the vastus medialis.

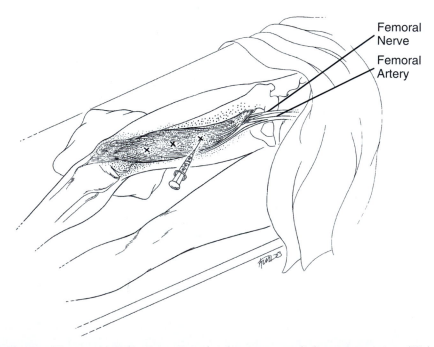

Femoral
Nerve

Femoral
Artery

FIG 10–17. Vastus medialis. Injection of right vastus medialis trigger points *(X's)*. The patient is supine with a pillow under the knee. The leg is slightly externally rotated with flexion of the hip. Trigger point pain pattern is shown by *stippling*. Anatomic landmarks are noted including the femoral artery and nerve.

Differential Diagnosis

- Internal derangement of the knee.
- Chondromalacia.
- Arthritis of the knee.

Anatomy

Origin: intertrochanteric line, medial linea aspera.
Insertion: common tendon of the quadriceps to the medial side of the patella, through the patellar ligament to the tubercle of the tibia.
Action: extends leg.

Noninvasive Therapy

The post–trigger point injection follow-up program described in Chapter 9 is recommended as a conservative therapeutic treatment approach. Noninvasive therapy can include:

- Physical therapy modalities (e.g., electrical stimulation and warm packs; see Chapter 15).
- Manual physical therapy techniques (e.g., massage and the Trager Approach; see Chapters 13 and 14).
- Active and passive stretching and limbering of muscles with or without the use of vapocoolant spray or ice. Active exercise is part of the stretch-and-spray technique. Limbering and relaxation are necessary prior to stretching. Contract-relax techniques may be used.
- Stretch and spray: Bring the knee into flexion using vapocoolant spray or ice. Spray the trigger point area and referred areas of pain. The extensor muscles are lengthened by progressively flexing the knee. Electrical stimulation, limbering of muscles, and warm packs should precede stretch and spray to relax the muscles. Stretching of muscle is also accomplished actively and with assistance during the exercise program. Active exercise is part of the stretch-and-spray technique.
- Exercise and a home program for the lower extremity and knee and hip exercises are prescribed (see Chapter 12). Exercise programs include relaxation, limbering, stretching, and strengthening. When the patient is free of pain and full motion has been achieved, progress to strength and endurance programs.

Injection of Trigger Points

Injection may be given with the patient supine, with the leg outstretched or in slight flexion, abduction, and external rotation, depending on the findings, patient's comfort, and ease of the injection (see Fig 10–17). Palpate all neighboring muscles for additional trigger points. Perform multiple needling to determine the presence of other trigger points which may not have been found with palpation.
Needle size: 1.5, 2.0, 3.0 in., 21 gauge. Length of needle depends on patient's size.

Solution: Any one of the following solutions may be used: 0.5% procaine; 1.0% lidocaine; saline and dry needling in case of allergy. Do not use epinephrine.

Precautions

- Avoid the femoral artery.
- Always aspirate before injecting (see Fig 10–17).

Postinjection Physical Therapy Follow-Up Program

Follow-up program requires 3 to 4 consecutive days of follow-up treatment. Physical therapy should include electrical stimulation, relaxation, limbering of muscles, and stretching of the involved muscles using vapocoolant spray or ice as needed combined with and followed by an exercise program. Active and active-assisted exercises are an integral part of the physical therapy program. When the lower extremities are injected the patient should use crutches for 2 days to avoid full weightbearing and prevent limping and muscle spasm. Following 3 to 4 days of physical therapy the patient is then placed on a progressive exercise program (see Chapter 9 for details).

Exercise and Home Program

Exercises for the knee are prescribed. Exercises should at first be performed under the guidance of a therapist. When the patient is free of pain and full motion has been achieved, progress to strength and endurance programs. Begin and end exercise sessions with stretching and relaxation (see Chapter 12 for exercise details).

Corrective and Preventive Measures

- Check for malalignment of lower extremities, e.g., genu varus, genu valgus, or foot abnormalities (e.g., flatfoot).
- Prescribe orthoses as indicated.

VASTUS INTERMEDIUS

Symptoms and Pain Pattern

- Pain in the thigh is noted with activity (Fig 10–18).
- Pain may be present at rest.

Findings

- Tender trigger points on palpation of the vastus intermedius together with vastus medialis, vastus lateralis, and femoris.
- Trigger points in these muscles cause shortening which inhibits flexion of the knee.

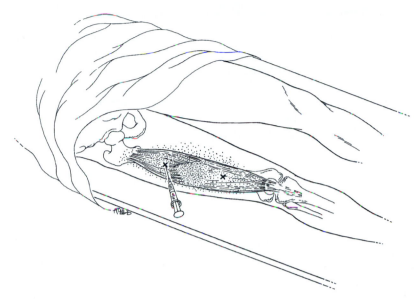

FIG 10–18. Vastus intermedius. Injection of trigger points *(X's)* in the right vastus intermedius with the patient supine. The leg is in neutral position. Trigger point pain is shown by *stippling*. Muscle origin and insertion are noted.

Differential Diagnosis

- Osteoarthritis of the hip.
- Neuralgia paresthetica.
- Herniated lumbar disc.

Anatomy

Origin: upper anterior aspect of the shaft of the femur.

Insertion: common tendon of quadriceps through the patellar ligament to the tubercle of the tibia.

Action: extends leg.

Injection of Trigger Points

With the patient in the supine position identify trigger points by palpation. Trigger points in a deep-lying muscle may be difficult to palpate. The vastus intermedius is covered by the rectus femoris. A needle that is long enough to penetrate the covering musculature should be used. Multiple needle entries along the length of the muscle are indicated in order to find all trigger points (see Fig 10–17, and Chapter 9 for injection technique).

Needle size: 1.5–3.0 in., 21 gauge, depending on thigh musculature.

Solution: Any one of the following solutions may be used: 0.5% procaine; 1.0% lidocaine; saline and dry needling in case of allergy. Do not use epinephrine.

Noninvasive Therapy

The post–trigger point injection follow-up program described in Chapter 9 is recommended as a conservative therapeutic treatment approach. Noninvasive therapy can include:

- Physical therapy modalities (e.g., electrical stimulation and warm packs; see Chapter 15).
- Manual physical therapy techniques (e.g., massage and the Trager Approach; see Chapters 13 and 14).
- Active and passive stretching and limbering of muscles with or without the use of vapocoolant spray or ice. Active exercise is part of the stretch-and-spray technique. Limbering and relaxation are necessary prior to stretching. Contract-relax techniques may be used.
- Stretch and spray: Electrical stimulation, limbering of muscles, and warm packs should precede stretch and spray to relax the muscles prior to stretching. Flexion of the knee is performed passively and actively. The pelvis is stabilized. This can be performed both in the supine and sitting positions. Full range of motion of the knee is accomplished by stretching the extensors. Use vapocoolant spray or ice as necessary. Stretching of the muscle is also accomplished actively and with assistance during the exercise program. Active exercise is part of the stretch-and-spray technique.
- Exercise and a home program for the hip and knee are prescribed (see Chapter 12). Exercise programs include relaxation, limbering, stretching, and strengthening. When the patient is free of pain and full motion has been achieved, progress to strength and endurance programs.

Injection of Trigger Points

With the patient in the supine position identify trigger points by palpation. Trigger points in a deep-lying muscle may be difficult to palpate. The vastus intermedius is covered by the rectus femoris. A needle that is long enough to penetrate the covering musculature should be used. Multiple needle entries along the length of the muscle are indicated in order to find all trigger points (see Fig 10–18, and Chapter 9 for injection technique).

Needle size: 1.5–3.0 in., 21 gauge, depending on thigh musculature.

Solution: Any one of the following solutions may be used: 0.5% procaine; 1.0% lidocaine; saline and dry needling in case of allergy. Do not use epinephrine.

Postinjection Follow-Up Physical Therapy Program

Patient should receive 3 to 4 consecutive days of treatment. Physical therapy should include electrical stimulation, relaxation, limbering, and stretching of the involved muscle using vapocoolant spray or ice as needed combined with and followed by an exercise program. Active and active-assisted exercises are an integral part of the physical therapy program (see Chapter 9 for details).

Exercise and Home Program

Exercises for hip and knee are prescribed. Exercises should at first be performed under the guidance of a therapist. When the patient is free of pain and full motion has been achieved, progress to strength and endurance programs. Begin and end exercise sessions with stretching and relaxation. (See Chapter 12 for exercise details.)

Corrective and Preventive Measures

- Check for malalignment of the lower extremities, including genu varus or valgus.
- Check for foot abnormalities such as flatfoot.
- Prescribe orthoses as indicated.

VASTUS LATERALIS

Symptoms and Pain Pattern

- Pain over the lateral aspect of the thigh which may radiate to the knee (Fig 10–19).
- Pain when lying directly on the trigger point.[4, 19]
- Myofascial trigger points in the distal end of the vastus lateralis can cause a completely locked patella which will immobilize the knee joint.[46]

Findings on Examination

- Tenderness on palpating trigger points over the vastus lateralis.
- Pain may be limited to the area of palpation or may radiate distally to the knee.

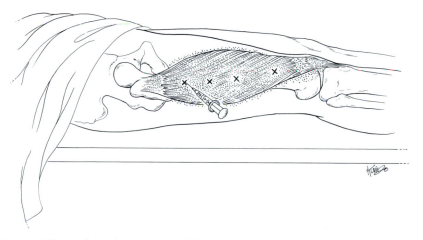

FIG 10–19.   Vastus lateralis. Injection of trigger points *(X's)* in the right vastus lateralis with the patient supine. Trigger point pain pattern is shown by *stippling*. Muscle origin and insertion are noted.

Differential Diagnosis

- Neuralgia paresthetica.
- Trochanteric bursitis.
- Herniated lumbar disc.
- Internal derangement of the knee.

Anatomy

Origin: lateral lip of linea aspera, front of base of greater trochanter.

Insertion: common tendon of quadriceps, lateral part of patellar ligament to the tibial tubercle.

Action: extends leg.

Noninvasive Therapy

The post–trigger point injection follow-up program described in Chapter 9 is recommended as a conservative therapeutic treatment approach. Noninvasive therapy can include:

- Physical therapy modalities (e.g., electrical stimulation and warm packs; see Chapter 15).
- Manual physical therapy techniques (e.g., massage and the Trager Approach; see Chapters 13 and 14).
- Active and passive stretching and limbering of muscles with or without the use of vapocoolant spray or ice. Active exercise is part of the stretch-and-spray technique. Limbering and relaxation are necessary prior to stretching. Contract-relax techniques may be used.
- Stretch and spray: The knee is flexed to extend the shortened extensor muscle. The thigh extensors may be stretched in both the lying-down and sitting positions. Electrical stimulation, limbering of muscles, and warm packs may precede stretch and spray to relax the muscles. Stretching of the muscle is also accomplished actively and with assistance during the exercise program. Active exercise is part of the stretch-and-spray technique.
- Exercise and a home program for the vastus lateralis are prescribed (see Chapter 12 for exercises for the knee and hip). Exercise programs include relaxation, limbering, stretching, and strengthening. When the patient is free of pain and full motion has been achieved, progress to strength and endurance programs.

Injection of Trigger Points

In the supine position, palpation for trigger points is performed from the most proximal part of the muscle (area of greater trochanter) to its insertion in the patellar ligament. All tender trigger points are injected (see Chapter 9 for technique). Perform multiple needle entries over the entire length of the muscle. Multiple needling may encounter trigger points that were missed on palpation. Most trigger points are found in the areas of origin and insertion (see Fig 10–19).

Needle size: 2, 3 in., 21 gauge. The length of needle depends on the patient's size.

Solution: Any one of the following solutions may be used: 0.5% procaine; 1.0% lidocaine; saline and dry needling in case of allergy. Do not use epinephrine.

Postinjection Follow-Up Program

The patient should use crutches for 24 hours to avoid pain and limping. The patient should receive 3 to 4 consecutive days of treatment. Physical therapy should include electrical stimulation, relaxation, limbering, and stretching of the involved muscle using vapocoolant spray or ice as needed combined with and followed by an exercise program. Active and active-assisted exercises are an integral part of the physical therapy program (see Chapter 9 for details).

Exercise and Home Program

Exercises for the hip and knee are prescribed. Exercises should at first be performed under the guidance of a therapist. When the patient is free of pain and full motion has been achieved, progress to strength and endurance programs. Begin and end exercise session with stretching and relaxation (see Chapter 12 for exercise details).

Corrective and Preventive Measures

- Check for malalignment of the lower extremities, e.g., genu varus, genu valgus, or foot abnormalities such as flatfoot.
- Prescribe orthoses as indicated.

GRACILIS

Symptoms and Pain Pattern

- Pain over the inner aspect of the thigh over the gracilis (Fig 10–20).
- Pain may be described as hot or stinging.[18, 45]

Findings on Examination

- Tender trigger points along the gracilis, especially at its insertion at the medial upper aspect of the tibia.
- The patient demonstrates restriction in abduction of the thigh and knee extension.

Anatomy

Origin: lower symphysis pubis arch.
Insertion: upper medial tibia.
Action: adduction of the thigh, flexion of the knee.

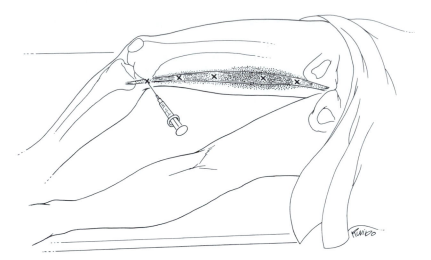

FIG 10–20.   Gracilis. Injection of trigger points in the right gracilis *(X's)*. Note trigger points in the area of origin and insertion. The patient is in the supine position with the thigh in flexion, external rotation, and abduction. Trigger point pain pattern is shown by *stippling*.

Differential Diagnosis

- Pes anserinus bursitis.
- Osteitis pubis.
- Hip joint abnormality.

Noninvasive Therapy

The post–trigger point injection follow-up program described in Chapter 9 is recommended as a conservative therapeutic treatment approach. Noninvasive therapy can include:

- Physical therapy modalities (e.g., electrical stimulation and warm packs; see Chapter 15).
- Manual physical therapy techniques (e.g., massage and the Trager Approach; see Chapters 13 and 14).
- Active and passive stretching and limbering of muscles with or without the use of vapocoolant spray or ice. Active exercise is part of the stretch-and-spray technique. A self-stretch can be performed in the same manner with the patient in the standing position flexing the knee, and pulling the heel toward the buttock, while the opposite hand holds a table the wall for balance. Hold the stretch for 10 seconds. Relax and repeat. Limbering and relaxation are necessary prior to stretching. Contract-relax techniques may be used.
- Stretch and spray. Use vapocoolant spray or ice. Stretching should be performed by abducting the hip with the knee in extension. Spray the area of the gracilis muscle. Spray the trigger area and the length of the muscle. Follow stretch and spray with passive and active range-of-motion exercises as tolerated. Electrical stimulation, limbering of muscles, and warm packs should precede stretch and spray to relax muscles.

• Exercise and home program (see Chapter 12 for exercises for the hip and knee). Exercise programs include relaxation, limbering, stretching, and strengthening. When the patient is free of pain and full motion has been achieved, progress to strength and endurance programs.

Injection of Trigger Points

The gracilis muscle is superficial. In addition to the localized tender point or trigger point, the entire muscle body should be examined. Trigger points are most often found in the areas of origin and insertion. Injection is given with the patient in the supine position. The thigh is flexed, externally rotated, and abducted (see Fig 10–20, and Chapter 9 for injection technique).

Needle size: 1.5–2.0 in., 21 gauge.

Solution: Any one of the following solutions may be used: 0.5% procaine; 1.0% lidocaine; saline and dry needling in case of allergy. Do not use epinephrine.

Postinjection Follow-Up Program

The patient should receive 3 to 4 consecutive days of treatment. Physical therapy should include electrical stimulation, relaxation, limbering, and stretching of the involved muscle using vapocoolant spray or ice as needed combined with and followed by an exercise program. Active and active-assisted exercises are an integral part of the physical therapy program (see Chapter 9 for details).

Exercise and Home Program

Exercises for the hip and knee are prescribed. Exercises should at first be performed under the guidance of a therapist. When the patient is free of pain and full motion has been achieved, progress to strength and endurance programs. Begin and end exercise sessions with stretching and relaxation. (See Chapter 12 for exercise details).

Corrective and Preventive Causes

• Avoid prolonged adduction and flexion of the thigh.

SARTORIUS

Symptoms and Pain Pattern

• Thigh pain extending medially along the course of the sartorius extending to the medial aspect of the knee[20] (Fig 10–21).
• Symptoms of lateral femoral cutaneous entrapment consisting of pain and numbness over the anterolateral aspect of the thigh have been reported to be relieved by trigger point injection. Injecting the trigger point in the region of the nerve may have released muscle tension in the entrapment area.[15, 20, 46]

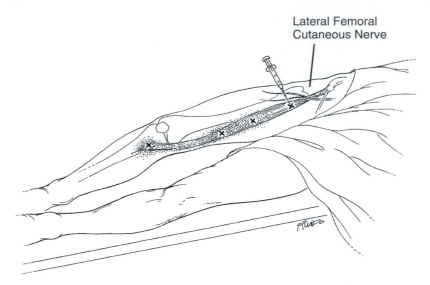

FIG 10–21.   Sartorius muscle. Injection of trigger points in the right sartorius muscle *(X's)*. Anatomic landmarks are noted including the lateral femoral cutaneus nerve. The patient is supine. Pain pattern is shown by *stippling*. Multiple trigger points are noted.

Findings on Examination

- Trigger point tenderness may be found in various areas extending from the origin to the insertion of the muscle.

Differential Diagnosis

- Osteoarthritis of the hip.
- Knee joint abnormality.

Anatomy

Origin: anterior superior iliac spine.
Insertion: upper medial tibia.
Action: flexion, abduction, external rotation of thigh, flexion of the knee.

Noninvasive Therapy

The post–trigger point injection follow-up program described in Chapter 9 is recommended as a conservative therapeutic treatment approach. Noninvasive therapy can include:

- Physical therapy modalities (e.g., electrical stimulation and warm packs; see Chapter 15).
- Manual physical therapy techniques (e.g., massage and the Trager Approach; see Chapters 13 and 14).
- Active and passive stretching and limbering of muscles with or without the use of vapocoolant spray or ice. Active exercise is part of the stretch-and-spray technique. Limbering and relaxation are necessary prior to stretching. Contract-relax techniques may be used.

- Stretch and spray for the sartorius is performed by extension, adduction, and internal rotation of the hip and extension of the knee (see Chapter 9 for spray-and-stretch technique). The patient is moved forward to the edge of the foot of the table. The pelvis should be stabilized. The leg is held free and supported by the therapist off the examining table for the stretch maneuvers. Electrical stimulation, limbering of muscles, and warm packs should precede stretch and spray to relax the muscles prior to stretching. Stretching of muscle is also accomplished actively and with assistance during the exercise program. Active exercise is part of the stretch-and-spray technique.
- Exercises and a home program for the hip and knee are prescribed (see Chapter 12). Exercise programs include relaxation, limbering, stretching, and strengthening. When the patient is free of pain and full motion has been achieved, progress to strength and endurance programs.

Injection of Trigger Points

Injection is performed with the patient supine. Palpable tender areas are identified. Multiple needling along the length of the muscle is indicated. Needling is not limited to the initial area of tenderness. Look for additional trigger points along the muscle belly. Other neighboring thigh muscles such as the rectus femoris and vastus medialis may also have trigger points and should be carefully examined. The sartorius muscle is superficial. The needle may be angled and need not penetrate too deeply (see Fig 10–21).

Needle length: One may use a 1.5- or 2.0-in. needle length, 21 gauge.

Solution: Any one of the following solutions may be used: 0.5% procaine; 1.0% lidocaine; saline and dry needling in case of allergy. Do not use epinephrine.

Postinjection Follow-Up Physical Therapy Program

The patient should avoid prolonged sitting, walking, or standing. The patient should receive 3 to 4 consecutive days of treatment. Physical therapy should include electrical stimulation, relaxation, limbering, and stretching of the involved muscle using vapocoolant spray or ice as needed combined with and followed by an exercise program. Active and active-assisted exercises are an integral part of the physical therapy program (see Chapter 9 for details).

Exercise and Home Program

Exercises for the hip and knee are prescribed. Exercises should at first be performed under the guidance of a therapist. When the patient is free of pain and full motion has been achieved, progress to strength and endurance programs. Begin and end exercise sessions with stretching and relaxation. (See Chapter 12 for exercise details.)

Corrective and Preventive Measures

- Correct leg length inequality, e.g., with a heel lift.
- Avoid sitting cross-legged with the knees flexed and hips externally rotated and abducted.

ADDUCTOR MAGNUS

Symptoms and Pain Pattern

- Patients may complain of pain in the groin in addition to the anteromedial aspect of the thigh[18, 20, 28] (Fig 10–22).
- Intrapelvic referred pain has been reported (e.g., rectum or vagina).[45]
- Athletic activities frequently cause active trigger points in the adductor muscles which are a cause of prolonged complaints when untreated.

Findings on Examination

- Trigger points are felt posteromedially in the region of the ischium as well as midthigh in the area of the muscle insertion.
- Limitation in lateral rotation, flexion, and adduction of the hips may be present and restriction in motion may be accompanied by pain.
- Look for trigger points in neighboring muscles (e.g., the adductor longus and adductor brevis).

Differential Diagnosis

- Hip joint abnormality.
- Intrapelvic disease.[44]

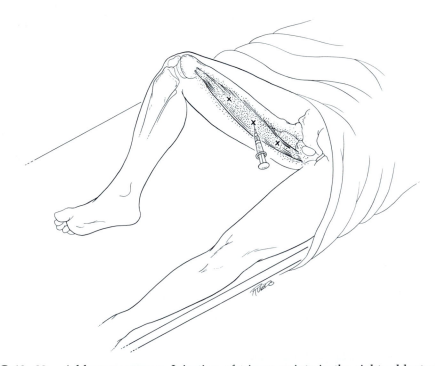

FIG 10–22.   Adductor magnus. Injection of trigger points in the right adductor magnus (*X's.*) The patient is supine with slight flexion, abduction, and external rotation of the leg. Anatomic landmarks are noted. Pain pattern is shown by *stippling*.

Anatomy

Origin: inferior ischiopubic rami, outer inferior ischial tuberosity.

Insertion: medial gluteal tuberosity, medial linea aspera.

Action: adduction and extension of hip joint; the ischial head acts as a hamstring muscle.

Noninvasive Therapy

The post–trigger point injection follow-up program described in Chapter 9 is recommended as a conservative therapeutic treatment approach. Noninvasive therapy can include:

- Physical therapy modalities (e.g., electrical stimulation and warm packs; see Chapter 15).
- Manual physical therapy techniques (e.g., massage and the Trager Approach; see Chapters 13 and 14).
- Active and passive stretching and limbering of muscles with or without the use of vapocoolant spray or ice. Active exercise is part of the stretch-and-spray technique. Contract-relax techniques may be used.
- Stretch and spray for the adductor magnus is performed by stretching in hip abduction and flexion. Limbering and relaxation is necessary prior to stretching. Electrical stimulation, limbering of muscles, and warm packs should precede stretch and spray to relax muscles.
- Exercise and a home program for the adductor magnus are prescribed (see Chapter 12 for exercises for the hip). Exercise programs include relaxation, limbering, stretching, and strengthening. When the patient is free of pain and full motion has been achieved, progress to strength and endurance programs.

Injection of Trigger Points

With the patient supine the length of the muscle is best examined for trigger points with the thigh in flexion, abduction, and external rotation (see Fig 10–22). Multiple needle entries are performed along the length of the muscle in addition to specific tender areas. Multiple needling may identify trigger points that are not found on palpation (see Fig 10–22). Palpate neighboring muscles for trigger points. Most trigger points are found in the region of origin (ischial area).

Needle size: 2.0, 3.0 in., 21 gauge.

Solution: Any one of the following solutions may be used: 0.5% procaine; 1.0% lidocaine; saline and dry needling in case of allergy. Do not use epinephrine.

Postinjection Follow-Up Physical Therapy Program

The patient should receive 3 to 4 consecutive days of treatment. Physical therapy should include electrical stimulation, relaxation, limbering, and stretching of the involved muscle using vapocoolant spray or ice as needed combined with and followed by an exercise program. Active and active-assisted exercises are an integral part of the physical therapy program.

Exercise and Home Program

Exercises for the hip are prescribed (see Chapter 12). Exercises should at first be performed under the guidance of a therapist. When the patient is free of pain and full motion has been achieved, progress to strength and endurance programs. Begin and end exercise sessions with stretching and relaxation.

Corrective and Preventive Measures

- Correct leg length inequalities (e.g., with a shoe lift).
- Avoid prolonged adduction and flexion of the thigh.
- Avoid overstretch of adductors (e.g., athletic injury). Emphasize the importance of proper stretching before and after athletic activities.

ADDUCTOR LONGUS AND ADDUCTOR BREVIS

Symptoms and Pain Pattern

- Pain in the groin may radiate to the medial thigh and knee and leg[19, 20, 29, 45] (see Fig 10–23).
- Trigger points in the adductor muscles are frequently caused by athletic injuries and remain a source of prolonged complaints when left untreated.

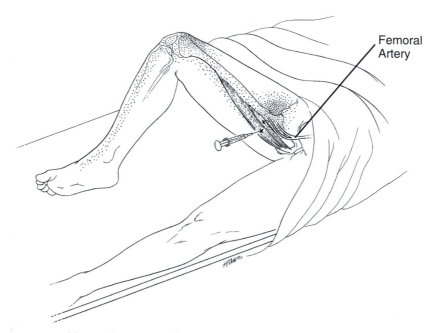

FIG 10–23.   Adductor longus and brevis. Injection of trigger points in the right adductor longus and brevis (*X's*). The femoral artery lies deep to the sartorius and is lateral to the long and short adductor muscles. The patient is positioned with the hip and knee flexed. The leg is externally rotated with slight abduction. Pain pattern is noted by *stippling*.

Findings on Examination

- Trigger point tenderness is found on palpation of the adductor longus.
- Pain of the trigger point may cause the pain to radiate to the lower portion of the thigh to the knee.
- Pain and tightness of the adductor muscles may limit lateral rotation and abduction.
- The Fabere test is often painful and limited.
- The adductor brevis muscle, which is under the adductor longus, demonstrates the same clinical picture.

Differential Diagnosis

- Hip disease (e.g., arthritis of the hip).
- Herniated disc L3–4.
- Strain of the adductor muscles.
- Osteitis pubis.

Anatomy

Adductor Longus
Origin: front of pubis.
Insertion: linea aspera.
Action: adduction and medial rotation of the thigh.

Adductor Brevis
Origin: inferior pubic ramus.
Insertion: linea aspera.
Action: adduction and flexion of the hip.

Treatment

Noninvasive Therapy

The post–trigger point injection follow-up program described in Chapter 9 is recommended as a conservative therapeutic treatment approach. Noninvasive therapy can include:

- Physical therapy modalities (e.g., electrical stimulation and warm packs; see Chapter 15).
- Manual physical therapy techniques (e.g., massage and the Trager Approach; see Chapters 13 and 14).
- Active and passive stretching and limbering of muscles with or without the use of vapocoolant spray or ice. Active exercise is part of the stretch-and-spray technique by stretching in hip abduction and flexion. Electrical stimulation, limbering of muscles, and warm packs should precede stretch and spray to relax muscles. Limbering and relaxation are necessary prior to stretching. Contract-relax techniques may be used.
- Stretch and spray is performed with the leg in extension using gentle abduction. Add flexion, abduction, and external rotation as performed in

the Faber test. Increase abduction and external rotation. Use relaxation techniques. Follow with passive and active range-of-motion exercises as tolerated. Electrical stimulation, limbering of muscles, and warm packs should precede stretch and spray to relax muscles.
- Exercise and a home program for the hip and knee are prescribed (see Chapter 12). Exercise programs include relaxation, limbering, stretching, and strengthening. When the patient is free of pain and full motion has been achieved, progress to strength and endurance programs.

Injection of Trigger Point

Trigger points are best palpated with the hip and knee in flexion, the hip abducted and externally rotated (Fabere position) (see Fig 10–23). Examine the adductor longus for trigger points beginning at its origin in the groin and progressing along the inner side of the thigh. The adductor longus is superficial to the adductor brevis. Look for multiple trigger point areas by palpation and multiple needling. Most frequently trigger points will be found proximally at the adductor longus origin. Neighboring muscles, such as the adductor brevis, adductor magnus, pectineus, and gracilis may demonstrate trigger points.

Needle size: 1.5, 2.0, 3.0 in., 22 gauge.

Solution: Any one of the following solutions may be used: 0.5% procaine; 1.0% lidocaine; saline and dry needling in case of allergy. Do not use epinephrine.

Precautions

- Identify and avoid the femoral artery (see Fig 10–23). The femoral artery lies lateral to the adductor muscle in the thigh.
- Aspirate prior to injection.

Postinjection Follow-Up Physical Therapy Program

The patient is advised to avoid prolonged standing, sitting, or walking, and to use crutches for 2 days. The patient should receive 3 to 4 consecutive days of treatment. Physical therapy should include electrical stimulation, relaxation, limbering, and stretching of the involved muscle using vapocoolant spray or ice as needed combined with and followed by an exercise program. Active and active-assisted exercises are an integral part of the physical therapy program (see Chapter 9 for details).

Exercise and Home Program

Exercises for the adductor muscles are prescribed. Exercises should at first be performed under the guidance of a therapist. When the patient is free of pain and full motion has been achieved, progress to strength and endurance programs. Begin and end exercise sessions with stretching and relaxation. (See Chapter 12 for exercise details.)

Corrective and Preventive Measures

- Avoid prolonged adduction and flexion of the thigh.
- Emphasize proper warm-up prior to athletic activities to avoid muscle injury. Proper warm-up prior to athletic activities will prevent strains and sprains leading to trigger point formation or activation of latent trigger points. Close athletic activities with stretching and relaxation.

PECTINEUS

Symptoms and Pain Pattern

- Patients with pectineus muscle trigger points may complain of pain in the hip joint, groin area, or over the medial aspect of the upper thigh (Fig 10–24).
- The patient may experience pain and limitation in the groin area with abduction of the hip.
- Pain may radiate from the groin down the inner side of the thigh.[45]

Findings on Examination

- Tenderness on palpation of the pectineus. The pectineus is best palpated with the leg in abduction. Palpate the femoral artery. The pectineus is medial to the artery and lateral to the adductor brevis and adductor longus.

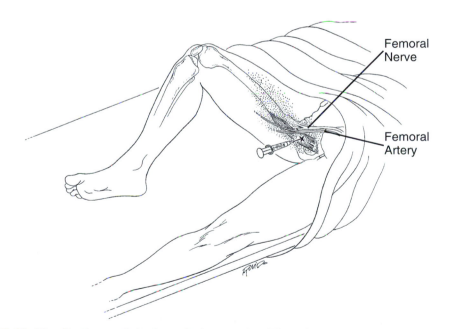

Femoral
Nerve

Femoral
Artery

FIG 10–24. Pectineus. Injection of trigger point *(X)* in the right pectineus. Patient is supine, the thigh in slight flexion, abduction, and external rotation. Avoid the femoral artery. Anatomic landmarks, including the femoral artery and nerve, are noted. Trigger point pain pattern is shown by *stippling*.

- Neighboring groups of muscles (e.g., adductors) should be examined for trigger points.

Differential Diagnosis

- Arthritis of the hip.
- Osteitis pubis.
- Obturator nerve entrapment.[15]

Anatomy

Origin: superior ramus of the pubis.
Insertion: upper portion of the pectineal line below the lesser trochanter.
Action: flexes thigh, adducts and laterally rotates thigh.

Noninvasive Therapy

The post–trigger point injection follow-up program described in Chapter 9 is recommended as a conservative therapeutic treatment approach. Noninvasive therapy can include:

- Physical therapy modalities (e.g., electrical stimulation and warm packs; see Chapter 15).
- Manual physical therapy techniques (e.g., massage and the Trager Approach; see Chapters 13 and 14).
- Active and passive stretching and limbering of muscles with or without the use of vapocoolant spray or ice. Active exercise is part of the stretch-and-spray technique. Limbering and relaxation are necessary prior to stretching. Contract-relax techniques may be used.
- Stretch and spray: Stretching should include abduction and extension of the hip. Neighboring muscles of similar function must be evaluated and often will require treatment (see Chapter 8). Electrical stimulation, limbering of muscles, and warm packs should precede stretch and spray to relax the muscles prior to stretching. Stretching of muscle is also accomplished actively and with assistance during the exercise program.
- Exercise and a home program for the pectineus and adductors are prescribed (see Chapter 12). Exercise programs include relaxation, limbering, stretching, and strengthening. When the patient is free of pain and full motion has been achieved, progress to strength and endurance programs.

Injection of Trigger Point

Trigger points in the pectineus are best injected with the patient supine, the thigh in slight flexion, abduction, and external rotation with flexion of the knee (see Chapter 9 for injection technique). Palpate the femoral artery which lies over the pectineus and direct the needle medial to the artery. Aspirate before injection (see Fig 10–24). If the artery is entered, remove the needle and apply compression.

Needle size: 1.5, 2.0 in., 21 gauge.
Solution: Any one of the following solutions may be used: 0.5% procaine;

1.0% lidocaine; saline and dry needling in case of allergy. Do not use epinephrine.

Precautions

- Avoid the femoral artery.

Postinjection Follow-Up Physical Therapy Program

The patient should receive 3 to 4 consecutive days of treatment. Physical therapy should include electrical stimulation, relaxation, limbering, and stretching of the involved muscle using vapocoolant spray or ice as needed combined with and followed by an exercise program. Active and active-assisted exercises are an integral part of the physical therapy program (see Chapter 9 for details).

Exercise and Home Program

Exercises should at first be performed under the guidance of a therapist. When the patient is free of pain and full motion has been achieved, progress to strength and endurance programs. Begin and end exercise sessions with stretching and relaxation. (See Chapter 12 for exercise details.)

Corrective and Preventive Measures

- Avoid prolonged flexion and adduction of the hip.
- Correct leg length inequality. Use a heel lift if necessary.
- Correct pelvic asymmetry, e.g., a patient with a small hemipelvis or scoliosis may require a buttock lift (cushion) to improve alignment.

ILIOPSOAS   PSOAS MAJOR, ILIACUS

Symptoms and Pain Pattern

Patients complain of pain in the low back, groin, and thigh. Symptoms may be aggravated by activity and relieved with rest (Fig 10–25). A vertically oriented pattern of pain has been described in the low back in addition to pain in the front of the thigh.[44]

Findings on Examination

- Shortening of the iliaopsoas muscle causes inability to extend the hip, increasing lordosis. To test for iliopsoas shortening the patient flexes the uninvolved hip, flattening the lumbar spine. The involved hip will remain in flexion with the knee in flexion, indicating involvement of both one joint and two joint hip flexors. If the knee joint is permitted to extend and the hip extends normally, the one joint hip flexor muscle of the iliopsoas is normal, but the rectus femoris and probably the tensor fasciae latae are shortened.[14]
- Trigger points may be found in the area of the insertion at the lesser trochanter area of the femur, the medial wall of the femoral triangle, and

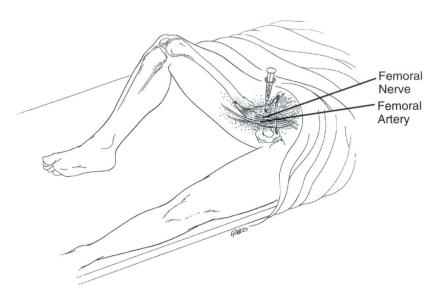

Femoral Nerve
Femoral Artery

FIG 10–25. Iliopsoas. Injection of trigger point *(X)* in the right iliopsoas. The patient is supine with the thigh flexed, abducted, and externally rotated. Anatomic landmarks are noted, including the inguinal ligament, femoral artery, and femoral nerve. Trigger point pain pattern is shown by *stippling*.

behind the anterior superior iliac spine behind the brim of the pelvis. Trigger points may also be found on palpation of the abdomen below the umbilicus lateral to the rectus abdominis.

Anatomy

Psoas Major
Origin: Transverse processes of L1–5, and vertebral bodies of T12–L5.
Insertion: lesser trochanter.
Action: flexes thigh, rotates thigh laterally, flexor of the spine and lateral bending.

Iliacus
Origin: iliac fossa, iliac crest, anterior sacroiliac ligaments at base of sacrum.
Insertion: tendon of psoas major into lesser trochanter.
Action: flexes and laterally rotates thigh.

Differential Diagnosis

- Kidney abnormality.
- Iliopsoas bursitis.
- Neuralgia paresthetica.
- Low back syndrome.

Noninvasive Therapy

The post–trigger point injection follow-up program described in Chapter 9 is recommended as a conservative therapeutic treatment approach. Noninvasive therapy can include:

- Physical therapy modalities (e.g., electrical stimulation and warm packs; see Chapter 15).
- Manual physical therapy techniques (e.g., massage and the Trager Approach; see Chapters 13 and 14).
- Active and passive stretching and limbering of muscles with or without the use of vapocoolant spray or ice. Active exercise is part of the stretch-and-spray technique. Electrical stimulation, limbering of muscles, and warm packs should precede stretch and spray to relax muscles. Limbering and relaxation are necessary prior to stretching. Contract-relax techniques may be used.
- Stretch and spray (see Chapter 9): Extend and medially rotate the hip area. Spray includes abdomen, groin, lower back, and area of referred pain as necessary.
- Exercise and a home program for low back pain and the hip are described in Chapter 12. Exercise program includes relaxation, limbering, stretching, and strengthening. When the patient is free of pain and full motion has been achieved, progress to strength and endurance programs.

Trigger Point Injection

With the patient in the supine position the right hip is abducted, flexed, and externally rotated. Palpate the femoral artery. Inject lateral to the femoral artery (see Fig 10–25, and Chapter 9 for injection technique).

Needle size: 3 in., 20 gauge

Solution: Any one of the following solutions may be used: 0.5% procaine; 1.0% lidocaine; isotonic saline and dry needling in case of allergy. Do not use epinephrine.

Precautions

- Note neurovascular structures found in the femoral triangle.
- Avoid femoral artery and nerve.
- Aspirate prior to injection.
- Inject lateral to the artery.

Postinjection Follow-Up Physical Therapy Program

The patient should receive 3 to 4 consecutive days of treatment. Physical therapy should include electrical stimulation, relaxation, limbering, and stretching of the involved muscle using vapocoolant spray or ice as needed combined with and followed by an exercise program. Active and active-assisted exercises are an integral part of the physical therapy program (see Chapter 9 for details).

Exercises and Home Program

Stretching the iliopsoas muscle requires hip extension. Prescribe McKenzie-type extension exercises for the low back reminding the patient to keep the pelvis flat on the exercise mat. The patient lifts the upper body by extending the arms. Lumbar extension will stretch the iliopsoas. This should not be done if pain in the low back is aggravated. Home stretching and exercise programs are

prescribed. Exercises should at first be performed under the guidance of a therapist. When the patient is free of pain and full motion has been achieved,
progress to strength and endurance programs. Begin and end exercise sessions
with relaxation (see Chapter 13 for details).

Corrective and Preventive Measures

- Avoid prolonged sitting or lying with the hip in flexion. This can result
  from prolonged sitting in a wheelchair or bed rest.

TIBIALIS ANTERIOR

Symptoms and Pain Pattern

- Pain over the front of the leg along the path of the anterior tibial
  muscle[11, 12] (Fig 10–26).
- Pain may be aggravated with activity.
- Weakness in dorsiflexion of the ankle.
- Tenderness over the tibialis anterior with local pain. Pain may radiate to
  the anteromedial side of the leg and big toe.[34, 43, 45]
- Symptoms are aggravated by walking or running.

Findings on Examination

- Examination may reveal tender trigger points in the tibialis anterior in addition to a referred pain pattern.

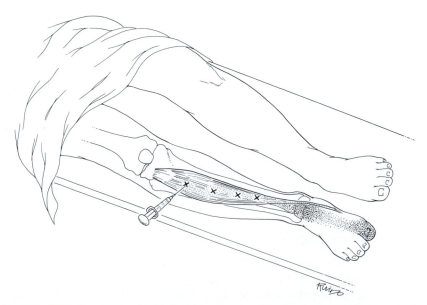

FIG 10–26.   Tibialis anterior. Injection of trigger points in the right tibialis anterior with
the patient supine. Multiple trigger points *(X's)* are noted. Anatomic landmarks are
noted. Trigger point pain pattern is shown by *stippling*.

- A degree of dorsiflexion weakness and limitation in plantarflexion may be present.

Differential Diagnosis

- Anterior compartment syndrome.
- Lumbar radiculopathy.
- Shin splints.
- Tibial stress fracture.

Anatomy

Origin: lateral tibial condyle, lateral tibia interosseous membrane.
Insertion: medial side of the first cuneiform, base of the first metatarsal.
Action: dorsiflexes foot, inverts foot.

Noninvasive Therapy

The post–trigger point injection follow-up program described in Chapter 9 is recommended as a conservative therapeutic treatment approach. Noninvasive therapy can include:

- Physical therapy modalities (e.g., electrical stimulation and warm packs; see Chapter 15).
- Manual physical therapy techniques (e.g., massage and the Trager Approach; see Chapters 13 and 14).
- Active and passive stretching and limbering of muscles with or without the use of vapocoolant spray or ice. Active exercise is part of the stretch-and-spray technique. Limbering and relaxation are necessary prior to stretching. May use contract-relax technique.
- Stretch-and-spray technique: plantarflex the ankle and pronate the foot. Electrical stimulation, limbering of muscles, and warm packs should precede stretch and spray to relax the muscles prior to stretching. Stretching of the muscle is also accomplished actively as well as with assistance during the exercise program. Active exercise is part of the stretch-and-spray technique (see Chapter 9).
- Exercise and home program for the ankle are prescribed (see Chapter 12). Exercise programs include relaxation, limbering, stretching, and strengthening. When the patient is free of pain and full motion has been achieved, progress to strength and endurance programs.

Injection of Trigger Points

Trigger points are identified. Injection is performed with the patient in the supine position. Use multiple injection and needling technique (see Chapter 9). Look for additional trigger points over the length of the anterior tibial muscle by means of palpation and needle probing (see Fig 10–26).
Needle size: 1.5, 2.0 in., 21 gauge.
Solution: Any one of the following solutions may be used: 0.5% procaine; 1.0% lidocaine; saline and dry needling in case of allergy. Do not use epinephrine.

Precautions

- Aspirate before injection.
- Avoid anterior tibial artery and deep peroneal nerve.

Postinjection Follow-Up Physical Therapy Program

The patient is to use crutches to avoid full weightbearing for 24 hours. The patient should receive 3 to 4 consecutive days of treatment. Physical therapy should include electrical stimulation, relaxation, limbering, and stretching of the involved muscle using vapocoolant spray or ice as needed combined with and followed by an exercise program. Active and active-assisted exercises are an integral part of the physical therapy program (see Chapter 9 for details).

Exercise and Home Program

Home program: Continue exercises and stretching. Encourage plantarflexion and pronation. Exercises should at first be performed under the guidance of a therapist. When the patient is free of pain and full motion has been achieved, progress to strength and endurance programs. Begin and end exercise sessions with stretching and relaxation (see Chapter 12 for exercise details).

Corrective and Preventive Measures

- Avoid overuse syndromes (e.g., unaccustomed prolonged walking or running).
- Avoid walking on uneven surfaces for prolonged periods.
- Correct foot abnormalities, e.g., flatfoot, Morton's foot.
- Prescribe orthoses as needed.

PERONEAL MUSCLES
Peroneus longus, peroneus brevis, peroneus tertius

Symptoms and Referred Pain Pattern

- Pain over the lateral aspect of the ankle and lateral dorsum of the foot[20] (Fig 10–27).
- Muscle weakness of the ankle.[18, 43]

Findings

- Tenderness on palpation of peroneal muscles.
- Tightness of the peroneal muscles will restrict inversion.
- The peroneus tertius is a dorsiflexor. Shortening of the peroneus tertius will limit plantarflexion.

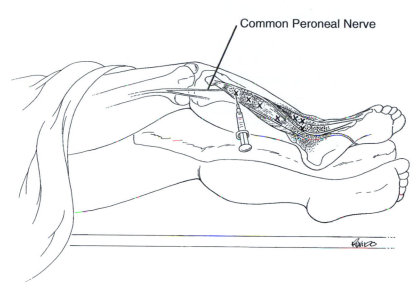

Common Peroneal Nerve

FIG 10–27. Peroneal muscles. Injection of trigger points *(X's)* in the right peroneal muscles. Patient is positioned lying on the uninvolved side. Anatomic landmarks are noted. Avoid the common peroneal nerve. Pain pattern is shown by *stippling*. Multiple trigger points are noted.

- Muscle testing may reveal a weakness in plantarflexion, dorsiflexion, and eversion.
- Palpation of trigger point may elicit distal referred pain over the lateral aspect of the ankle and lateral dorsum of the foot.

Differential Diagnosis

- Lumbar herniated disc.
- Common peroneal nerve entrapment.
- Peroneal muscle spasm due to foot abnormalities (flatfoot).
- Arthritis of the ankle.

Anatomy

Peroneus Longus
Origin: fibular head and proximal two thirds of fibula.
Insertion: base of first metatarsal and first cuneiform.
Action: plantarflexion and eversion of the foot.

Peroneus Brevis
Origin: middle lateral aspect of the fibula.
Insertion: dorsal surface of fifth metatarsal.
Action: plantarflexion and eversion of the foot.

Peroneus Tertius
Origin: distal fibula.
Insertion: base of fifth metatarsal.
Action: dorsiflexion of the foot.

Noninvasive Therapy

The post–trigger point injection follow-up program described in Chapter 9 is recommended as a conservative therapeutic treatment approach. Noninvasive therapy can include:

- Physical therapy modalities (e.g., electrical stimulation and warm packs; see Chapter 15).
- Manual physical therapy techniques (e.g., massage and the Trager Approach; see Chapters 13 and 14).
- Active and passive stretching and limbering of muscles with or without the use of vapocoolant spray or ice. Active exercise is part of the stretch-and-spray technique. Limbering and relaxation are necessary prior to stretching. Contract-relax techniques may be used.
- Stretch and spray with vapocoolant or ice. Stretch of the peroneus longus and brevis requires inversion and dorsiflexion. To stretch the peroneus tertius, plantarflexion is performed. Electrical stimulation, limbering of muscles, and warm packs should precede stretch and spray to relax the muscles. Stretching of muscle is also accomplished actively and with assistance during the exercise program.
- Exercise and a home program for the ankle are prescribed (see Chapter 12). Exercise programs include relaxation, limbering, stretching, and strengthening. When the patient is free of pain and full motion has been achieved, progress to strength and endurance programs.

Trigger Point Injection Technique

Trigger points are identified with the patient supine or lying on the uninvolved side. Multiple needling entry sites are usually necessary to locate additional trigger points which are not found on palpation (see Fig 10–27; see Chapter 9 for technique).

Needle size: 1.5 in., 22 gauge.

Solution: Any one of the following solutions may be used: 0.5% procaine; 1.0% lidocaine; saline and dry needling in case of allergy. Do not use epinephrine.

Precautions

- Avoid the common peroneal nerve.[15]

Postinjection Follow-Up Program

The patient should receive 3 to 4 consecutive days of treatment. Therapy should include electrical stimulation, relaxation, limbering, and stretching of the involved muscle using vapocoolant spray or ice as needed combined with and followed by an exercise program.

Exercise and Home Program

Exercises for the foot and ankle are prescribed (see Chapter 12). Instruct the patient on a daily exercise program for the foot and ankle. Exercise programs include relaxation, limbering, stretching, and strengthening. When the patient is free of pain and full motion has been achieved, progress to strength and endurance programs. Begin and end exercise sessions with relaxation and stretching.

Corrective and Preventive Measures

- Correct foot abnormalities such as flatfoot and Morton's foot. Prescribe orthoses as indicated.
- Avoid running on uneven surfaces.

GASTROCNEMIUS MUSCLE GROUP
Gastrocnemius, medial and Gastrocnemius, lateral

Symptoms and Pain Pattern

- Pain in the calf and back of the knee which may radiate to the lower thigh[18, 28] (Fig 10–28).
- Trigger points in the medial gastrocnemius may also refer pain to the plantar surface of the foot.[4, 45]
- Trigger points have been reported as a frequent cause of nocturnal calf cramp and intermittent claudication.[33, 35, 45]
- Pain may be referred to the Achilles tendon and the heel.[33, 35]

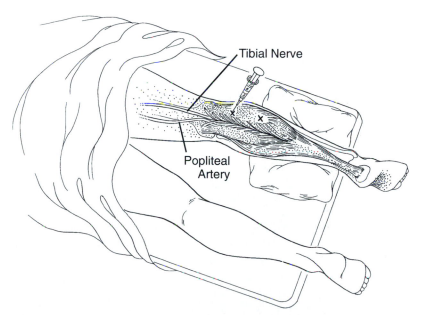

FIG 10–28. Gastrocnemius. Injection of trigger points *(X's)* in the lateral head of the right gastrocnemius. Trigger point pain pattern *stippling* is characteristic of both medial and lateral head trigger points. Only one side of the gastrocnemius is injected at a time when both are involved. The popliteal artery and tibial nerve are noted.

Findings on Examination

- With the patient prone or sitting, tender trigger points are best palpated with the knee flexed and the ankle plantarflexed.
- Palpate the entire length of the medial and lateral gastrocnemius muscle. Local tenderness and referred pain may be elicited.
- Trigger points may be found frequently in both the medial and lateral heads of the gastrocnemius as well as along the midline.

Differential Diagnosis

- Tennis leg (plantaris tendon rupture, gastrocnemius rupture).
- Herniated lumbar disc.
- Phlebitis.
- Spinal stenosis.
- Intermittent claudication.

Anatomy

Gastrocnemius, Medial
Origin: medial femoral condyle.
Insertion: on the calcaneus as part of the Achilles tendon.
Action: flexes the leg, plantarflexes the foot.

Gastrocnemius, Lateral
Origin: lateral femoral condyle.
Insertion: on the calcaneus as part of the Achilles tendon.
Action: flexes the leg, plantarflexes the foot.

Noninvasive Therapy

The post–trigger point injection follow-up program described in Chapter 9 is recommended as a conservative therapeutic treatment approach. Noninvasive therapy can include:

- Physical therapy modalities (e.g., electrical stimulation and warm packs; see Chapter 15).
- Manual physical therapy techniques (e.g., massage and the Trager Approach; see Chapters 13 and 14).
- Active and passive stretching and limbering of muscles with or without the use of vapocoolant spray or ice. Active exercise is part of the stretch-and-spray technique. Limbering and relaxation are necessary prior to stretching. Contract-relax techniques may be used.
- Stretch and spray (see Chapter 9): Extend the knee and dorsiflex the foot with the help of vapocoolant spray or ice, as needed, to regain full muscle length. Stretch is performed with the patient in the prone position with the feet off the examining table, as well as in the supine position. Electrical stimulation, limbering of muscles, and warm packs may precede stretch and spray to relax the muscles. Relaxation is accomplished prior to stretching. Stretching of the muscle is also accomplished actively as well

as with assistance during the exercise program. Active exercise is part of the stretch-and-spray technique.

- Exercise and home program for the knee and ankle (see Chapter 12). Exercise programs include relaxation, limbering, stretching, and strengthening. When the patient is free of pain and full motion has been achieved, progress to strength and endurance programs. Begin and end exercise sessions with relaxation and stretching.

Injection of Trigger Points

If trigger points are found in both gastrocnemius muscles they should be injected on separate occasions 2 or 3 days apart. Multiple injections cause muscle soreness and spasm. Injection may be performed with the patient in the prone or side-lying position. The knee is relaxed. Trigger points are identified by palpation and needling. Use a multiple needling technique covering the length of the muscle (see Fig 10–28 and Chapter 9 for injection technique).

Needle size: 1.5, 2.0 in., 22 gauge.

Solution: Any one of the following solutions may be used: 0.5% procaine; 1.0% lidocaine (approximately 2–10 mL); saline and dry needling in case of allergy. Do not use epinephrine.

Precautions

- Avoid the popliteal artery when injecting in the popliteal region. Aspirate prior to injection.

Postinjection Follow-Up Program

Crutches are used for 24 hours following the injection to avoid pain, muscle spasm, and limping. The patient should receive 3 to 4 consecutive days of treatment. Physical therapy should include electrical stimulation, relaxation, limbering, and stretching of the involved muscle using vapocoolant spray or ice as needed combined with and followed by an exercise program. Active and active-assisted exercises are an integral part of the physical therapy program (see Chapter 9 for details).

Exercise and Home Program

Exercises for the ankle and knee are prescribed. Exercises should at first be performed under the guidance of a therapist. When the patient is free of pain and full motion has been achieved, progress to strength and endurance programs. Begin and end exercise session with relaxation (see Chapter 12 for exercise details).

Corrective and Preventive Measures

- Avoid overuse syndrome, e.g. unaccustomed prolonged walking and athletic activity.
- Correct foot deformities, e.g., flatfoot. Prescribe orthoses as necessary.
- Avoid walking or running for prolonged periods on uneven surfaces.

- Short gastrocnemius muscles are frequently found in women associated with prolonged use of high heels.
- Relaxation and stretching exercises prior to and after athletic activities.

PLANTARIS

Symptoms and Referred Pain Pattern

- Symptoms may present as pain in the back of the knee and upper calf.
- Pain is aggravated by walking and running.

Findings on Examination

- Anatomically, trigger points are difficult to diagnose. Findings and symptoms may resemble those related to the soleus and gastrocnemius muscles.
- Pain may be aggravated with dorsiflexion of the foot.

Differential Diagnosis

- Tear of gastrocnemius muscle.
- Rupture of the plantaris tendon (tennis leg).
- Trigger points may result from rupture of the plantaris tendon.

Anatomy

Origin: lateral supracondylar line of the femur, popliteal ligament.
Insertion: calcaneal tendon, medial side and posterior part of the calcaneus.
Action: the plantaris muscle crosses two joints; therefore, it flexes the knee and plantarflexes the foot.

Noninvasive Therapy

The post–trigger point injection follow-up program described in Chapter 9 is recommended as a conservative therapeutic treatment approach. Noninvasive therapy can include:

- Physical therapy modalities (e.g., electrical stimulation and warm packs; see Chapter 15).
- Manual physical therapy techniques (e.g., massage and the Trager Approach; see Chapters 13 and 14).
- Active and passive stretching and limbering of muscles with or without the use of vapocoolant spray or ice. Active exercise is part of the stretch-and-spray technique. Limbering and relaxation are necessary prior to stretching. Contract-relax techniques may be used.
- Stretch and spray: Extend the knee and dorsiflex the foot with the help of vapocoolant spray or ice. Electrical stimulation, limbering of muscles, and warm packs should precede stretch and spray to relax the muscles.

Stretching of muscle is also accomplished actively and with assistance during the exercise program. Active exercise is part of the stretch-and-spray-technique.

- Exercise and home program: Exercises for heel cord stretching and exercises for the ankle and foot are prescribed (see Chapter 12). Exercise programs include relaxation, limbering, stretching, and strengthening. When the patient is free of pain and full motion has been achieved, progress to strength and endurance programs.

Injection of Trigger Points

Trigger points are treated similarly to treatment of the lateral head of the gastrocnemius (see Fig 10–28) and soleus (see Fig 10–29).

Needle size: 1.5 or 2.0 in., 22 gauge.

Solution: Any one of the following solutions may be used: 0.5% procaine; 1.0% lidocaine; saline and dry needling in case of allergy. Do not use epinephrine.

Postinjection Follow-Up Program

The patient should receive 3 to 4 consecutive days of treatment. Physical therapy should include electrical stimulation, relaxation, limbering, and stretching of the involved muscle using vapocoolant spray or ice as needed combined with and followed by an exercise program. Active and active-assisted exercises are an integral part of the physical therapy program (see Chapter 9 for details).

Exercise and Home Program

Heel chord stretching, range-of-motion exercises for the knee and ankle, and exercises for the plantaris muscle are prescribed. Exercises should at first be performed under the guidance of a therapist. When the patient is free of pain and full motion has been achieved, progress to strength and endurance programs. Begin and end exercise sessions with relaxation (see Chapter 12 for exercise details).

Corrective and Preventive Measures

- Relaxation and stretching exercises prior to and after athletic activities will prevent plantaris and gastrocnemius muscle tears as well as trigger point formation and activation of latent trigger points.

SOLEUS

Symptoms and Pain Pattern

- Pain in the calf and posterior aspect of the ankle (Fig 10–29).
- Pain may be referred to the plantar aspect of the heel and to the area of the sacroiliac joint.[45]

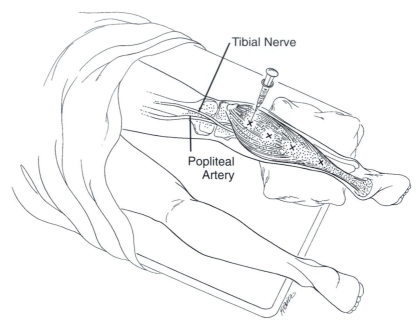

FIG 10–29.   Soleus. Injection of trigger points *(X's)* in the right soleus muscle. The patient is in the prone position with a pillow under the leg for slight knee flexion. All trigger points are injected. Trigger point pain pattern is shown by *stippling*. The popliteal artery and tibial nerve are noted. Aspirate prior to injection.

- Pain is aggravated with weightbearing.
- Heel pain may be mistaken for heel bursitis.

Findings on Examination

- The patient may be examined in the prone or side-lying position.
- The gastrocnemius muscle covers the soleus making palpation of the soleus difficult.
- Relax the gastrocnemius by flexing the knee.
- It may be difficult to distinguish between trigger points in the gastrocnemius and soleus.
- Shortening of the soleus together with the gastrocnemius may cause a restriction in full dorsiflexion.
- To test for triceps surae strength, which would include the gastrocnemius and soleus muscles, ask the patient to stand on one leg while holding onto an object for balance and to lift his or her body weight by raising up on the toes by plantarflexing the foot. Difficulty rising on the toes indicates weakness of the triceps surae.
- In the standing position weakness of the soleus and gastrocnemius can be differentiated. If the soleus is weak, the knee joint will flex and the ankle joints will dorsiflex. If the gastrocnemius is weak, the knee joints will tend to hyperextend and the ankle joints will plantarflex.[14]
- With the patient prone, ask the patient to hold the foot plantarflexed with the knee flexed. Place pressure against the calcaneus pulling the heel plantarward. The patient will not be able to hold the foot in plantarflexion against resistance when the muscles are weak.[14]

Differential Diagnosis

- Thrombophlebitis.
- Heel bursitis, heel spur.
- Herniated lumbar disc (lumbar radiculopathy).
- Tennis leg (tear of gastrocnemius or plantaris).
- Achilles tendonitis.

Anatomy

Origin: head and upper fibula, upper midtibia.
Insertion: through the Achilles tendon to the calcaneus bone.
Action: plantarflexes the foot.

Noninvasive Therapy

The post–trigger point injection follow-up program described in Chapter 9 is recommended as a conservative therapeutic treatment approach. Noninvasive therapy can include:

- Physical therapy modalities (e.g., electrical stimulation and warm packs; see Chapter 15).
- Manual physical therapy techniques (e.g., massage and the Trager Approach; see Chapters 13 and 14).
- Active and passive stretching and limbering of muscles with or without the use of vapocoolant spray or ice. Active exercise is part of the stretch-and-spray technique. Limbering and relaxation are necessary prior to stretching. Contract-relax techniques may be used.
- Stretch and spray: Dorsiflex the foot and ankle with the knee in flexion using vapocoolant spray or ice, as needed. Electrical stimulation, limbering of muscles, and warm packs may precede stretch and spray to relax the muscles. Stretching of muscle is also accomplished actively with assistance during the exercise program. Active exercise is part of the stretch-and-spray technique.
- Exercises and a home program for the knee and ankle are prescribed (see Chapter 12). Exercise programs include relaxation, limbering, stretching, and strengthening. When the patient is free of pain and full motion has been achieved, progress to strength and endurance programs. Begin and end exercise sessions with relaxation and stretching.

Injection of Trigger Point

The patient should be prone or side-lying with the knee flexed. Identify trigger points. Use sterile technique (see Chapter 9 for injection technique). In the lower half of the calf the soleus is covered by the gastrocnemius. The medial and lateral aspects are more accessible to injection than the covered midportion of the muscle (see Fig 10–29).

Needle size: 1.5, 2.0 in., 22 gauge (3 in., 21 gauge may be necessary).

Solution: Any one of the following solutions may be used: 0.5% procaine; 1.0% lidocaine; saline and dry needling in case of allergy. Do not use epinephrine.

Precautions

- Aspirate before injection.
- Avoid posterior tibial artery and nerve which lie deep to the soleus muscle.

Postinjection Follow-Up Physical Therapy Program

The patient should receive 3 to 4 consecutive days of treatment. Physical therapy should include electrical stimulation, relaxation, limbering, and stretching of the involved muscle using vapocoolant spray or ice as needed combined with and followed by an exercise program. Active and active-assisted exercises are an integral part of the physical therapy program (see Chapter 9 for details).

Exercise and Home Program

Exercises for the lower extremity include the knee, ankle and foot. Exercises for heel chord stretching are prescribed. Exercises should at first be performed under the guidance of a therapist. When the patient is free of pain and full motion has been achieved, progress to strength and endurance programs. Begin and end exercise session with relaxation and stretching (see Chapter 12 for exercise details).

Corrective and Preventive Measures

- Avoid overuse syndrome (e.g., unaccustomed prolonged walking and running).
- Prevent prolonged plantarflexion (e.g., use of high heels).
- Avoid direct pressure on the calf muscles.
- Avoid running on uneven surfaces.
- Correct foot deformities (e.g., flatfoot, Morton's foot).
- Prescribe orthoses as necessary.
- Perform relaxation and stretching exercises prior to and after athletic activities.

TIBIALIS POSTERIOR

Symptoms and Referred Pain Pattern

- Patient may complain of localized calf pain.
- Pain may be referred to the Achilles tendon, extending to the sole of the foot and toes.[45] (Fig 10–30).
- Symptoms are aggravated by prolonged walking and running.

Findings on Examination

- Shortening of the tibialis posterior or spasm promotes limitation in pronation, abduction, and eversion of the foot.
- Tenderness may be palpated through the overlying muscles.
- In areas of deep tenderness it is difficult to distinguish between gastrocnemius or soleus muscle trigger points.

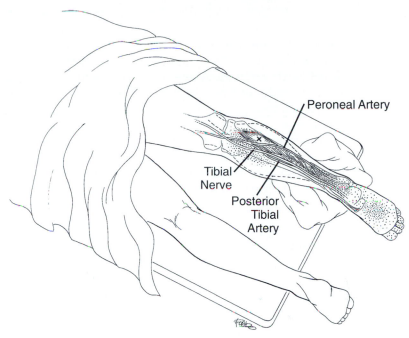

FIG 10–30. Tibialis posterior. Trigger point *(X)* and referred pain pattern *(stippling)* are noted. Trigger point injection is not recommended. Anatomic relations of the tibialis posterior and neurovascular structures (posterior tibial artery and tibial nerve) are noted.

Differential Diagnosis

- Phlebitis.
- Lumbar radiculopathy.
- Achilles tendonitis.
- Pain due to structural foot deficiencies. e.g., flatfoot, Morton's foot.
- Heel bursitis.
- Posterior tibial tendonitis.

Anatomy

Origin: the interosseous membrane, posterior surface of the body of the tibia, upper two thirds of the medial surface of the fibula.

Insertion: tuberosity of the navicula, sustentaculum tali, cuneiforms, cuboid, bases of metatarsals 2 and 3.

Action: plantarflexes, adducts, and inverts foot.

Noninvasive Therapy

The post–trigger point injection follow-up program described in Chapter 9 is recommended as a conservative therapeutic treatment approach. Noninvasive therapy can include:

- Physical therapy modalities (e.g., electrical stimulation and warm packs; see Chapter 15).
- Manual physical therapy techniques (e.g., massage and the Trager Approach; see Chapters 13 and 14).
- Active and passive stretching and limbering of muscles with or without

the use of vapocoolant spray or ice. Active exercise is part of the stretch-and-spray technique. Limbering and relaxation are necessary prior to stretching. Contract-relax techniques may be used.

- Stretch and spray: Assess limitation in motion. With the foot everted and dorsiflexed, spray the trigger point area and referred pain area including the heel and foot (see Chapter 9). Electrical stimulation, limbering of muscles, and warm packs should precede stretch and spray to relax muscles.
- Exercises and a home program for the lower extremities and ankle are described in Chapter 12. Exercise programs include relaxation, limbering, stretching, and strengthening. When the patient is free of pain and full motion has been achieved, progress to strength and endurance programs. Begin and end exercise sessions with stretching and relaxation.

Injection of Trigger Point

The surrounding muscle and bone make the precise localization of trigger points unlikely. This uncertainty in diagnosis coupled with the danger of injuring neurovascular structures in the area makes injection therapy an unwise approach; the risk of vascular injury outweighs the chance of benefiting from the trigger point injection. Injection therapy is therefore not described (see Fig 10–30). I agree with Travell and Simons who do not recommend injecting the tibialis posterior.[45] Although one can attempt the trigger point injection a description of the injection technique is omitted to discourage this temptation. Steroid injections are commonly given for posterior tibial tendonitis in the area of the ankle and foot. Tendon rupture, however, can result from steroid injection.

Exercise and Home Program

Exercises for the lower extremity include the knee, ankle, and foot. Exercises for heel chord stretching are prescribed. Exercises should at first be performed under the guidance of a therapist. When the patient is free of pain and full motion has been achieved, progress to strength and endurance programs. Begin and end exercise sessions with relaxation and stretching (see Chapter 12 for exercise details).

Corrective and Preventive Measures

- Correction of foot deformities, e.g., flatfoot, Morton's foot. Prescribe orthoses as necessary.
- Avoid running on uneven surfaces (e.g., beach running).
- Avoid overuse syndrome (e.g., unaccustomed prolonged walking or running).
- Relaxation and stretching exercises prior to and after athletic activities.

POPLITEUS

Symptoms and Pain Pattern

- Pain in the back of the knee aggravated by activities such as walking or running (Fig 10–31).

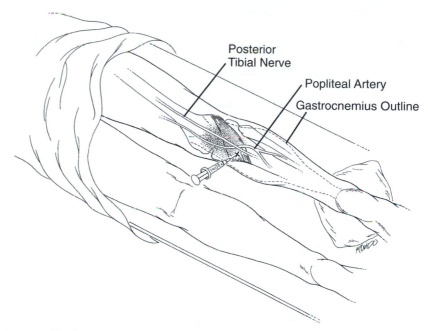

Posterior
Tibial Nerve

Popliteal Artery

Gastrocnemius Outline

FIG 10–31. Popliteus. Injection of popliteal muscle trigger point *(X)*. The patient is prone with slight flexion of the knee to relax structures in the popliteal area. The popliteal muscle is covered by the gastrocnemius. Aspirate prior to injection. The patient may be prone or side-lying. Trigger point pain pattern is noted by *stippling. Dashed line* represents the gastrocnemius.

Findings on Examination

- Trigger points are difficult to palpate in view of the overlying muscles; the gastrocnemius must be relaxed. The popliteus is more easily examined with the knee in flexion. The popliteus may be palpated medial to the lateral gastronemius on the lateral side. The semimembranosus and semitendinosus must be relaxed in order to palpate the medial aspect of the popliteus.
- Shortening of the popliteus results in some restriction in lateral rotation of the tibia on the femur. This is noted with flexion of the knee.
- Shortening of the popliteus will also limit extension of the knee.

Differential Diagnosis

- Popliteal tendinitis.
- Tear of posterior horn of the lateral meniscus.
- Baker's cyst.

Anatomy

Origin: popliteal surface of tibia above the soleal line.
Insertion: lateral femoral condyle, the medial half of the muscle into the lateral meniscus.
Action: rotates knee (femur laterally or tibia medially), flexes the leg.

Noninvasive Therapy

The post–trigger point injection follow-up program described in Chapter 9 is recommended as a conservative therapeutic treatment approach. Noninvasive therapy can include:

- Physical therapy modalities (e.g., electrical stimulation and warm packs; see Chapter 15).
- Manual physical therapy techniques (e.g., massage and the Trager Approach; see Chapters 13 and 14).
- Active and passive stretching and limbering of muscles with or without the use of vapocoolant spray or ice. Active exercise is part of the stretch-and-spray technique. Limbering and relaxation are necessary prior to stretching. Contract-relax techniques may be used.
- Stretch and spray for the popliteus is performed by laterally rotating the knee while the joint is relaxed in flexion. Follow with spray and stretch in medial rotation and extension of the knee. Use vapocoolant spray or ice as indicated. Electrical stimulation, limbering of muscles, and warm packs should precede stretch and spray to relax muscles.
- Exercise and home program for the knee are described in Chapter 12. Exercise programs include relaxation, limbering, stretching, and strengthening. When the patient is free of pain and full motion has been achieved, progress to strength and endurance programs.

Injection of Trigger Points

Palpate trigger points with the patient in the prone position and the knee slightly flexed to relax the popliteal region. Palpate the popliteal artery (see Fig 10–31).

Size of needle: 1.5–2.0 in., 21 gauge.

Solution: Any one of the following solutions may be used: 0.5% procaine; 1.0% lidocaine; isotonic saline and dry needling in case of allergy. Do not use epinephrine.

Precautions

- Avoid the popliteal artery and vein and tibial nerve (see Fig 10–31).
- Aspirate prior to injection.

Postinjection Follow-Up Physical Therapy Program

The patient should receive 3 to 4 consecutive days of treatment. Physical therapy should include electrical stimulation, relaxation, limbering, and stretching of the involved muscle using vapocoolant spray or ice as needed combined with and followed by an exercise program (see Chapter 9). Active and active-assisted exercises are an integral part of the physical therapy program. Crutches are used for 24 hours following the injection to avoid pain, muscle spasm, and limping.

Exercise and Home Program

Exercises should at first be performed under the guidance of a therapist. When the patient is free of pain and full motion has been achieved, progress to strength and endurance programs. Begin and end exercise sessions with stretching and relaxation (see Chapter 13 for exercise details).

LONG EXTENSORS OF THE TOES
Extensor digitorum longus, Extensor hallucis longus

Symptoms and Pain Patterns

- Pain is experienced over the lower third of the leg, both laterally and anteriorly. Pain may radiate distally to the foot.[18]
- Referred pain to the dorsum of the foot and middle three toes by the extensor digitorum longus. The extensor hallucis longus refers pain to the dorsum of the foot and metatarsophalangeal joint area of the big toe to the tip of the big toe[22, 43] (Fig 10–32).
- Weakness of extension of the toes may occur with trigger points.
- Marked weakness may occur with entrapment of the deep peroneal nerve.

Findings on Examination

- Tenderness on palpation of trigger points with referred pain patterns involving the foot and toes.
- Weakness on testing dorsiflexors of the ankle and toes.

Differential Diagnosis

- Herniated lumbar disc.
- Morton's neuroma.
- Gout.

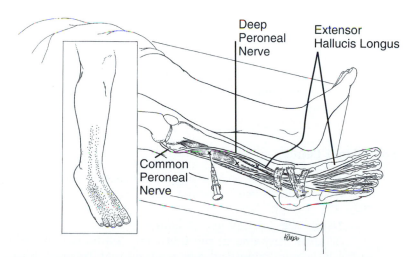

FIG 10–32.   Long extensors of the toes. Injection of trigger points (*X's*) in the right extensor digitorum longus with the patient supine. Anatomic landmarks are noted, including the deep peroneal nerve. Aspirate prior to injection. Avoid the deep peroneal nerve and anterior tibial vessels. Localize trigger points by means of palpation prior to injection. Do not use multiple probing. *Inset,* trigger point pain pattern (*stippling*).

Anatomy

Extensor Digitorum Longus

Origin: lateral condyle of the tibia, proximal three fourths of the fibula, interosseous membrane.

Insertion: dorsum of the middle and the distal phalanx of the four lateral toes.

Action: extends toes, dorsiflexes the foot, everts the foot.

Extensor Hallicus Longus

Origin: middle anterior aspect of the fibula and interosseous membrane.

Insertion: base of distal phalanx of the big toe.

Action: extends the big toe, everts the foot.

Noninvasive Therapy

The post–trigger point injection follow-up program described in Chapter 9 is recommended as a conservative therapeutic treatment approach. Noninvasive therapy can include:

- Physical therapy modalities (e.g., electrical stimulation and warm packs; see Chapter 15).
- Manual physical therapy techniques (e.g., massage and the Trager Approach; see Chapters 13 and 14).
- Active and passive stretching and limbering of muscles with or without the use of vapocoolant spray or ice. Active exercise is part of the stretch-and-spray technique. Limbering and relaxation is necessary prior to stretching. Contract-relax techniques may be used.
- Stretch and spray is performed by plantarflexing the ankle, inverting the foot, and flexing the toes. Use vapocoolant or ice as necessary. Electrical stimulation, limbering of muscles, and warm packs may precede stretch and spray to relax the muscles. Stretching of muscle is also accomplished actively and with assistance during the exercise program. Active exercise is part of the stretch-and-spray technique.
- Exercises and a home program for the ankle, foot, and toes are prescribed (see Chapter 12). Exercise program includes relaxation, limbering, stretching, and strengthening. When the patient is free of pain and full motion has been achieved, progress to strength and endurance programs.

Injection of Trigger Points

With the patient supine trigger points are identified. Injection is performed for well-localized trigger points (see Chapter 9). Multiple needling is not used (see Fig 10–32).

Needle size: 1.5–2.0 in., 21 gauge.

Solution: Any one of the following solutions may be used: 0.5% procaine; 1.0% lidocaine; saline and dry needling may be used in case of allergy. Do not use epinephrine.

Precautions

- Avoid multiple needling because of neurovascular structures.
- Aspirate before injection.
- Avoid the deep peroneal nerve and anterior tibial vessels.

Postinjection Follow-Up

The patient should receive 3 to 4 consecutive days of treatment. Physical therapy should include electrical stimulation, relaxation, limbering, and stretching of the involved muscle using vapocoolant spray or ice as needed combined with and followed by an exercise program. Use crutches (partial weightbearing) for 24 hours to avoid limping, pain, and muscle spasm.

Exercise and Home Program

Exercises for the ankle, foot, and toes are prescribed. Exercises should at first be performed under the guidance of a therapist. When the patient is free of pain and full motion has been achieved, progress to strength and endurance programs. Begin and end exercise sessions with relaxation and stretching (see Chapter 12 for exercise details).

Corrective and Preventive Measures

- Avoid overuse syndromes, e.g., unaccustomed prolonged walking or jogging.
- Avoid jogging on uneven surfaces.
- Avoid positions of prolonged dorsiflexion of the foot and toes.
- Prescribe orthoses for flatfoot and Morton's foot as indicated.
- Continue home program for exercises for ankle, foot, and toes.

LONG FLEXOR MUSCLES OF THE TOES
Flexor digitorum longus, Flexor hallucis longus

Symptoms and Pain Pattern

- Calf pain with walking or running.[19]
- Referred pain to the bottom of the foot and toes by the flexor digitorum longus.[45] (Fig 10–33)
- Referred pain to the plantar aspect of the big toe and metatarsal head area by the flexor hallucis longus.[22, 45]

Findings on Examination

- Trigger points are found by palpating the flexor digitorum longus on the medial side of the leg, anteromedial to the medial gastrocnemius.
- The flexor hallucis longus is palpated on the lateral side of the middle lower portion of the leg.

- Overlying muscles make palpation of the long flexor muscles of the toes difficult.
- Look for local pain and referred pain pattern.

Differential Diagnosis

- Phlebitis.
- Tennis leg (plantaris tendon rupture, gastrocnemius rupture).
- Radiating pain of tarsal tunnel syndrome.
- Plantar fasciitis.
- Peripheral neuropathy.

Anatomy

Flexor Digitorum Longus
Origin: posterior tibia.
Insertion: base of distal phalanx, and second, third, fourth, and fifth toes.
Action: flexes the toes, plantarflexes the foot, inverts the foot.

Flexor Hallucis Longus
Origin: posterior fibula, interroseous membrane.
Insertion: base of distal phalanx of big toe.
Action: flexes the distal phalanx, plantarflexes the foot, inverts the foot.

Noninvasive Therapy

The post–trigger point injection follow-up program described in Chapter 9 is recommended as a conservative therapeutic treatment approach. Noninvasive therapy can include:

- Physical therapy modalities (e.g., electrical stimulation and warm packs; see Chapter 15).
- Manual physical therapy techniques (e.g., massage and the Trager Approach; see Chapters 13 and 14).
- Active and passive stretching and limbering of muscles with or without the use of vapocoolant spray or ice. Active exercise is part of the stretch-and-spray technique. Limbering and relaxation are necessary prior to stretching. Contract-relax techniques may be used.
- Stretch and spray for the long flexors of the toes is performed with the toes dorsiflexed and the foot everted. Use vapocoolant spray or ice as indicated.
- Exercises and a home program for the toes and ankle are described in Chapter 12. Exercise programs include relaxation, limbering, stretching, and strengthening.

Injection of Trigger Point

With the patient in the prone position, identify trigger points. Trigger points are usually found in the upper lateral aspect of the leg for the flexor digitorum longus and over the medial aspect of the lower third of the leg for the flexor hallucis longus. In performing the injection the needle should be placed directly into the area of the trigger point. Palpate the medial edge of the midshaft of the tibia, inserting the needle just posterior to the medial edge. The needle will then enter the flexor digitorum longus (Fig 10–33). (See Chapter 9 for injection technique.)

Needle size: 1.5, 2.0, 3.0 in., 21 gauge.

Solution: Any one of the following solutions may be used: 0.5% procaine; 1.0% lidocaine; use saline and dry needling in case of allergy. Do not use epinephrine.

Precautions

- Inject isolated, well-localized trigger points.
- Do not use a fanning, circular technique or multiple needling techniques.
- Aspirate prior to injecting. The posterior tibial artery, vein, and tibial nerve and peroneal vessels lie between the long flexor muscles.

Postinjection Follow-Up Physical Therapy Program

The patient should receive 3 to 4 consecutive days of treatment. Physical therapy should include electrical stimulation, relaxation, limbering, and stretching of the involved muscle using vapocoolant spray or ice as needed combined with and followed by an exercise program. Active and active-assisted exercises are an integral part of the physical therapy program. Use crutches (partial weightbearing) for 24 hours to avoid limping, pain, and muscle spasm. (See Chapter 9 for program details.)

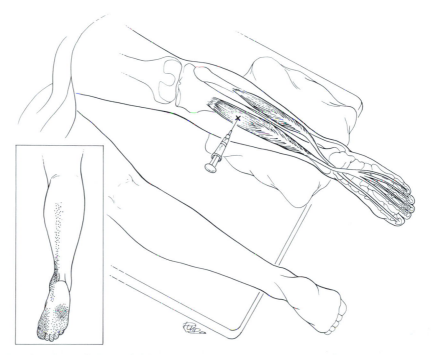

FIG 10–33. Long flexors of the toes. Injection of trigger point *(X)* in the flexor digitorum longus. Anatomic landmarks are noted for the flexor digitorum longus and flexor hallucis longus. Inject directly into the palpated trigger point. Insert needle just posterior to the medial border of the tibia for the flexor digitorum longus. *Inset,* trigger point pain pattern *(stippling).*

Exercise and Home Program

Exercises should at first be performed under the guidance of a therapist. When the patient is free of pain and full motion has been achieved, progress to strength and endurance programs. Begin and end exercise sessions with relaxation and stretching (see Chapter 12 for exercise details).

Corrective and Preventive Measures

- Orthoses for foot abnormalities, e.g., flatfoot, Morton's foot.
- Avoid running on uneven surfaces.

SUPERFICIAL INTRINSIC FOOT MUSCLES
Extensor digitorum brevis, Extensor hallucis brevis, Abductor hallucis, Flexor digitorum brevis, Abductor digiti minimi

Symptoms and Pain Pattern

Trigger points in the muscles of the foot may cause pain on the sole or dorsum of the foot, or both. The following referred pain patterns have been described[45] (Fig 10–34).

FIG 10–34.   Superficial intrinsic muscles of the foot. **A,** abductor halllucis longus; **B,** abductor digiti minimi; **C,** flexor digitorum brevis; **D,** extensor hallucis brevis and extensor digitorum brevis. Trigger points *(X's)* are identified. Needling is performed directly into the trigger point area. Trigger point pain patterns are shown by *stippling.*

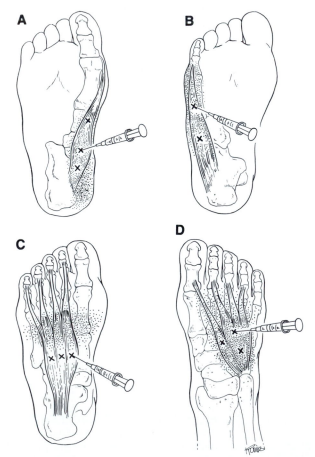

- The extensor hallucis brevis and extensor digitorum brevis refer pain to the dorsum of the foot.[13]
- The abductor hallucis refers pain to the medial side of the heel and instep.
- The abductor digiti minimi refers pain to the plantar aspect of the fifth metatarsal head.
- The flexor digitorum brevis refers pain to the heads of the second, third, fourth, and fifth metatarsals.

Findings on Examination

- Local tenderness over the above muscles.
- Examination may find foot abnormalities that contribute to the development of trigger points, e.g., Morton's foot, flatfoot, calcaneovalgus.

Differential Diagnosis

- Ligamentous foot strain.
- Plantar fasciitis.
- Flatfoot.
- Metatarsalgia.
- Tarsal tunnel syndrome.

Anatomy

Abductor Digiti Ouinti (Minimi)
Origin: lateral and medial process of the tuberosity of the calcaneus.
Insertion: lateral surface of the proximal phalanx of the small toe.
Action: flexes and abducts the proximal phalanx of the small toe.

Abductor Hallucis Longus
Origin: medial tuberosity of the calcaneus.
Insertion: Medial side and base of the proximal phalanx of the big toe.
Action: flexes and abducts the big toe.

Flexor Digitorum Brevis
Origin: medial tubercle of the calcaneus, plantar aponeurosis.
Insertion: plantar surface of base of the middle phalanx of the second, third, fourth, and fifth toes.
Action: flexes toes.

Extensor Digitorum Brevis
Origin: upper lateral surface of the calcaneus.
Insertion: proximal phalanx of the great toe and tendon of the extensor digitorum longus of the second, third, and fourth toes.
Action: extends big toe, second, third, and fourth toes.

Extensor Hallucis Brevis
Origin: anterior fibula and interosseous membrane.
Insertion: base of the distal phalanx of the big toe.
Action: extends the big toe, everts the foot.

Noninvasive Therapy

The post–trigger point injection follow-up program described in Chapter 9 is recommended as a conservative therapeutic treatment approach. Noninvasive therapy can include:

- Physical therapy modalities (e.g., electrical stimulation and warm packs; see Chapter 15).
- Manual physical therapy techniques (e.g., massage and the Trager Approach; see Chapters 13 and 14).
- Active and passive stretching and limbering of muscles with or without the use of vapocoolant spray or ice. Active exercise is part of the stretch-and-spray technique. Limbering and relaxation are necessary prior to stretching. Contract-relax techniques may be used.
- Stretch and spray: Stretch opposite the direction of muscle function. Stretch the extensors by flexing the toes and inverting the foot. Flexor muscles are stretched in the direction of extension. (See Chapter 9 for stretch-and-spray technique.) Electrical stimulation, limbering of muscles, and warm packs may precede stretch and spray to relax the muscles. Stretching of muscles is also accomplished actively and with assistance during the exercise program. Active exercise is part of the stretch-and-spray technique.
- Exercise and a home program to increase strength and flexibility of toe extensors are described in Chapter 12. Exercise program includes relaxation, limbering, stretching, and strengthening.

Injection of Trigger Point

With the patient in the supine position trigger points are identified. Use multiple needling or fanning technique to find all trigger points in the area of the muscles involved (see Chapter 9). (Figure 10–34 demonstrates trigger point areas, muscular attachments, and pain patterns.)

Needle size: 1.5, 2.0 in., 22–25 gauge.

Solution: Any one of the following solutions may be used: 0.5% procaine; 1.0% lidocaine; saline and dry needling in case of allergy. Do not use epinephrine.

Postinjection Follow-Up Physical Therapy Program

The patient should receive 3 to 4 consecutive days of treatment. Physical therapy should include electrical stimulation, relaxation, limbering, and stretching of the involved muscle using vapocoolant spray or ice as needed combined with and followed by an exercise program. Active and active-assisted exercises are an integral part of the physical therapy program (see Chapter 9 for details).

Exercise and Home Program

Exercises to increase strength and flexibility of the toes are prescribed (see Chapter 12). Exercises should at first be performed under the guidance of a therapist.

Corrective and Preventive Measures

- If foot deformities are present (e.g., Morton's foot, flatfoot, calcaneovalgus), prescribe orthoses as indicated.
- Treat metatarsalgia with metatarsal bars or orthoses.
- Correct source of foot pain, e.g., hammer toes, plantar callosities.
- Lower extremity casts should be applied so that free range of motion of the toes is possible to avoid muscle trigger points and joint stiffness.
- Avoid running on uneven surfaces.
- Wear properly sized shoes.

DEEP INTRINSIC FOOT MUSCLES

Quadratus plantae, Lumbricals, second, third, and fourth, Adductor hallucis, oblique head, Adductor hallucis, transverse head, Flexor hallucis brevis, Interossei

Symptoms and Pain Pattern

- Pain on the sole and dorsum of the foot with weightbearing.
- Patterns of numbness in the toes due to interrossei trigger points which may be mistaken for Morton's neuroma.
- The quadratus plantae and lumbricals refer pain to the plantar surface of the heel.
- The adductor hallucis, oblique and transverse heads, refers pain to the plantar surface of the forefoot.[45]
- The flexor hallucis brevis refers pain to the head of the first metatarsal, and the medial and plantar aspects of the first and second toes.[13, 44]
- The interossei may refer pain and numbness to the side of the toe and dorsum of the foot.[18]
- The quadratus plantae refers pain to the bottom of the heel[44] (Fig 10–35).

Findings on Examination

Tender trigger points cause local and referred pain patterns. Examination may reveal foot abnormalities, e.g., flatfoot, Morton's foot, calcaneovalgus, which contribute to the formation of trigger points and symptoms.

Differential Diagnosis

- Morton's neuroma.
- Heel bursitis.
- Metatarsalgia due to foot deformity.
- Foot strain.
- Stress fracture.

Anatomy

Quadratus Plantae
Origin: calcaneus.
Insertion: lateral border of the long flexor tendons.
Action: flexes toes.

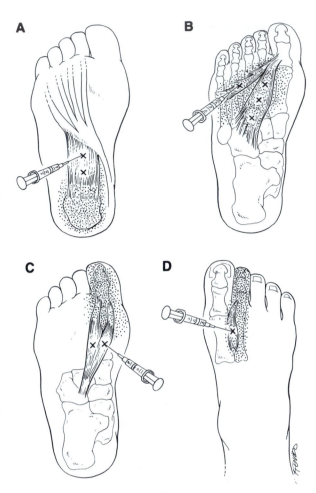

FIG 10–35. Deep intrinsic foot muscles. **A,** injection of trigger points *(X's)* in the quadratus plantae. The foot may be dorsiflexed or turned to the side. The needle may be directed perpendicular to the quadratus plantae or tangentially. **B,** injection of trigger points *(X's)* in the adductor hallucis, transverse and oblique heads. Injection is given into the plantar surface. **C,** injection of trigger points *(X's)* in the flexor hallucis brevis. Injection is given into the plantar space. **D,** injection of trigger point *(X)* in the right first dorsal interosseus. Injection is performed through the dorsum of the foot between the first and second metatarsals. The foot is in neutral position or slight plantarflexion. **D, A–D,** *stippling* shows pain patterns.

Lumbrical, First
Origin: medial side of the first long flexor tendon.
Insertion: proximal phalanx and extensor tendons of the second toe.
Action: flexes the proximal phalanx, extends the distal phalanx.

Lumbricals, Second, Third, and Fourth
Origin: long flexor tendons (second, third, and fourth)
Insertion: proximal phalanx and extensor tendons (third, fourth, and fifth).
Action: flexes the proximal phalanx, extends the distal phalanx.

Adductor Hallucis, Oblique Head
Origin: peroneus longus sheath; base of second, third, and fourth metatarsals.
Insertion: lateral aspect of the base of the proximal phalanx of the big toe.

Adductor Hallucis, Transverse Head
Origin: capsules of third, fourth, and fifth metatarsophalangeal joints.
Insertion: lateral aspect of the base of the proximal phalanx of the big toe.
Action: adducts and flexes the proximal phalanx of the big toe.

Flexor Hallucis Brevis

Origin: cuboid and lateral cuneiform.
Insertion: medial and lateral sides or proximal phalanx of the great toe.
Action: flexes the proximal phalanx of the big toe.

Interossei

Origin: three plantar interossei from the base and medial sides of the third, fourth, and fifth metatarsal bones; four dorsal interossei each arise by two heads from adjacent sides of metatarsal bones.

Insertion: base of proximal phalanges and dorsal digital expansions to the second, third, fourth, and fifth toes.

Action: adducts toes, flexes the proximal phalanx, extends the distal phalanx of the third, fourth, and fifth toes.

Noninvasive Therapy

The post–trigger point injection follow-up program described in Chapter 9 is recommended as a conservative therapeutic treatment approach. Noninvasive therapy can include:

- Physical therapy modalities (e.g., electrical stimulation and warm packs; see Chapter 15).
- Manual physical therapy techniques (e.g., massage and the Trager Approach; see Chapters 13 and 14).
- Active and passive stretching and limbering of muscles with or without the use of vapocoolant spray or ice. Active exercise is part of the stretch-and-spray technique. Limbering and relaxation are necessary prior to stretching. Contract-relax techniques may be used.
- Stretch and spray (see Chapter 9): Vapocoolant spray or ice may be used to aid in extension and abduction of toes. Movements should be both active and passive. Heat, massage, and ischemic pressure can be used. Electrical stimulation, limbering of muscles, and warm packs should precede stretch and spray to relax muscles.
- Exercises and a home program for flexion and extension of the toes are described in Chapter 12. Exercise program includes relaxation, limbering, stretching, and strengthening. When the patient is free of pain and full motion has been achieved, progress to strength and endurance programs.

Injection of Trigger Points

With the patient in the supine position trigger points are identified. Trigger points may be found both locally and in the referred pain area. Injections may be given with the patient supine with the foot in dorsiflexion or in the side-lying position (see Fig 10–35).

Needle size: 1.5 in., 22 gauge.

Solution: Any one of the following solutions may be used: 0.5% procaine; 1.0% lidocaine; saline and dry needling in case of allergy. Do not use epinephrine.

Postinjection Follow-Up Program

The patient should receive 3 to 4 consecutive days of treatment. Physical therapy should include electrical stimulation, relaxation, limbering, and stretching of the involved muscle using vapocoolant spray or ice as needed combined with and followed by an exercise program.

Exercise and Home Program

Exercises to encourage toe flexion are prescribed. Exercises should at first be performed under the guidance of a therapist. When the patient is free of pain and full motion has been achieved, progress to strength and endurance programs. Begin and end exercise sessions with stretching and relaxation (see Chapter 12 for exercise details).

Corrective and Preventive Measures

- Correct foot deformities such as flatfoot and calcaneovalgus.
- Prescribe orthoses if necessary.
- The patient should be aware of his or her proper shoe size and avoid tight shoes.
- Avoid unaccustomed prolonged walking or running, i.e., the overuse syndrome.
- Avoid running on uneven surfaces.
- Lower extremity casts should be applied so that full range of motion of the toes is possible.

Cervical and Upper Dorsal Muscles

STERNOCLEIDOMASTOID

Symptoms and Pain Pattern

- The sternocleidomastoid muscle consists of a more superficial sternal division and a deeper clavicular division (Fig 10–36).
- The sternal portion of the muscle may refer pain to the cheek, temporomandibular joint area, supraorbital ridge, occipital area, and orbit. Autonomic symptoms such as lacrimation and coryza may occur on the same side as the trigger points.[20, 43, 46]
- The clavicular component may refer pain to the occipital area and across the forehead.[43]
- Symptoms may include dizziness, vertigo, and problems with equilibrium.
- Eye symptoms may include blurred vision.[44]
- Referred pain may involve the ear, jaw, and neck area.[3, 4]

Findings on Examination

- Tender trigger points on palpation of the sternocleidomastoid causing local or referred pain patterns, or both.

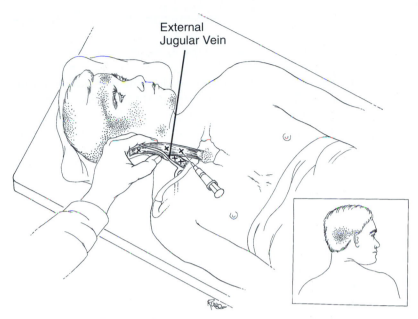

FIG 10–36.   Sternocleidomastoid. Injection of right sternocleidomastoid trigger points (*X's*). The patient is supine, the head tilted toward the same side, the chin directed to the opposite shoulder. The muscle is grasped between the thumb, index, and middle fingers. Anatomic landmarks are noted. Avoid the jugular vein. Avoid deep penetration in the area of the clavicle. Pain pattern is shown by *stippling*.

- May be a cause of torticollis with muscle shortening.
- Lacrimation, rhinitis may be present.

Differential Diagnosis

- Tension headache.
- Atypical facial neuralgia.
- Meniere's disease.
- Temporomandibular joint dysfunction.

Anatomy

Origin: sternum and clavicle.
Insertion: mastoid process.
Action: bends the head to the same side, rotates head and raises the chin to the opposite side; both right and left sternocleidomastoid muscles working together bend the head forward and also elevate the chin.

Noninvasive Therapy

The post–trigger point injection follow-up program described in Chapter 9 is recommended as a conservative therapeutic treatment approach. Noninvasive therapy can include:

- Physical therapy modalities (e.g., electrical stimulation and warm packs; see Chapter 15).
- Manual physical therapy techniques (e.g., massage and the Trager Approach; see Chapters 13 and 14).

- Active and passive stretching and limbering of muscles with or without the use of vapocoolant spray or ice. Active exercise is part of the stretch-and-spray technique. Limbering and relaxation of muscles are necessary prior to stretching. Contract-relax techniques may be used.
- Stretch and spray: Bend head to the opposite side, raising the chin to the same side. Include rotation, raising the chin on the shoulder, flexion, and extension of the head. Treat both sides to achieve full range of motion.
- Exercises and a home program for the cervical area are described in Chapter 12 (exercises for the neck.) Exercise program includes relaxation, limbering, stretching, and strengthening. When the patient is free of pain and full motion has been achieved, progress to strength and endurance programs.

Injection of Trigger Points

With the patient supine, tilt the chin to the opposite side and bend the head toward the side to be injected. The muscle is grasped between the thumb and index finger. All trigger points are injected and needled. Look for trigger points in the areas of origin and insertion. Avoid deep penetration in the area of the clavicle to avoid a pneumothorax. (See Chapter 9 for injection technique.)

Needle size: 1.5 in., 22–25 gauge

Solution: Any one of the following solutions may be used: 0.5% procaine; 1.0% lidocaine; saline and dry needling in case of allergy. Do not use epinephrine.

Precaution

- Avoid the external jugular vein; aspirate prior to injection
- Avoid deep penetration in the area of the clavicle to prevent puncturing the lung apex.

Postinjection Follow-Up Physical Therapy Program

The patient should receive 3 to 4 consecutive days of treatment. Physical therapy should include electrical stimulation, relaxation, limbering, and stretching of the involved muscle using vapocoolant spray or ice as needed combined with and followed by an exercise program. Active and active-assisted exercises are an integral part of the physical therapy program (see Chapter 9 for details).

Exercise and Home Program

Exercises should at first be performed under the guidance of a therapist. Begin and end exercise sessions with relaxation and stretching. (See Chapter 12 for exercise details.)

Corrective and Preventive Measures

- Avoid maintaining rotational positions of the neck for long periods, e.g., sitting in an airplane engaged in prolonged conversations with the head turned.

- Correct faulty posture, e.g., head-forward posture (see Chapters 12 and 13).
- Correct poor work postural attitudes, e.g., holding the telephone between the ear and shoulder to free both hands; avoid poor sitting and standing postures (see Chapter 16).

SCALENE MUSCLE GROUP
Scalenus anterior, Scalenus medius, Scalenus posterior

Symptoms and Pain Pattern

- Pain in the upper arm radiating to the forearm and hand (Fig 10–37).
- Referred pain to the interscapular area, medial scapular border, upper back, upper chest, and radial side of the hand.[18, 43, 46]
- Symptoms of neurovascular entrapment indicative of thoracic outlet syndrome may include numbness in the fourth and fifth fingers.[28]

Findings on Examination

- On examination, tenderness over the scalene muscles producing local pain or referred pain patterns, or both.
- If trigger points cause neurovascular entrapment, Adson's sign may be positive in addition to diminished sensation of the fourth and fifth fingers and swelling of the hand.

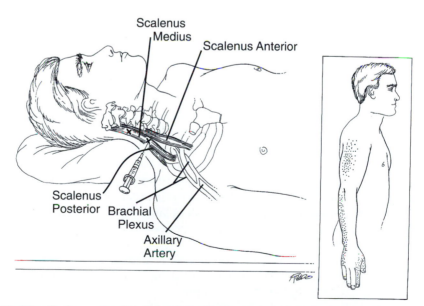

FIG 10–37. Scalene muscles. Injection of the scalenus medius muscle trigger points (*X's*). The patient is supine, the head turned away from the area of pain. Anatomic landmarks are noted, including axillary artery and lateral chord. Referred pain pattern is shown by *stippling*.

Anatomy

Scalenus Anterior
Origin: tubercles of the transverse processes of C3–6.
Insertion: scalene tubercle on inner border of the first rib.
Action: flexion and lateral flexion of the neck, elevation of first rib.

Scalenus Medius
Origin: transverse processes of C2–6.
Insertion: upper surface of the first rib.
Action: lateral flexor of the neck and elevator of the first rib.

Scalenus Posterior
Origin: transverse processes of C5–7.
Insertion: outer surface of second rib.
Action: lateral flexor of the neck and elevator of second rib.
    The brachial plexus and subclavian artery exit between the scalenus anterior and scalenus medius.

Differential Diagnosis

- Thoracic outlet syndrome.
- Cervical herniated disc.
- Carpal tunnel syndrome.
- Cervical sprain.

Noninvasive Therapy

    The post–trigger point injection follow-up program described in Chapter 9 is recommended as a conservative therapeutic treatment approach. Noninvasive therapy can include:

- Physical therapy modalities (e.g., electrical stimulation and warm packs; see Chapter 15).
- Manual physical therapy techniques (e.g., massage and the Trager Approach; see Chapters 13 and 14).
- Active and passive stretching and limbering of muscles with or without the use of vapocoolant spray or ice. Active exercise is part of the stretch-and-spray technique. Limbering and relaxation of muscles are necessary prior to stretching. Contract-relax techniques may be used.
- *Stretch and spray:* Use vapocoolant or ice. Stretch by extending the neck and tilting the neck to the opposite side. Electrical stimulation, limbering of muscles, and warm packs may precede stretch and spray to relax the muscles. Stretching of muscle is also accomplished actively and with assistance during the exercise program. Active exercise is part of the stretch-and-spray technique.
- Exercises and a home program for the neck are prescribed. (see Chapter 12). Exercise programs include relaxation, limbering, stretching, and strengthening.

Injection of Trigger Points

Identify the anterior border of the levator scapulae and the posterior border of the sternocleidomastoid. Trigger points are palpated with the patient supine (see Fig 10–37). The head is turned away from the area of pain. The trigger point is isolated between two fingers. Maintain a distance of more than 1.5 in. above the clavicle to avoid the apex of the lung. The scalenus posterior is approached with the patient lying on the uninvolved side.

Needle size: Small-sized needles are used (1.0–1.5 in., 23–25 gauge).

Solution: Any one of the following solutions may be used: 0.5% procaine; 1.0% lidocaine; saline and dry needling in case of allergy. Do not use epinephrine.

Precautions

- Avoid the brachial plexus by isolating the trigger points between two fingers while controlling needle direction.
- Transient numbness and weakness may occur following injection.
- An injection performed too deeply may cause a stellate ganglion block.

Postinjection Follow-Up Physical Therapy Program

The patient should receive 3 to 4 consecutive days of treatment. Physical therapy should include electrical stimulation, relaxation, limbering, and stretching of the involved muscle using vapocoolant spray or ice as needed combined with and followed by an exercise program. Active and active-assisted exercises are an integral part of the physical therapy program (see Chapter 9 for details).

Exercise and Home Program

Exercises for the cervical spine are prescribed. Exercises should at first be performed under the guidance of a therapist. When the patient is free of pain and full motion has been achieved, progress to strength and endurance programs. Begin and end exercise sessions with stretching and relaxation (see Chapter 12 for exercise details).

Corrective and Preventive Measures

- Postural correction, e.g., correct forward head position.
- Correct poor reading habits, e.g., reading in bed holding a book with outstretched arms, and tilting the neck owing to poor lighting (see Chapter 17).
- Avoid holding the telephone between the ear and shoulder which may cause and activate trigger points.
- Avoid paradoxical respiration which has been noted as a cause of scalene overload.[45]

TRAPEZIUS
Upper trapezius, Middle trapezius, Lower part of trapezius

Symptoms and Pain Pattern

- The trapezius muscle is the most common muscle in the body to harbor trigger points. They are often found incidentally in asymptomatic persons.[37, 38]
- Upper trapezius trigger points may involve pain in the cervical area in addition to referred pain to the ear region, face, and frontal area. Headaches may be noted in the temporal area. Patients may present with symptoms of dizziness and vertigo[6] in addition to pilomotor activity involving the upper arm.[44]
- Trapezius trigger points in the area of the midscapula may cause symptoms of brachial neuralgia and subdeltoid bursitis.[7, 13]
- Symptoms referable to the lower trapezius trigger points may refer pain to the paradorsal, high cervical area, medial border of the scapula, and acromion[4, 11–13, 19, 25, 28, 44] (Fig 10–38).

Findings on Examination

- Local tenderness over trigger points. Trigger points are most commonly located in the upper two thirds of the muscle.[35]
- Limitation in range of motion of the cervical spine.

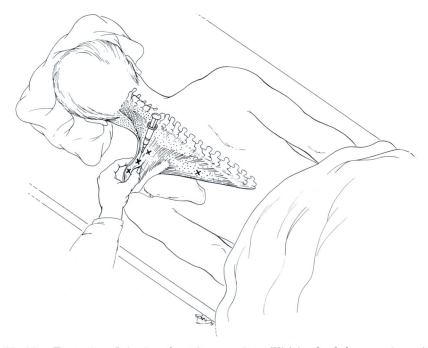

FIG 10–38. Trapezius. Injection for trigger points *(X's)* in the left trapezius with the patient prone. The upper portion of the left trapezius is grasped between the thumb, index, and middle fingers and elevated to avoid penetrating the apex of the lung. Several entries are usually necessary to treat all trigger points that are present. Aspirate prior to injection. Pain pattern is shown by *stippling.*

- Pain with cervical rotation, flexion, and with shoulder shrug.
- Elevation of the arms and abduction may be limited by muscle shortening and pain.
- Trigger point palpation may give rise to referred pain patterns.

Differential Diagnosis

- Cervical disc.
- Temporomandibular joint dysfunction.
- Trapezius muscle sprain.

Anatomy

Upper Trapezius
Origin: occipital bone (ligamentum nuchae).
Insertion: outer one third of the clavicle.
Action: upper fibers elevate the shoulder (shrugging), rotates scapula, draws head to the same side, turns face to the opposite side; both trapezius muscles working together extend the head.

Middle Trapezius
Origin: spinous processes of C7 and C8 and upper thoracic vertebrae.
Insertion: spine of the scapula and acromion.
Action: adduction of the scapula.

Lower Part of Trapezius
Origin: spinous processes of lower thoracic vertebra.
Insertion: spine of the scapula.
Action: lowers and pulls the scapula down.

Noninvasive Therapy

The post–trigger point injection follow-up program described in Chapter 9 is recommended as a conservative therapeutic treatment approach. Noninvasive therapy can include:

- Physical therapy modalities (e.g., electrical stimulation and warm packs; see Chapter 15).
- Manual physical therapy techniques (e.g., massage and the Trager Approach; see Chapters 13 and 14).
- Active and passive stretching and limbering of muscles with or without the use of vapocoolant spray or ice. Limbering and relaxation of muscles are necessary prior to stretching. Contract-relax techniques may be used for muscle lengthening.
- Stretch and spray: Stretch in the opposite direction of the muscle pull. Stretch the head gently toward the opposite side for stretch of the upper trapezius fibers. Adduct the arms across the chest, with flexion of the cervical area and upper back to stretch the mid and lower portion of the trapezius. Trapezius muscle trigger points are often accompanied by neighboring trigger points found in the infraspinatus, supraspinatus, and levator scapulae.

- Exercise program: Exercises for the neck and shoulder (see Chapter 12) include relaxation, limbering, stretching, and strengthening. When the patient is free of pain and full motion has been achieved, progress to strength and endurance programs.

Injection of Trigger Point

With the patient in the supine position, trigger points are identified and injected under sterile precautions (see Chapter 9 for trigger point injection technique). The upper trapezius is held between the thumb, index, and middle fingers and lifted slightly (see Figs 10–38 and 9–13) This helps control the depth of needle penetration to avoid the apex of the lung. Trigger points in the middle and lower fibers may sometimes be palpated best with the patient in the side-lying position. Trigger points should be well localized and held between two fingers during injection and needling in the chest wall area. Care must be taken that the direction of injection and needling is tangential to the thorax. The needle should avoid the intercostal space. Injections in the thoracic area are best given with the needle caudally directed to avoid entering the intercostal spaces.

Needle size: 1.5, 2.0 in., 21 gauge.

Solution: Any one of the following solutions may be used: 0.5% procaine; 1.0% lidocaine; saline and dry needling in case of allergy. Do not use epinephrine.

Precautions

- Elevate muscle to avoid puncturing the pleura (pneumothorax) (see complications in Chapter 9).
- Aspirate prior to injection and needling.

Postinjection Follow-Up Physical Therapy Program

The patient should receive 3 to 4 consecutive days of treatment. Physical therapy should include electrical stimulation, relaxation, limbering, and stretching of the involved muscle using vapocoolant spray or ice as needed, combined with and followed by an exercise program. Active and active-assisted exercises are an integral part of the physical therapy program (see Chapter 9 for details).

Exercise and Home Program

Exercises for neck and shoulder are prescribed. Exercises should at first be performed under the guidance of a therapist. When the patient is free of pain and full motion has been achieved, progress to strength and endurance programs. Begin and end exercise sessions with stretching and relaxation (see Chapter 12 for exercise details).

Corrective and Preventive Measures

- Avoid maintaining rotational positions of the cervical region for long periods, e.g., sitting in an airplane engaged in prolonged conversations with the head turned.

- Holding the telephone between the ear and shoulder to free the arms is a common cause of neck pain.
- Sitting in chairs with no armrests; patients with short arms require elevation of the arms to a proper height to avoid stress on the trapezius area. Correct sitting posture (see Chapter 16).
- Avoid reading and watching television in bed.
- Do not use a firm pillow. The pillow should be soft (e.g., stuffed with feathers) so that it contours to the neck area.

SPLENIUS CAPITIS AND SPLENIUS CERVICIS

Symptoms and Pain Pattern

- Patient may complain of headache.
- Pain in the posterior cervical area (Fig 10–39).
- Pain in the head and face.[35]
- The splenius capitis may refer pain to the top of the head (vertex), with blurring of vision on the same side.[46]
- The splenius cervicis refers pain to the occiput and back of the eye on the same side.[43, 44]

Findings on Examination

- Pain in the cervical area with rotation and flexion of the spine.
- Limitation in range of motion with rotation to the same side.
- Tender trigger points may cause local and referred pain.
- The splenius capitis can be palpated between the trapezius, which is behind the muscle, and the sternocleidomastoid in front.

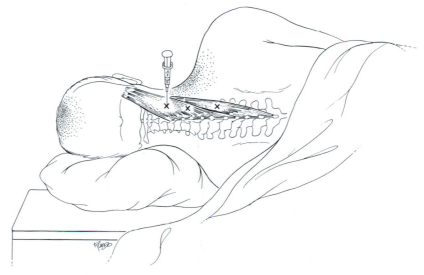

FIG 10–39. Splenius capitis and splenius cervicis. Injection of trigger points (*X's*) in the right splenius capitis and cervicis with the patient lying on the uninvolved side. Avoid the vertebral artery. Aspirate prior to injection. Anatomic landmarks are noted. Trigger point pain pattern is shown by *stippling*.

- The splenius cervicis is palpated between the upper trapezius and levator scapulae.
- Neighboring trigger points (both active and latent) occur frequently with all neck muscles, e.g., the upper trapezius, levator scapulae.

Differential Diagnosis

- Cervical arthritis.
- Cervical disc herniation.
- Additional causes of headaches, e.g., tension, tumor.

Anatomy

Splenius Capitis
Origin: ligamentum nuchae and spinous processes of C7, T1–3.
Insertion: lateral part of occipital bone, and mastoid of the temporal bone.

Splenius Cervicis
Origin: spinous processes of T3–6.
Insertion: transverse processes of C1–3.
Action: the splenius capitis and cervicis extend the head, bend the head laterally, and rotate the face to the same side.

Noninvasive Therapy

The post–trigger point injection follow-up program described in Chapter 9 is recommended as a conservative therapeutic treatment approach. Noninvasive therapy can include:

- Physical therapy modalities (e.g., electrical stimulation and warm packs; see Chapter 15).
- Manual physical therapy techniques (e.g., massage and the Trager Approach; see Chapters 13 and 14).
- Active and passive stretching and limbering of muscles with or without the use of vapocoolant spray or ice. Active exercise is part of the stretch-and-spray technique. Limbering and relaxation of muscles are necessary prior to stretching. Contract-relax techniques may be used.
- Stretch and spray: Stretching is accomplished by flexion of the head, bending the head laterally to the opposite side, and rotating the face to the opposite side. Stretches are done with the patient in the sitting position. Electrical stimulation, limbering of muscles, and warm packs should precede stretch and spray to relax muscles.
- Exercises and home program for the splenius muscles (see Chapter 12 for neck exercises). Exercise programs include relaxation, limbering, stretching, and strengthening. When the patient is free of pain and full motion has been achieved, progress to strength and endurance programs.

Injection of Trigger Point

With the patient in the side-lying position, the trigger point is well localized (see Chapter 9 for technique). Awareness of the posterior occipital triangle is necessary to avoid injecting in the area of the vertebral artery (see Posterior Cervical Muscles, below).

Needle size: 1.5 in., 22–25 gauge.

Solution: Any one of the following solutions may be used: 0.5% procaine; 1.0% lidocaine; saline and dry needling in case of allergy. Do not use epinephrine.

Precautions

- Aspirate prior to injection.
- Avoid the vertebral artery.
- Avoid area of the posterior occipital triangle.

Postinjection Follow-Up Physical Therapy Program

The patient should receive 3 to 4 consecutive days of treatment. Physical therapy should include electrical stimulation, relaxation, limbering, and stretching of the involved muscle using vapocoolant spray or ice as needed combined with and followed by an exercise program. Active and active-assisted exercises are an integral part of the physical therapy program (see Chapter 9 for details).

Exercise and Home Program

Exercises for the cervical area are described in Chapter 12. Exercises should at first be performed under the guidance of a therapist. When the patient is free of pain and full motion has been achieved, progress to strength and endurance programs. Begin and end exercise sessions with stretching and relaxation.

Corrective and Preventive Measures:

- Correct poor posture (forward head and neck position).
- Avoid occupational neck strain, e.g., place a computer screen and work activities and tools properly to avoid constant rotation of the cervical area (see Chapter 16).
- Use a soft pillow for sleeping (i.e., one that will contour to the neck). Prescribe a cervical pillow if necessary.
- Proper use and prescription of bifocal eyeglasses to avoid head-forward posture.
- Avoid chilling of the neck area, e.g., as often caused by an air conditioner directly above the patient.
- Continue the home exercise program.

POSTERIOR CERVICAL MUSCLES
Semispinalis capitis, Semispinalis cervicis, Multifidi

Symptoms and Pain Pattern

- Trigger points in the posterior cervical muscles cause pain in the posterior cervical area.[19, 28]

- Different pain patterns have been described depending on the position of trigger points.
- Three trigger point locations were described with individual pain patterns.[43, 44]
- The more distal trigger points, which lie in the deeper muscles, refer pain to the occipital area, neck, and vertebral body of the scapula.
- More proximal and superficial trigger points refer pain to the occipital area extending around the skull to the forehead and above the eye.
- Occipital nerve entrapment may occur causing symptoms of occipital neuralgia and headaches (Fig 10–40).

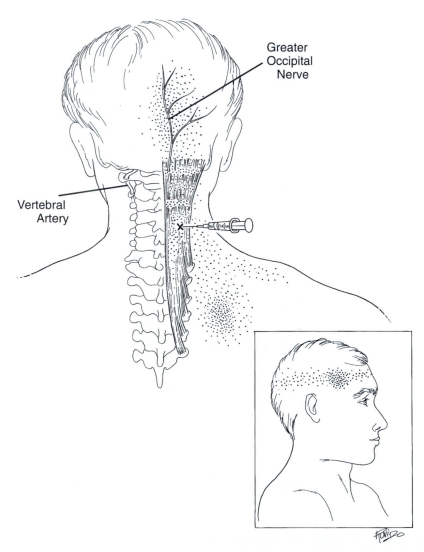

FIG 10–40.   Posterior cervical muscles (semispinalis and multifidi). Injection of trigger point in the right posterior cervical muscles. The greater occipital nerve is visualized. Anatomic landmarks are noted in addition to visualization of the left vertebral artery. Avoid the vertebral artery by injecting above or below the vertebral artery area. Aspirate prior to injection. Pain pattern is shown by *stippling.*

Findings on Examination

- Tender trigger points cause local or referred pain.
- Restricted cervical spine motion is limited, mostly in flexion and extension.
- All motions may be restricted, especially with involvement of neighboring muscles.

Differential Diagnosis

- Cervical sprain.
- Cervical radiculopathy.
- Other causes of headache.

Anatomy

Semispinalis Capitis
Origin: transverse processes of C7–T7, articular processes of C4–6.
Insertion: occipital bone.
Action: extends the head, rotates the head and face to the opposite side.

Semispinalis Cervicis
Origin: transverse processes of T1–6.
Insertion: spinous processes of C2–5.
Action: extends the vertebral column and rotates the cervical spine to the opposite side.

Multifidi (Cervical)
Origin: articular processes of C4–7.
Insertion: fibers of the multifidi pass up and into the sides of the spines of the vertebrae above, skipping two to four vertebrae.
Action: the multifidus muscle rotates the spine, flexes the vertebral column laterally, and rotates it to the opposite side; when acting together the multifidi extend the cervical dorsal area.

Noninvasive Therapy

The post–trigger point injection follow-up program described in Chapter 9 is recommended as a conservative therapeutic treatment approach. Noninvasive therapy can include:

- Physical therapy modalities (e.g., electrical stimulation and warm packs; see Chapter 15).
- Manual physical therapy techniques (e.g., massage and the Trager Approach; see Chapters 13 and 14).
- Active and passive stretching and limbering of muscles with or without the use of vapocoolant spray or ice. Active exercise is part of the stretch-and-spray technique. Limbering and relaxation of muscles are necessary prior to stretching. Contract-relax techniques may be used.
- Stretch and spray: Stretching of restricted range of motion is accom-

plished by flexing the head and rotating the head and face to the same side. If lateral flexion is restricted, stretch and spray is performed by stretching the cervical area to the opposite side. Vapocoolant is applied to the trigger point and referred pain area.

- Exercises and a home program for the cervical area are described in Chapter 12. Exercise programs include relaxation, limbering, stretching, and strengthening.

Injection of Trigger Point

The patient may be injected in the prone or side-lying position. Be aware of the location of the vertebral artery. The injection may be given above or below the area of the vertebral artery (suboccipital) (see Fig 10–40). (See Chapter 9 for injection technique.)

Needle size: 1.5–2.0 in., 22–25 gauge.

Solution: Any one of the following solutions may be used: 0.5% procaine; 1.0% lidocaine; saline and dry needling in case of allergy. Do not use epinephrine.

Precautions

- Inject trigger points above and below the area of the vertebral artery to avoid puncturing the artery or causing vertebral artery spasm (see Fig 10–39).
- Aspirate prior to injection.

Postinjection Follow-Up Physical Therapy Program

The patient should receive 3 to 4 consecutive days of treatment. Physical therapy should include electrical stimulation, relaxation, limbering, and stretching of the involved muscle using vapocoolant spray or ice as needed combined with and followed by an exercise program. Active and active-assisted exercises are an integral part of the physical therapy program (see Chapter 9 for details).

Exercise and Home Program

Exercises should at first be performed under the guidance of a therapist. Begin and end exercise sessions with relaxation and stretching. (See Chapter 12 for exercise details.)

Corrective and Preventive Measures

- Avoid flexion, extension, and rotation of the cervical area for long periods.
- Do not use a firm pillow. The pillow should be soft (e.g., stuffed with feathers) so that it can contour to the neck area.
- Avoid reading and viewing television in bed.
- Correct poor postural habits, e.g., the head-forward posture (see Chapter 16).

SUBOCCIPITAL MUSCLES
Obliquus capitis inferior, Obliquus capitis superior, Rectus capitis posterior major, Rectus capitis posterior minor, Suboccipital triangle

Symptoms and Pain Pattern

- Trigger points in the suboccipital muscles are a frequent cause of headaches in addition to neck pain.[11, 12]
- Pain may be referred from the occipit to the forehead, including the area of the orbit[44] (Fig 10–41).

Findings on Examination

- Local tenderness in the suboccipital region.
- Patients are often able to identify the trigger point.

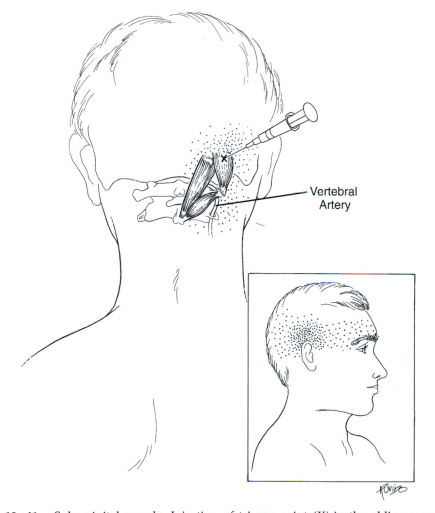

FIG 10–41. Suboccipital muscle. Injection of trigger point (X) in the obliquus capitis superior muscle with the patient in the prone position. Injection is localized directly over the trigger point and the superior portion of the occipital area to avoid the vertebral artery. The occipital triangle and vertebral artery are noted. Pain pattern is shown by *stippling*.

- Trigger points may be well isolated and respond well to injection and needling.
- Trigger points occur frequently in neighboring muscles (e.g., the posterior cervical muscles).
- Pain in the upper cervical area with flexion, extension, and rotation movements.
- Restricted motion in flexion and rotation.

Differential Diagnosis

- Cervical sprain.
- Headaches due to other causes.

Anatomy

Obliquus Capitis Inferior
Origin: spinous process of the axis.
Insertion: back of the transverse process of the atlas.
Action: rotates the skull, turning the face to the same side.

Obliquus Capitis Superior
Origin: transverse process of the atlas.
Insertion: occipital bone between the superior and inferior nuchal lines.
Action: extends the head, pulls the head to the same side.

Rectus Capitis Posterior Major
Origin: spinous process of the axis.
Insertion: occipital bone below the inferior nuchal line.
Action: extends the head.

Rectus Capitis Posterior Minor
Origin: posterior tubercle on the arch of the atlas.
Insertion: medial area of the occipital bone below the inferior nuchal line.
Action: extends the head.

Suboccipital Triangle
The three sides of the suboccipital triangle are made up of the rectus capitis posterior major, obliquus capitis superior, and obliquus capitis inferior muscles. The floor of the triangle contains the posterior arch of the atlas and the vertebral artery. The greater occipital nerve crosses over the suboccipital triangle (see Fig 10–40 and 10–41).

Noninvasive Therapy

The post–trigger point injection follow-up program described in Chapter 9 is recommended as a conservative therapeutic treatment approach. Noninvasive therapy can include:

- Physical therapy modalities (e.g., electrical stimulation and warm packs; see Chapter 15).
- Manual physical therapy techniques (e.g., massage and the Trager Approach; see Chapters 13 and 14).

- Active and passive stretching and limbering of muscles with or without the use of vapocoolant spray or ice. Active exercise is part of the stretch-and-spray technique. Limbering and relaxation of muscles are necessary prior to stretching. Contract-relax techniques may be used.
- Stretch and spray for the suboccipital muscles is performed. Stretching is performed opposite the pull of shortened muscles. Stretch will usually be performed in the direction of flexion and rotation to the opposite side.
- Exercises and a home program for the cervical area are prescribed (see Chapter 12). Exercise program includes relaxation, limbering, stretching, and strengthening.

Injection of Trigger Point

With the patient in the prone position the trigger point is carefully identified. Injection is localized directly over the trigger point in the superior portion of the occipital area to avoid the vertebral artery (see Fig 10–41). (See Chapter 9 for injection technique.)

Needle size: 1.5 in., 25 gauge.

Solution: Any one of the following solutions may be used: 0.5% procaine; 1.0% lidocaine; saline and dry needling in case of allergy. Do not use epinephrine.

Precautions

- Avoid the vertebral artery. Spasm of the vertebral artery may cause cerebral ischemia.
- Aspirate prior to injection.

Postinjection Follow-Up Physical Therapy Program

The patient should receive 3 to 4 consecutive days of treatment. Physical therapy should include electrical stimulation, relaxation, limbering, and stretching of the involved muscle using vapocoolant spray or ice as needed combined with and followed by an exercise program. Active and active-assisted exercises are an integral part of the physical therapy program (see Chapter 9 for details).

Exercise and Home Program

Exercises for the suboccipital muscles are prescribed. Exercise should at first be performed under the guidance of a therapist. Begin and end exercise sessions with stretching and relaxation (see Chapter 12 for details).

Corrective and Preventive Measures

- Avoid flexion, extension, and rotation of the cervical area for prolonged periods.
- Do not use a firm pillow. The pillow should be soft (e.g., stuffed with feathers) so that it can contour to the neck area.
- Avoid reading and viewing television in bed (see Chapter 16).
- Correct poor sitting and standing postures, e.g., the head-forward position.

RHOMBOID MAJOR AND RHOMBOID MINOR

Symptoms and Pain Pattern

- Pain in the dorsal region between the vertebral body of the scapula and paraspinal muscles[18, 28] (Fig 10–42).
- Pain may be present at rest.
- Pain may be aggravated with motions of the shoulder.
- Trigger points may result from a dorsal sprain or prolonged strain due to chronic tension related to poor posture (e.g., the round-shouldered position with prolonged reading).

Findings on Examination

- Palpation may be performed with the patient sitting, standing, or in the prone position.
- Tender trigger points are found medial to the vertebral body of the scapula.
- Pain may be aggravated with motions of the shoulder.

Anatomy

Rhomboid Major
Origin: spinous processes of T2–5.
Insertion: vertebral border of the scapula, between the spine and inferior angle.
Action: adducts and rotates the scapula.

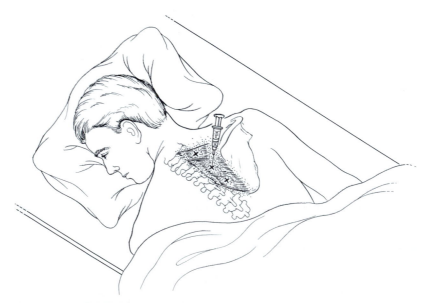

FIG 10–42.   Rhomboid major and minor. Injection of trigger points (*X's*) in the right rhomboid muscles. Direct the needle tangentially and caudally to avoid entering the intercostal space. Anatomic landmarks are noted. Pain pattern is shown by *stippling.*

Rhomboid Minor

Origin: lower part of ligamentum nuchae, spinous processes of C7 and T1.
Insertion: vertebral border of scapula opposite the root of the spine.

Action: the rhomboid muscles brace the back of the shoulder holding the scapula to the chest, and raise the scapula tilting the lower inferior angle medially.

Differential Diagnosis

- Dorsal sprain.
- Intrathoracic disease.
- Cervical disc herniation.

Noninvasive Therapy

The post–trigger point injection follow-up program described in Chapter 9 is recommended as a conservative therapeutic treatment approach. Noninvasive therapy can include:

- Physical therapy modalities (e.g., electrical stimulation and warm packs; see Chapter 15).
- Manual physical therapy techniques (e.g., massage and the Trager Approach; see Chapters 13 and 14).
- Active and passive stretching and limbering of muscles with or without the use of vapocoolant spray or ice. Active exercise is part of the stretch-and-spray technique. Limbering and relaxation of muscles are necessary prior to stretching. Contract-relax techniques may be used.
- Stretch and spray (see Chapter 9): The scapula must be brought forward. This is best done with the patient sitting. The bend sitting exercise position is appropriate for stretch and spray. Vapocoolant or ice over the trigger point areas and referred pain area are used as needed. Perform bending with the arms between the knees as well as side-to-side bending as illustrated for active stretch (see Chapter 12). Electrical stimulation, limbering of muscles, and warm packs may precede stretch and spray to relax the muscles. Stretching of muscle is also accomplished actively and with assistance during the exercise program. Active exercise is part of the stretch-and-spray technique.
- Exercises and a home program for the shoulders and cervical and dorsal areas are described in Chapter 12. Instruct the patient in correct posture. Exercise programs include relaxation, limbering, stretching, and strengthening. When the patient is free of pain and full motion has been achieved, progress to strength and endurance programs.

Injection of Trigger Point

With the patient prone trigger points are identified. Identify bony landmarks. Palpate the entire muscle for multiple trigger points. Use multiple needle entries along the muscle belly. Angle the needle tangentially. Use sterile precaution. (See Chapter 9 for injection technique.)

Needle size: 1.5 in., 21 gauge.

Solution: Any one of the following solutions may be used: 0.5% procaine; 1.0% lidocaine; saline and dry needling may be used in case of allergy. Do not use epinephrine.

Precautions

- Angle the needle tangentially to avoid entering the chest cavity.
- Aspirate prior to injection.

Postinjection Follow-Up Physical Therapy Program

The patient should receive 3 to 4 consecutive days of treatment. Physical therapy should include electrical stimulation, relaxation, limbering, and stretching of the involved muscle using vapocoolant spray or ice as needed combined with and followed by an exercise program. Active and active-assisted exercises are an integral part of the physical therapy program (see Chapter 9 for details).

Exercise and Home Program

Instruct the patient in correct posture and use of lumbar supports to improve spinal alignment and decrease stress in the intrascapular area. Exercises for the shoulders and cervical and dorsal area are described in Chapter 12. Exercises should at first be performed under the guidance of a therapist. When the patient is free of pain and full motion has been achieved, progress to strength and endurance programs. Begin and end exercise sessions with relaxation.

Corrective and Preventive Measures

- Eliminate causes related to posture and tension, e.g., correct poor sitting posture. Chairs should have proper back supports and armrests (see Chapter 16).
- Change position often.
- Instruct patient in a daily program of exercise and stretching.

LEVATOR SCAPULAE

Symptoms and Pain Pattern

- Pain over the medial border of the scapula extending upward to the base of the occiput[25, 37] (Fig 10–43).
- Generalized headaches.
- Pain may radiate to the head and shoulder.[18, 43]
- Pain may be noted around the ear.[35]
- Levator scapulae muscle pain is often involved in chronic cervical conditions.[35]
- Patients complain of limitation in rotation of the neck.

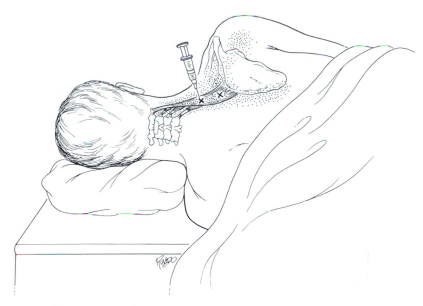

FIG 10–43. Levator scapulae. Injection of trigger points *(X's)* in the right levator scapulae. Aspirate prior to injection. Avoid the intercostal space and direct the needle tangentially to the frontal plane of the patient. Trigger point pain pattern is shown by *stippling.*

Findings on Examination

- Trigger points are most frequently found at the attachment of the muscle on the upper medial border of the scapula (the greatest point of mechanical stress).[38]
- In 200 asymptomatic persons examined for shoulder girdle muscle trigger points (100 male, 100 female) the levator scapulae was implicated in 19.7% of the patients, second in frequency to the trapezius (34.7%). The trigger points found most frequently in symptomatic persons were in the levator scapulae and infraspinatus. The trapezius was not implicated as often in symptomatic patients (2% vs. 55% for the levator scapulae, and 31% for the infraspinatus).[38]
- Trigger points may be palpated in the upper portion of the levator scapulae at the base of the neck. Palpation is more easily achieved when the anterior border of the trapezius can be relaxed and retracted medially.
- Tenderness and referred pain may be produced on palpation of trigger points.
- Limited rotation of the neck to the opposite side. Limitation in lateral flexion to the opposite side.

Differential Diagnosis

- Cervical disc herniation.
- Scapulocostal syndrome.
- Cervical sprain.
- Neck and shoulder pain due to trigger points in neighboring muscles (e.g., trapezius, supraspinatus, rhomboids).

Anatomy

Origin: transverse processes of C1–4.

Insertion: medial border of the scapulae between the superior angle and root of the spine.

Action: with the origin fixed, the levator scapulae elevates the scapulae and rotates the glenoid cavity caudally; with the insertion fixed, acting unilaterally, the levator scapulae flexes and rotates the cervical vertebrae to the same side; acting bilaterally, the muscle acts as an extensor of the cervical spine.

Noninvasive Therapy

The post–trigger point injection follow-up program described in Chapter 9 is recommended as a conservative therapeutic treatment approach. Noninvasive therapy can include:

- Physical therapy modalities (e.g., electrical stimulation and warm packs; see Chapter 15).
- Manual physical therapy techniques (e.g., massage and the Trager Approach; see Chapters 13 and 14).
- Active and passive stretching and limbering of muscles with or without the use of vapocoolant spray or ice. Active exercise is part of the stretch-and-spray technique. Limbering and relaxation of muscles are necessary prior to stretching. Contract-relax techniques may be used.
- Stretch and spray is performed by means of flexion, lateral stretch, and rotation to the opposite side of the symptoms. Electrical stimulation, limbering of muscles, and warm packs should precede stretch and spray to relax muscles. Limbering and relaxation of muscles are necessary prior to stretching.
- Exercises and a home program for the cervical area are described in Chapter 12. The exercise program includes relaxation, limbering, stretching, and strengthening. When the patient is free of pain and full motion has been achieved, progress to strength and endurance programs.
- Prevention and correction of contributing factors.

Injection of Trigger Points

Injection of trigger points is accomplished with the patent lying on the uninvolved side (see Fig 10–43). Palpate for both upper and lower trigger points. Relaxation of the upper border of the trapezius permits better exposure of the levator scapulae. (See Chapter 9 for injection technique.)

Needle size: 1.5–2.0 in., 22–24 gauge.

Solution: Any one of the following solutions may be used: 0.5% procaine; 1.0% lidocaine; saline and dry needling in case of allergy. Do not use epinephrine.

Precautions

- Aspirate prior to injection.
- Avoid entering the chest cavity.

- The angle of the needle should be directed tangentially when in the region of the scapulae and chest cavity.

Postinjection Follow-Up Physical Therapy Program

The patient should receive 3 to 4 consecutive days of treatment. Physical therapy should include electrical stimulation, relaxation, limbering, and stretching of the involved muscle using vapocoolant spray or ice as needed combined with and followed by an exercise program. Active and active-assisted exercises are an integral part of the physical therapy program (see Chapter 9 for details).

Exercise and Home Program

Exercises for the cervical area are prescribed. Exercises should at first be performed under the guidance of a therapist. When the patient is free of pain and full motion has been achieved, progress to strength and endurance programs. Begin and end exercise sessions with stretching and relaxation (see Chapter 12 for details).

Corrective and Preventive Measures

- Avoid maintaining the cervical area in rotated postures for prolonged periods of time (e.g., as in conversation on an airplane with the head turned toward the interlocutor; improper placement of work tools necessitating the head and neck to be repeatedly rotated (see Chapter 16).
- Chairs should have armrests high enough to permit relaxation and support of the cervical and shoulder muscles.
- Patient should continue exercises stressing relaxation, flexibility, and stretching.
- Avoid cervical strain by wearing proper eyeglasses.
- Avoid reading and viewing television in bed.
- The pillow used at night should be soft to contour to the neck area. Avoid the use of two pillows which encourages cervical strain and a head-forward neck posture.
- Prescribe a cervical pillow if necessary.

Muscles of the Upper Extremities

DELTOID

Symptoms and Pain Pattern

- Pain over the shoulder, either the anterior or posterior aspect, or both[4, 30] (Fig 10–44).
- Pain in the upper back, neck, and arm.[28]
- Pain with abduction, forward flexion, and elevation of the shoulder.

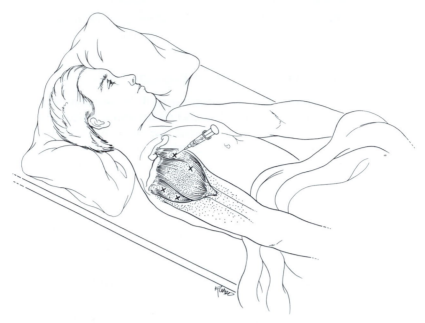

FIG 10–44. Deltoid. Injection of trigger points in the right deltoid muscle. Trigger points *(X's)* are noted in the posterior and anterior deltoid. Patient is in the side-lying position. Anatomic landmarks are noted. Pain pattern is shown by *stippling*.

Findings on Examination

- Tender trigger points may be found over the anterior, middle, or posterior aspect of the deltoid.
- Limitation in shoulder point motion.
- Pain with abduction and elevation.

Anatomy

Origin: anterior border of the clavicle, outer border of the acromion, lower edge of the spine of the scapula.

Insertion: outer side of the humerus.

Action: abducts the arm to the horizontal position, anterior fibers flex the shoulder, posterior fibers extend the arm at the shoulder joint.

Differential Diagnosis

- Cervical radiculopathy.
- Shoulder bursitis.
- Bicipital tendonitis.
- Rotator cuff injury.

Noninvasive Therapy

The post–trigger point injection follow-up program described in Chapter 9 is recommended as a conservative therapeutic treatment approach. Noninvasive therapy can include:

- Physical therapy modalities (e.g., electrical stimulation and warm packs; see Chapter 15).
- Manual physical therapy techniques (e.g., massage and the Trager Approach; see Chapters 13 and 14).
- Active and passive stretching and limbering of muscles with or without the use of vapocoolant spray or ice. Active exercise is part of the stretch-and-spray technique. Limbering and relaxation are necessary prior to stretching. Contract-relax techniques may be used.
- Stretch and spray for the deltoid muscle is performed with the aid of vapocoolant or ice. For anterior fibers abduct and extend the arm. For posterior fibers flex the shoulder and adduct the arm across the chest. (see Chapter 9). Electrical stimulation, limbering of muscles, and warm packs may precede stretch and spray to relax the muscles. Stretching of muscle is also accomplished actively and with assistance during the exercise program. Active exercise is part of the stretch-and-spray technique.
- Exercises and a home program for the shoulder muscles are prescribed (see Chapter 12). The exercise program includes relaxation, limbering, stretching, and strengthening. When the patient is free of pain and full motion has been achieved, progress to strength and endurance programs.

Injection of Trigger Points

The patient may be injected for the anterior and middle deltoid in the supine position. The side-lying position can expose both the anterior and posterior aspects of the deltoid (see Fig 10–44). All palpable trigger points are injected. Multiple needle entries are important to find those trigger points that are not recognized by palpation.

Needle size: 1.5 or 2.0 in., 21 gauge.

Solution: Any one of the following solutions may be used: 0.5% procaine; 1.0% lidocaine; saline and dry needling in case of allergy. Do not use epinephrine.

Postinjection Follow-Up Physical Therapy Program

The patient should receive 3 to 4 consecutive days of treatment. Physical therapy should include electrical stimulation, relaxation, limbering, and stretching of the involved muscle using vapocoolant spray or ice as needed combined with and followed by an exercise program. Active and active-assisted exercises are an integral part of the physical therapy program (see Chapter 9 for details).

Exercise and Home Program

Exercises for the shoulder are prescribed. Exercises should at first be performed under the guidance of a therapist. When the patient is free of pain and full motion has been achieved, progress to strength and endurance programs. Begin and end exercise sessions with relaxation and stretching. (See Chapter 12 for exercise details.)

Corrective and Preventive Measures

- Avoid repetitive activities involving shoulder joint motion, e.g., practicing tennis serves.
- Continue daily stretching activities.
- Do warm-up exercises before activities which stress the shoulder joint area.

SUPRASPINATUS

Symptoms and Pain Pattern

- Pain with abduction and elevation of the arm.
- Pain is noted over the posterior aspect of the shoulder and referred to the deltoid region, upper arm, lateral epicondyle, and forearm[11, 12, 28, 43, 45, 46] (Fig 10–45).

Findings

- Local trigger point tenderness or referred pain pattern to the upper extremity.
- Limited range of motion of the shoulders.
- Often accompanied by trigger points in neighboring muscles, e.g., the trapezius and infraspinatus.

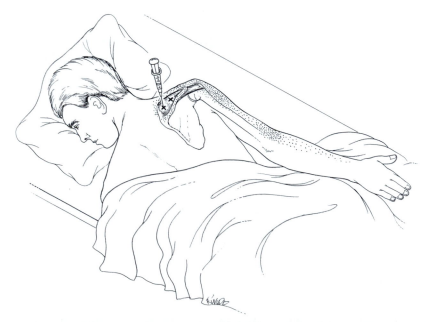

FIG 10–45. Supraspinatus. Injection of trigger points (*X's*) in the right supraspinatus with the patient prone. The needle is directed directly over the supraspinous fossa of the scapula to avoid penetrating the rib cage. Anatomic landmarks are noted. Pain pattern is shown by *stippling*.

Differential Diagnosis

- Deltoid bursitis.
- Cervical herniated disc.
- Cervical radiculopathy.
- Bicipital tendonitis.

Anatomy

Origin: supraspinous fossa.

Insertion: greater tuberosity of the humerus; the supraspinatus tendon is aligned with the lateral part of the upper part of the capsule of the shoulder joint.

Action: abductor and lateral rotator, helps as a fixator of the shoulder joint.

Noninvasive Therapy

The post–trigger point injection follow-up program described in Chapter 9 is recommended as a conservative therapeutic treatment approach. Noninvasive therapy can include:

- Physical therapy modalities (e.g., electrical stimulation and warm packs; see Chapter 15).
- Manual physical therapy techniques (e.g., massage and the Trager Approach; see Chapters 13 and 14).
- Active and passive stretching and limbering of muscles with or without the use of vapocoolant spray or ice. Active exercise is part of the stretch-and-spray technique. Limbering and relaxation are necessary prior to stretching. May use contract-relax techniques.
- Stretch and spray for the supraspinatus muscle: Stretch in the direction of shoulder internal rotation and adduction using vapocoolant or ice as needed. Electrical stimulation, limbering of muscles, and warm packs should precede stretch and spray to relax the muscles. Stretching of muscle is also accomplished actively as well as with assistance during the exercise program. Active exercise is part of the stretch-and-spray technique.
- Exercises and a home program for the shoulder are prescribed (see Chapter 12). Exercises for the shoulder begin with relaxation, limbering, and stretching. Stretch in the direction of elevation, adduction, and internal rotation. Begin strengthening exercises as symptoms decrease. When the patient is free of pain and full motion has been achieved, progress to strength and endurance programs.

Trigger Point Injection

Injection may be performed with the patient in the prone or side-lying position (see Fig 10–45). It is important that the needle be introduced directly over the supraspinous fossa of the scapula to avoid penetrating the rib cage. Injecting at the muscle insertion, directing the needle under the acromion, may be necessary in addition to multiple needling involving the area of the supraspinous fossa.

Needle size: 1.5 in., 21 gauge.

Solution: Any one of the following solutions may be used: 0.5% procaine; 1.0% lidocaine; saline and dry needling in case of allergy. Do not use epinephrine.

Precautions

- Identify anatomic landmarks prior to injection.
- Inject over the scapular area to avoid a pneumothorax.
- Insert the needle tangentially to avoid entering the chest wall.

Postinjection Follow-Up Physical Therapy Program

The patient should receive 3 to 4 consecutive days of treatment. Physical therapy should include electrical stimulation, relaxation, limbering, and stretching of the involved muscle using vapocoolant spray or ice as needed combined with and followed by an exercise program. Active and active-assisted exercises are an integral part of the physical therapy program.

Exercise and Home Program

Exercises for the shoulder are prescribed. Exercises should at first be performed under the guidance of a therapist. When the patient is free of pain and full motion has been achieved, progress to strength and endurance programs. Begin and end exercise sessions with relaxation and stretching. (See Chapter 12 for exercise details.)

Corrective and Preventive Measures

- Avoid overuse syndromes, e.g., prolonged activities involving elevation of the arms, overhead movements, or excessively repetitive motions such as practicing a tennis serve or throwing a ball.
- Perform warm-up exercises prior to activities which use repetitive shoulder motions, e.g., painting or tennis.

INFRASPINATUS AND TERES MINOR

Symptoms and Pain Pattern

- Pain over the posterior aspect of the shoulder and upper dorsal and cervical area.
- Referred pain pattern to the front of the shoulder, radiating pain to the front and lateral aspect of the arm and forearm extending to the radial aspect of the hand[25, 39, 45, 46] (Fig 10–46).
- Referred pain may be noted over the lateral anterior aspect of the shoul-

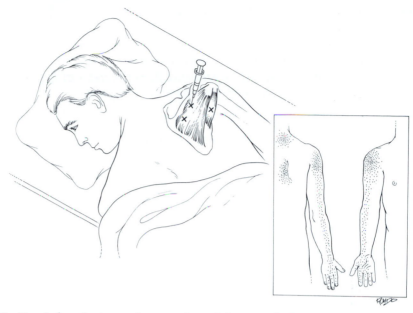

FIG 10–46. Infraspinatus and teres minor. Injection of trigger points *(X's)* in the right infraspinatus and teres minor. The patient is in the prone position. Anatomic landmarks are noted. *Inset,* pain pattern *(stippling).* Observe precautions to avoid entering the chest cavity.

der and anterior chest, together with sympathetic hyperactivity which may contribute to dystrophy-like syndromes—shoulder girdle fatigue, weakness of grip, hyperhidrosis, and skin temperature changes.[39]
- Limited motion in activities which require placing the hand behind the back (internal rotation) and forward flexion.

Findings on Examination

- Local tenderness from trigger points occur most frequently along the lateral border of the scapula.[37, 38]
- Restriction in internal rotation may be present.
- Palpation of the trigger points may elicit a referred pain pattern.
- Pain as well as muscle shortening may restrict elevation of the shoulder and internal rotation.
- When examining for trigger points the teres minor muscle appears anatomically as an extension of the infraspinatus. The teres minor is inferior to the infraspinatus. Because of their proximity they are treated together and are difficult to distinguish when one palpates the lateral aspect of the infraspinatus (see Fig 10–46).

Differential Diagnosis

- Deltoid bursitis.
- Frozen shoulder (adhesive capsulitis).
- Cervical radiculopathy.

Anatomy

Infraspinatus
Origin: infraspinous fossa.
Insertion: greater tuberosity of humerus.
Action: lateral rotator and stabilizes the head of the humerus in the glenoid cavity during movements of the shoulder joint.

Teres Minor
Origin: upper part of dorsal aspect of the axillary border of the scapula.
Insertion: greater tuberosity.
Action: lateral rotator and fixator, stabilizes the head of the humerus in the glenoid cavity during movements of the shoulder joint.

Noninvasive Therapy

The post–trigger point injection follow-up program described in Chapter 9 F is recommended as a conservative therapeutic treatment approach. Noninvasive therapy can include:

- Physical therapy modalities (e.g., electrical stimulation and warm packs; see Chapter 15).
- Manual physical therapy techniques (e.g., massage and the Trager Approach; see Chapters 13 and 14).
- Active and passive stretching and limbering of muscles with or without the use of vapocoolant spray or ice. Active exercise is part of the stretch-and-spray technique. Limbering and relaxation are necessary prior to stretching. Contract-relax techniques may be used.
- Stretch and spray for the infraspinatus and teres minor is performed by stretching in the direction of shoulder internal rotation and adduction.
- Exercises and a home program for the shoulder are prescribed (see Chapter 12). The exercise program includes relaxation, limbering, stretching, and strengthening. When the patient is free of pain and full motion has been achieved, progress to strength and endurance programs.

Injection of Trigger Point

With the patient in the prone or side-lying position, trigger points are identified and isolated between two fingers for injection. Further palpation of the muscle throughout its length is done to explore for additional trigger points. Multiple needling should be performed to identify those trigger points not found on palpation (see Fig 10–46; see Chapter 9 for injection technique).
Needle size: 1.5 in., 21 gauge.
Solution: Any one of the following solutions may be used: 0.5% procaine; 1.0% lidocaine; saline and dry needling in case of allergy. Do not use epinephrine.

Precautions

- Identify bony landmarks.
- Aspirate prior to injection and needling.
- With needling stay within the borders of the scapula over the infraspina-

tus to avoid penetrating the thorax. Angle the needle tangentially when injecting and needling to avoid entering the chest wall (see Chapter 9 for complications).

Postinjection Follow-Up Physical Therapy Program

The patient should receive 3 to 4 consecutive days of treatment. Physical therapy should include electrical stimulation, relaxation, limbering, and stretching of the involved muscle using vapocoolant spray or ice as needed combined with and followed by an exercise program. Active and active-assisted exercises are an integral part of the physical therapy program (see Chapter 9 for details).

Exercise and Home Program

Exercises for the shoulder are prescribed. Exercises should at first be performed under the guidance of a therapist. When the patient is free of pain and full motion has been achieved, progress to strength and endurance programs. Begin and end exercise session with stretching and relaxation (see Chapter 12 for exercise details).

Corrective and Preventive Measures

- Avoid repetitive shoulder motions.
- Do warm-up exercises to include relaxation and stretching prior to activities involving shoulder motion, e.g., painting or tennis.
- Relaxation and stretching after athletic activities.
- Correct poor working habits, e.g., use a stool for overhead activities (see Chapter 16).

SUBSCAPULARIS

Symptoms and Pain Pattern

- Pain in the shoulder area is most pronounced over the posterior deltoid with referred pain to the upper arm (Fig 10–47).
- Pain may be felt in the wrist.[20, 43]
- Patients complain of pain with motions that require external rotation and abduction.
- Limited motion in abduction and lateral rotation.

Findings

- Palpate trigger points with the patient in the supine position. Abduct the arm and extend the examining finger anterior to the latissimus dorsi to palpate the axillary border of the scapula.
- Patients may complain of local and referred pain.
- Range of motion assessment may demonstrate limitation in abduction and lateral rotation.

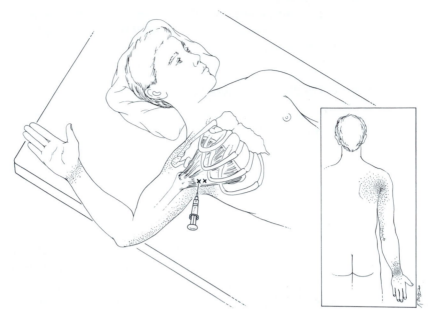

FIG 10–47. Subscapularis. Injection of trigger points *(X's)* in the right subscapularis with the patient supine. The arm is abducted. The axillary border of the scapula is palpated. Trigger points should be well localized by palpation prior to injection. The needle is directed into the trigger point area away from the chest wall to avoid puncturing the pleura. Pain pattern is shown by *stippling*.

Differential Diagnosis

- Cervical radiculopathy.
- Cervical spondylosis.
- Cervical disc herniation.
- Periadhesive capsulitis (frozen shoulder).

Anatomy

> *Origin:* subscapular fossa.
> *Insertion:* lesser tuberosity of humerus and shaft.
> *Action:* medial rotator and shoulder fixator.

Noninvasive Therapy

The post–trigger point injection follow-up program described in Chapter 9 is recommended as a conservative therapeutic treatment approach. Noninvasive therapy can include:

- Physical therapy modalities (e.g., electrical stimulation and warm packs; see Chapter 15).
- Manual physical therapy techniques (e.g., massage and the Trager Approach; see Chapters 13 and 14).
- Active and passive stretching and limbering of muscles with or without the use of vapocoolant spray or ice. Active exercise is part of the stretch-

and-spray technique. Limbering and relaxation are necessary prior to relaxation. May use contract-relax technique.

- Stretch and spray: Stretching is performed in the direction of external rotation, abduction, and elevation. Use vapocoolant spray or ice as needed. Electrical stimulation, limbering of muscles, and warm packs may precede stretch and spray to relax the muscles. Stretching of muscle is also accomplished actively and with assistance during the exercise program.
- Exercises and home program. Exercises for the shoulder and neck are described in Chapter 12. Exercise programs include relaxation, limbering, stretching, and strengthening. When the patient is free of pain and full motion has been achieved, progress to strength and endurance programs.

Injection of Trigger Points

With the patient in the supine position the arm is abducted (see Fig 10–47). Palpate the axillary border of the scapula by abducting and elevating the arm. Inject those trigger points that can be palpated and localized. Observe precautions. (See Chapter 9 for injection technique.)

Needle size: 1.5–2.0 in., 21 gauge.

Solution: Any one of the following solutions may be used: 0.5% procaine; 1.0% lidocaine; saline and dry needling in case of allergy. Do not use epinephrine.

Precautions

- The needle should be directed tangentially and away from the chest wall to avoid pneumothorax. Inject only those trigger points which are palpated. The needle should be placed directly into the trigger points. Do not use the needle to explore for trigger points.
- Aspirate prior to injection.

Postinjection Follow-Up Physical Therapy Program

The patient should receive 3 to 4 consecutive days of treatment. Physical therapy should include electrical stimulation, relaxation, limbering, and stretching of the involved muscle using vapocoolant spray or ice as needed combined with and followed by an exercise program. Active and active-assisted exercises are an integral part of the physical therapy program (see Chapter 9 for details).

Exercise and Home Program

Exercises for the shoulder and neck are prescribed. Exercises should at first be performed under the guidance of a therapist. When the patient is free of pain and full motion has been achieved, progress to strength and endurance programs. Begin and end exercise sessions with stretching and relaxation (see Chapter 12 for details).

Corrective and Preventive Measures

- Avoid prolonged positions of adduction.
- Stretching exercises should be performed prior to and after athletic activities.
- Prevent the development of joint adhesions, muscle shortening, and trigger points by maintaining active and passive range of motion in patients who have injuries and paralysis of the upper extremity, e.g., stroke patients.

BICEPS BRACHII

Symptoms and Pain Pattern

- Pain in the front of the shoulder, upper arm, and suprascapular region[7, 31] (Fig 10–48).
- Pain at rest as well as with abduction and elevation of the shoulder.

Findings on Examination

- Tenderness along the biceps extending from the upper portion to the elbow.
- Pain in the upper arm with flexion and supination of the forearm.

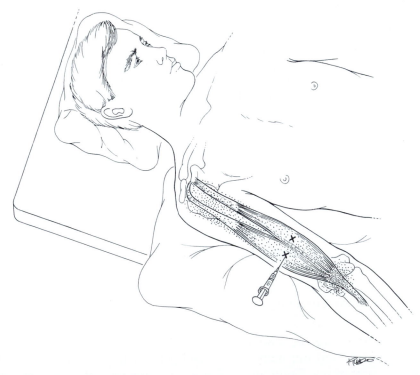

FIG 10–48.   Biceps brachii. Injection of trigger points *(X's)* in the right biceps brachii. The patient is supine with slight abduction of the arm. Anatomic landmarks are noted. Pain pattern is shown by *stippling.*

- Painful limited adduction and elevation of the shoulder.
- Limitation in extension and pronation of the elbow.

Differential Diagnosis

- Bicipital tendonitis
- Cervical radiculopathy

Anatomy

Origin: short head of the biceps from the tip of the coracoid process, long head from the supraglenoid tubercle of the scapula; the two heads join together about the middle of the upper arm.

Insertion: back of the tuberosity of the radius, the bicipital aponeurosis to the subcutaneous border of the ulna.

Action: supinates forearm, flexes elbow and shoulder.

Noninvasive Therapy

The post–trigger point injection follow-up program described in Chapter 9 is recommended as a conservative therapeutic treatment approach. Noninvasive therapy can include:

- Physical therapy modalities (e.g., electrical stimulation and warm packs; see Chapter 15).
- Manual physical therapy techniques (e.g., massage and the Trager Approach; see Chapters 13 and 14).
- Active and passive stretching and limbering of muscles with or without the use of vapocoolant spray or ice. Active exercise is part of the stretch-and-spray technique. Limbering and relaxation are necessary prior to stretching. Contract-relax technique may be used.
- Stretch and spray for the biceps brachii is performed with the elbow extended and pronated and the shoulder abducted and extended. The area of trigger point and referred pain is sprayed with vapocoolant (see Chapter 9). Electrical stimulation, limbering of muscles, and warm packs should precede stretch and spray to relax muscles.
- Exercise and home program for the shoulder and elbow are prescribed (see Chapter 12). Exercise programs include relaxation, limbering, stretching, and strengthening. When the patient is free of pain and full motion has been achieved, progress to strength and endurance programs.

Injection of Trigger Points

Position the patient in the supine position (see Fig 10–48). Trigger points are identified. As much of the muscle as possible is palpated for trigger points. Multiple needling along the body of the biceps brachii is usually required. Multiple needling may find trigger points not found on palpation. Trigger points may be held between the thumb and index finger or isolated between the index and middle fingers. (See Chapter 9 for injection technique.)

Needle size: 1.5, 2.0 in., 21 gauge.

Solution: Any one of the following solutions may be used: 0.5% procaine; 1.0% lidocaine; saline and dry needling in case of allergy. Do not use epinephrine.

Precautions

- Avoid median and radial nerves.

Postinjection Follow-Up Physical Therapy Program

The patient should receive 3 to 4 consecutive days of treatment. Physical therapy should include electrical stimulation, relaxation, limbering, and stretching of the involved muscle using vapocoolant spray or ice as needed combined with and followed by an exercise program. Active and active-assisted exercises are an integral part of the physical therapy program (see Chapter 9 for details).

Exercise and Home Program

Exercises for the shoulder and elbow are prescribed. Exercises should at first be performed under the guidance of a therapist. When the patient is free of pain and full motion has been achieved, progress to strength and endurance programs. Begin and end exercise sessions with stretching and relaxation (see Chapter 12 for details).

Corrective and Preventive Measures

- Home exercise program for shoulder and elbow.
- Relaxation and stretching exercises prior to and after strenuous activities, e.g., athletics, work activities requiring upper extremity effort.

CORACOBRACHIALIS

Symptoms and Referred Pain Pattern

- Pain over the anterior aspect of the shoulder (Fig 10–49).
- Referred pain to the posterior part of the arm, forearm, and dorsum of the hand.[44]
- Pain with abduction, extension, and elevation of the arms.

Findings

- Local trigger point tenderness, especially over the area of muscle insertion and origin.
- Limitation in abduction and elevation.
- Pain with abduction, internal rotation, and elevation.
- Referred pain pattern may be elicited on palpation.
- Weakness in shoulder forward flexion may be noted in movements requiring simultaneous elbow flexion and supination, e.g., hair combing.[14]

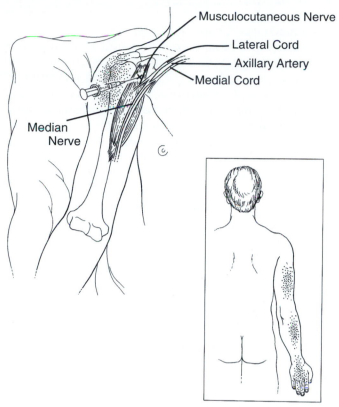

FIG 10–49. Coracobrachialis. Injection of trigger point (X) in the right coracobrachialis with the patient supine, the arm slightly externally rotated and abducted. Anatomic landmarks are noted including neurovascular structures and the musculocutaneus nerve. Pain pattern is shown by *stippling*.

Differential Diagnosis

- Cervical radiculopathy.
- Subdeltoid bursitis.

Anatomy

Origin: apex of the coracoid of the scapula.

Insertion: medial aspect of the humerus, at the level of the middle of the humerus shaft.

Action: flexes and adducts the arm.

Noninvasive Therapy

The post–trigger point injection follow-up program described in Chapter 9 is recommended as a conservative therapeutic treatment approach. Noninvasive therapy can include:

- Physical therapy modalities (e.g., electrical stimulation and warm packs; see Chapter 15).

- Manual physical therapy techniques (e.g., massage and the Trager Approach; see Chapters 13 and 14).
- Active and passive stretching and limbering of muscles with or without the use of vapocoolant spray or ice. Active exercise is part of the stretch-and-spray technique. Limbering and relaxation are necessary prior to stretching. Contract-relax techniques may be used.
- Stretch and spray for the coracobrachialis is performed with the shoulder in abduction and elevation. Electrical stimulation, limbering of muscles, and warm packs should precede stretch and spray to relax muscles.
- Exercises and a home program for the shoulder are prescribed (see Chapter 12). The exercise program includes relaxation, limbering, stretching and strengthening. When the patient is free of pain and full motion has been achieved, progress to strength and endurance programs.

Injection of Trigger Point

Trigger points are often found near the origin of the coracobrachialis at the coracoid process. Note the proximity of the musculocutaneous nerve (see Fig 10–49). The coracoid process and coracobrachialis muscle are covered by the anterior deltoid. The lower portion of the coracobrachialis is covered by the pectoralis major. With the patient supine identify the trigger point. This may require the arm to be slightly externally rotated and abducted. The trigger point is maintained between two fingertips and the needle is inserted directly into the area of maximum tenderness. (See Chapter 9 for injection technique.)

Needle size: 1.5 in., 21 gauge.

Solution: Any one of the following solutions may be used: 0.5% procaine; 1.0% lidocaine; saline and dry needling may be used in case of allergy. Do not use epinephrine.

Precautions

The musculocutaneous×[001b] nerve at first lies medial to the coracolateralis on the lateral side of the axillary artery. Aspirate prior to injection. Infiltration of the nerve may cause temporary weakness of the coracobrachialis, biceps, and brachialis, and anesthesia of the ball of the thumb and lower third of the back of the forearm.

Postinjection Follow-Up Physical Therapy Program

The patient should receive 3 to 4 consecutive days of treatment. Physical therapy should include electrical stimulation, relaxation, limbering, and stretching of the involved muscle using vapocoolant spray or ice as needed combined with and followed by an exercise program. Active and active-assisted exercises are an integral part of the physical therapy program (see Chapter 9 for details).

Exercise and Home Program

Exercises for the shoulder are prescribed. Exercises should at first be performed under the guidance of a therapist. When the patient is free of pain and full motion has been achieved, progress to strength and endurance programs.

Begin and end exercise sessions with stretching and relaxation (see Chapter 12 for exercise details).

Corrective and Preventive Measures

- Relaxation and stretching exercises prior to and after athletic activities involving the upper extremities.
- Continue home exercise programs.
- Avoid repetitive activities involving the shoulder area, e.g., prolonged practicing of one's tennis serve.

BRACHIALIS

Symptoms and Pain Pattern

- Pain due to trigger points in the brachialis muscle may be experienced in the upper arm and front of the elbow. Referred pain may include the base of the thumb and dorsum of the web space between the thumb and index finger[32] (Fig 10–50).
- Pain is noted with flexion and extension of the elbow.
- Paresthesia over the dorsum of the thumb has been reported due to entrapment of the sensory branch of the radial nerve[45] (see Fig 10–50).

Findings

- Palpate trigger points by flexing the elbow and relax the biceps muscle which covers the brachialis.

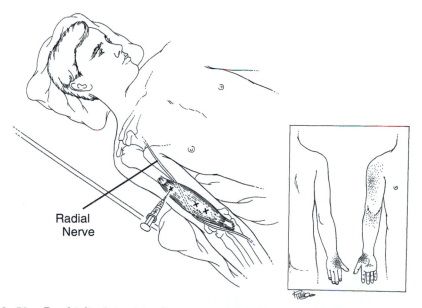

Radial
Nerve

FIG 10–50. Brachialis. Injection of trigger points in the right brachialis muscle (*X's*) with the patient supine. Anatomic landmarks, including the radial nerve, are noted. Exposure of the brachialis is best obtained if the biceps is shifted medially. *Inset*, pain pattern (*stippling*).

- Trigger points may cause local pain as well as referred pain to the elbow and base of the thumb.
- Flexion and extension of the elbow both actively and passively may cause pain.
- Hypoesthesia of the dorsum of the thumb.

Anatomy

Origin: front of the lower half of the shaft of the humerus and intermuscular septum.

Insertion: coronoid process and tuberosity of the ulna.

Action: flexes the elbow.

Differential Diagnosis

- Cervical radiculopathy.
- Radial nerve entrapment.
- Muscle strain, e.g., acute or overuse syndrome.

Noninvasive Therapy

The post–trigger point injection follow-up program described in Chapter 9 is recommended as a conservative therapeutic treatment approach. Noninvasive therapy can include:

- Physical therapy modalities (e.g., electrical stimulation and warm packs; see Chapter 15).
- Manual physical therapy techniques (e.g., massage and the Trager Approach; see Chapters 13 and 14).
- Active and passive stretching and limbering of muscles with or without the use of vapocoolant spray or ice. Active exercise is part of the stretch-and-spray technique. Limbering and relaxation are necessary prior to stretching. Contract-relax techniques may be used.
- Stretch and spray for the brachialis muscle using vapocoolant or ice is performed in the direction of elbow extension. Electrical stimulation, limbering of muscles, and warm packs should precede stretch and spray to relax muscles.
- Exercises and a home program for the shoulder and elbow are prescribed (see Chapter 12). Exercise programs include relaxation, limbering, stretching, and strengthening. When the patient is free of pain and full motion has been achieved, progress to strength and endurance programs.

Injection of Trigger Point

Injection is performed with the patient supine. The trigger point is injected under sterile technique (see Fig 10–50). Greater exposure of the brachialis is obtained by moving the biceps medially (see Chapter 9 for injection technique).

Needle size: 1.5, 2.0 in., 21 gauge.

Solution: Any one of the following solutions may be used: 0.5% procaine; 1.0% lidocaine; saline and dry needling in case of allergy. Do not use epinephrine.

Precautions

- Avoid the radial nerve which is superficial in the area of the brachialis as it passes to the front of the lateral epicondyle between the brachialis medially and the brachioradialis laterally (see Fig 10–50).

Postinjection Follow-Up Physical Therapy Program

The patient should receive 3 to 4 consecutive days of treatment. Physical therapy should include electrical stimulation, relaxation, limbering, and stretching of the involved muscle using vapocoolant spray or ice as needed combined with and followed by an exercise program. Active and active-assisted exercises are an integral part of the physical therapy program (see Chapter 9 for details).

Exercise and Home Program

Exercises for the elbow are prescribed. Exercises should at first be performed under the guidance of a therapist. When the patient is free of pain and full motion has been achieved, progress to strength and endurance programs. Begin and end exercise sessions with stretching and relaxation. (See Chapter 12 for exercise details.)

Corrective and Preventive Measures

- Do not maintain the elbow in flexion for prolonged periods. Learn to change position and relax the extremity.
- Instruct the patient in relaxation and stretching exercises.
- All neighboring muscles should be examined for trigger points.

SUPINATOR

Symptoms and Pain Pattern

- Pain over the outer aspect of the elbow, upper forearm, and lateral epicondyle[1, 13, 28] (Fig 10–51).
- Radiation of pain to the dorsal web space of the thumb.[32]
- Pain resulting from trigger points is noted with flexion and extension of the fingers, handshaking, and is classically associated with tennis elbow related to poor tennis technique, and overuse syndromes related to work and athletic activities.
- Muscle weakness may result from entrapment of the deep radial nerve due to trigger points.[15, 44]

Findings

- Tenderness over the lateral epicondyle, typical of tennis elbow.
- Tenderness over the lateral upper forearm involving the extensor muscles.
- Limitation in full elbow extension.
- Pain with wrist extension and supination.

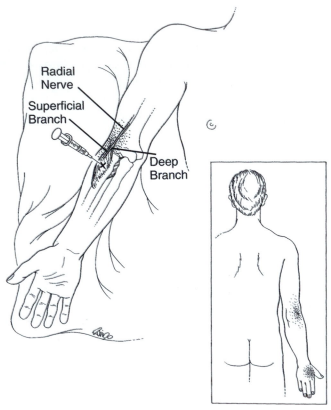

FIG 10–51. Supinator. Injection of trigger point (X) in the right supinator. The forearm is supinated with slight elbow flexion to relax the forearm muscles. Anatomic landmarks, including the deep branch of the radial nerve, are noted. Pain pattern is shown by *stippling*.

Differential Diagnosis

- Tendonitis involving the extensor forearm muscles.
- Lateral epicondylitis.
- Muscle strain of supinator and extensor muscles of the forearm.

Anatomy

Origin: deep fibers from the supinator crest just below the radial notch of the ulna; oblique fibers more superficial from the back of the lateral epicondyle, lateral ligament of elbow, and annular ligament.

Insertion: neck and shaft of the radius.

Action: supination of the radius.

Noninvasive Therapy

The post–trigger point injection follow-up program described in Chapter 9 is recommended as a conservative therapeutic treatment approach. Noninvasive therapy can include:

- Physical therapy modalities (e.g., electrical stimulation and warm packs; see Chapter 15).
- Manual physical therapy techniques (e.g., massage and the Trager Approach; see Chapters 13 and 14).
- Active and passive stretching and limbering of muscles with or without the use of vapocoolant spray or ice. Active exercise is part of the stretch-and-spray technique. Limbering and relaxation are necessary prior to stretching. Contract-relax techniques may be used.
- Stretch and spray for the supinator muscle: Bring the wrist into pronation with elbow extension. Use vapocoolant as needed. Electrical stimulation, limbering of muscles, and warm packs may precede stretch and spray to relax the muscles. Stretching of muscle is also accomplished actively as well as with assistance during the exercise program. Active exercise is part of the stretch-and-spray technique.
- Exercise and home program. Exercises for the shoulder, elbow, and wrist are described in Chapter 12. Exercise programs include relaxation, limbering, stretching, and strengthening. When the patient is free of pain and full motion has been achieved, progress to strength and endurance programs.

Trigger Point Injection

Injection is performed with the patient supine. The forearm is supinated with slight elbow flexion to relax the forearm muscles. Identify the trigger point. Inject medial to the brachioradialis (see Fig 10–51). (See Chapter 9 for injection technique).

Needle size: 1.5 in., 21 gauge.

Solution: Any one of the following solutions may be used: 0.5% procaine; 1.0% lidocaine; saline and dry needling in case of allergy. Do not use epinephrine.

Precaution

Avoid the radial nerve when injecting the trigger point (see Fig 10–51).

Postinjection Follow-Up Physical Therapy Program

The patient should receive 3 to 4 consecutive days of treatment. Physical therapy should include electrical stimulation, relaxation, limbering, and stretching of the involved muscle using vapocoolant spray or ice as needed combined with and followed by an exercise program. Active and active-assisted exercises are an integral part of the physical therapy program (see Chapter 9 for details).

Exercise and Home Program

Increase flexibility, range of motion, and strengthening. After full range is obtained, strengthen the forearm muscles by means of isotonic exercise beginning with light weights (1 or 2 lb) and progressing gradually without overstressing the muscle. Dorsiflexion, volarflexion, pronation, and supination of the wrist are performed with the elbow stabilized in flexion.

The patient is placed on a home exercise program. Exercises should at first be performed under the guidance of a therapist. When the patient is free of pain and full motion has been achieved, progress to strength and endurance programs. Begin and end exercise sessions with stretching and relaxation (see Chapter 12 for exercise details).

Corrective and Preventive Measures

- Avoid overuse syndromes, whether athletic or occupational.
- Correct tennis technique. This will usually concern one's backhand and serve. Proper athletic equipment is essential. The patient may require a lighter, more flexible racquet with a proper grip. Tennis handle grips that are too small contribute to the development of tennis elbow. Physical therapy or surgery will not solve the tennis elbow problem if technique and athletic equipment are not corrected.
- Perform warm-up relaxation and stretching exercises (shoulder, elbow, wrist) prior to playing, and stretching and relaxation after exercise.

PALMARIS LONGUS AND PRONATOR TERES

PALMARIS LONGUS
Symptoms and Pain Pattern

- Pain is produced by gripping any firm object in the palm.
- Referred pain pattern includes characteristic prickling and needling pain over the palm referred from a trigger point in the upper midforearm in the palmaris longus[44] (Fig 10–52).
- Local tenderness resulting from trigger points in the palm.

Findings on Examination

- Tenderness in the palm.
- Tender trigger points in the midportion of the palmaris longus and the palm.
- Contracture of the palmar fascia.[44]

Anatomy

Origin: common flexor origin.
Insertion: proximal end of palmar aponeurosis.
Action: flexes the wrist.
The palmaris longus may be absent in 10% of patients.

Differential Diagnosis

- Strain of forearm muscles.
- Palmar fibrosis.

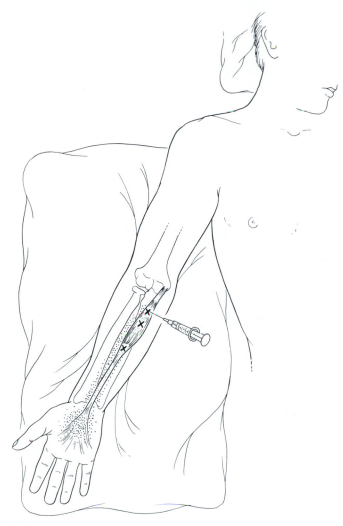

FIG 10–52. Palmaris longus. Injection of trigger points *(X's)* in the right palmaris longus. The patient is supine with the forearm supinated. Trigger point pain pattern is shown by *stippling.*

PRONATOR TERES
Symptoms and Pain Pattern

- Pain in the upper forearm at rest and with forearm motion.
- Pain radiating to the forearm and wrist.

Findings

- Tenderness in upper forearm.
- Pain with restriction in supination.

Differential Diagnosis

- Strain in forearm muscles

Anatomy

Origin: common flexor origin, front of medial epicondyle of the humerus, medial aspect of the coronoid process of the ulna.
Insertion: middle aspect of radius.
Action: flexion and pronation of the forearm.

Noninvasive therapy

The post–trigger point injection follow-up program described in Chapter 9 is recommended as a conservative therapeutic treatment approach. Noninvasive therapy can include:

- Physical therapy modalities (e.g., electrical stimulation and warm packs; see Chapter 15).
- Manual physical therapy techniques (e.g., massage and the Trager Approach; see Chapters 13 and 14).
- Active and passive stretching and limbering of muscles with or without the use of vapocoolant spray or ice. Active exercise is part of the stretch and spray technique. Limbering and relaxation are necessary prior to stretching. Contract-relax techniques may be used.
- Stretch-and-spray techniques using vapocoolant spray or ice: Stretching of the palmaris longus is performed by extending the wrist and fingers with the elbow extended. Stretch for pronator trigger points is performed by supination with the elbow extended. Electrical stimulation, limbering of muscles, and warm packs may precede stretch and spray to relax the muscles. Stretching of muscle is also accomplished actively as well as with assistance during the exercise program. Active exercise is part of the stretch-and-spray technique.
- Exercises and a home program for the elbow, wrist, and fingers are prescribed (see Chapter 12). Exercise programs include relaxation, limbering, stretching, and strengthening. When the patient is free of pain and full motion has been achieved, progress to strength and endurance programs.

Injection of Trigger Point

With the patient positioned comfortably in the supine position, the arm is supinated. The trigger point in the palmaris longus is identified (see Fig 10–52). Multiple needling should be performed over the muscle area to identify trigger points not diagnosed by palpation.

Needle size: 1.5 in., 21 gauge.

Solution: Any one of the following solutions may be used: 0.5% procaine; 1.0% lidocaine; saline and dry needling in case of allergy. Do not use epinephrine.

Postinjection Follow-Up Physical Therapy Program

The patient should receive 3 to 4 consecutive days of treatment. Physical therapy should include electrical stimulation, relaxation, limbering, and stretching of the involved muscle using vapocoolant spray or ice as needed combined with and followed by an exercise program. Active and active-assisted exercises are an integral part of the physical therapy program (see Chapter 9 for details).

Exercise and Home Program

Exercises for the elbow, wrist, and fingers are described in Chapter 12. Exercises should at first be performed under the guidance of a therapist. When the patient is free of pain and full motion has been achieved, progress to strength and endurance programs. Begin and end exercise sessions with relaxation and stretching.

Corrective and Preventive Measures

- Instruct patient in home exercise program and stretching.
- Avoid grasping firm objects in the palm for prolonged periods, e.g., a screwdriver, hedge clippers.
- Edges of casts applied for fractures should be well padded to avoid pressure areas in the palm and forearm. Casts should be trimmed to allow full range of motion of the fingers and thumb.
- Avoid prolonged repetitive pronation, occupational or athletic (excessive topspin stroke in tennis).

WRIST, HAND, AND FINGER FLEXORS

Flexor carpi ulnaris, Flexor carpi radialis, Flexor digitorum superficialis, Flexor digitorum profundus, Flexor pollicis longus

Symptoms and Pain Pattern

- Wrist flexors refer pain to the lower aspect of the wrist.[4]
- Trigger points in the wrist and finger flexors may refer pain to the medial aspect of the elbow ("medial tennis elbow"). Muscle weakness in the forearm and hand together with symptoms of numbness or paresthesia in the hand and fingers may be due to trigger points in muscles which originate in the flexor region of the medial epicondyle as well as from trigger points originating in extensor forearm muscles from the lateral epicondyle.
- Pain in the fingers and wrists may be due to myofascial trigger points in the flexor carpi radialis, flexor carpi ulnaris, flexor digitorum superficialis, (Fig 10–53) flexor digitorum profundus, flexor pollicis longus, and pronator teres. Finger flexors refer pain to their respective fingers; the flexor pollicis longus refers pain to the thumb.[44]
- Myofascial trigger points in the region of the medial epicondyle may be a cause of ulna nerve entrapment, a mechanism similar to the radial nerve entrapment seen on the lateral aspect of the elbow.[15, 44]

Findings on Examination

- Local tenderness over the muscle belly with or without referred pain.
- Trigger points may be primary or secondary.
- Look for trigger points in neighboring muscles.
- Pain with active and passive motion of involved muscles.

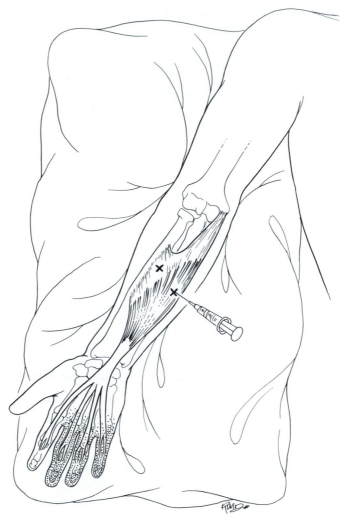

FIG 10–53. Injection of trigger points *(X's)* in the right flexor digitorum superficialis. The forearm is supinated and extended for easy access. Anatomic landmarks are noted. Pain pattern is shown by *stippling*.

Differential Diagnosis

- Forearm muscle strain.
- Carpel tunnel syndrome.
- Ulnar nerve entrapment.
- Cervical radiculopathy.

Anatomy

Flexor Carpi Radialis
Origin: medial epicondyle.
Insertion: base of second and third metacarpals.
Action: abductor and flexor of the wrist, wrist stabilizer.

Flexor Carpi Ulnaris
Origin: common flexor origin, upper two thirds of the border of the ulna.
Insertion: piriform bone, hook of hamate, fifth metacarpal.
Action: ulnar flexion and adduction of the wrist, wrist stabilizer.

Flexor Digitorum Superficialis
Origin: common flexor origin, coranoid process, anterior surface shaft of the radius.
Insertion: the sides of the middle phalanx of each finger.
Action: flexor of the middle phalanx and secondarily of the wrist.

Flexor Digitorum Profundus
Origin: front and medial surface of shaft of the ulna and olecranon.
Insertion: terminal phalanges of the finger.
Action: flexor of terminal phalanx, secondarily flexion of other joints and fingers and wrist.

Flexor Pollicis Longus
Origin: anterior aspect of shaft of the radius.
Insertion: front of base of the terminal phalanx of the thumb.
Action: flexion of the thumb.

Noninvasive Therapy

The post–trigger point injection follow-up program described in Chapter 9 is recommended as a conservative therapeutic treatment approach. Noninvasive therapy can include:

- Physical therapy modalities (e.g., electrical stimulation and warm packs; see Chapter 15).
- Manual physical therapy techniques (e.g., massage and the Trager Approach; see Chapters 13 and 14).
- Active and passive stretching and limbering of muscles with or without the use of vapocoolant spray or ice. Active exercise is part of the stretch-and-spray technique. Limbering and relaxation are necessary prior to stretching. Contract-relax techniques may be used.
- Stretch and spray for the finger flexors is performed by extending the fingers and wrist with the help of vapocoolant spray or ice. Passive stretching as well as active motion should be performed. Electrical stimulation, limbering of muscles, and warm packs should precede stretch and spray to relax the muscles. Stretching of muscle is also accomplished actively as well as with assistance during the exercise program. Active exercise is part of the stretch and spray technique (see Chapter 9).
- Exercises and a home program for the wrist and finger flexors are described in Chapter 12. The exercise program includes relaxation, limbering, stretching, and strengthening.

Injection of Trigger Point

Identify trigger points in the forearm. Trigger points are injected with the patient supine, and the forearm supinated. The position may be changed according to the muscle to be injected. Figure 10–53 demonstrates trigger points in the flexor digitorum superficialis. (See Chapter 9 for injection technique.)

Needle size: 1.5 in., 22 gauge

Solution: Any one of the following solutions may be used: 0.5% procaine; 1.0% lidocaine; saline and dry needling in case of allergy. Do not use epinephrine.

Postinjection Follow-Up Program

The patient should receive 3 to 4 consecutive days of physical therapy. Therapy should include electrical stimulation, relaxation, limbering, and stretching of the involved muscle using vapocoolant spray or ice as needed combined with and followed by an exercise program.

Exercise and Home Program

Exercises for wrist and fingers are described in Chapter 12. Exercises should at first be performed under the guidance of a therapist. Begin and end exercise sessions with stretching and relaxation.

Corrective and Preventive Measures

- Avoid overuse syndrome related to excessive flexion of the fingers, e.g., using scissors, gardening shears, excessive writing.
- Avoid repetitive occupational tasks requiring wrist flexion.

TRICEPS

Symptoms and Referred Pain Pattern

- Pain due to trigger points may be present over the posterior aspect of the upper arm and forearm in addition to pain over the shoulder, scapula, and trapezius area (Fig 10–54).
- Pain over the medial and lateral aspect of the elbow with radiation to the fourth and fifth fingers.[31]

Findings on Examination

- Tenderness on palpation of the medial, long, or lateral head of the triceps.
- Lack of full extension of the elbow, shoulder, or both.
- Lack of full extension of the elbow is noted in patients with a long history of tennis elbow. All neighboring muscles surrounding the elbow contribute to the condition of tennis elbow, e.g., trigger points in the anconeus muscle, which arises from the posterior surface of the lateral epicondyle of the humerus, may contribute to lateral tennis elbow.

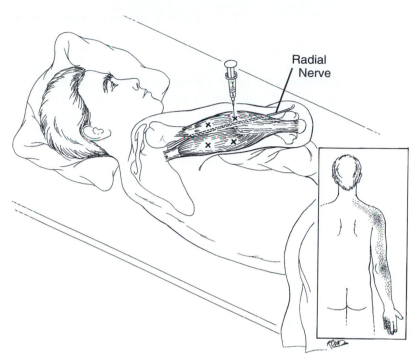

FIG 10–54.   Triceps. Injection of trigger points *(X's)* in the right triceps brachii. The position of the patient is determined by the position of the trigger point to be injected. Pain pattern is noted by *stippling*. The radial nerve may be encountered with deep probing of the needle.

Differential Diagnosis

- Cervical radiculopathy.
- Medial or lateral epicondylitis.
- Thoracic outlet syndrome.

Anatomy

Origin: the long head from the infraglenoid tubercle of the scapula; the medial head from the posterior surface of the humerus below the spiral groove from the medial and lateral intermuscular septa; the lateral head from the ridge on back of the humerus above the musculospiral groove.

Insertion: by means of a conjoint tendon into the olecranon process of the ulna.

Action: extension of the elbow; the long head stabilizes the shoulder joint in abduction.

Noninvasive therapy

The post–trigger point injection follow-up program described in Chapter 9 is recommended as a conservative therapeutic treatment approach. Noninvasive therapy can include:

- Physical therapy modalities (e.g., electrical stimulation and warm packs; see Chapter 15).

- Manual physical therapy techniques (e.g., massage and the Trager Approach; see Chapters 13 and 14).
- Active and passive stretching and limbering of muscles with or without the use of vapocoolant spray or ice. Active exercise is part of the stretch-and-spray technique. Limbering and relaxation are necessary prior to stretching. Contract-relax techniques may be used.
- Stretch-and-spray techniques using vapocoolant spray or ice in the direction of flexion of the elbow and extension of the shoulder. Vapocoolant spray is used in the trigger point and referred pain areas. Electrical stimulation, limbering of muscles, and warm packs may precede stretch and spray to relax the muscles. Stretching of muscle is also accomplished actively as well as with assistance during the exercise program. Active exercise is part of the stretch-and-spray technique.
- Exercises and a home program for the elbow and shoulder are prescribed (see Chapter 12). Exercise programs include relaxation, limbering, stretching, and strengthening. When the patient is free of pain and full motion has been achieved, progress to strength and endurance programs.

Injection of Trigger Point

The position of the patient on the table is determined by the site of the trigger point to be injected. Trigger points may involve the lateral head, medial head, or long head. They may be positioned for easy access to the individual trigger point areas. This could require internally rotating or externally rotating the arm. Injection is not limited to the area of tenderness. Multiple insertions along the muscle belly of the triceps are necessary to localize trigger points that may be missed on palpation (see Fig 10–54). (See Chapter 9 for injection technique.)

Needle size: 1.5, 2.0 in., 21 gauge

Solution: Any one of the following solutions may be used: 0.5% procaine; 1.0% lidocaine; saline or dry needling in case of allergy. Do not use epinephrine.

Precautions

The radial nerve, which is found between the long head and the medial head of the triceps passing deep to the lateral head of the triceps and descending in the spiral groove behind the humerus, may be encountered with deep probing of the needle.

Postinjection Follow-Up Physical Therapy Program

The patient should receive 3 to 4 consecutive days of treatment. Physical therapy should include electrical stimulation, relaxation, limbering, and stretching of the involved muscle using vapocoolant spray or ice as needed combined with and followed by an exercise program. Active and active-assisted exercises are an integral part of the physical therapy program. (See Chapter 9 for program details.)

Exercise and Home Program

Exercises should at first be performed under the guidance of a therapist. When the patient is free of pain and full motion has been achieved, progress to strength and endurance programs. Begin and end exercise sessions with relaxation and stretching. (See Chapter 12 for exercise details.)

Corrective and Preventive Measures

- Avoid overuse syndromes, e.g., overzealous athletic activity for which the patient is not prepared.
- Encourage the patient to continue the exercise program.
- Relaxation and stretching exercises prior to and after athletic and strenuous work activities.

EXTENSOR MUSCLES OF THE WRIST AND BRACHIORADIALIS

Extensor carpi ulnaris
Extensor carpi radialis brevis

Extensor carpi radialis longus
Brachioradialis

Symptoms and Referred Pain Pattern

- Pain in the upper forearm and lateral epicondyle. Trigger points in this area are frequently overlooked as a cause of tennis elbow symptoms[18] (Fig 10–55).
- Trigger points in the extensor carpi radialis may refer pain to the lateral epicondyle and dorsum of the hand.[43] This muscle, together with the brachioradialis and supinator (see above), contributes to the pain experienced over the lateral epicondyle area diagnosed frequently in patients as tennis elbow. Omitting trigger point management and directing treatment only to the area of the lateral epicondyle often results in poor therapeutic results.
- Pain may be experienced over the dorsum of the forearm, hand, and wrist.[6, 7, 13]
- Inhibition of grip strength due to pain (e.g., difficulty with grasp and handshaking).
- Pain is referred to the ulnar aspect of the wrist by the extensor carpi ulnaris, to the radial side by muscles on the radial side of the forearm. The brachioradialis refers pain to the wrist and base of the thumb and web space.[7, 43, 44]
- Trigger points may cause a tightening of the fibrous edge of the extensor carpi radialis brevis and supinator. When the extensor origin tightens it can compress both the deep radial nerve and its recurrent epicondylar branch. The mechanism of this nerve entrapment caused by supination, dorsiflexion, or radial deviation against resistance has been recognized as a possible cause of tennis elbow pain.[15]

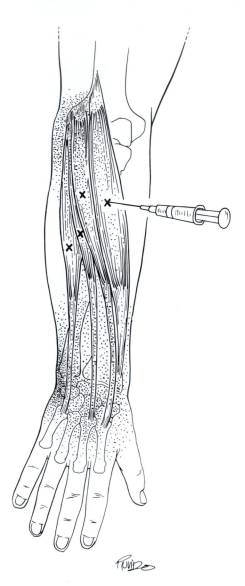

FIG 10–55.   Extensor muscles of the wrist and the brachioradialis. Injection of a trigger point *(needle X)* in the brachioradialis. Trigger points in the extensor carpi radialis longus and brevis and extensor carpi ulnaris *(X's)* are shown also. The forearm is pronated. Anatomic landmarks are noted. Trigger point pain pattern is shown by *stippling*.

Findings on Examination

- Local tenderness and referred pain on trigger point palpation of the forearm muscles.
- When trigger points are in neighboring fingers the patient may experience pain with extension and flexion of the fingers (e.g., handshaking, repeated gripping).
- Pain with active wrist extension and when maintaining extension against resistance.
- Pain with supination, dorsiflexion.
- Local tenderness over the lateral epicondyle area as well as the extensor forearm muscles.

Differential Diagnosis

- Tenosynovitis of extensor forearm muscles.
- de Quervain's disease.
- Arthritis of the wrist.
- Arthritis of the carpometacarpal joint of the thumb.
- Strain of extensor forearm muscles.
- Lateral epicondylitis.

Anatomy

Extensor Carpi Radialis
Origin: lower one third of the lateral supercondylar ridge.
Insertion: back of the second metacarpal bone.
Action: extensor of the wrist and fixator of the wrist joint.

Extensor Carpi Radialis Brevis
Origin: common extensor origin
Insertion: styloid process of base of the third metacarpal.
Action: extensor of the wrist and fixator of the wrist.

Extensor Carpi Ulnaris
Origin: common extensor origin, and aponeurosis attached to the subcutanous border of the ulna.
Insertion: dorsal aspect of the base of the fifth metacarpal.
Action: extension and adduction of the hand; fixator of the wrist.

Brachioradialis
Origin: upper two thirds of the lateral supracondylar ridge of the humerus.
Insertion: outer side of the base of the radial styloid process.
Action: flexion of the elbow when the forearm is midway between supination and pronation.

Noninvasive Therapy

The post–trigger point injection follow-up program described in Chapter 9 is recommended as a conservative therapeutic treatment approach. Noninvasive therapy can include:

- Physical therapy modalities (e.g., electrical stimulation and warm packs; see Chapter 15).
- Manual physical therapy techniques (e.g., massage and the Trager Approach; see Chapters 13 and 14).
- Active and passive stretching and limbering of muscles with or without the use of vapocoolant spray or ice. Active exercise is part of the stretch-and-spray technique. Limbering and relaxation are necessary prior to stretching. Contract-relax techniques may be used.
- Stretch and spray is accomplished by flexing the wrists, thereby stretching the extensors. Muscles that cross the elbow joint (extensor carpi radialis longus, brachioradialis) require the elbow to be extended when the wrist is flexed. Stretching of the extensor carpi ulnaris may be accom-

plished with the elbow in flexion. Brachioradialis stretch includes extension of the elbow and pronation. Electrical stimulation, limbering of muscles, and warm packs should precede stretch and spray to relax muscles.

- Exercises and home program: The patient is instructed in exercises for the upper extremities and stretching exercises for the elbow and wrist, as described in Chapter 12. Exercise programs include relaxation, limbering, stretching, and strengthening. When the patient is free of pain and full motion has been achieved, progress to strength and endurance programs.

Injection of Trigger Points

With the patient in the supine position, trigger points are isolated between two fingers or the index finger and thumb. Injection is given directly into the trigger point. The entire muscle and neighboring muscles are palpated for possible trigger points. (See Chapter 9 for injection technique.)

Needle size: 1.5, 2.0 in., 21 gauge

Solution: Any one of the following solutions may be used: 0.5% procaine; 1.0% lidocaine; saline and dry needling in case of allergy. Do not use epinephrine.

Postinjection Follow-Up Physical Therapy Program

The patient should receive 3 to 4 consecutive days of treatment. Physical therapy should include electrical stimulation, relaxation, limbering, and stretching of the involved muscle using vapocoolant spray or ice as needed combined with and followed by an exercise program. Active and active-assisted exercises are an integral part of the physical therapy program. (See Chapter 9 for program details.)

Exercise and Home Program

Exercises should at first be performed under the guidance of a therapist. When the patient is free of pain and full motion has been achieved, progress to strength and endurance programs. Begin and end exercise sessions with stretching and relaxation. (See Chapter 12 for exercise details.)

Corrective and Preventive Measures:

- Prescribe a wrist splint to prevent excessive flexion if the patient is symptomatic.
- Avoid activities which promote inflammation and pain (e.g., excessive handshaking).
- Correct faulty tennis stroke technique and inappropriate tennis equipment. The patient should use a proper grip and a lightweight racquet. A stiff racquet should be avoided. The use of a tennis elbow band may relieve symptoms not only during the athletic activity of tennis but also during certain occupational activities that require stress on the extensor forearm muscles.
- Avoid overuse syndromes (prolonged unaccustomed activity in occupational and athletic activities).

EXTENSOR MUSCLES OF THE FINGERS AND THUMB
Extensor digitorum communis, Extensor indicis, Extensor digiti minimi, Extensor pollicis longus, Extensor pollicis brevis, Abductor pollicis longus

Symptoms and Referred Pain Pattern

- Local pain limited to the forearm (Fig 10–56).
- Pain at rest as well as with activity, e.g., handshaking, playing a musical instrument, typing.
- Complaint of grip weakness is usually a result of pain.
- Referred pain to the dorsum of the hand and less frequently to the fingers of individual tendons.[13, 44]
- Pain in the thenar area of the palm and base of the thumb referred from the abductor pollicis longus.[11, 12]

Findings on Examination

- Local or referred pain on palpation of trigger points.
- Limitation in flexion of proximal interphalangeal (PIP) joints due to short-

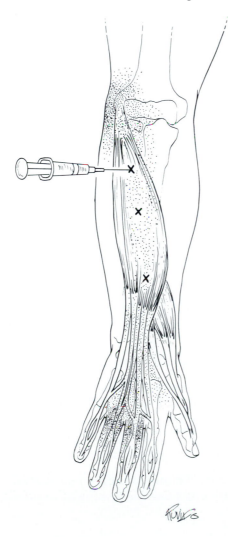

FIG 10–56. Extensor muscles of the fingers and thumb. Injection of trigger points *(X's)* in the extensor digitorum communis. The patient is supine. Neighboring muscles are noted which may also harbor trigger points. Pain pattern is shown by *stippling*.

ening of the extensors. Pain and limitation are elicited with flexion of the PIP joint while making a fist as well as with flexion of PIP joints with the metacarpophalangeal joints maintained in extension.
- Weakness of grip.
- Trigger points are most easily detected in the extensor digitorum communis.

Differential Diagnosis

- Tennis elbow.
- Arthritis of wrist or fingers.
- Tenosynovitis of extensor tendons.

Anatomy

Extensor Digitorum Communis
Origin: lateral epicondyle of the humerus.
Insertion: middle base of the second and third phalanges of index, middle, ring, and fifth fingers.
Action: extension of the fingers and wrist.

Extensor Indicis
Origin: dorsal shaft of the ulna.
Insertion: joins the dorsal extension on the index finger, extends and adducts the index finger.

Extensor Digiti Minimi
Origin: common extensor tendon.
Insertion: extensor expansion of the little finger.
Action: extends the fifth finger.

Extensor Pollicis
Origin: lateral side of dorsal surface of the ulna.
Insertion: dorsum of base of the distal phalanx of the thumb.
Action: extends the distal phalanx of the thumb.

Extensor Pollicis Brevis
Origin: dorsum of the radius and interosseus membrane.
Insertion: base of the proximal phalanx of the thumb.
Action: extends the proximal phalanx, may also act as an abductor of the wrist.

Abductor Pollicis Longus
Origin: dorsum of the ulna, interosseus membrane of dorsum of the radius.
Insertion: lateral aspect of the base of the first metacarpal of the thumb.
Action: abducts thumb and hand.

Noninvasive Therapy

The post–trigger point injection follow-up program described in Chapter 9 is recommended as a conservative therapeutic treatment approach. Noninvasive therapy can include:

- Physical therapy modalities (e.g., electrical stimulation and warm packs; see Chapter 15).
- Manual physical therapy techniques (e.g., massage and the Trager Approach; see Chapters 13 and 14).
- Active and passive stretching and limbering of muscles with or without the use of vapocoolant spray or ice. Active exercise is part of the stretch-and-spray technique. Limbering and relaxation are necessary prior to stretching. Contract-relax techniques may be used.
- Stretch and spray is accomplished by flexing the fingers and hand simultaneously. The elbow is held in extension. The elbow may be flexed when stretching the thumb muscles, stabilizing the wrist. Thumb muscles are stretched in the direction of flexion of the interphalangeal and metacarpophalangeal joints. The thumb is adducted in addition to adduction of the wrist to stretch the abductor pollicis longus. Electrical stimulation, limbering of muscles and warm packs should precede stretch and spray to relax muscles.
- Exercises and a home program for the elbow, wrist, and fingers are described in Chapter 12. The exercise program includes relaxation, limbering, stretching, and strengthening. When the patient is free of pain and full motion has been achieved, progress to strength and endurance programs.
- Prevention and correction of contributing factors.

Injection of Trigger Point

With the patient supine, trigger points are identified. Trigger points may be isolated between two fingers when possible. Injection is given directly into the trigger point in addition to needling of the *immediate surrounding area* (see Chapter 9 for injection technique). Palpate the entire muscle and neighboring muscles for additional trigger points (see Fig 10–56 for injection of trigger points in the extensor digitorum communis. Look for trigger points in neighboring muscles. Trigger points in the extensor forearm muscles are usually treated as a group when involving the finger extensors together with the extensor carpi radialis longus and brevis. This is often seen in symptoms related to tennis elbow.

Needle size: 1.5, 2.0 in., 21 gauge

Solution: Any one of the following solutions may be used: 0.5% procaine; 1.0% lidocaine; saline and dry needling in case of allergy. Do not use epinephrine.

Precautions

- When injecting the extensor forearm muscles, avoid the superficial and deep branch of the radial nerve.

Postinjection Follow-Up Physical Therapy Program

The patient should receive 3 to 4 consecutive days of treatment. Physical therapy should include electrical stimulation, relaxation, limbering, and stretching of the involved muscle using vapocoolant spray or ice as needed combined with and followed by an exercise program. Active and active-assisted exercises are an integral part of the physical therapy program (see Chapter 9 for details).

Exercise and Home Program

Exercises should at first be performed under the guidance of a therapist. When the patient is free of pain and full motion has been achieved, progress to strength and endurance programs. Begin and end exercise sessions with stretching and relaxation (see Chapter 13 for exercise details.)

Corrective and Preventive Measures

- Avoid overuse syndromes (e.g., excessive writing, typing). Musicians may require limitation in practice sessions and correction in fingering technique as well as instrumental mechanical adjustments which can be made to decrease the demands on the wrist and fingers.
- Perform stretching and relaxation exercises for upper extremities, including hands and fingers.
- Both in occupational and athletic activities tools and athletic equipment should be of the appropriate size to avoid stress on the fingers and wrist, e.g., a hammer handle or tennis racquet that is too large or too small may cause tension in the forearm and hand muscles.

ADDUCTOR POLLICIS AND OPPONENS POLLICIS

Symptoms and Pain Pattern

- Pain over the palmar aspect of the thumb (Fig 10–57).
- Pain is aggravated with motions of the thumb.

FIG 10–57. Adductor pollicis and opponens pollicis. Injection of trigger points in the adductor pollicis and adductor opponens pollicis *(X's)*. The hand is supinated. The needle is inserted into the opponens pollicis trigger point. Trigger points may be approached from the palmer surface. The adductor muscle may be approached from the palm or dorsum between the first and second metacarpal bones. Anatomic landmarks are noted. Pain pattern is shown by *stippling*.

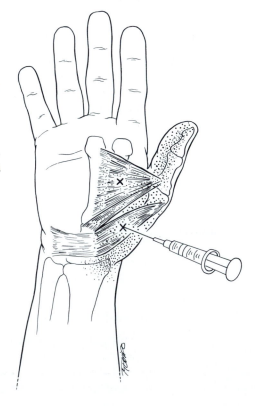

- Pain over the volar aspect of the wrist.
- Shortening of the muscles together with pain may decrease dexterity.[43]

Findings on Examination

- Tenderness over the adductor pollicus noted on palpation of the web space.
- Tenderness over the thenar eminence (opponens pollicis).
- Trigger points may cause restriction of full motion due to pain and muscle shortening.

Differential Diagnosis

- Carpal tunnel syndrome.
- Osteoarthritis of the thumb (e.g., carpometacarpal joint).

Anatomy

Adductor Pollicis
Origin: the oblique head from the front of the base of the second and third metacarpals, capitate, and trapezoid; the transverse head from the distal two thirds of the front of the third metacarpal.
Insertion: both oblique and transverse heads join to insert into the medial aspect base of the proximal phalanx of the thumb.
Action: adduction of the thumb.

Opponens Pollicis
Origin: trapezium.
Insertion: lateral side of the length of the first metacarpal.
Action: brings the tip of the thumb to the tip of the fifth finger.

Noninvasive therapy

The post–trigger point injection follow-up program described in Chapter 9 is recommended as a conservative therapeutic treatment approach. Noninvasive therapy can include:

- Physical therapy modalities (e.g., electrical stimulation and warm packs; see Chapter 15).
- Manual physical therapy techniques (e.g., massage and the Trager Approach; see Chapters 13 and 14).
- Active and passive stretching and limbering of muscles with or without the use of vapocoolant spray or ice. Active exercise is part of the stretch-and-spray technique. Limbering and relaxation are necessary prior to stretching. Contract-relax techniques may be used.
- Stretch and spray (see chapter 9): Stretching is performed in the opposite direction of muscle shortening by stretching the web space. Abduction and extension of the thumb are performed passively and actively with the help of vapocoolant spray or ice. Electrical stimulation, limbering of muscles, and warm packs may precede stretch and spray to relax the muscles. Stretching of muscle is also accomplished actively as well as

with assistance during the exercise program. Active exercise is part of the stretch-and-spray technique. Contract-relax techniques may be used. Exercises and a home program for the adductor and opponens pollicis are prescribed (see Chapter 12). The exercise program includes relaxation, limbering, stretching, and strengthening. When the patient is free of pain and full motion has been achieved, progress to a strengthening program.

Injection of Trigger Points

Trigger points are identified. Injection is performed directly into the trigger point area in the opponens pollicis (see Chapter 9 for technique). The adductor pollicis may be approached from the palm or dorsum of the hand in the web space between the first and second metacarpals (see Fig 10–57).

Needle size: 1.5, 1.0 in., 22 or 25 gauge.

Solution: Any one of the following solutions may be used: 0.5% procaine; 1.0% lidocaine; saline and dry needling in the case of allergy. Do not use epinephrine.

Postinjection Follow-Up Physical Therapy Program

The patient should receive 3 to 4 consecutive days of treatment. Physical therapy should include electrical stimulation, relaxation, limbering, and stretching of the involved muscle using vapocoolant spray or ice as needed combined with and followed by an exercise program. (See Chapter 9 for details.)

Exercise and Home Program

Exercises should at first be performed under the guidance of a therapist. Begin and end exercise sessions with relaxation and stretching. (See Chapter 12 for exercise details.)

Corrective and Preventive Measures

- Prevent repetitive adduction, opposition, and pinch movements.
- Avoid specific occupational stress which may occur with constant use of the thumb and fingers. Interrupt work routine for relaxation and stretching of muscles.

INTEROSSEI AND LUMBRICAL MUSCLES
Dorsal interossei, volar interossei, lumbrical muscles

Symptoms and Referred Pain Pattern

- Pain in the palm with radiation to the fingers[18] (Fig 10–58).
- Pain may occur on the dorsum or palmar aspect accompanied by stiffness.
- Pain may occur at rest as well as with finger motion.
- Heberden's nodes have been associated with interosseous trigger points.[44]

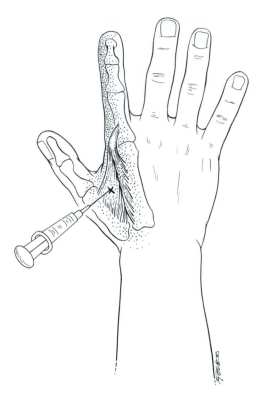

FIG 10–58. Interossei. Injection of trigger point *(X)* in the first interosseous muscle of the right hand. The injection approach for the first dorsal interosseous is from the dorsum of the hand. Trigger point pain pattern of the first dorsal interosseous is shown by *stippling.*

Findings on Examination

- Local tenderness on palpation of interossei.
- Local tenderness may cause referred pain to the fingers.
- Trigger points may cause hypoesthesia involving one side of the finger.

Differential Diagnosis

- Carpel tunnel syndrome.
- Digital neuroma.

Anatomy

Dorsal Interossei
Origin: each arises from the adjacent sides of two metacarpals.

Insertion: the first, into the radial side of the proximal phalanx of the second digit; the second, into the radial side of the proximal phalanx of the third digit (middle finger); the third, into the ulnar side of the proximal phalanx of the middle finger; the fourth, into the ulnar side of the proximal phalanx of the ring finger.

Action: abduction of the index, middle, and ring fingers from the midline.

Volar Interossei
Origin: the first, from the ulnar side of the second metacarpal; the second, from the radial side of the fourth metacarpal; the third, from the radial side of the fifth metacarpal.

Insertion: the first, into the ulnar side of the proximal phalanx of the second digit; the second, into the radial side of the proximal phalanx of the fourth digit; the third, into the radial side of the proximal phalanx of the fifth digit.

Action: each muscle adducts the fingers to the midline.

Lumbrical Muscles

Origin: the four lumbricals arise from tendons of the flexor digitor profundus, the first and second from the radial sides of the first and second tendons, and the third and fourth from the adjacent sides of the second, third, and fourth tendons.

Insertion: each inserts into the dorsal expansion on the middle phalanx together with tendons of the extensor digitorum and interossei into bases of terminal phalanges of the middle four fingers.

Action: flexes the metacarpophalangeal joint and extends the interphalangeal joint.

Noninvasive Therapy

The post–trigger point injection follow-up program described in Chapter 9 is recommended as a conservative therapeutic treatment approach. Noninvasive therapy can include:

- Physical therapy modalities (e.g., electrical stimulation and warm packs; see Chapter 15).
- Manual physical therapy techniques (e.g., massage and the Trager Approach; see Chapters 13 and 14).
- Active and passive stretching and limbering of muscles with or without the use of vapocoolant spray or ice. Active exercise is part of the stretch-and-spray technique. Limbering and relaxation are necessary prior to stretching. Use contract-relax technique.
- Stretch and spray for the interrossei and lumbricals is performed. Both abduction and adduction may be required depending on the muscles involved and the restrictions and symptoms noted. Perform extension of the metacarpal joints and flexion of the interphalangeal joints for the lumbricals. Use vapocoolant spray or ice as necessary. Electrical stimulation, limbering of muscles, and warm packs may precede stretch and spray to relax the muscles. Stretching of muscle is also accomplished actively as well as with assistance during the exercise program. Active exercise is part of the stretch-and-spray technique. Contract-relax techniques may be used.
- Exercises and a home program for the wrist and hand are described in Chapter 12. Hand exercises should include range-of-motion exercises involving all the muscles of the hand. Add exercises for the wrist. Prescribe the use of clay or putty to strengthen the fingers. Exercise programs include relaxation, limbering, stretching, and strengthening.

Injection of Trigger Points

Identify the trigger point by palpation. Inject directly into the trigger point area (see Chapter 9 for technique). Needling of the lumbrical muscles is performed on the palmar side of the hand. Figure 10–58 demonstrates injection of the first dorsal interosseus trigger point and pain pattern.

Needle size: 1.0, 1.5 in., 25 gauge.

Solution: Any one of the following solutions may be used: 0.5% procaine; 1.0% lidocaine; saline and dry needling in case of allergy. Do not use epinephrine.

Postinjection Follow-Up Physical Therapy Program

The patient should receive 3 to 4 consecutive days of treatment. Physical therapy should include electrical stimulation, relaxation, limbering, and stretching of the involved muscle using vapocoolant spray or ice as needed combined with and followed by an exercise program. Active and active-assisted exercises are an integral part of the physical therapy program.

Exercise and Home Program

Exercises for the hand and wrist are prescribed. Clay or putty is used to improve finger strength. Exercises should at first be performed under the guidance of a therapist. The exercise program includes relaxation, limbering, stretching, and strengthening. Begin and end exercise sessions with stretching and relaxation. (See Chapter 12 for exercise details.)

Corrective and Preventive Measures

- Avoid activities that require a prolonged pinching action of the fingers.
- Patients in occupations requiring repetitive use of the fingers must learn to relax the hand to avoid constant tension. Provide for periods of relaxation and stretching of muscles.

REFERENCES

1. Barton PM, Grainger RW, Nicholson RL, et al: Toward a rational management of piriformis syndrome (abstract), *Arch Phys Med Rehabil* 69:784, 1988.
2. Epstein SE, Gerber LH, Borer JS: Chest wall syndrome: A common cause of unexplained cardiac pain, *JAMA* 241:2793–2797, 1979.
3. Fricton JR, Auvinen MD, Dykstra D, et al: Myofascial pain syndrome: Electromyographic changes associated with local twitch response, *Arch Phys Med Rehabil* 66:314–317, 1985.
4. Good MG: Rheumatic myalgias, *Practitioner* 146:167–174, March 1941.
5. Good MG: Diagnosis and treatment of sciatic pain, *Lancet* 21:597–598, 1942.
6. Good MG: What is "fibrositis?", *Rheumatism* 5:117–123, 1949.
7. Gutstein M: Diagnosis and treatment of muscular rheumatism, *Br J Phys Med* 1:302–321, 1938.
8. Hallin RP: Sciatic pain and the piriformis muscle, *Postgrad Med* 74:69–72, 1983.
9. Hinks AH: Further aid for piriformis muscle syndrome, *J Am Osteopath Assoc* 74:93, 1974.
10. Hoppenfeld S: *Physical examination of the spine and extremities*, New York, Appleton-Century-Crofts 1976.
11. Kellgren JH: A preliminary account of referred pains arising from muscle, *Br Med J* 2:325–327, 1938.
12. Kellgren JH: Observations on referred pain arising from muscle, *Clin Sci* 3:175–190, 1938.
13. Kelly M: The relief of facial pain by procaine (Novocaine) injections, *J Am Geriatr Soc* 11:586–596, 1963.
14. Kendall FP, McCreary EK: *Muscle testing and function*, ed 3, Baltimore, 1983, Williams & Wilkins.

15. Kopell W, Thompson AL: *Peripheral entrapment neuropathies*, Baltimore, 1963, William & Wilkins.
16. Kraus H: Prevention of low back pain, *J Am Podiatr Med Assoc* 6:12–15, 1952.
17. Kraus H: "Pseudo-disc," *South Med J* 60:416–418, 1967.
18. Kraus H: *Clinical treatment of back and neck pain*, New York, 1970, McGraw-Hill.
19. Kraus H, editor: *Diagnosis and treatment of muscle pain*, Chicago, 1988, Quintessence.
20. Lang M: Die Muskelhärten (Myogelosen), Munich, 1931, JF Lehmann.
21. Lutz EG: Credit card–wallet sciatica (letter to the editor), *JAMA* 240:738, 1978.
22. Macdonald AJR: Abnormally tender muscle regions and associated painful movements, *Pain* 8:197–205, 1980.
23. Melnick J: Treatment of trigger point mechanisms in gastrointestinal disease. *NY State J Med* 54:1324–1330, 1954.
24. Melnick J: Trigger areas and refractory pain in duodenal ulcer, *NY State J Med* 57:1073–1076, 1957.
25. Pace JB: Commonly overlooked pain syndromes responsive to simple therapy, *Postgrad Med* 58:107–113, 1975.
26. Pace JB, Nagle D: Piriform syndrome, *West J Med* 124:435–439, 1976.
27. Puranen J, Orava S: The hamstring syndrome. A new diagnosis of gluteal sciatic pain, *Am J Sports Med* 16:517–521, 1988.
28. Rachlin ES: Musculofascial pain syndromes, *Medical Times* January 1984, pp 34–47.
29. Rachlin ES: Musculofasical pain syndromes. In Kraus H, editor. *Diagnosis and treatment of muscle pain*, Chicago, 1988, Quintessence, pp 8.
30. Reynolds MD: Myofascial trigger points in persistent posttraumatic shoulder pain, *South Med J* 77:1277–1280, 1984.
31. Simons DG: Myofascial pain syndrome. In Basmajian JV, Kirby RL, editors: *Medical rehabilitation*, Baltimore, 1984, Williams & Wilkins.
32. Simons DG: In Goodgold J, editor: *Rehabilitation medicine*, St Louis, 1988, Mosby–Year Book, 686–723.
33. Slocumb JC: Neurological factors in chronic pelvic pain: Trigger points and the abdominal pelvic pain syndrome, *Am J Obstet Gynecol* 149:536–543, 1984.
34. Sola AE: Treatment of myofascial pain syndromes. In Benedetti C, Chapman R, Moriocca G, editors: *Advances in pain research and therapy*, vol 7, New York, 1984, Raven Press, pp 467–485.
35. Sola AE: Trigger point therapy. In Robers JR, Hooges JR, editors: *Clinical procedures in emergency medicine* Philadelphia, 1985, WB Saunders.
36. Sola AE, Kuitert JH: Quadratus lumborum myofascitis, *Northwest Med* 53:1003–1005, 1954.
37. Sola AE, Kuitert JH: Myofascial trigger point pain in the neck and shoulder girdle, *Northwest Med* 54:980–984, 1955.
38. Sola AE, Rodenberger MS, Gettys BB: Incidence of hypersensitive areas in posterior shoulder muscles: A survey of two hundred young adults, *Am J Phys Med* 34:585–590, 1955.
39. Sola AE, Williams RL: Myofascial pain syndromes, *Neurology* 6:91–95, 1956.
40. Steiner C, Staubs C, Ganon M, et al: Piriformis syndrome: Pathogenesis, diagnosis, and treatment, *J Am Osteopath Assoc* 87:318–323, 1987.
41. Synek VM: The piriformis syndrome: Review and case presentation, *Clin Exp Neurol* 23:31–37, 1987.
42. TePoorten BA: The piriformis muscle, *J Am Osteopath Assoc* 69:150–160, 1969.
43. Travell J, Rinzler SH: The myofascial genesis of pain, *Postgrad Med* 11:425–434, 1952.
44. Travell JG, Simons DG: *Myofascial pain and dysfunction: The trigger point manual*, vol 1, Baltimore, 1983, Williams & Wilkins.
45. Travell JG, Simons DG: *Myofascial pain and dysfunction: The trigger point manual* vol 2, *The lower extremities*, Baltimore 1992, Williams & Wilkins.
46. Wyant GM: Chronic pain syndromes and their treatment II. Trigger points, *Canad Anaesth Soc J* 26:216–219, 1979.

Chapter 11

Diagnosis and Management of Facial Pain

Harold V. Cohen, D.D.S.
Richard A. Pertes, D.D.S.

Pain is the primary reason that patients seek medical or dental attention. When the craniofacial area is involved, the pain may take on even greater significance for the patient because of the psychological importance of the face. Craniofacial pain, especially if the problem is chronic, presents a diagnostic and management challenge to all health care practitioners. Multiple processes can coexist. For the doctor who treats facial pain complaints, a thorough knowledge of the sensory innervation of this area is essential in analyzing the chief complaint. The finite neural circuitry of the trigeminal nerve (cranial nerve V), which provides sensory innervation to most of the head, creates a complex clinical challenge in the diagnosis and management of these problems.

TRIGEMINAL SENSORY FUNCTION

Sensory information from the trigeminal (V) nerve distribution passes through the main gasserian ganglion in the pons and enters the central nervous system (CNS) in a manner similar to other afferent fibers of the peripheral nervous system. The sensory dorsal horn site for the first synapse is an elongate structure known as the V spinal nucleus. This structure extends from the pontine level caudally to cervical segments C2–3. It is within this relay center that there is pain and temperature integration from the face, dura mater, large blood vessels of the brain, eyeball (cornea), ear, paranasal sinuses, oral cavity, tongue, and cervical spine structures.[5] Included in this intermix is a barrage of signals from the mouth, teeth, facial muscles, and temporomandibular joint (TMJ). This amazingly complex convergence of sensory information then ascends to thalamic and cortical levels. Projection at the cortical level can lead to patient misinterpretation of the pain source. The doctor must be aware of this intricate neurophysiology and apply the caveat of viewing subjective pain complaints as often unknowingly misdirected by the patient (Fig 11–1).

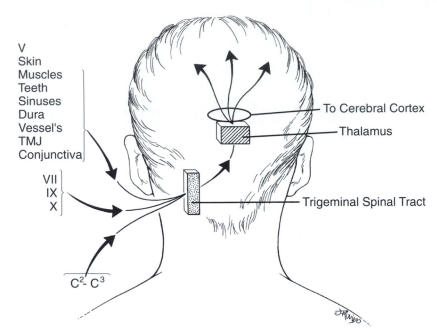

V
Skin
Muscles
Teeth
Sinuses
Dura
Vessel's
TMJ
Conjunctiva

VII
IX
X

To Cerebral Cortex

Thalamus

Trigeminal Spinal Tract

C^2- C^3

FIG 11–1.   Schematic of sensory convergence to the trigeminal spinal nucleus.

THE RELATIONSHIP OF CERVICAL SPINE DISORDERS TO FACIAL PAIN

It is well documented both clinically and scientifically that disorders of the cervical spine can produce pain within the cranial and orofacial regions. There is controversy, however, as to the exact anatomic/physiologic basis of this pain relationship. Three theories have been proposed to account for this connection: (1) direct connections through myofascial or neural structures; (2) convergence within the V spinal nucleus; and (3) functional connections mediated through enlarged receptive fields and central neuronal changes.

Cervical muscle pain associated with persistent headache syndromes is a common but controversial issue. The pain can be viewed as emanating from the cervical musculature as the primary process. Others describe a physiologically related neurogenic phenomenon whereby the headache process is related to a functional disturbance within the CNS which can affect multiple areas. Another viewpoint is that cervical muscle pain is due to a reflex contraction subsequent to the stress from the persistent headache discomfort.

DIFFERENTIAL DIAGNOSIS OF FACIAL PAIN

Dental and periodontal assessment should be the first evaluation in the differential diagnosis of pain in the orofacial area (Table 11–1). Most facial pain originates in the teeth and supporting periodontal and alveolar structures. Difficulties can be encountered in the localization of dental pain and this can be further complicated by pain referral patterns within the V spinal nucleus. Acute dental pain can mimic neuralgic phenomena whereas chronic dental disease may have characteristics of low-grade muscular pain.

Temporomandibular disorders (TMDs) are a group of related conditions in the masticatory system and should not be viewed as a single syndrome. Much of the population exhibits signs or symptoms of a temperomandibular joints (TMJ)

TABLE 11–1.

Differential Diagnosis of Facial Pain: Structural
and Functional Categories

Extracranial:
  Teeth and supporting structures
  Temporomandibular disorders
    Temporomandibular joints
    Masticatory musculature
Eyes, ears, nose, throat, sinuses, tongue,
  glandular tissue
Intracranial disease
  Neoplasm
  Arteriovenous malformations
Vascular
  Migrainous headache, cluster headache
    Giant cell arteritis
Neurogenic
  Paroxysmal disorders
  Continuous disorders
Psychogenic
  Endogenous disorders
  Reactive processes

---

or masticatory muscle problem during their lifetime. However, most people do not require treatment, and of those persons who do seek treatment, females far outnumber males. TMD classifies as a somatic pain problem with characteristics of myofascial and articular disease. TMDs can be divided into those disorders involving the structures of the TMJ and those affecting the masticatory musculature. The etiology of TMD can be multifactorial.

1. Macrotrauma.
2. Microtrauma—bruxism, major occlusal discrepancies.
3. Emotional tension.
4. Systemic arthritides.

Most commonly, oral parafunctional habits are prime contributors to these disorders. These deleterious habits include tooth clenching, tooth grinding (bruxism), nail or cuticle biting, gum chewing, and sustained muscle tension within the masticatory muscles from stress or other provocations. These cause repetitive microtrauma to the TMJs; the persistent adverse loading can cause adaptive and degenerative changes in the TMJs and also produce a painful masticatory muscle disorder.

Macrotrauma sustained in a mandibular injury can also lead to TMJ arthropathies. Additionally, as listed below in the TMD classification, there can be congenital, developmental, and acquired defects in this articular complex.

Clenching, Bruxism, and the Role of Emotional Tension in Temporomandibular Disorders

Tooth clenching is the habit of persistent gritting of the teeth without lateral sliding. If lateral grinding does occur, this is called bruxism and is usually evidenced by the presence of marked occlusal wear or flattening of the chewing surfaces of the back teeth. These deleterious habits usually occur repeatedly during a 24-hour cycle, but seem to cause the most symptomatic effects after sleep periods. These patients will generally report stiffness or pain of the face on arising in the morning. A good differential approach during the patient interview would be to ask if there is difficulty in opening the jaws to brush the teeth or if discomfort is felt while eating breakfast. Some patients will not report pain on arising, but rather will complain of late-day facial discomfort. These symptoms correlate with minimal tooth clenching at night but do imply a stress-oriented facial muscle tightening during the day.

Some diagnosticians consider the presence of wear facets on the teeth as correlating with these deleterious habits. However, the presence of wear facets in an *asymptomatic* dental population raises a doubt as to their diagnostic significance. Of clinical interest is the fact that most patients who do clench or grind during the daytime hours do not realize it and once asked to do self-monitoring will usually (suprisingly) become aware of this habit. Emotional tension is very frequently associated with TMD. The tensional issue may stem from an endogenous psychological problem or it may be a concomitant of a legitimate pain process. In either case, elevated facial muscle stress levels ensue and are commonly (but not always) accompanied by clenching or bruxism, or both, and subsequent TMD.

The Relationship of Malocclusion and Other Dental Disorders to the Etiology of Temporomandibular Disorders

Dental malocclusion has long been the subject of controversy as to its role in masticatory muscle and TMJ problems. Genetic malocclusion (as commonly assessed in the pediatric or adolescent dental patient) should not be considered a cause of myofascial dysfunction. Anecdotal reports of this interrelationship have not held up when subjected to scientific scrutiny.

The presence of missing teeth is not a specific correlate to TMD; however missing dental units can be a predisposing or complicating factor in TMD. This occurs because of chewing difficulties or inadequate dental arch support to the TMJs when joint pressure is increased as occurs in traumatic or bruxism situations. Recent changes in the dental occlusion (as with new bridgework) can trigger dysfunctional pain problems, but these complaints may be due to patient inability to accommodate and should not necessarily be ascribed to faulty restorations.

Dental disease can also affect the temporomandibular complex indirectly. The presence of loose or tender teeth may lead to altered chewing patterns. Periodontal or tooth pulpal disease can also lead to compromised jaw function along with referred dental pain throughout the face. Patients with dental problems may develop defensive chewing patterns that can also be contributory to TMD.

Other Causes of Facial Pain

Paranasal sinus disease can be a common cause of facial pain. Clinical characteristics are a constant, mild, nonpulsatile, or aching pain which can extend from the maxillary canine area to the third molars. As opposed to dental pain, this type of discomfort rarely refers to the mandibular arch. The patient commonly has a history of a recent upper respiratory infection which was antecedent to the development of the facial pain. Although the symptoms can include frontal headache, ear pain, fullness over the sinus, and nasal discharge, it is common that the only reported symptom is tenderness of the teeth and a postnasal drip. The diagnostician can assume that pain in this area *not associated with a recent cold* or active drainage probably implies a cause unrelated to the paranasal sinuses. (An exception to this would be a neoplasm or other structural disorder within a sinus cavity.) Because of the possibility of coexisting problems, a history of a recent respiratory infection should *not* preclude performance of a dental examination.

Intracranial lesions can also cause facial pain. The patient may not present with obvious neurologic signs or deficits; the pain can be referred to the dental arches and thus be confused with toothache. Patients with intracranial lesions such as neoplasm or arteriovenous malformation may first appear at the dental office complaining of pain within a dental arch. Referral for a neurologic assessment should be a strong consideration, especially for the mature or geriatric patient.

Vascular pain disorders, most commonly migraine and cluster headache, can also be expressed as facial pain. Tension-type headaches, usually described by the patient as the nonprogressive day-after-day headache, are included in this grouping because current research suggests a neurophysiologic relationship between these headaches and migrainous syndromes. Acute headache discomfort can also lead to reflex muscle tightening within the face which creates more pain. This self-sustaining loop creates diagnostic difficulty for the clinician as both the headache and muscular processes must be analyzed and treated.

Neurogenous disorders exhibit temporal pain qualities that can be grouped as either paroxysmal or continuous. Paroxysmal neurogenous pain can be initiated by a primary functional disturbance within the nervous system (e.g., trigeminal neuralgia, glossopharyngeal neuralgia). However, neuralgic episodes can also be associated with neoplasms or demyelinating disease.

Neuropathic discomfort may also be triggered by a traumatic episode (deafferentation process). This vague, intractable, chronic facial pain syndrome will often have overlying muscular responses. Here again, the astute clinician must sort out both the primary and secondary processes.

Psychological factors can create endogenous facial pain or can be considered as a reactive process to a legitimate pain complaint. Psychogenic pain has a psychological base as a causative factor. These patients will have an emotional or personality disorder and complaints do not follow reasonable biological principles. As in any medical work-up, a thorough examination is mandatory as more than one of the above disorders can be present at any one time. TMDs are classified as follows:

Classification of Temperomandibular Disorders[2]
TMJ Arthropathies

A. Noninflammatory.
  1. Disc displacements.
     a. With reduction.
     b. With intermittent jaw locking.
     c. Without reduction (closed lock).
  2. Deviations in form.
     a. Bony articular surface defect.
     b. Articular disc thinning and perforation.
  3. Displacements of disc-condyle complex.
     a. Hypermobility.
     b. Dislocation.
  4. Adhesions.
  5. Ankylosis.

        a. Fibrous.
        b. Bony.
   B. Inflammatory.
        1. Capsulitis, synovitis.
        2. Retrodiskitis.
   C. Arthritides.
        1. Osteoarthrosis.
        2. Osteoarthritis.
        3. Systemic arthritides.

The TMJ is also subject to additional congenital, developmental, and acquired disorders as are other orthopedic joints. This includes condylar hyperplasia, hypoplasia, aplasia, condylolysis, neoplasms, and fractures.

Disc Displacements of the TMJ

A common finding in patients is the presence of jaw clicking emanating from one or both TMJs. Clicking is usually indicative of anterior displacement of the articulating disc, whereby the mandibular condyle must traverse over the back end of the disc in order to accomplish the opening movement; it will than slip off the back end of this disc as the jaw closes to full occlusion. The clicking noises occur when the condyle jumps over the back end of the disc on opening and when it slips off the back end on jaw closure. The opening noise is more commonly heard than the closing noise and the sounds can be intermittent. This sequence of events is termed "anterior disc displacement with reduction."

In some patients, this is a painless process, as the tissues adapt well to the altered disc-condyle relationship. However, many patients experience pain in the TMJ because the cushioning effect of the displaced disc is lost and the tissues now supporting the mandibular condyle do not adapt but rather stay persistently inflamed and painful. *The clinician must realize that the presence of TMJ noise does not mandate corrective therapy unless it is accompanied by pain and/or intolerable or progressive dysfunction* (Fig 11–2).

Patients may also report episodes of persistent interference on opening as more advanced disc displacement starts to interfere with mandibular translation and the condyle cannot slip over the back end of the disc. The patient can usually maneuver the mandible to slip onto the disc, thus allowing for continued jaw translation. In the advanced degenerative stage, the articular disc may displace to a point at which it permanently interferes with mandibular opening. This sudden event is termed "anterior disc displacement without reduction," or "closed lock," and will require more aggressive therapies by the dentist.

Masticatory Muscle Disorders

Masticatory muscle disorders of the face may be classified as acute or chronic: *Acute disorders* include myositis, reflex muscle splinting, and muscle spasm. *Chronic disorders* include myofascial pain, muscle contracture, and myalgia secondary to systemic disease.

Acute
Myositis. Myositis is local inflammation due to trauma, acute muscle strain, a surgical procedure, or spread of infection from a nearby structure. This

Normal

Slight Displacement

Advanced Displacement

FIG 11–2. Variations of temporomandibular joint disc position.

is accompanied by pain, tenderness, restricted mandibular movement, and possible swelling. Clinically the patient may report a change in the bite along with difficulty in chewing.

Reflex Muscle Splinting. This is characterized by reflex rigidity of a muscle in an attempt to avoid pain by stabilizing and protecting the part from further damage. It can occur as a normal reaction to trauma, from a change in the bite, or as a response to a TMJ internal derangement. The patient usually presents with limited range of mandibular motion due to pain rather than a structural alteration.

Muscle Spasm. Muscle spasm is characterized by a sudden involuntary contraction of a muscle or group of muscles that are functionally related. It may occur as a result of overstretching a previously weakened muscle, overuse of the muscle, parafunctional activity such as bruxism, or in response to a TMJ injury. It is usually accompanied by pain and interference with function.

Chronic
Myofascial Pain. A *trigger point* is defined as "a focus of hyperirritabilty in a tissue, that when compressed, is locally tender, and if sufficiently hypersensitive, can give rise to referred pain and tenderness, and sometimes to referred autonomic phenomena and distortion of proprioception."[6] These trigger points can be found in a firm band of skeletal muscle, its fascial sheath, or its tendinous attachment.

Muscle Contracture. Muscle contracture is characterized by shortening of muscle due to excess fibrous tissue within the muscle or its sheath. It may occur as a result of trauma, infection, or prolonged hypomobility. Masticatory muscle contracture results in painless, limited mandibular opening unless an attempt is made to force the mandible open.

Myalgia Secondary to Systemic Disease.   Many rheumatic and collagen diseases can cause generalized pain and diffuse tenderness. Myalgia may then be associated with chronic inflammation of synovial membranes of joints or be the result of pathology within muscle.

All of the above entities can be associated with both pain and altered function. The general clinical presentation includes chief complaints of pain on mandibular movement, limited range of mandibular motion in the opening, lateral, and protrusive excursions, and a deep, diffuse aching pain which is usually aggravated by jaw movement. The muscle pain can be spontaneous even when the muscles are at rest. Discomfort is usually bilateral with one side predominating.

Trigger points can develop in the masticatory and associated head and neck musculature secondary to prolonged muscle tension, protracted muscle spasm, forward head posture, parafunctional habits, and trauma.[4]

The oral musculature is particularly susceptible to the deleterious effects of the parafunctions and the clinician would be remiss in not questioning the patient carefully for the presence of these habits.

In the final analysis, a firm TMD diagnosis, be it muscle or joint-related, should only be accepted after ruling out other possible medical and dental disorders. Classical TMD, although painful and at times disabling, is essentially a benign disorder. The clinician is at risk by not performing adequate differential diagnosis to rule out causes which may underlie or mimic TMD.

EXAMINATION OF THE PATIENT WITH TEMPOROMANDIBULAR DISORDER

As in other medical conditions, an adequate TMD assessment is based upon specific diagnostic steps. Because the bilateral TMJs are connected by a one-piece mandibular bone, joint and muscle evaluations are done bilaterally to allow for comparison of sides.

Steps in a TMD Examination

1. A thorough history includes a review of the patient's medical status. This should include a personal history, a review of the chief complaints, and a history of the present illness

2. Clinical examination. TMJ—palpation, auscultation, functional movements, diagnostic anesthetic blocks; muscles—palpation, functional testing, diagnostic anesthetic blocks.

3. Radiographic studies. Baseline views in the generalist's office would include a panoramic study and possible transcranial oblique films of both TMJs.

4. Bite analysis (through direct examination or plaster molds of the teeth).

5. Cervical and postural evaluation.

6. Psychometric screening examination.

7. Referral for additional imaging studies or medical testing.

Although the above steps involve an extended period of time, the practitioner can perform a rapid office screening examination to assess the presence of a

TMD. Patient complaints of recurrent facial pain with jaw function, clicking or locking of the jaw joints, and limited opening should alert the examiner to do further evaluation. The patient will usually react to palpation of the masseter or temporalis muscles, which are commonly tender in these disorders. Placement of the examiner's fingertips over the preauricular area (not in the external auditory meatus) will allow for superficial assessment of disc disorders of the TMJs. Positive responses to these brief tests could indicate an active TMD. It is important to note that many patients will present with nonprogressive TMJ noise that is *not* accompanied by pain or dysfunction. These patients may not require TMD therapy.

THE PRIMARY MASTICATORY MUSCLES: ANATOMY AND PHYSIOLOGY

The facial muscle complex consists of the muscles of mastication and the accessory muscles of facial expression. The primary muscles of mastication are the masseter, temporalis, medial pterygoid, and lateral pterygoid. The digastric and mylohyoid muscles are also involved in mandibular function but are usually not considered primary masticatory muscles and tend to be less involved in painful states. (However, they can be sources of orofacial pain and mandibular dysfunction.) In the assessment of orofacial-myofascial disorders, most attention should be directed toward the primary masticatory muscles and the associated trigeminal innervation.

These main masticatory muscles are involved in providing mandibular movement for opening, closing, mastication, and speech. The articulations around which these muscles function are the bilateral TMJs. This arrangement is unique in that the two joints are intimately connected in function through the body of the mandible; muscular effects on one joint are reflected in compensating stresses or movements in the other. In addition, because of the day-long habits of breathing, swallowing, chewing, and talking, the temporomandibular articulation is rarely at rest.

Masseter Muscle

The masticatory muscle most commonly involved in myofascial problems is the masseter muscle (Fig 11–3). Its prime function is to elevate the mandible and bring the teeth to maximum contact. It consists of two segments. One part is the *superficial belly* which originates on the zygomatic arch and inserts on the external surface of the angle of the mandible and the lower half of the ramus. A second portion, the *deep belly,* also originates on the zygomatic arch and inserts on the superior half of the ramus.[7] Muscle fibers from the deep belly have been found within the capsule of the TMJ and this may account for some of the confusion in differentiating facial myofascial pain from TMJ arthralgia.

Patients who present with limited opening, and pain with mandibular function, invariably have a component of a masseter problem. In the symptomatic patient, it is rare that palpation is negative for masseter pain.

Temporalis Muscle

This large fan-shaped muscle originates on the temporal bone and temporal fascia in the temporal fossa and inserts on the coronoid process of the man-

MASSETER MUSCLE-
SUPERFICIAL & DEEP BELLIES

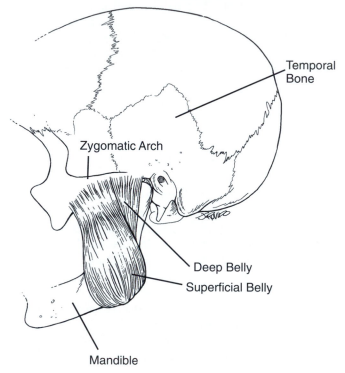

FIG 11–3. Masseter muscle.

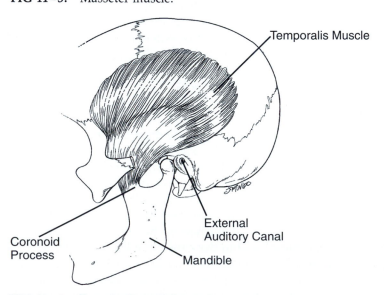

FIG 11–4. Temporalis muscle.

dible (Fig 11–4).[7] It functions to elevate and retract the mandible. Temporalis trigger points are commonly associated with masseter myofascial triggers. Pain in this muscle is often interpreted by the patient as "headache." Differentiating myofascial trigger points from a primary headache process is essential as different therapeutic approaches are indicated for each condition.

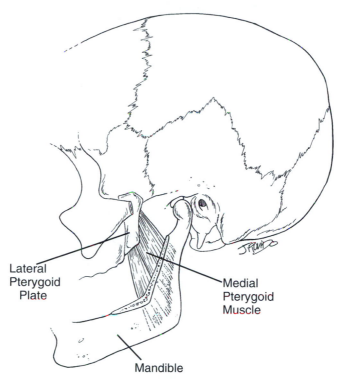

Lateral
Pterygoid
Plate

Medial
Pterygoid
Muscle

Mandible

FIG 11–5. Medial pterygoid muscle.

Medial Pterygoid Muscle

The medial pterygoid muscle originates on the lateral pterygoid plate and attaches at the angle of the mandible (Fig 11–5). It functions to elevate the jaw and assist in lateral and protrusive motions. This muscle, when symptomatic, can contribute to restricted jaw opening, but usually will be accompanied by masseter symptoms, the latter predominating.

Lateral Pterygoid Muscle

The lateral pterygoid muscle consists of two bellies that affect mandibular movement (Fig 11–6). The inferior belly functions to depress the mandible on jaw opening (along with the digastric). This portion originates on the lateral pterygoid plate and inserts on the neck of the mandible. The superior belly originates on the sphenoid bone and inserts into the anterosuperior portion of the condylar neck just below the condyle, with attachment fibers also inserting into the articular disc. The two muscle bellies function reciprocally. The inferior belly protrudes and depresses the mandible when contraction is bilateral. When contraction is unilateral, the *inferior belly* moves the mandible to the opposite side; this occurs because of the medial position of the inferior belly. The *superior belly* contracts as the teeth come to maximum intercuspation serving to "brace" the mandible against the articular disc and glenoid fossa.

Intraoral palpation of this muscle is difficult because of its high and medial position. Functional manipulation, as described by Bell,[1] provides the most consistent diagnostic approach to assessing this muscle.

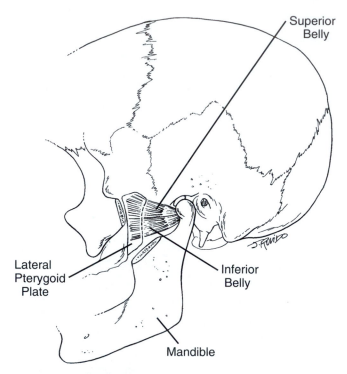

FIG 11–6.   Lateral pterygoid muscle.

CERVICAL MUSCLES AND OROFACIAL-MYOFASCIAL PROBLEMS

The muscles of the neck have a strong relationship to facial function and pain patterns. Cervical posture and pain referral patterns are factors which should always be assessed during analysis of facial complaints.

The cervical spine as part of the upper quarter (head, neck, and shoulder girdles) has the potential of causing pain in an adjacent or functionally related area. Forward head posture can disrupt the high degree of finely coordinated muscle balance necessary to support the head and neck. This is usually accompanied by referral of muscular trigger point pain to the face, the physiology of which is mediated through the V spinal nucleus. The clinician needs only to provoke a trapezius trigger point to have the patient report ipsilateral temporal pain. The sternocleidomastoid muscle is a common referrer of myofascial pain to multiple areas of the face. Therefore, differential diagnosis of nonspecific orofacial complaints may often involve diagnostic anesthetic injection of cervical muscles. Secondary or satellite trigger points in the face may occur as a product of continuous input from the cervical region and treatments addressing only the secondary sites may not resolve the patient's complaints.

CLINICAL FINDINGS IN TEMPOROMANDIBULAR DISORDERS

"It hurts when I chew!" "I can't open my jaw all the way!" "My jaws hurt when I talk a lot and I have a persistent headache!" These quotes represent the usual complaints given by patients with facial myofascial trigger points. Although pain can be present when the jaws are not used, most commonly it is jaw function that elicits the complaint. Restricted vertical range of mandibular motion accompanied by pain on jaw movement is a consistent finding in patients with facial trigger points. The patient often has an associated TMJ disorder which can contribute to the limitation as a primary or secondary factor.

The patient with muscle pain (myalgia) from guarding or spasm may also present with limited opening. Differentiating myalgic pain from trigger point discomfort can be difficult; as a general rule, the sore muscle has a generalized aching pattern without the presence of the taut bands or twitch responses commonly found in trigger points. Well-defined pain referral patterns are more common with trigger point provocation.

For both the myalgic and trigger point pain patient, reasonable opening range is attainable after pain reduction through the use of anesthetic injection, vapocoolant spray, or medications. These diagnostic and therapeutic steps can help in differentiating muscle-induced restraint from intracapsular TMJ restrictions due to disc interferences.

Examination of the masticatory muscles is done by direct palpation of accessible areas and functional manipulation of deeper-lying muscles. Because of the unique bilateral nature of the mandibular attachment to the maxilla, examination should include both the side ipsilateral to the chief pain complaint and also the contralateral musculature. Mandibular functional and pain patterns are the sum total of multiple bilateral structures. Treatments should encompass both sides.

Masseter pain is commonly felt locally under the examiner's hand or it may exhibit trigger point referral patterns to the teeth, maxilla, mandible, and temples. Referred pain patterns from the deep belly of the masseter are commonly felt in the periauricular area and can be mistaken for TMJ arthralgia or otalgia. Clinical signs will be limited opening, usually accompanied by pain, discomfort on chewing, and a fatigued feeling after brief jaw use, particularly after meals.

Temporalis pain is also readily palpable by the examiner and may exhibit trigger point referral patterns to the vertex, maxilla, and upper teeth. The tendinous insertion on the coronoid process is often sore to intraoral finger palpation. Because this area has little submucosal tissue, examination should be done judiciously as the mucosa is tightly attached to the underlying bone and can be exquisitely sensitive to excessive finger pressure. Temporalis trigger points can cause pain described as "headache," and soreness in the temples on opening, chewing, or talking.

Medial pterygoid assessment is more of a challenge as many patients will manifest a gag response to the examiner's finger. However, notable tender differences between sides are often reported by the patient. Here again, the patient may describe a deeper soreness with mandibular use and a sense of having a sore throat. Pain on opening and hard biting, which is not palpable externally, implicates the medial pterygoid.[2] Pain deep to the ear can also be reported. Pain at the inferior border of the mandible can be reported in the area of the medial pterygoid attachment, but may be difficult to differentiate from soreness at the masseter insertion. It is *not* common to find the medial pterygoid as a primary sore muscle in a facial trigger point analysis; masseter discomfort is invariably present and usually predominates.

The lateral pterygoid muscle is not readily accessible for palpation; techniques of functional manipulation allow for indirect assessment of this muscle while differentiating which of the reciprocally functioning bellies is responsible for the trigger point pain. Pain initiated by resisted protrusion and clenching that is reduced by biting against a tongue blade identifies inferior lateral pterygoid pain. Pain from clenching the teeth or clenching on a tongue blade that does not occur with resisted protrusion or opening widely identifies superior lateral pterygoid pain.[1]

THERAPIES FOR OROFACIAL MYOFASCIAL TRIGGER POINTS

Diagnostic and therapeutic approaches to orofacial myofascial trigger points can be frustrating to both the clinician and the patient. The bilateral influence of multiple muscles creates complex pain and functional patterns which can be difficult to assess. In addition, as previously stated, the mandible is rarely at rest as normal functional demands of chewing and talking are often complicated by dysfunctional habits (clenching). The latter problem often continues uncontrolled throughout the sleep period. The therapeutic approaches to orofacial myofascial disorders are:

1. Injections—anesthetic, dry needling.
2. Physical therapy.
3. Intraoral orthotics.
4. Pharmacologic management.
5. Behavioral modification.

Treatment sequencing of the above steps will vary depending on the severity of the initial symptom presentation and whether the problem is acute or chronic. Acute episodes can be aborted with physical therapy approaches accompanied by insertion of an intraoral orthosis and the use of adjunctive short-term medication. Intramuscular injections can also be used to eradicate trigger points and restore more comfortable functional patterns. Behavioral modification can then be added to prevent recurrence. Chronic facial pain issues are understandably more difficult to manage. As expressed by Sternbach, acute pain is a symptom of disease whereas chronic pain is a disease unto itself.[6]

Injection Techniques

Injection of facial muscle trigger points provides a rapid and convenient approach to management. Physicians tend to be more comfortable with extraoral injections, whereas dentists are understandably more at home with the intraoral route. Extraoral techniques are preferable because they allow access to all four of the primary masticatory muscles and enable manipulation of the syringe at various angles.

Few patients look forward to the discomfort usually associated with intraoral injections for dental treatment. Although most patients are initially alarmed at the thought of receiving injections to the external face, the pain experienced tends to be less than that of intraoral injections. Once the initial anesthetic is deposited, the clinician will be surprised at patient tolerance to prolonged manipulation of the syringe following needle entry.

General Considerations in Facial Injections

Risks of untoward side effects in masticatory muscle injections are relatively low. By applying anatomic considerations for each masticatory muscle being treated, problems can be kept to a minimum. The occurrence of hematoma and prolonged muscle inflammatory response is not unusual and is easily managed. Important considerations for the outpatient are cosmetic disturbances due to the injections and anesthetic effects which may affect the patient's ability to drive from the office. As in any medical or dental technique, *informed consent* is mandatory.

Armamentarium

Because masticatory muscle mass is small in comparison to other major body muscles, a 25-gauge needle is sufficiently wide to provide for trigger point needling without excessive muscle tissue damage. Smaller-gauge needles will deflect in these muscles and not allow for operator control; also, false-negative aspiration is more likely with the narrower gauge. The masseter and temporalis muscles are amenable to needles of 1½-in. length, whereas muscles medial to the mandible, the medial and lateral pterygoid, may require a longer needle to access them from the extraoral route. The shorter-length needle will suffice for intraoral approaches.

Recommended syringe techniques for trigger point ablation usually include injection of anesthetic, saline, or no solution at all (dry needling technique). Because of the sensitive nature of the face and the proximity of critical structures, local anesthetic is the preferred vehicle as the numbness will allow for needle manipulation without the potential danger of face or eye injury due to patient movement.

Anesthetics of choice are those *without vasoconstrictor*, most commonly mepivacaine, lidocaine, or bupivacaine. Mepivacaine and lidocaine are readily available in multidose vials or dental cartridges and will provide sufficient facial anesthesia for trigger point needling and increased range of mandibular motion in the absence of pain. The duration of action for mepivacaine and lidocaine is short. This feature may be valuable as temporary anesthesia of the facial nerve commonly occurs as a side effect of solution dispersion and this may compromise the patient's ability to drive home (see below). Bupivacaine can be used for prolonged anesthesia, but patients should be accompanied by another adult if they are to leave the office after the procedure.

Skin preparation before needle penetration can be accomplished with povidone-iodine (Betadine) wipes. Patients will appreciate removal of the orange color with an additional alcohol wipe. Surfaces are then sprayed to an initial frost using a vapocoolant spray such as fluorimethane spray (Gebalier Pharmaceutical Co., Cleveland, Ohio). Because of the proximity of the eye and ear

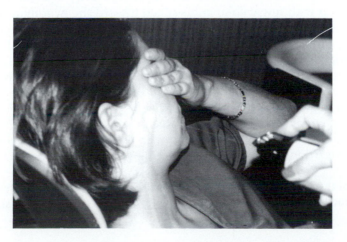

FIG 11–7. Application of vapocoolant spray prior to needle insertion.

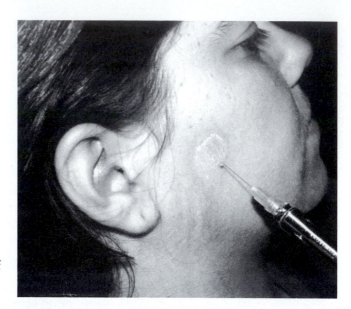

FIG 11–8. Insertion of needle at point of skin frosting.

to the refrigerant stream, the operator or assistant should provide hand protection to both these structures (Fig 11–7).

Needle penetration at the site of the frost is usually painless, and a small amount of anesthetic solution is deposited followed by a pause to allow for initial localized numbness (Fig 11–8).

Initial aspiration is done and is repeated throughout the injection process. The needle can then be advanced slowly while expressing anesthetic solution to further widen the anesthetized area. The pause is repeated and this can then be followed by fanning out with the syringe and needling of trigger points. On completion of the injection-needling procedure, pressure is applied to promote hemostasis and a small bandage is placed over the site of needle penetration. This is followed by bilateral stretch and spray of the involved muscles. The patient should be kept in the office under observation for at least 30 minutes and anti-inflammatory medication should be prescribed for 1 to 3 days. The patient is then referred for physical therapy management starting on the following day.

Masseter Muscle

The size and superficial location of this muscle allows for efficient trigger point injection procedures. Pain in the superficial belly is usually reported in the midportion with fewer complaints noted toward the zygomatic origin or insertion point on the mandibular border. Because of the relatively large size of this muscle, multiple sore areas will be found and the clinician will have to differentiate trigger point sites from surrounding myalgia. When the deep belly is symptomatic, the patient usually reports marked pain on palpation just inferior to the tragus.

For needle insertion into the superficial belly, the patient is asked to open the mouth as wide as possible and the doctor's free hand index finger is placed intraorally to locate the anterior border of this belly. This should provide a guide for needle insertion that will prevent needle entrance into the oral cavity (Fig 11–9).

If the patient cannot open, direct insertion of the needle to contact the mid-lateral surface of the mandibular ramus will provide a sufficient starting land-

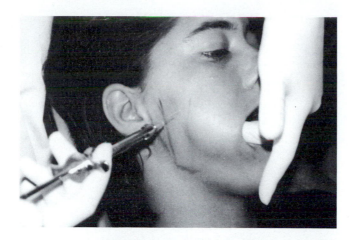

FIG 11–9. Needle insertion into superficial belly of masseter muscle.

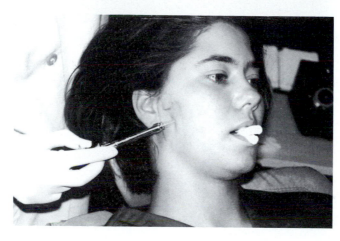

FIG 11–10. Fanning of needle within masseter muscle to disrupt trigger points.

mark. After superficial deposition of anesthetic, the needle is rapidly advanced to contact the bony ramus. The importance of making this contact is to be sufficiently deep within the muscle area, thus avoiding injection into the parotid gland. The needle is then fanned out through the large muscle belly to break up trigger points (Fig 11–10). The facial artery and the parotid gland are the prime structures to avoid. For deep belly needle insertion, the prime landmark is the posterior border of the condylar neck just below the ear. The needle is inserted just anterior to this until bony contact with the neck or lateral surface of the ramus is reached (Fig 11–11).

Having the patient open slightly may allow for better palpation of landmarks. It is essential to contact bony landmarks thus avoiding untoward injection into the coronoid notch of the mandible or deeper soft tissue structures within the neck.

The most common, usually benign, side effect of masseter injection is that associated with anesthesia of the facial nerve as it passes through the parotid gland. This is more common with deep belly injection and the patient should be advised before starting the procedure that he or she may lose the ability to close or blink the ipsilateral eye for about 40 minutes subsequent to the injection. In order to protect conjunctival and corneal structures, the patient should be given safety glasses or the eye should be taped closed for the duration of anesthesia. The patient should then wait in the office until motor function returns.

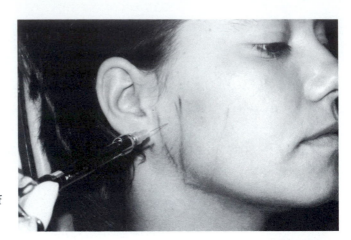

FIG 11–11.   Injection of deep belly of masseter muscle.

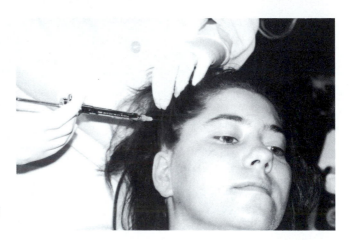

FIG 11–12.   Injection of temporalis muscle.

Temporalis Muscle

Most trigger point pain in the temporalis muscle will be felt in the middle portion and is easily provoked by palpation. Tenderness in this muscle can be confused with a potential headache process of central origin. It is not routine practice to shave this area before injection, and surface wiping with disinfectant will not totally clean epithelial surfaces below the hair. However, the potential for complications from a compromised surface preparation is low. The clinician should insert the syringe fully until contacting the bony surface of the temporal bone and then withdraw the needle followed by a subsequent fanning-out motion to broach trigger points. The superficial temporal artery is the main complicating anatomic part to be avoided (Fig 11–12).

Medial Pterygoid

Intraoral trigger point injection of the medial pterygoid muscle is feasible but can present difficulties because of restricted opening range, the gag reflex, and limited ability to manipulate the needle. If the intraoral route is desired, the patient is asked to open the mouth as wide as possible and a prop is than inserted between the teeth on the opposite side to stabilize the mandible. The needle is inserted just medial to the pterygomandibular raphe about midway between the upper and lower teeth. The needle should also be held horizontal and parallel to the ramus.[2] After insertion into the muscle, trigger points can

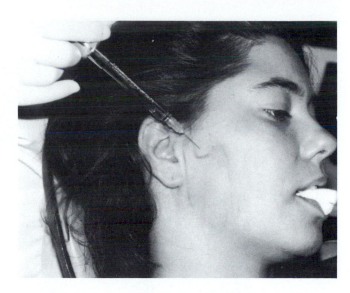

FIG 11–13. Injection of medial pterygoid muscle.

be approached by redirecting the needle, although syringe manipulation may be limited by space available in the oral cavity.

There are two extraoral techniques for injection of the medial pterygoid. The inferior portion may be approached under the inferior ramus of the mandible just anterior to the angle of the jaw.[2] Injecting through the coronoid notch of the mandible provides direct access to the muscle belly, especially when the patient presents with severely restricted opening.[6] The mouth is propped open if possible, and the needle is inserted through the coronoid notch in an inferior and slightly caudad direction until the muscle belly is penetrated. The pterygoid plexus of veins lies just medial to the mandible and lateral to the lateral pterygoid muscle; hemorrhage can be avoided by smoothly and rapidly passing the needle through this plexus (Fig 11–13).

Lateral Pterygoid Muscle

Intraoral approaches to injection of the lateral pterygoid muscle are not recommended as the high and medial position of this large muscle body prevents direct access with the needle. The extraoral route through the coronoid notch provides good access to both bellies of the lateral pterygoid. The patient's mouth is propped open and the syringe is passed through the coronoid notch in an upward direction until contact with the lateral pterygoid plate is made. The needle is withdrawn slightly and the inferior and lateral bellies may be injected by altering needle direction. Again, rapidly passing the needle through the pterygoid plexus will prevent a bleeding episode. The other possible vascular event may be nicking of the maxillary artery which runs in close proximity to the muscle bellies. Because of the size and deep location of this muscle, false-negative results may occur with injection techniques (Fig 11–14).

Physical Therapy

Physical therapy care is mandatory for both short- and long-term management of chronic myofascial trigger points. Stretch and spray techniques using vapocoolant are effective in eliminating trigger points and can be first-line therapy to obviate the need for needling procedures.[3] Restoration of reasonable jaw function and continued management for recurrent muscular pain problems

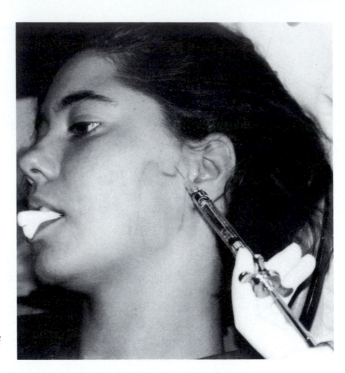

FIG 11–14. Injection of lateral pterygoid muscle.

can be accomplished within the physical therapy setting, perhaps avoiding the necessity of further injections or medication treatments.

Intraoral Orthotics

Adjunctive care to facial trigger point management should include possible insertion of an intraoral plastic orthosis to help manage parafunctional habits. This appliance is similar to an orthodontic retainer except that it covers the occlusal surfaces of the teeth with a thin layer of plastic. The appliance is placed preferably over the maxillary teeth, but can be placed on the mandibular arch. The result is usually a reduction in clenching habits and some reflex relaxation of the masticatory musculature. These orthoses provide varying degrees of improvement in different patients. However, when successful, the relief provided may obviate the need for supplemental medications.

If the patient has a major TMJ disc displacement disorder which interferes with jaw opening, repositioning of the mandible with the bite plate may allow for more acceptable joint function (Fig 11–15). This is accomplished by changing the bite pattern on the orthosis so as to make the lower teeth meet the bite plate in a more anterior position. This brings the mandible forward, thus moving the condyle forward onto the displaced articular disc. However, wearing this orthosis for extensive time periods can lead to irreversible tooth movement and a permanent change in mandibular position, necessitating additional dental rehabilitation procedures. As in any arthropathy that is refractory to nonsurgical management, arthroscopic or open joint surgery remains an option.

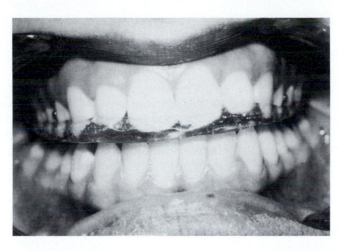

FIG 11–15. Intraoral bite plate: maxillary flat plane design.

Pharmacologic Management

Medications are a valuable adjunct in the management of myofascial trigger point pain. Drug selection is based on the pharmacologic objective and the length of time the patient will be taking the medication. Medications include nonsteroidal anti-inflammatory drugs (NSAIDs), anxiolytics, skeletal muscle relaxants, and antidepressants.

Nonsteroidal Anti-inflammatory Drugs

NSAIDs can have both short-term and long-term application within trigger point management. For brief periods of acute pain, NSAID management can provide sufficient analgesia to allow for better mandibular function. They should be prescribed routinely after trigger point injections to reduce postoperative discomfort. Longer-term use may be indicated for prolonged problems, but this will require blood monitoring and the added risk of adverse gastrointestinal side effects. Pregnancy, asthma, and a history of gastrointestinal disorders are major medical considerations in use of these drugs.

Anxiolytics

Anxiolytic medication provides more predictable muscle relaxation effects than that attained by use of skeletal muscle relaxants. The γ-aminobutyric acid (GABA)–enchancing limbic effects are anxiolytic by pharmacologic mechanisms, and this creates a reflex muscle relaxation effect in many patients. The benzodiazepines are most commonly prescribed, but long-term use is contraindicated because of their addiction potential.

Skeletal Muscle Relaxants

These medications do not seem to have marked effect on myofascial trigger point pain. They do not work directly on the motor end plate but apparently exert their influence on local reflex arcs within the spinal cord and on the reticular activating system. Some of their analgesic effect may be due to sedation.

Antidepressant Medication

Antidepressants are better suited for longer-term use on the chronic myofascial pain patient. The therapeutic window for pain management generally requires dose amounts below that commonly used for behavioral therapy. In addition to their neurohumoral pain-reducing mechanisms, they also tend to improve sleep in chronic pain patients.

Behavioral Modification

Behavioral approaches for patient management fall into two categories. The first concerns itself with the psychological manifestations of the patient's pain syndrome (see Chapter 4). Whether the problems are endogenous or reactive, functional difficulties due to behavioral input will affect the course of treatment and this level of care should be instituted when indicated.

The second approach involves the use of biofeedback training. As stated previously, oral parafunctional habits are common in patients with orofacial myofascial trigger points. A biofeedback therapist may be able to effect a reduction in these deleterious habits and educate the patient in self-modulation of facial muscle tension.

SUMMARY

As documented in this chapter, the complexities encountered in analyzing and managing facial pain challenge the practitioner in multiple areas of diagnosis and treatment. The clinician must be sure that facial myofascial trigger points are the primary disorder and are not associated with another pathologic process. Use of testing procedures where indicated along with medical and dental consult should allow for defining the specific problem. There is often difficulty in long-term management of masticatory muscle problems owing to patient inability to control etiologic factors. However, levels of improvement to allow for daily functional comfort are usually attainable. Careful diagnosis and adequate technique should provide pain management in an area of the human soma that is critical to the day-to-day comfort and function of most individuals.

REFERENCES

1. Bell WE: *Temporomandibular disorders: Classification diagnosis,* management, ed 3, St Louis, 1990, Mosby–Year Book.
2. Fricton JR, Kroening RJ, Hathaway KM: *TMJ and craniofacial pain: Diagnosis and management,* ed 1, St Louis, Ishiyaku EuroAmerican.
3. Pertes R, Cohen H: Clinical management of temporomandibular disorders: Part 2, *Compendium Continuing Education Dent* 12:270, 410, 1992.
4. Pertes R, Heir G: Chronic orofacial pain—A practical approach to differential diagnosis, *Den Clin North Am* 35:30, 1991.
5. Sigiura K, Robinson G, Stuart D: *Illustrated guide to the central nervous system,* St Louis, 1989, Ishiyaku EuroAmerica, p 114.
6. Sternbach RA, Chronic pain as a disease entity, *Triangle* 20:27-32.
7. Travell J, Simons D: *Myofascial pain and dysfunction. The trigger point manual,* Baltimore, 1983, Williams & Wilkins, pp 4, 221, 236, 255–258.

PART *III*

PHYSICAL THERAPY AND REHABILITATION

Chapter *12*

Muscle Deficiency

Hans Kraus, M.D.

MYOFASCIAL PAIN

Myofascial pain can be categorized into four types: (1) muscle spasm, (2) muscle tension, (3) muscle deficiency, and (4) trigger points.

Medical literature tends to concentrate on trigger points and injection therapy to the exclusion of the other types of myofascial pain. The clinical facts contradict such emphasis. I can find no better way to clarify this than to describe my own experience with the history of myofascial pain.

When I was a resident in 1931 at the fracture service of Vienna University's Department of Surgery, it was the custom to treat acute muscle spasm—following sprain, strain, or fracture—with either immobilization or traction. My coach, Heinz Kowalski, taught me differently. The way he treated an injured extremity was to wrap it in towels soaked with alcohol, expose it to live steam, and follow up with gentle limbering movements. This method produced much more rapid and satisfactory results than our usual immobilization.

Taking a cue from Kowalski, I used the same treatment on two skiers with sprained ankles and was surprised to find how quickly their pain was relieved and full function restored. Later, in an attempt to improve on this cumbersome method involving alcohol and live steam, I experimented with various fluids. Eventually, I hit on ethyl chloride as the most effective means of relieving discomfort and facilitating movement.[7, 8] Ethyl chloride is superior to procaine (Novocain) injections because it does not mask pathologic conditions; the hypoesthesia it produces is only temporary and does not affect major injuries. With ethyl chloride I began to obtain consistently favorable results in treating sprains, muscle strains, partial ligament tears, back pain, and certain types of impacted fractures.[16]

I followed the above treatment with exercises to strengthen, limber, and stretch the affected muscles. Not only was the period of disability shortened considerably but improvement was usually permanent. I became so involved in therapeutic exercise that I established an exercise department adjacent to the fracture service. However, while exercise helped increase function, I discovered this same treatment frequently to be ineffective in alleviating chronic pain.

Fortunately, I came across a book written in 1931 by Max Lange,[19] with a lengthy description of "myogelosis" or muscle hardening, which he treated with deep point massage or glucose injections. Lange's co-workers, Glogowsky and Wallraff,[4] biopsied these tender spots and found them to be degenerated areas of muscle tissue. In 1959, Steindler[25] described these tender nodules as trigger points. Lange discussed not only all the most common trigger points; he also indicated their locations at the myofascial or myotendinous junction. After studying his book, I added trigger point injections and needling to my treatment of chronic muscle pain. Later, I discovered that gentle relaxing and limbering exercises, in combination with ethyl chloride spray and 15 minutes of sinusoidal current, were an important follow-up to injection and notably improved the chances of success.

I was now aware of three types of muscle pain: muscle deficiency (weakness and stiffness), muscle spasm, and trigger points.

Between 1940 and 1946, at the Posture Clinic at Columbia Presbyterian Hospital in New York, Dr. Sonya Weber and I developed a test chart to appraise faulty posture and scoliosis.[13] This chart included six tests for strength and flexibility of key posture muscles. In 1946, we used these so-called Kraus-Weber tests to evaluate patients in a multidisciplinary back clinic organized by Dr. Barbara Stimson at the same hospital. Eighty-two percent of the 3,000 back patients we saw in the clinic had no pathologic condition;[3] their back pain was of postural or muscular origin. These patients often turned out to be deficient in one or more of the six key posture muscles. An exercise program aimed at correcting these deficiencies obtained satisfactory results.[8] I was now even more convinced of the value of properly prescribed therapeutic exercise.

Since back pain was endemic in the United States, we wondered how children would fare on the Kraus-Weber tests. Although children rarely suffer from backache, the unfitness of their trunk muscles seemed to prognosticate future problems. Accordingly, we examined 5,000 youngsters between 5 and 16 years of age. Almost 60% failed one or more of the tests.[15] This result seemed to explain the frequency of back pain among adults.

To verify these facts, we traveled to Europe in 1951 to test 1,000 children each in Switzerland, Austria, and Italy. We selected these countries because at that time they had a much smaller incidence of back pain than the United States. Fewer than 10% failed the tests.[15] In fact, none failed more than one of the six components of the test, whereas our children frequently failed two or three components. Our children were better nourished but sat much more than their European counterparts, who had to walk everywhere. The American children spent more time watching television than engaging in active play. Schools concentrated their physical education efforts on sports and games that involved the fittest children while neglecting the others.

When President Eisenhower was informed of the unfit condition of American children, he established the President's Council on Youth Fitness, since renamed the President's Council on Physical Fitness and Sports.

We found the same kind of sedentary lifestyle in our adult back pain population, who were also exposed to tension-creating stress. Suppression of the normal biological fight-or-flight response[1] meant that people had no physical release for stress. Tension thus appeared to form another link in the pathogenesis of myofascial pain. We recognized tension as the fourth important cause of muscle pain. The absence of a normal response to stress and the role of underexercise in the development of balanced physiology became important aspects of our approach to treating myofascial pain.

Myofascial back and neck pain may frequently be one indication of hypokinetic disease (disease produced by stress and lack of exercise).[18] It has been shown that duodenal ulcers, coronary heart disease, overweight, diabetes, and emotional problems may be due, at least in part, to the imbalance between stress and physical release.[18]

It is obvious that injections alone will not help a person who has no physical outlet, exhibits weakness and stiffness of key postural muscles, and leads a tension-filled life. A concerted effort is required to manage muscle deficiency with exercise and to manage tension in various ways: with relaxation exercise, medication, biofeedback, and psychiatry, where needed. A patient's lifestyle, working posture, and physical activities may require modification.

Injecting trigger points is important in chronic cases. The use of surface anesthesia (cold) and gentle motion is essential for breaking spasm in the acute phase. In chronic cases, all four types of myofascial pain may be present. The patient may present with acute muscle spasm. When spasm is relieved, we may find trigger points, muscle deficiency, tension, or any combination of these. We then proceed with trigger point injections, exercises directed at muscle deficiency, and relaxation. Merely relieving pain is simplistic. Any treatment which does not include specific exercises and relaxation training and fails to modify pathogenic activities and lifestyle will yield only temporary results.

TREATMENT

The best way of treating muscle deficiency, which is the diminution of strength or flexibility, or both, is with exercise. Exercise is also an essential element in treating tension, muscle spasm, and the aftereffects of trigger point injection.

Exercise is the most effective and frequently needed modality in managing myofascial pain. Unfortunately, it is prescribed cavalierly. Few physicians know the basic principles of exercise. Even fewer are familiar with the details.

When properly prescribed and executed, exercise can be a very important therapeutic agent. It deserves the same careful attention as prescribing medication. This includes the correct indication, type, and quality of exercise. No physician would consider prescribing "heart medicine" as such, and yet therapeutic exercise is often prescribed as "back exercise" and its execution left haphazardly to a therapist. Therapists are frequently trained to give a standard set of exercises to all comers, regardless of the complaint.

In order to prescribe exercise properly, one has to evaluate the patient's individual needs. This is achieved by testing strength and flexibility.[10] The basic qualities of muscle function are contraction, strength, and flexibility. Flexibility consists of two parts: (1) physiologic elasticity, i.e., the ability to relax, give up tension, and decontract; and (2) mechanical elasticity, i.e., yielding to active or passive stretch.

How can muscle strength be gauged? For the extremities we advocate the old Lovett[21] approach, which is still useful and does not require any machines. The Lovett scale tests 0, if the muscle cannot contract at all; 1, if it can contract but cannot produce movement; 2, if it can contract and move with assistance; 3, if it can move against gravity and minimal resistance; 4, if it can overcome gravity and increased resistance to 70% of normal function; and 5, if it has full strength in comparison with the contralateral side or the patient's previous ability.

To assess strength and flexibility of key posture muscles, we use the Kraus-Weber tests[13, 14] (see Figs 12–1,A–F). The most common findings in back problems are stiffness of back and hamstring muscles and weakness of abdominal muscles.

To test total flexibility of a joint, we first appraise the patient's ability to relax. When the patient has relaxed as much as possible, we ask him or her to extend the joint to full range. We measure the excursion with a goniometer. In the Kraus-Weber tests, we gauge flexibility by noting the difference between the spontaneous floor reach and the floor reach after the patient is told not to try hard but to let go. The increased reach correlates with tension.

There are two types of strengthening exercises: anisometric and isometric.[6, 20] In anisometric exercise, the patient goes through the full range of motion. This means contracting or gradually lengthening against weight or resistance. Anisometric exercises are the most frequently used exercises, especially gradual shortening against resistance (concentric contraction). In isometric exercise, the muscle is tightened against resistance but without movement. Isometric exercises can be useful as part of a program, but should never be attempted without warm-up, relaxation, and stretching before and after.

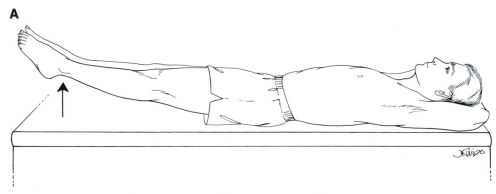

A

FIG 12–1.   **A,** the patient is supine, hands behind the neck, and legs extended with the knees straight. The patient is asked to lift both feet 10 in. off the table, holding that position for 10 seconds. This is a test for hip flexor muscles. **B,** test no. 2 is a test for hip flexors and abdominal muscles. Keeping the hands behind the neck, the patient is asked to roll up to a sitting position, with the legs straight, and the ankles held down. The *arrow* indicates the point at which the patient's body is stabilized by another person. **C,** this is a test for the abdominal muscles. With the patient in the supine position, hands behind the neck, with knees flexed, the examiner holds the patient's feet down on the table (indicated by *arrow*). The patient is asked to "roll up to a sitting position." **D,** test for upper back muscles. Lying prone with a pillow under the hips, the hands behind the neck and the feet and hips held down, the patient is asked to raise the trunk and hold for 10 seconds. *Arrows* indicate point at which the patient's body is stabilized by another person. **E,** with the patient in the same position as in D, the examiner holds the shoulders and hips down (indicated by *arrows*). The patient is asked to raise both legs and hold for 10 seconds. This tests the muscles of the lower back. **F,** this is a test for muscle flexibility and muscle tension. With the patient standing erect with the feet together, the knees extended, and his hands at his sides, he is asked to try to touch the floor with the fingertips. If the patient cannot touch the floor he is asked to try again, this time being asked to relax, drop the head forward, and try to let the torso "hang" from the hips. The patient is told not to try hard but to let go. The increased reach on the second attempt correlates with the presence of muscle tension.

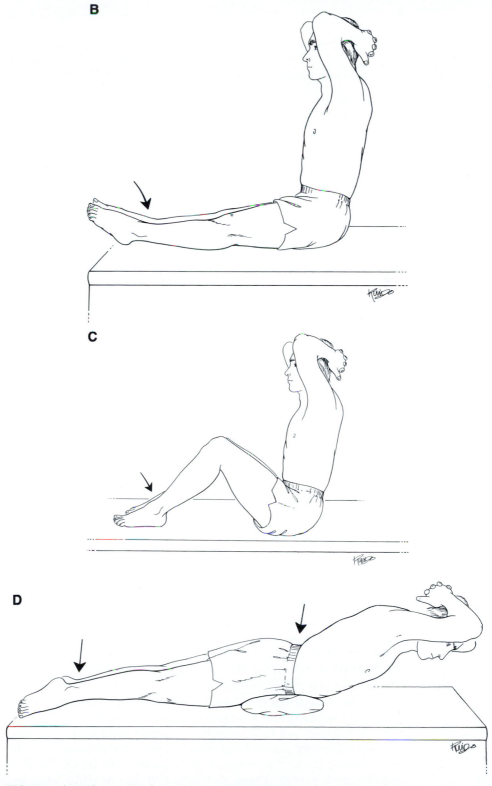

FIG 12–1 (cont.).   —For legend see opposite page.

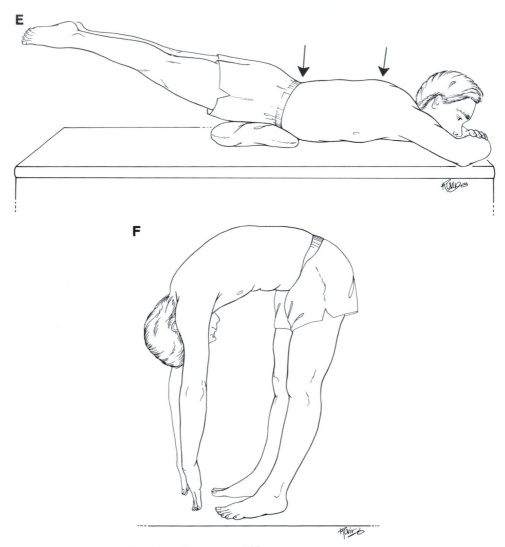

FIG 12–1 (cont.). — For legend see page 388.

We always give the muscle sufficient rest between movements. In the case of the extremities, we first have the patient warm up with general exercises for the whole extremity, then concentrate on the muscle group that needs strengthening. We never give multirepetitions but have the patient perform various movements in turn. If the extremity is weak, we work each muscle group three or four times, then proceed to the next group, and the next, before returning to the first. When we notice that the patient is beginning to tire, we stop. Gradually we add more demanding exercises.

In our back program,[11] we try to alternate prone and supine exercises in which, by working the antagonists, we give the muscles alternate chances to rest. Here again, we limit ourselves to three repetitions at a time.

The successful possibilities of such a program are evidenced by the "Y's Way to a Healthy Back"[22] program, which we devised in 1972 and which operated until December 1986. These exercises were intended to address the main deficiencies seen in our population at the Columbia Presbyterian Hospital's back clinic.[9] The program included strengthening abdominal muscles and limbering, relaxing, and stretching back muscles and hamstrings. In a one-on-one situation in private practice, we add further exercises, if needed. For example, we may work at strengthening upper or lower back muscles, although these muscles are seldom weak enough to require such exercises.

Thanks to the work of its organizer, Mr. Alexander Melleby, the "Y's Way to a Healthy Back" was eventually offered in a thousand YMCAs and YWCAs throughout the country. Six thousand physical educators were trained in a program that developed trainers as well as exercise instructors. All were taught to give the same exercises in a standardized way. At its height, the program functioned in the United States, Canada, Japan, Taiwan, and Australia.

The results of these original exercises were reviewed in a study of 11,809 participants,[17] who were tested with the Kraus-Weber tests before and after taking part. Of these, 80.7% said they felt better after completing the exercise series, which consisted of two sessions a week for 6 weeks.

Unfortunately, when Mr. Melleby retired, his successors found it necessary to alter the exercises and to leave out some essential movements and alternating positions. The program was gradually used less and less. In my opinion it cannot be as effective as the original program.

When administering strengthening exercises, we must be aware of just how much the patient can tolerate. While it is necessary to give an "overload,"[5] i.e., somewhat more than the patient can accomplish easily, working to fatigue is contraindicated.

Peder Palmen[23] showed that fatigue exercises for healthy young athletes result in declining performance. Improvement takes place only after 4 days of exercise during which performance decreases. If you put a patient's weak muscles onto a similar regimen, he or she will not be able to perform at all and will require a few days of rest, after which you will have to start all over again. If the same process is repeated, the same result will occur. In other words, in order to strengthen a weak muscle, we have to increase our demands gradually instead of working to maximum capacity. This precept is often overlooked.

In the case of patients who have had a leg encased in plaster following surgery or injury to knee or ankle, the muscles tend to be quite weak. Nonetheless, patients are often instructed to walk as much as possible. The result is stiffness, pain, and the frequent development of trigger points.

Before addressing flexibility, we must first treat the tension that is inherent to some degree in almost everyone. For this reason, we begin all flexibility exercises with relaxation. Next, we treat mechanical flexibility by stretching the muscle, first actively, by using the antagonists to gain full range, and then passively, by stretching the muscle gently. Before giving passive stretch, we often use "reflex relaxation,"[24] giving resistance to the antagonist of the tight muscle. For example, we give resistance to extensors, which causes the flexors to relax, or vice versa. Reflex relaxation increases muscle range. When the patient cannot go beyond that range, the therapist helps with passive stretching.

Passive stretching or violent active stretching without prior relaxation and warm-up can lead to muscle strain and diminished range. Just as we do not work to full capacity in our strengthening exercises, we do not attempt to obtain maximum range in our flexibility treatment. Maximum stretch will cause discomfort and result in limited rather than increased range. The basic rule is never to exceed existing pain limits. In stretching, however, we sometimes have to raise the pain threshold by using cold (ethyl chloride spray or ice).

After the patient has been fully rehabilitated, he or she should continue therapeutic exercises, to which can be added more strenuous physical activities like swimming, fast walking, bicycling, or jogging. Demanding exercises have a relaxing effect that can be measured by electromyogram. De Vries and Adams[2] have shown that exercises which raise the heartbeat to 100 or 120 beats/min produce greater relaxation than 500 mg of meprobamate.

The most common mistakes incurred in prescribing therapeutic exercises are the following:[11, 12]

1. Prescribing a program without previous muscle testing.
2. Omitting warm-up and cool-down exercises, which should include relaxing and limbering.
3. Handing out an exercise sheet, thereby leaving the entire treatment to the patient.
4. Giving multirepetition exercises.
5. Prescribing isometric exercises as the main part of the program, without stressing relaxation and stretching of the same muscle groups.
6. Giving too many or too strenuous exercises instead of gradually adding more demanding ones.
7. Doing the exercises in rapid succession without relaxing between movements.
8. Omitting the home program, which the patient should perform daily.
9. Discharging the patient too soon, i.e., before he or she is fully capable of resuming all normal activities. This means strengthening the muscles far above their minimal ability.

One back patient whom we saw had a job which required him to lift 200-lb weights. After treatment, his lifting ability was only 100 lbs. His insurance carrier insisted against our advice that he return to work and that he perform weightlifting exercises until he regained his former strength. After a few weeks, the patient returned with the same injury.

In treating acute muscle spasm, we give the first three or four exercises of the respective program (back, shoulder, neck, etc.), while relieving pain with electrotherapy and ethyl chloride spray. We have the patient perform these exercises frequently at home, using ice. We avoid bed rest and immobilization whenever possible.

The following is a list of exercises we have used for many years, first in rehabilitation fracture patients at the Vienna University Medical School, later in treating posture and back patients at Columbia Presbyterian Hospital with Dr. Barbara Stimson, and in over 50 years of private practice.

Exercise for the Extremities

In the acute phase: Perform only the first two or three exercises, using ice or ethyl chloride spray. Gradually increase the number and intensity of exercises.

In the chronic phase: Always relax between movements. Provide resistance to antagonists in order to achieve reflex relaxation. Stretch gently, always within pain limits.

Begin all exercises with relaxation. Have the patient lie on his or her back with a pillow under the knees (Fig 12–2). Tell the patient to close the eyes, take a

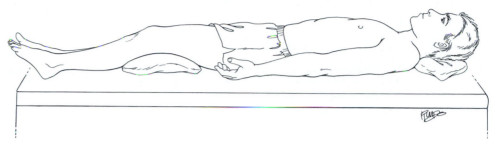

FIG 12–2.

deep breath, exhale slowly, drop the head to the left, then to the right, pull up the shoulders, and let go. Continue until the patient is relaxed. Perform the first four relaxation exercises of the neck program.

Exercises should be performed no more than three times in succession, with rest between each movement. Perform each series in sequence, forward and backward, several times. *The most frequent mistakes are:*

- Starting antigravity exercises before the patient is adequately strengthened.
- Giving too strenuous resistance or stretching.
- Using wall climbing or pendulum exercises (the latter are insufficient to increase range or strength).
- Omitting relaxation.
- Giving isometric exercises alone, without the full program.

Exercises for the Upper Extremities

Shoulder. The first five exercises should first be performed lying down, then sitting up.

1. Close the fist, touch the shoulder, and extend and unclench the fist (Fig 12–3).
2. With hands on chest, abduct, sliding the elbows upward, and then bring them back to the original position (Fig 12–4).
3. Extend arm straight up, bring it down, and relax (Fig 12–5).
4. Bring the arm across the chest and return to the starting position (Fig 12–6).
5. Join hands, bring them down, forward the legs, and raise the arms above the head (Fig 12–7).

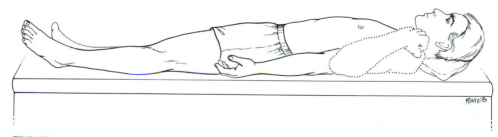

FIG 12–3.

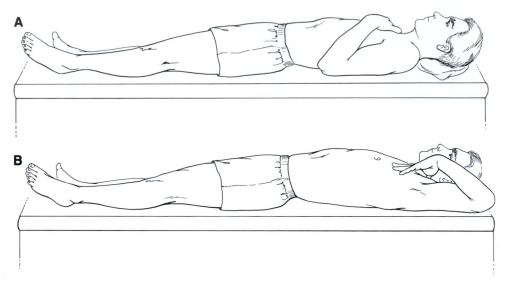

FIG 12–4.

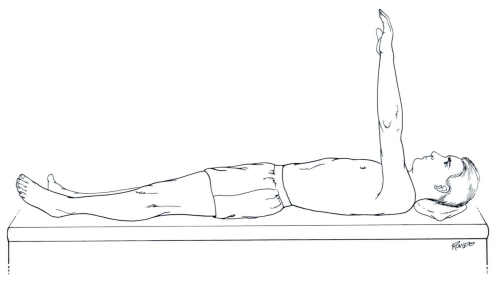

FIG 12–5.

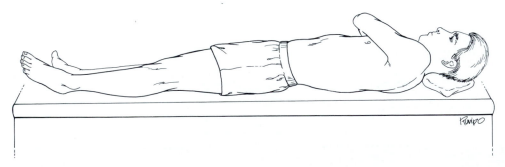

FIG 12–6.

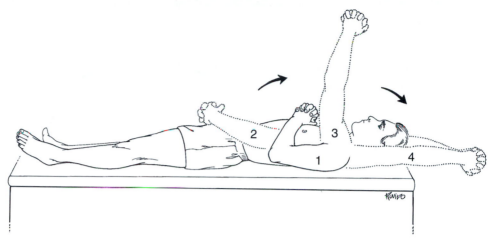

FIG 12–7.

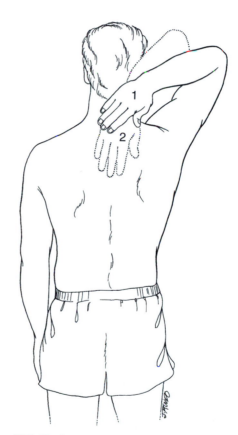

FIG 12–8.

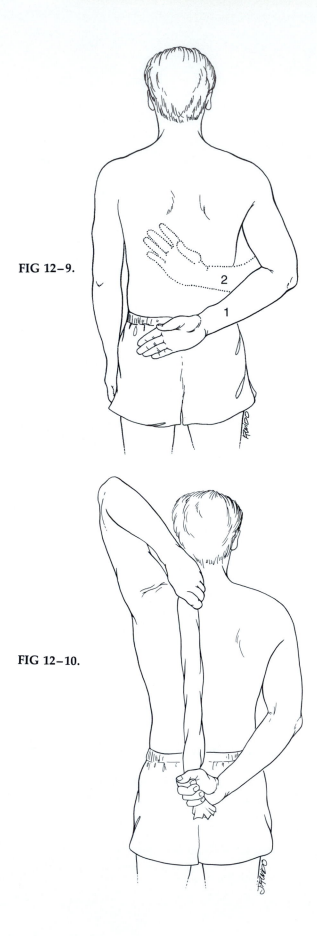

FIG 12–9.

FIG 12–10.

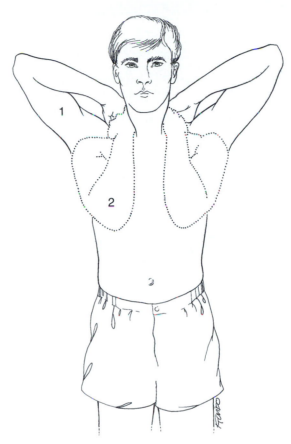

FIG 12–11.

The following exercises should be performed sitting up or standing:

6. Touch the back of the neck reaching down as far as possible (Fig 12–8).
7. Touch the lower back and slide the hand up as far as possible (Fig 12–9).
8. Continue the previous exercise by pulling the hand up with the help of the injured arm or by pulling the end of a towel (Fig 12–10).
9. Fold the arms behind the neck and bring the elbows back. Bring elbows forward, then relax (Fig 12–11).

Elbow. Use shoulder exercises as warm-up. All exercises are first performed lying down, then sitting or standing:

10. Bend and extend the elbow with the palm facing up and then with the palm facing down (Fig 12–12).
11. Bring the hand across the chest to the opposite shoulder; turn out, turn in (Fig 12–13).
12. To stretch elbow flexors, join hands, raise to shoulder height, pronate, and extend as far as possible, using the good hand to increase range (Fig 12–14).

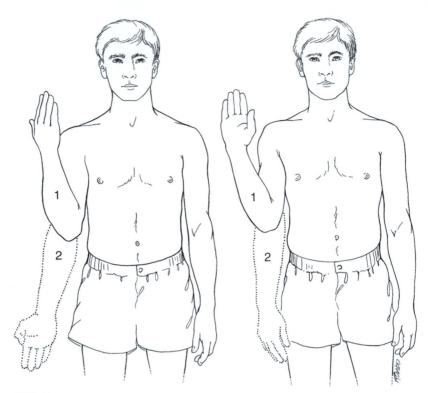

FIG 12–12.

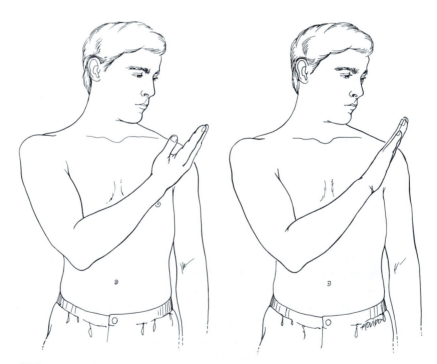

FIG 12–13.

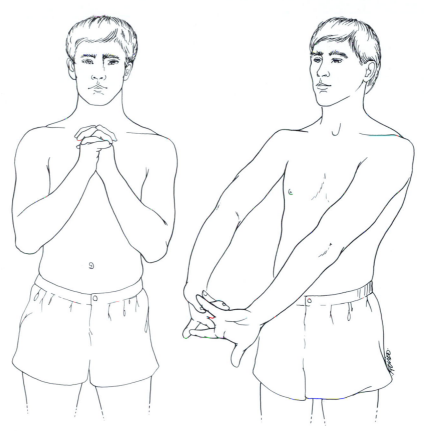

FIG 12–14.

Wrist and Hand.   Use shoulder and elbow exercises as warm-up. The following exercises may be performed sitting.

13. Flex and extend the wrist over the edge of a table or pillow.
14. Use exercise 11 for supination and pronation.
15. Close and open the fist, first with the thumb inside the fingers, then with the thumb outside.
16. Spread and close the fingers.
17. Knead clay or putty to increase the strength of the flexors.

Exercises for the Lower Extremities
Begin with relaxation exercises (exercises 50–53), as above. Perform each exercise in a sequence of three. At first, while there is discomfort and the leg is weak, all lower extremity exercises should be done lying down. Slide the leg along the surface in the beginning. Later, lift against gravity. As the patient gets stronger, use the entire exercise program as a warm-up and follow with specific exercises and gradually increasing resistance. Lastly, use weights for work at home.

Hip

18. Lying on the back, bring the knee to the chest, then straighten out. Relax (Fig 12–15,A).

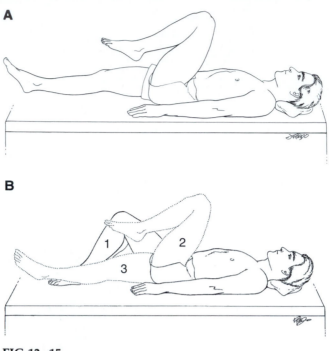

FIG 12–15.

19. Lying on the back with the knees flexed, bring the knee to the chest, slide to full extension, and return to the flexed position. Alternate with the other knee (Fig 12–15,B).
20. Perform the same movement while lying on the side. Alternate legs (Fig 12–16).
21. Prone, tighten buttocks, and relax (Fig 12–17).
22. Again supine, abduct and adduct extending the legs (Fig 12–18).
23. Supine, with knee flexed, abduct and adduct (Fig 12–19).
24. Lying on the side, abduct with a straight leg, lower it, and relax (Fig 12–20).
25. Lying on the side, abduct with flexed knee.

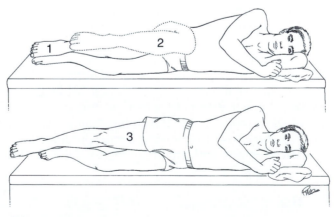

FIG 12–16.

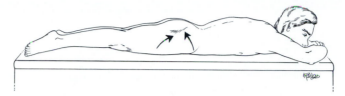

FIG 12–17.

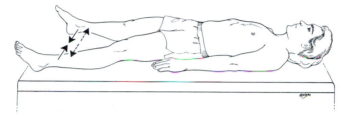

FIG 12–18.

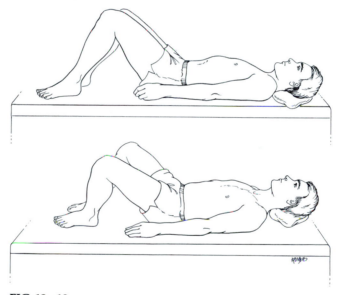

FIG 12–19.

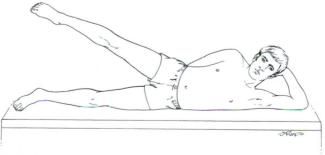

FIG 12–20.

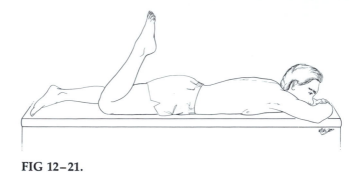

FIG 12–21.

The last two exercises should be performed with a therapist's assistance. The patient should not attempt them at home until he or she can do so without strain or discomfort. The following four exercises are all performed prone.

26. Flex and extend the knee (Fig 12–21).
27. Flex knees and rotate hips out and in (Fig 12–22).
28. Flex the knee and lift the leg (Fig 12–23).
29. Repeat exercise 28, with the knee extended.
30. Sitting with the legs hanging over the edge of the table, with the good leg resting on the floor or a stool, bring the affected knee to the chest, bring the leg down, and relax (Fig 12–24).
31. Sitting in the same position, extend the knee fully. Keep foot outwardly rotated in order to strengthen the vastus medialis (Fig 12–25).

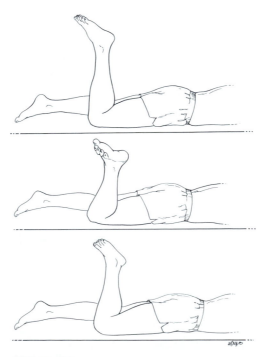

FIG 12–22.

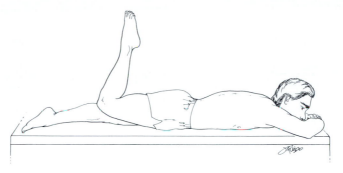

FIG 12–23.

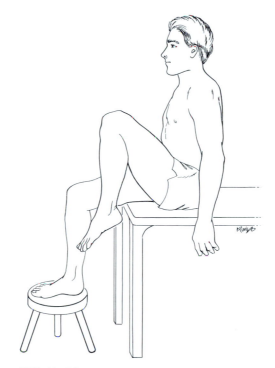

FIG 12–24.

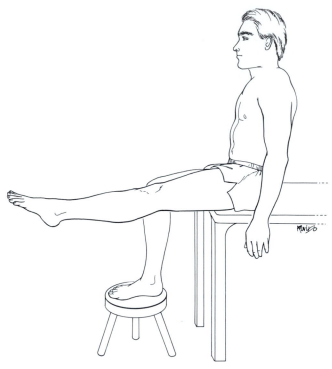

FIG 12–25.

Knee

32a. Supine, gently bend and extend the injured knee (Fig 12–26).
32b. Supine with the knees flexed, extend the knee, and flex back to the starting position (Fig 12–27).
32c. Supine, with the knees flexed, bring the knee to the chest, extend, and return to flexed position.
33. With a pillow under the knee, extend the leg (Fig 12–28).
34. Tighten quadriceps and let go.
35. Prone, flex and extend the knee (see Fig 12–21).
36. Supine, do bicycle stretch. Bring knee to chest, extend toward ceiling, stretch out, and slowly return to the flexed position. Do this first with the toes pointed, then with the heel first (Fig 12–29).
37. Sitting with the legs hanging over the edge of the table, with the good leg supported, extend the knee. Hold foot in outward rotation. The patient may add weights when flexibility is achieved and the pain is gone (see Fig 12–25).

    Isometric exercises:
38. Supine, with the leg straight and outwardly rotated (held down by the therapist or by a heavy piece of furniture), tighten the quadriceps and attempt to raise the leg against resistance. Hold for 10 seconds and release.
39. Repeat exercise 38, holding the leg extended for 10 seconds against resistance.

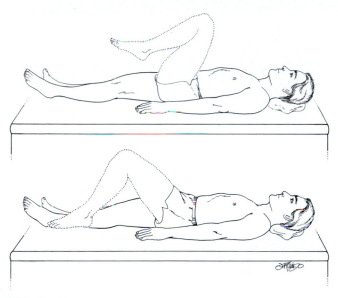

FIG 12–26.

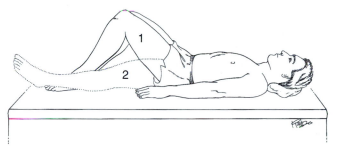

FIG 12–27.

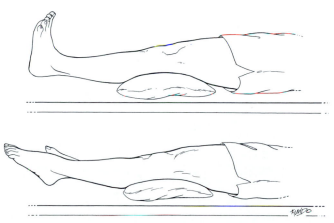

FIG 12–28.

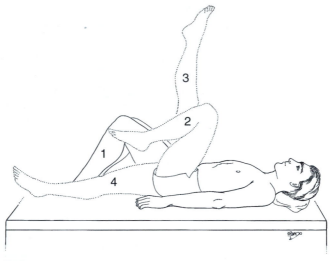

FIG 12–29.

Ankle

40. Supine, with the knees straight, dorsiflex and plantarflex ankle.
41. Repeat, with the knees flexed.
42. With the knees straight, pronate and supinate (Fig 12–30,A).
43. Sitting with the legs hanging over the edge of the table, dorsiflex and plantarflex.

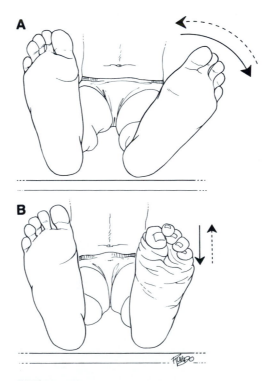

FIG 12–30.

44. Repeat, with pronation and supination.
45. Flex and extend the toes (Fig 12–30,B).

The following four exercises are performed standing:

46. Holding on to the table, stand on toes and increase lifting body weight as tolerated (Fig 12–31).
47. Holding on to the table, bend the knees, keeping the heels on the floor.
48. Holding on to a table or leaning against a wall, with heels on floor, lean forward from the hips (Fig 12–32).
49. Stand on the outside, then on the inside, of the foot, holding on to a table if necessary.

The most common mistakes in lower extremity exercises are:

• Permitting walking and weightbearing when these cause pain or limping.
• Administering antigravity exercises too soon.
• Performing multirepetition straight leg raises, which can produce backache and tight quadriceps.

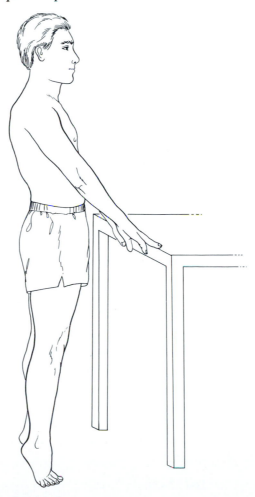

FIG 12–31.

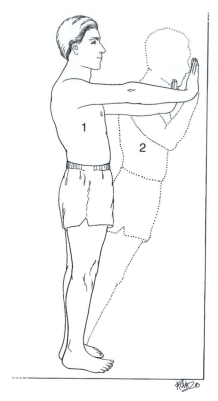

FIG 12–32.

Neck Exercises

The basic position is supine with the knees flexed. Exercises should always be done slowly, with rest between movement. No exercise is performed more than three times in succession. The exercise order is reversed as a cool-down.

50. The patient, positioned comfortably in the supine position with the knees flexed, takes a deep breath and exhales slowly with the eyes closed. Slide one leg out and slide it back, alternating legs. Tighten both fists, then let go and take another deep breath. Bring up the shoulders and let go. Breathe in when shrugging up, exhale when letting go of the shrug. Drop the head to the left, return to the normal position, then permit the head to drop to the right. Repeat until completely relaxed (Fig 12–33).

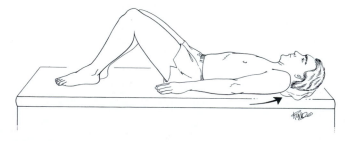

FIG 12–33.

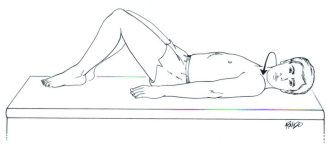

FIG 12–34.

51. Turn the head to the left, return to a normal position in front followed by rotation to the right, returning to the normal front and center position (Fig 12–34).
52. Tilt the head to the left, then to the right.
53. Pull the shoulder blades together; relax.

Repeat the above movements sitting up. In addition, flex and extend the neck. Add gentle passive and active stretching, first supine, then sitting.

Back Exercises*

54. Perform the first four relaxation exercises of the neck program.
55. Supine, with the knees flexed, bring the knee to the chest, extend, and return to the flexed position. When extending the leg the foot is returned to the floor permitting the leg to slide out and slide back (see Fig 12–15,B).
56. Repeat, alternately lying on either side. Remember to slide the leg when it is extended. Do not tense the top leg. The leg should be "dead weight" (see Fig 12–16).
57. Prone, tighten buttocks and relax (see Fig 12–17).
58. In the basic position, bring both knees to the chest, then return to the basic position. Do not raise the hips off the floor (Fig 12–35).
59. On hands and knees, arch back, then collapse to swayback position ("cat back") (Fig 12–36).

*A videotape, *Say Goodbye to Back Pain,* including neck exercises, is available by calling 1-800-383-8811.

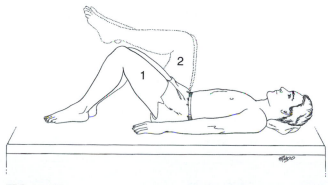

FIG 12–35.

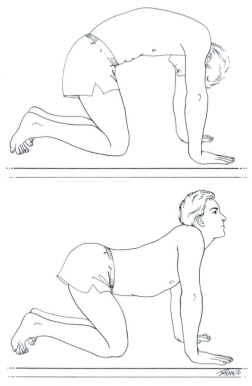

FIG 12–36.

60. In the basic position, raise the head and shoulders reaching toward the knees. Perform the exercise slowly. Relax (Fig 12–37).
61. Kneeling with the forearms resting on a plinth, slowly slide hands forward, stretching the pectoral muscles. Maintain the thighs perpendicular to the floor (Fig 12–38).
62. Sitting on the edge of a table or chair with the feet on the floor or a stool, slowly drop the head and arms between the legs. Return to the upright position and relax (Fig 12–39).
63. In the basic position, with the feet held down, slowly curl up to a sitting position. If the patient has weak abdominal muscles, begin with the hands along the sides. Later, the hands can be crossed over the stomach, then over the chest, and lastly behind the neck (Fig 12–40).
64. Sitting as in exercise 62, twist the trunk to the left, dropping the head and arms, and then straighten up and repeat to the right (Fig 12–41).
65. Bicycle stretch: Bring the knee to the chest, extend toward the ceiling,

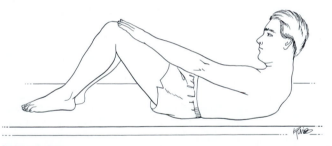

FIG 12–37.

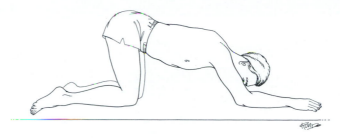

FIG 12–38.

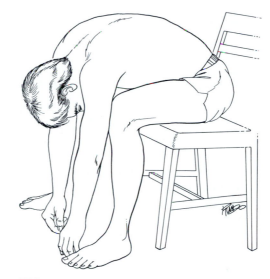

FIG 12–39.

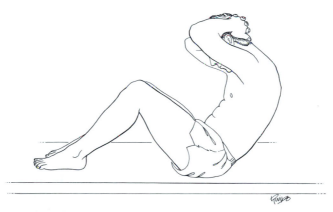

FIG 12–40.

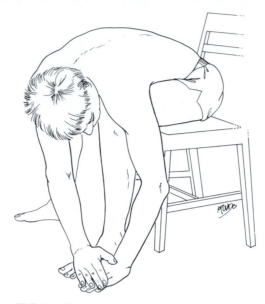

FIG 12–41.

stretch out, and return to the flexed position, first with the toes pointed, then with the heel first (see Fig 12–29).

66. Straight leg stretch: From the basic position, straighten the leg, raise as high as possible, lower, and return to the basic position. Do this first with pointed toes, then with the ankle in dorsiflexion (Fig 12–42).

67. Standing with the hands joined behind the back and the arms straight, slowly bend forward as far as possible from the waist until you feel stretching in the back of the legs. Keep your back and neck straight when bending forward from the hips (Fig 12–43).

68. Calf muscle stretch: Holding on to a table or leaning against a wall, with the heels on the floor, lean forward from the hips (see Fig 12–32).

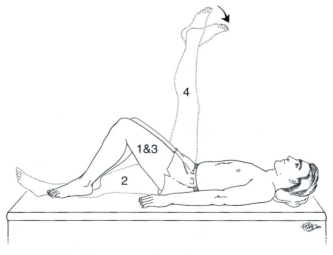

FIG 12–42.

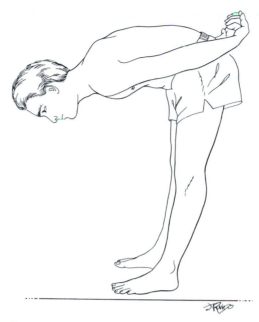

FIG 12–43.

69. Standing with the feet together and the knees straight, slowly reach toward the floor (see Fig 12–1,F).

These standard exercises will suffice in most cases. If the Kraus-Weber tests show weakness of the upper or lower back, the following exercises should be added to the previous program:

Lower Back Weakness

70. Lying prone with a pillow under the hips, raise and lower each leg in turn, relaxing between movements.
71. When stronger, in the same position as exercise 70, raise both legs simultaneously, lower them and relax (see Fig 12–1,E).

Upper Back Weakness

72. Prone with a pillow under the hips, raise the arms and shoulders; lower them and relax. Repeat with the other arm (Fig 12–1,D).
73. In the same position as exercise 72, with the legs stabilized, raise the head, shoulders, and upper back while the arms are held alongside the body. Relax. When stronger, perform the same movement with the hands clasped behind the neck.

In acute cases of back pain, begin with exercises 54 through 57, gradually adding others as tolerated. Always keep within pain limits. The *most frequent mistakes are:*

- Neglecting relaxation.
- Omitting warm-up and cool-down.
- Giving multirepetition exercises.

- Giving too many exercises too soon, or giving exercises that are too demanding.
- Handing out written exercise sheets instead of teaching and monitoring the patient.
- Forgetting to use ice or ethyl chloride to relieve discomfort.

REFERENCES

1. Cannon WB: *Bodily changes in pain, hunger, fear and rage,* ed 2, New York, 1929, Appleton-Century-Crofts.
2. DeVries HA, Adams GM: Electromyographic comparison of single doses of exercise and meprobamate as to effect of muscular relaxation.
3. Gaston S, Personal communication, 1946.
4. Glogowsky G, Wallraff J: Ein Beltrag zur Klinik und Histologie der Muskelhärten (Myogelosen), *Z Orthop* 80:237–268, 1951.
5. Hellbrandt FA: Application of the overload principle to muscle training in man, *Am J Phys Med* 35:278–283, 1958.
6. Hettinger T, Muler EA: Muskelleistung und Muskeltraining, *Arbeltsphysiologie* 15:111–126, 1953.
7. Kraus H: New treatment for injured joints (abstract), *JAMA* 104:1261, 1935.
8. Kraus H: Use of surface anesthesia in the treatment of painful motion, *JAMA* 116:2582–2583, 1941.
9. Kraus H: Diagnosis and treatment of low back pain, *Gen Pract* 5:55–60, 1952.
10. Kraus H: *Therapeutic exercise,* Springfield, Ill, 1963, Charles C Thomas.
11. Kraus H: *Clinical treatment of back and neck pain,* New York, 1970, McGraw-Hill.
12. Kraus H, editor: *Diagnosis and treatment of muscle pain,* Chicago, 1988, Quintessence.
13. Kraus H, Eisenmenger-Weber S: Quantitative tabulation of postural evaluation (report), *Physiother Rev* 26:235–242, 1946.
14. Kraus H, Eisenmenger-Weber S: Fundamental considerations of postural exercises, *Physiother Rev* 27:361–368, 1947.
15. Kraus H, Hirschland RP: Minimum muscular fitness tests in school children, *Res Q* 25:178–188, 1954.
16. Kraus H, Mahoney JW: Fracture Rehabilitation. In Covalt DA, editor: *Rehabilitation in industry,* New York, 1958, Grune & Stratton.
17. Kraus H, Nagler W, Melleby Al: Evaluation of an exercise program for back pain, *Fam Physician,* 28:153–158, 1983.
18. Kraus H, Raab W: *Hypokinetic disease—Diseases produced by lack of exercise,* Springfield, Ill, 1961, Charles C Thomas.
19. Lange M: *Die Muskelhärten (Myogelosen),* Munich, 1931, Lehmann.
20. Liberson WT: Brief isometric exercises. In Basmajian JV, editor: *Therapeutic exercise,* ed 4, Baltimore, 1984, Williams & Wilkins.
21. Lovett RW: *The treatment of infantile paralysis,* Philadelphia, 1916, Lea & Febiger.
22. Melleby A: *The Y's way to a healthy back,* Piscataway, NJ, 1982, New Century.
23. Palmen P: Über die Bedeutung der Nährung für die Erholung der Leistungsfähigkeit der Muskeln, *Scand Arch Physiol* 24:174, 1911.
24. Sherrington CS: Reciprocal innervation of antagonist muscles: 14th note on double reciprocal innervation, *Proc R Soc Lond [Biol]* 81:249–268, 1909.
25. Steindler A: *Lectures on the interpretation of pain in orthopedic practice,* Springfield, Ill, 1959, Charles C Thomas.

Chapter 13

Manual Therapy Treatment of Myofascial Pain and Dysfunction

Brian Miller, P.T.

According to Lewit, "The structure in the motor system that reacts most to stimuli and is the effector of the nervous system is the muscle. As a result, it is also the structure that most regularly and intensively expresses pain."[37] In other words, myofascial tissue, partly owing to its dynamic and mutable nature, is highly susceptible to dysfunction and pain. This, fortunately, also makes it highly amenable to positive change via physical means of treatment, specifically orthopedic manual therapy. The exact nature of the pathologic changes in myofascial tissues has not been elucidated. There appears to be no simple answer and possibly a complex combination of factors is involved. This area is certainly one in urgent need of further research. We can, however, speculate about various hypothetical mechanisms of myofascial pain and dysfunction (MPD) and how they may relate to management of the problem.

These mechanisms can be categorized in various ways but I have found three main classifications helpful. This chapter is in no way offered as a comprehensive or scientifically exacting investigation of this area but provides a modicum of organization for directing future study.

The first category includes biomechanical influences. These range from simple mechanical inefficiency to actual muscle and connective tissue changes. Mechanical inefficiency can result from intratissue as well as intertissue and extratissue sources. Intratissue sources include increased muscle tension levels which can include tension increases from passive sources such as increased muscle edema[58] and also from active sources such as excessive muscle tonus (as indicated by elevated electromyographic [EMG] activity)[21] associated with dysponesis.[60] Intertissue sources involve increased friction or drag between adjacent structures (or even actual adherences) which are manifested in decreased layer mobility or decreased muscle play as defined by Johnson.[27] Myofascial tissue changes can include tissue dehydration (as occurs in many aging connective tissues), tissue or collagen creep (as occurs with diminished or absent movement), sources of tethering ranging from the microlevel (e.g., collagen cross-linking) to the macrolevel (e.g., posttraumatic scarring), and other constituent changes (e.g., alterations in the extracellular matrix, ground substance, etc.). These changes range from microscopic ultrastructural changes to macroscopic morphologic changes. Extratissue sources are discussed below.

The second category includes neurophysiologic influences. This category can include reflex action, cyclic stereotyped action, and habitual, conditioned action.[14] At the reflex level, such well-known reflexes as the stretch reflex or the Golgi tendon organ (GTO) reflex may be involved. Also, less well-known "reflexes" may be involved (which may possibly be classified as cyclic stereotyped action) such as the protective arthrokinematic reflex[3, 63] and the startle pattern.[52] Overlapping with this area are both conscious and unconscious aspects of instinctive and learned behavior. Since the musculature of the body is a primary means of emotional expression, emotional and cognitive states can have a profound influence upon neuromuscular behavior and contribute to MPD.

The third category involves fluidochemical influences. This category includes micro- and macrocirculatory changes affecting fluidochemical transport and exchange (such as altered chemical exchange on the cellular level, impaired lymphatic flow, vascular stasis or ischemia, etc.). Rolf[46] discussed changes in the chemical state of the muscle from a gel to a solid state, a hypothesis which has been shown to be invalid, yet which may offer insights into the nature of change in myofascial tissues. Various chemical substances may influence myofascial tissue such as metabolites (both substrates and byproducts), electrolytes, hormones, neurotransmitters, neurogenic and non-neurogenic pain mediators, etc. One or more of these chemicals may be lacking, overabundant, or present in imbalanced qualities. Tsujii[58] has shown the relationship of mechanical stimulation of polymodal receptors to neurogenically based inflammatory and immunologic activity.

Electrochemical influences may be involved as well since most essential biological functions are comprised of biochemical and bioelectric phenomena such as membrane depolarization and repolarization (with the accompanying production of weak electromagnetic fields). The interactive nature of biological tissues and electromagnetic fields is a fascinating area which is just beginning to be studied and could yield valuable information related to MPD as well as many other areas in medicine. In addition, such phenomena as the piezoelectric effect are well known in the physical sciences and there may be a parallel phenomenon in biological tissues. A mechanism similar to this phenomenon could explain why practitioners can touch tissues in different ways utilizing differing therapeutic forces but still produce similar beneficial effects when the touching is performed with a clear intention and purpose. Certainly this is an area worthy of investigation.

Obviously, these different categories and the proposed hypothetical mechanisms are not mutually exclusive but involve significant interaction and overlap. Both the mechanically based intention of orthopedic manual therapies and the reeducational emphasis of neurologic manual therapies can operate through any number of the above-proposed mechanisms.

This lack of precise knowledge regarding pathologic changes in myofascial tissues does not preclude effective treatment, however. Maitland discusses "not allowing theoretical knowledge (which in fact may be quite false), or lack of it, to obstruct seeing and finding clinical facts."[39] A balance of both the science and the art of myofascially directed manual therapy is needed. While science, in the laboratory and clinic, provides the framework and guidelines for treatment, historically, a large majority of scientific discoveries have been in accordance with the adage that "empiricism adjusts the path of science behind it."[24] Maitland states that "there is much in medicine that is still unknown, and although precise diagnosis is not always possible, this need be no bar to precise, effective, and informative manipulative treatment . . . ."[39] Herein enters the art of treatment, which ultimately determines how successfully (or unsuccessfully) this information is utilized.

The particular approach discussed in this chapter is eclectic but based heavily upon the functional orthopedic perspective developed by Johnson[27] and also influenced by the recent research of Tsujii.[58]

EVALUATION

Although MPD is wide-reaching in its scope and influence and can involve virtually any region in the body, I have chosen to select illustrative examples from the cervical region (the upper cervical region in particular). This choice was made so as adapt this information to the practical limits imposed by the necessity of confining it to a single chapter. The reader should keep in mind that in no way does this selective presentation indicate that the author advocates a reductionist approach whereby a region of the body is evaluated and treated in isolation. On the contrary, unless the therapist adopts a systems-based approach and looks at whole-body functioning in relationship to the symptomatic or dysfunctional area, it is likely that the patient's full rehabilitation potential will not be attained and therapeutic benefits will be both incomplete and temporary.

Subjective

Subjective evaluation has been very thoroughly presented by others and extensive discussion here would be redundant. Nevertheless, it should be emphasized that a methodical and meticulous subjective examination will provide the clinician with the majority of information necessary to obtain an accurate clinical impression. One point that deserves special mention is the importance of tracing the patient's actions as thoroughly as possible through the entire course of a typical day (and night). This process is indispensable in uncovering the habitual positions, postures, activities, or movements that contribute to the patient's problem. An outline of key points in taking a history follows:

I. Type of onset.
    A. Sudden.
        1. Nontraumatic.
        2. Traumatic.
            a. Microtraumatic.
            b. Macrotraumatic.
    B. Gradual or insidious.
        1. When was it first noticeable? Problematic?
        2. What was the time frame of its development?
II. Occurrence.
    A. First time.
    B. Occurred previously (episodic).
        1. Sporadically.
        2. Predictably.

    C. Past occurrence.
        1. Course of the problem.
        2. Response to treatment.
        3. Recovery time.
III. Symptom location.
    A. Pain.
        1. Body chart.
        2. Quality of location.
            a. Localized or diffuse.
            b. Superficial or deep.
        3. Does it change distribution (size, depth, etc.)?
            a. Location at its worst.
            b. Location at its best.
    B. Dysesthesias.
    C. Other symptoms.
        1. Stiffness or immobility.
        2. Weakness.
        3. Swelling.
        4. Instability, giving way.
        5. Locking.
        6. Other.
IV. Nature of pain.
    A. Pain quality.
 V. Presence.
    A. Constant.
        1. Fixed intensity.
        2. Variable intensity.
    B. Intermittent.
        1. Duration when present.
        2. Frequency of appearance.
VI. Quantitative ranking of intensity (on an analog scale).
    A. In last 24 hours.
    B. Since problem began.
        1. At its best.
        2. At its worst.
VII. Influence of motion and position.
    A. Aggravating factors.
    B. Easing factors.
        1. Activity level.
            a. Rest.
            b. Prolonged postures.
            c. Activity.
                (1) Dosage—how much?
        2. Posture.
            a. Recumbent.
                (1) Supine.
                (2) Side-lying.
                (3) Prone.
                (4) Other.
            b. Sitting.

             (1) Unsupported or supported.
             (2) Slouched or upright.
        c. Standing.
     3. Movements.
        a. Transfers.
             (1) Rolling over in bed.
             (2) Lying-to-sitting.
             (3) Sitting-to-standing.
        b. Stairs.
        c. Squatting.
        d. Bending.
        e. Lifting.
        f. Carrying.
        g. Twisting.
        h. Reaching.
     4. Cough, sneeze.
 VIII. Rest factors.
    A. Sleeping position.
    B. Bed.
     1. Type of bed.
     2. Side slept on.
     3. Position relative to bed partner.
    C. Pillow.
     1. Composition of pillow.
     2. Number and thickness of pillows.
     3. Positioning of pillows.
    D. Sleep quality.
     1. How much sleep.
     2. Quality of sleep.
     3. How easy to fall asleep and wake up.
    E. Pre- and postsleep activities.
     1. Activities just prior to sleeping.
     2. How one wakes up first thing in the morning.
     3. Activities just after awakening.
  IX. State of health.
    A. General appraisal of health.
    B. Recent weight change.
     1. Explained (dieting, stress, etc.).
     2. Unexplained.
    C. Medications.
     1. Contraindications to manual therapy.
        a. Steroids.
        b. Anticoagulants.
    D. Night pain.
     1. None noticed.
     2. Pain provoked with position change but then allows patient to fall asleep again.
     3. Pain keeps patient awake but patient can stay in bed.
     4. Pain keeps patient awake and requires that patient periodically get out of bed to obtain relief.

X. Personal information.
   A. Age and weight.
   B. Family and social factors.
XI. Personal habits.
   A. Bowel and bladder function.
   B. Menstruation.
   C. Sex.
   D. Diet.
XII. Lifestyle.
   A. Occupation.
      1. Physical demands.
      2. Workplace design.
      3. Psychological demands.
   B. Recreation.
      1. Leisure activities.
      2. Sports, performing arts, etc.
XIII. Test results.
   A. Imaging tests—radiographs, computed tomography (CT), magnetic resonance (MR), bone scans, etc.
   B. Blood tests.
   C. Electrodiagnostic tests.
   D. Others.
XIV. General leading questions.
   A. Are you under any unusual stresses?[43]
   B. Is there anything else I should know about?

Some excellent references in this area include the works of Maitland[39] and McKenzie.[43] Although these monographs are intended for joint-oriented therapies, their principles apply to myofascially directed therapies as well. Maitland's discussion of communication is particularly noteworthy and merits special attention. Refined communication skills are of fundamental value in the management of any neuromusculoskeletal condition. One of the most well-known and respected clinicians in this area of patient-clinician communication was Milton Erickson. Although he practiced psychiatry, the principles which he developed and expounded upon are applicable to myofascial and other musculoskeletal problems.[14] It behooves both the novice and the experienced practitioner to study works written by and particularly about this consummately skilled physician.

Information more specifically related to myofascial disorders is provided by the classic works of Travell and Simons.[56, 57] In particular, the stereotypic patterns of local and referred pain from myofascial tissues which these authors documented should be noted during the subjective aspect of the evaluation. For example, myofascial dysfunction in the suboccipital muscles such as the rectus capitus posterior major may cause local pain in the posterior suboccipital region as well as pain referred from the occipital to the orbital region.

Objective

Objective findings are obtained through both visual and tactile-kinesthetic means. One observes the patient's static structure and observes as well as feels the quantity, and particularly, the quality of his or her movements.

Observation

The therapist observes the patient's skeletal and soft tissue structure. In observing skeletal structure, the therapist views the patient as if possessing "x-ray eyes," noting the skeletal orientation, alignment, and position from an impression of the underlying skeletal configuration and visible bony landmarks. The skeleton should be aligned so that a vertical plumb line would bisect the skeleton symmetrically when viewed in the frontal plane. Left-right symmetry relative to this central bisecting line should also be noted. While lack of symmetry is not necessarily indicative of myofascial dysfunction (since asymmetry tends to be the norm in the human body), myofascial dysfunction is often reflected in structural asymmetry.[22]

Laterally, the alignment of bony parts and joints should match up with those parameters that have been established by other authors for so-called good posture.[21] This alignment involves the center of gravity of each body part being aligned vertically above the one below it. In addition to optimal *vertical* alignment of the axial skeleton (cranium, spine, and pelvis) and the limbs with the vertical line of gravity, the appendicular skeleton (shoulder and pelvic girdles) should be level *horizontally* as well. The ideal skeletal alignment would be that alignment assumed by a freely articulated skeleton if it were suspended from the cranium with its component parts hanging downward.

The three-dimensional position in space of each skeletal part should also be noted. Deviations from the normal can be expressed in biomechanical terms as rotations (Flexion-extension, left and right rotation, left and right side-bending) and translations (anterior-posterior positioning, left-right or medial-lateral positioning, and compressed-distracted positioning).[61] For example, common deviations noted in the position of the cranium are anterior translation (i.e., forward head), extension (usually in the upper and midcervical joints), and lateral translation (lateral shift).

In addition to the relationship of each skeletal part with the *whole-body* base of support (the feet in standing, and primarily the pelvis and thighs in sitting), each inferior part provides an *individual* base of support for the superior part. For example, the rib cage provides the base of support for the shoulder girdle. A forward shoulder position results in inadequate inferior support for the shoulder with the result that a large portion of the support comes through suspensory muscles such as the upper trapezius and the levator scapulae hanging from the cervical spine. The result is that not only are these muscles overstressed but also other synergistic supporting muscles in the kinetic chain, such as the posterior cervical muscles, are overloaded.

Another way of viewing the body has its origins in spatial aesthetic considerations (as opposed to traditional orthopedic considerations). With this spatial perspective in mind, the therapist notes the *dimensions* of a specific region of the body, i.e., its length, depth, and width. Since muscle overactivity involves a process of shortening, the resulting decrease in span can be readily detected by noting comparative differences in the dimensions of a body region. For example, cervical muscles that are in a chronic state of co-contraction will often pull the neck into a shortened configuration, roughly akin to a turtle withdrawing its head into a shell. Thus, the dimension which is diminished is length. Tight pectoral muscles will pull the shoulder girdles anteriorly and medially causing an anterior narrowing. In this instance, the decreased dimension is width. Noting these alterations in body dimensions can be a useful guide to identifying myofascial restriction and directing treatment.[27]

In addition to noting posture, the configuration and distribution of the myofascial tissue mass are observed. A two-dimensional perspective can be gained via an outline or "silhouette" view. This view is obtained by looking at a body part profile, or conversely, by observing the negative space around a body part. When an artist draws the human body, he composes it as an amalgam of ellipses. The curves in this profile view should present with that same elliptic quality. Overly flat curves suggest muscle underdevelopment or underuse while excessively rounded or bulging curves suggest overdevelopment or overuse. Since these patterns of myofascial development accurately reflect the patterns of use in the body, they enable the therapist to identify sites of stress and potential dysfunction in the body. This myofascial development can also be assessed three-dimensionally as a contour rather than simply a profile.[15]

One also needs to consider the proportions of muscle development, i.e., is a particular region of the body under-, over-, or appropriately developed relative to adjacent areas of the body? The junctions between disproportionately developed areas are prime sites for tissue overload and potential sites for future degenerative changes. An example of this is the patient with overdeveloped extensor muscles in the cervical spine and underdeveloped deep flexors. This person will probably develop an excessively lordotic cervical curve and eventually demonstrate degenerative changes in the posterior articular structures as well as other related problems.

While these observation schemes give us an indication of how the appearance of the body may deviate from the ideal, appearances can be deceptive. The patient can often be utilizing excessive effort to maintain what appears to be an ideal orthostatic position, but which is, in fact, inefficient and stressful. While the experienced eye can appreciate the degree of ease or effort in posture and movement, there is a subtleness to this quality that is difficult to convey verbally. It is, therefore, more concretely detected by the *feel* of resistance with the induction of small early-range passive motions (initiation feel) as described in the next paragraphs.

Motion Testing

The therapist assesses active motion from the micro- to the macrolevel noting (1) both spinal segmental motion and regional motion in the symptomatic region, (2) how that region participates in whole-body motion, and (3) how motion in other parts of the body relates to and affects the symptomatic region. Turning the head, for example, should involve not only cervical spine segmental rotation but for optimal efficiency should also involve the participatory action of the upper thoracic spine and rib cage, slight motion in the shoulder girdle (particularly the clavicle and the scapula), slight exhalation in the rib cage, a very subtle torsioning down through the torso, and a slight lateral weight shift in the base of support (Figs 13–1,A and B). If any one of these components demonstrates disturbed motion, the resulting inefficient motion contributes, either directly or indirectly, to overload of the myofascial tissues (as well as other structures such as the joints).

Both passive and active motions are examined. Active-assistive motions with the patient in a functional weightbearing position are of particular value. The therapist gently moves the body part a few degrees in each direction with light, gentle, slow movements, noting the patient's responsiveness to the movement, i.e., how readily, easily, and willingly the patient moves (Fig 13–2,A). This induced motion has the quality of a passive motion since it is manually initiated by the therapist, but it also has the quality of active motion since the

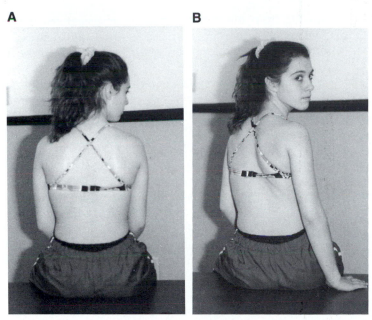

FIG 13–1. **A,** rotation of cervical spine performed in isolated fashion with lack of participation of inferior segments. **B,** rotation of cervical spine performed with integrated participation of pelvis, rib cage, and shoulder girdle, and utilization of weight-shifting.

patient actively goes along with the movement and does not remain totally passive. The feel of resistance to this movement is noted and can be described as an *initiation feel*[18, 44] (early-range). If the amplitude of motion is progressed further (into the midrange), a *through-range feel*[44, 48] is assessed (Fig 13–2,B). Both of these forms of motion resistance assessment offer information that differs

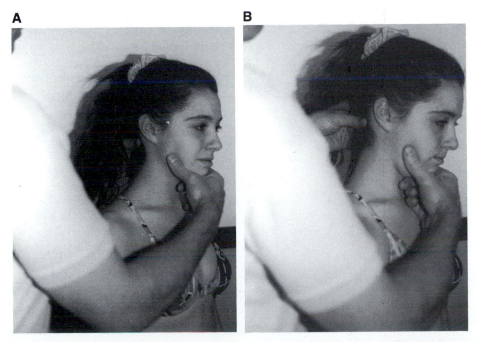

FIG 13–2. **A,** assessing initiation feel of head movements. **B,** assessing through-range feel of head movements.

somewhat from the more commonly assessed *end feel* (end-range). In general, active motions are assessed more easily in a functional weightbearing position whereas passive motions can often be assessed more accurately in a relaxed, nonweightbearing position.

One can also observe the length of individual muscles via well-documented muscle length tests[10, 15, 56, 57] involving combinations of various physiologic movements. One common error made by the novice is to assume that a muscle is normal simply because it can be stretched in one direction to its full range. A large percentage of muscles have a complex muscle fiber arrangement or unusual muscle belly morphology. Multiangular (as opposed to pure parallel) fiber direction may be present such as the twisted fibers in the levator scapulae. The levator scapulae has long, more vertically oriented, more superficial fibers, as well as shorter, more horizontally oriented, deeper diagonal fibers.[56] In other muscles, there are also pennate and bipennate muscle fiber arrangements to consider. Therefore, stretches, both for evaluation and treatment, will usually involve motion in an arcuate pathway that involves more than one plane of movement.

One can also assess the accessory lengthening ability (or extensibility) of soft tissues (including muscle, fascia, and neuromeningeal elements) by applying a light tensile load, sustaining it, and noting the resulting distribution of tensile deformation.[15, 59] One common way of assessing this is with the arm-pull technique (Fig 13–3). Restrictions are perceived as a remote "tethering," i.e., the tissue will fail to elongate in proportion to adjacent tissues. The restriction can be perceived along the linear extent of the upper quarter (in the neck region, shoulder, upper arm, etc.) as well as in the cross section of the upper limb and forequarter (anterior or posterior, superficial or deep, etc.). While this is a highly subjective method of assessment, it can often provide information that is unobtainable by other means. Also, correlating the therapist's findings with other motion tests and with direct palpation as well as with the patient's complaints can add to the validity and reliability of the information.

Observation and motion testing are valuable tools that are very useful for determining the structural or functional dysfunction that is the *cause* of the problem. In terms of localizing the *source* of the problem, however, they are rarely as specific as palpation. While these assessment tools may have the sensitivity

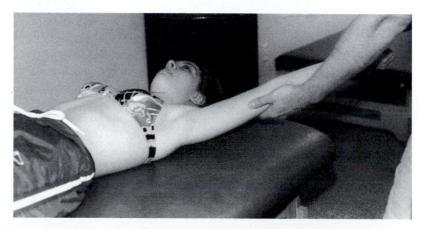

FIG 13–3. Assessing and treating muscle extensibility in forequarter region with arm-pull technique.

to determine what motion or muscle is affected, and possibly, why, only palpation is discriminating enough to determine exactly what *part* of the muscle is affected and to direct treatment accordingly.*

Palpation

The high degree of sensitivity and precision possible with palpation allows one to accurately locate an area with a lesion. Palpation can often detect subtle changes that would go undetected by observation alone. Witness one's ability to feel a hair beneath a sheet of paper, a perception that would go unnoticed with just simple observation.

The therapist first notes the subjective response to palpation. Is an area tender to palpation and if so, how easily is that area provoked? Is the area very sensitive and will light, superficial palpation provoke pain, or is firmer, deeper palpation necessary to provoke pain? How irritable is the area to palpation? Does the pain subside rapidly once pressure is withdrawn or does it linger for a considerable period of time afterward? With sustained pressure to the area (5–15 seconds) does the pain begin to spread and begin referring to another area, or does the pain remain local or even begin to abate?

Next, more objective findings are noted with palpation. Does the condition of the area suggest a more acute lesion (i.e., warmer with a sense of bogginess, congestion, swelling, or inflammation) or does it appear to be more chronic (i.e., cooler with a sense of "dryness," stringiness, ropiness, or hardness)? Does it have qualities of both (i.e., a harder, denser core surrounded by an outer "sheath" layer of apparent edema)? Is the location of the sensitive indurated area focal (i.e., resembles a discrete nodule), is it more linear (i.e., it resembles a band or fibril), or does it involve a more general area (i.e., an entire region of a muscle belly)? Does the sense of tenseness and fullness involve the entire muscle or just discrete areas of the muscle and does it resemble that of turgor (as would occur with intramuscular edema) or does it have a more elastic, "twangy" property (as would occur with muscle spasm and hypertonicity)? Does palpating the sensitive area provoke a local twitch response or a jump sign[56] suggesting high reactivity?

In assessing tenderness of an area, some additional points need to be clarified. While tenderness of a particular structure may be present in the majority of patients, tenderness should *not* be present in a healthy, optimally functioning structure. Consequently, while tenderness may be "the norm" for that person, it is not truly normal or an ideal state, and indicates, at the least, a subclinical dysfunction. However, in detecting dysfunction beyond the baseline level, one should check if this same level of tenderness is present on the contralateral side. Virtually every myofascial structure is represented bilaterally in the human body and therefore we have this basis of comparison available to us. To determine if a patient is unusually sensitive to palpation in general, we may also consider palpating a healthy muscle belly in an unrelated area and noting the patient's reaction to it.

---

*It is of vital importance to recognize that the *cause* of the problem may be distinctly different from the *source* of the problem. While myofascial pain arising from a one-time acute traumatic injury may respond to locally directed treatment of the *source* (i.e., the lesion), a longstanding chronic problem, particularly one of apparently insidious (but usually repetitive microtraumatic) onset, will usually require that the *cause* (i.e., the contributory whole-body structural or functional pattern or both), be treated via a systems approach. Therefore, for successful treatment of MPD, the thinking therapist always considers both the cause *and* the source in developing his or her treatment plan.

Additional tissue characteristics that have been well described by Johnson[27] are examined via palpation. The intrinsic mobility of the skin as detected by sliding one's finger through the tissue and noting its inherent extensibility (finger sliding), the sliding mobility of the skin in relationship to the underlying tissue (skin sliding to assess superficial fascial mobility), the side-to-side (i.e., lateral) mobility of a muscle and its freedom from adjacent structures (muscle play), and the texture and consistency of the muscle itself in response to focal, linear, and general pressures and frictioning (the latter indicating both muscle tonus and muscle condition) are the major categories that are noted. The reader should note that the distinct separation of these factors for didactic purposes should not be construed as being entirely accurate of the in vivo presentation (where, in fact, there is a considerable degree of mutual interdependency and fusion of characteristics).

ASSESSMENT

Once the examination is completed, the findings are sorted and correlated until a hypothesis is formed regarding the tissue(s) at fault and the causation of that tissue dysfunction. For example, if the posterior suboccipital muscles are found to be dysfunctional, a number of hypotheses may be considered. Some possibilities might include a somatic manifestation of systemic stress, abnormal use patterns related to improper head positioning, and disturbed neuromuscular or biomechanical relationships with other areas. Discussion of some of these possibilities follows as an illustration of the complexity involved in determining the cause.

Systemic stress can be manifested somatically in the form of the startle reflex as described by Kendall et al.[33] (Fig 13–4,A and B), sympatheticotonia as described by Korr,[34] Selye's general and local adaptation syndromes,[51] etc. Each of these physiologic occurrences is an explanation for increased local and general hypertonicity which could overstress the suboccipital region.

One set of abnormal use patterns in the cervical spine is related to how the head can be postured in various ways to accommodate vision. Prolonged work on a cathode-ray tube (CRT) with a fixed visual focus involves static contraction of the suboccipital muscles. The suboccipital muscles have approximately the same motor unit–nerve fiber ratio (5:1) as the ocular muscles, suggesting a strong functional connection, as indeed is aptly demonstrated with normal eye-head coordination. Any time we turn to look at something, the eye and neck movements are well synchronized. This static positioning at the CRT, the protracted position often adopted with strained vision, the forward tilt position that is necessary in using bifocals, and the backward tilt position that is often employed when using glasses that slide down one's nose are but a few of the aberrant use patterns that can contribute to pain and dysfunction in the cervical musculature, especially the suboccipital musculature.

The suboccipital region is related to other areas of the body, both neuromuscularly and biomechanically. Besides its direct relationship to the eyes discussed above, the suboccipital region is also related to the temporomandibular joint (TMJ) since an increase in tone in the masticatory muscles sets off a kinetic chain reaction involving other muscles (such as the hyoid muscles). This in turn requires a proportional increase in the suboccipital muscle tone to main-

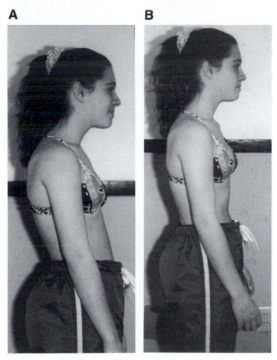

FIG 13–4. **A,** "startle" response or somatic retraction posture. Note the posterior inclination of the thorax and the withdrawn position of the sternum which dictate the dysfunctional shoulder girdle, neck, and head position. **B,** less overt, more subtle "startle" response posture.

tain a balanced, level position of the cranium in the sagittal plane. The sacroiliac joint is also related to the suboccipital region, especially the occipitoatlantal joint. The exact nature of this relationship is unclear—perhaps it has to do with horizontal balance in the axial skeleton. Nevertheless, it has been noted by numerous clinicians, including Grieve[20] and Lewit.[38] There are numerous other clinical situations that contribute to dysfunction in the suboccipital region. The examples given are a representative sampling of some of the more common possibilities.

In summary, both in elevation and treatment, a systems type of approach needs to be taken in addressing MPD. Otherwise, the practitioner is in danger of perpetually chasing symptoms but constantly overlooking the source of the problem. The postural, movement, and behavioral patterns of the entire system must be considered in determining causation. It will often be discovered that what, at first glance, appears to be a local myofascial problem is very commonly a problem involving the use pattern of the entire organism.

TREATMENT

I have found that a three-pronged approach to managing MPD is effective. This approach involves manual ("hands-on") therapy, movement and exercise therapy, and education (Fig 13–5). Manual therapy includes a host of tech-

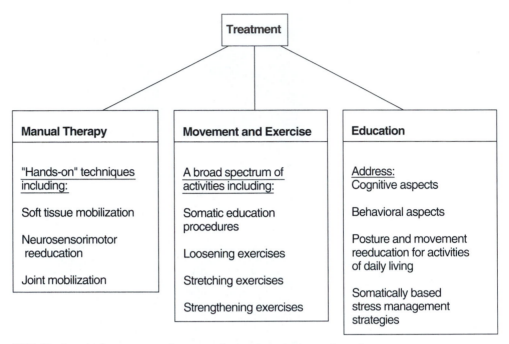

FIG 13–5.   A three-pronged approach to managing myofascial pain.

niques with primary emphasis on soft tissue mobilization, neurosensorimotor reeducation, and to a lesser extent, joint mobilization techniques. Movement and exercise therapy can include a broad spectrum of activities including somatic education procedures,[13, 30] and loosening exercises,[1, 9, 54] as well as more traditional stretching, strengthening, and conditioning exercises. Education involves both cognitive and behavioral aspects and can range from teaching improved rest and work positions to offering somatically based stress management strategies.

The intention of treatment is to restore normal intra- and intertissue mobility in the myofascial tissues. These forms of mobility are influenced by such factors as muscle play, condition, tone, length, control, and "strength" (meaning aspects of strength, power, endurance, and conditioning). Most of these factors are interrelated and to some extent inextricably intertwined. Separation is largely artificial and more for didactic purposes. From the standpoint of pure mechanics, the therapeutic goal is to improve biomechanical efficiency in the system, thereby reducing adverse "wear and tear" on the tissues and the pain that accompanies it.

This treatment philosophy addresses both pain and dysfunction. To treat pain exclusively leads one down a deceptive path, chasing pain here and there in the body, occasionally wining "battles" but ultimately always losing the "war." Failure results because symptoms of the problem are addressed rather than the problem itself and its cause. Conversely, treating dysfunction to the exclusion of pain can lead to an approach which is overly mechanistic and frequently interpreted by the patient as cold and insensitive. The latter situation may lead to a loss of rapport with the patient and a disappointing therapeutic outcome. Rather a balance between the two is sought, addressing both cause and symptoms, and addressing not only the problem but also the whole patient. The practitioner needs to be open-minded and flexible in his or her approach and have a wide variety of treatment options available. Particularly in dealing with chronic myofascial pain, a broad armamentarium of treatment principles and procedures can be invaluable since individual patient sensitivities and preferences often preclude "cookbook" or overly orthodox approaches.

Indications and Contraindications

The lack of normal soft tissue condition and mobility is the prime indication for treatment. While pain is what brings the patient to our clinic and it certainly guides the course of treatment, accurate and fruitful assessment requires that we have more objectively verifiable findings to base our treatment on. These findings consist of the structural (i.e., biomechanical) and functional (i.e., neuromuscular and behavioral) restrictions which make up soft tissue dysfunction.

I categorize the patient's problem according to the McKenzie[43] paradigm to decide the most appropriate form of treatment. The postural (or positional, or both) syndrome is well suited to a neurosensorimotor reeducation approach while the dysfunction syndrome lends itself well to a soft tissue mobilization approach. While the derangement syndrome *can* be addressed with either of these two manual approaches, it lends itself to more direct and rapid improvement with joint-oriented techniques involving repeated or sustained end-range positioning or joint mobilization and manipulation, individually or in combination. Obviously, such "cookbook" generalizations lend themselves to a certain degree of inaccuracy but they do provide a useful starting point for less experienced clinicians.

Contraindications are similar to those well documented with joint-oriented manual therapy[10] but soft tissue–oriented techniques are much safer. Conditions involving active infection, inflammation, neoplasia, or other dangerous disease processes; severe neurologic changes; instability; fresh tissue injury; and similar circumstances should be avoided. However, the actual extent of the above conditions, the specific way in which manual therapy is administered, and the practitioner's skills make many contraindications relative rather than absolute. Travell and Simons[56] mention the danger involved with pressure over the posterior triangle of the neck but I have never personally encountered a difficulty with this procedure and in informal surveys of fellow clinicians performing similar work, no difficulties of that specific type have been encountered. On three occasions, I have had patients experience mild autonomic reactions involving sweating, lightheadedness, and diffuse uneasiness, similar to an acute stress reaction, but these were transient reactions only. The patient was allowed to rest quietly in a recumbent position and was given a small amount of drink or food if requested. The problem passed within 30 minutes and the patient experienced no ill effects the following day.

Manual Therapy Options

The therapist is presented with various therapeutic dichotomies when selecting from among the different manual therapy options. For example, either a hypo- or a hyperstimulation approach may be used. A hypostimulation approach (light force and strong avoidance of any discomfort) has many applications but can be particularly useful for the anxious, sensitive, or more acute patient. A hyperstimulation approach[28, 58] (heavier force and some tolerance for producing moderate discomfort) is used far more sparingly but can often be of value for a more athletic or heavily muscled patient with tight or thick connective tissue, or for a chronically involved patient with lower levels of irritability (Fig 13–6).

One can also choose between sustained and rhythmic techniques. Sustained techniques can be useful if repetitive motion is irritating, while rhythmic techniques have a neuromodulatory influence and are useful for tonus and nonirritable pain reduction. Monophasic techniques are normally utilized, but polyphasic techniques (involving several simultaneous directions or rhythms of motion) can be employed when the need arises to disrupt dysponetic[60] patterns of muscle activity. Likewise, one can select between nonweightbearing and weightbearing treatment. Treatment in a nonweightbearing position facilitates overall relaxation while treatment in a weightbearing position simulates a more functional position.

Surprisingly, under certain circumstances, as when treating the neck, patients may actually feel more secure in a weightbearing position as opposed to a nonweightbearing position. This situation occurs since in the supine position, patients are obliged to surrender much of their muscular control in the neck to allow passive movement. If they fail to do so, they may experience even more pain with manual therapy than without. Similar dichotomies are specific vs. generalized treatment and an isolated vs. an integrated approach.

Of a more specific and practical nature, there are also numerous mechanical options in technique application. Therapeutic force can be applied tangentially to more superficial tissues or perpendicularly to deeper tissues; the contact area can be focal or broad; pressures can be light or firm, involve a moving contact and a stationary muscle, or a stationary contact and a moving muscle; the contact site can be fixed or variable; and movement rhythm can be sustained or intermittent. In addition, intermittent rhythms can range from slow repetitive (approximately 0.5 Hz), to medium rhythmic (approximately 0.5–2.0 Hz), to fast oscillatory (approximately 2–4 Hz) rhythms.

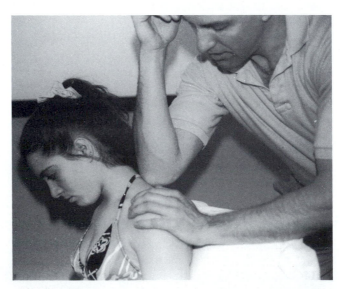

FIG 13–6. A hyperstimulation technique utilizing deep focal pressure technique in the left superomedial interscapular region with patient's upper quarter slumped into flexion, the cervical spine rotated mildly to the right, and the left arm hanging relaxed.

Soft Tissue Treatment Options

The number of techniques that can be applied is almost infinite, each individual technique being a composite of a number of variables depending upon the desired therapeutic effect. The following are some of the variables that can constitute the individual characteristics of specific techniques:

1. The particular soft tissue characteristic to be addressed.
   a. Layer mobility.
   b. Muscle play.
   c. Muscle tonus.
   d. Muscle condition.
   e. Myofascial length and extensibility (including muscular, fascial, neuro-meningeal, and other components).
2. The position of the patient.
   a. Supine, prone, side-lying, sitting, and other traditional positions.
   b. Nontraditional static positions such as those adopted from Rolfing, Feldenkrais, yoga, dance, and other nontraditional sources.
   c. Dynamic movements involving active motion adopted from Rolfing as well as newer bodywork approaches.
3. The anatomic region addressed.
   a. Specific.
   b. General.
4. The manual "tools" (and hence contact area and pressure).
   a. Combinations of fingers and thumbs.
   b. Knuckles.
   c. Handles.
   d. Elbows and forearms.
   e. Feet and other body parts.
5. The intensity of the technique.
   a. Hypostimulatory.
   b. Neutral.
   c. Hyperstimulatory.
6. The temporal nature of techniques.
   a. Sustained.
   b. Rhythmic and the variation of the rate.
   c. Monophasic or polyphasic activities.
7. The dynamics of the technique.
   a. Body part relatively stationary and manual contact moving.
   b. Manual contact relatively stationary and body part moving.
8. The topographic distribution of manual therapy attention.
   a. Isolated.
   b. Integrated and balanced.

The mechanical actions performed with soft tissue mobilization have been described as pressure, pressing, compressing, frictioning, cross-fiber stroking, snapping, strumming, rubbing, pumping, bending or breaking, stripping massage, light or firm stroking, jostling, shaking, kneading, ironing, effleurage, pétrissage, etc. The specific type of action depends upon the desired effect, the patient's response to the variety of tissue deformation being performed, the morphology of the muscle being treated, and so forth.

Layer Mobility

Techniques can be specific to tissue characteristics. In addressing layer mobility, one can treat restrictions both focally and generally. A focal technique, described by Johnson[27] as a superficial fascia technique, involves (1) locating a specific point and direction of maximum sliding restriction in the superficial plane of tissue, (2) applying a light sustained force with the fingertip(s) to that specific point in the specific planar direction of restriction, and (3) allowing soft tissue deformation to occur with the sustained application of this load (Fig 13–7). A general technique involves a broader contact such as the entire palmar surface of the hand and fingers and again involves sustained application of a low-level force in the superficial plane (Fig 13–8) with the addition of spiral twisting as an option. The spiral twist can be performed in the direction of maximum ease (for the indirect technique) or the direction of maximum bind (for the direct technique).

A common error made when addressing superficial fascial mobility is to note the amplitude of mobility rather than the quality of end feel. Just as amplitude of mobility can vary from joint to joint, so will the mobility of superficial fascia vary throughout the body (depending upon whether it is on a softer ventral surface or a tougher dorsal surface, whether it is in close proximity or distant from a bony attachment, etc.). Johnson[27] makes the important distinction of noting that the critical factor is an abrupt, harder end feel that exists with a restriction as opposed to a softer, more resilient end feel that is present in the absence of a restriction.

Muscle Play

In addressing muscle play, therapeutic force can be applied (1) transversely to the muscle fiber direction obtaining a perpendicular deformation of the muscle or (2) longitudinally alongside the muscle obtaining a parallel separation of the muscle from adjacent tissues. The transverse technique can be sustained or repetitive with either a slow rhythmic stretch or a more rapid oscillatory stretch. The contacts can be focal, allowing greater specificity (Fig 13–9), or broad, allowing more comfort and dispersal of possibly irritating forces (Fig

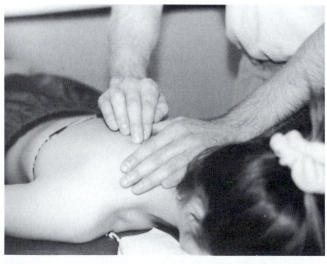

FIG 13–7. Treating focal superficial fascia layer mobility.

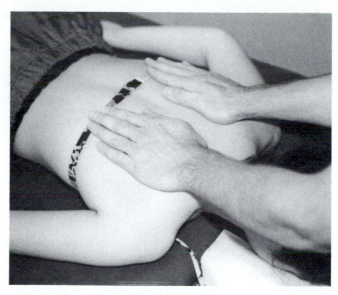

FIG 13–8. Treating generalized layer mobility of superficial fascia in the inferior direction.

13–10). The longitudinal technique may consist of long, continuous strokes, optimally suited for promoting fluid (i.e., lymphatic) flow, or it may consist of short, interrupted strokes designed to prevent the accumulation of annoying tissue tension (Fig 13–11). This longitudinal technique can be performed along the muscle belly or in a similar fashion along the bony attachments of the muscles, described by Johnson as a "bony contours" technique[27] (Fig 13–12). It

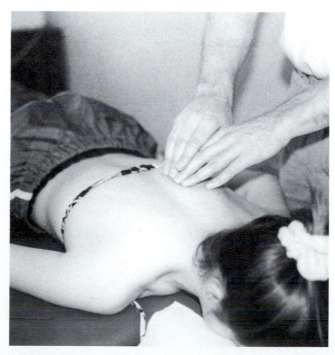

FIG 13–9. Soft tissue mobilization using focal contact in a transverse direction to improve the muscle play of the thoracic paraspinal muscles.

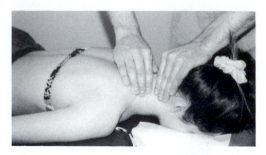

FIG 13–10. Using broad contact to effect gross muscle play in a posterior direction of the cervical extensors.

can function to separate muscles from adjoining muscles or other noncontractile soft tissues, or from adjacent bones or bony attachments. Johnson[27] makes the particularly important point of stressing the specific location, depth, and direction of the muscle play restriction. This in turn requires that the therapist position and angle the therapeutic pressures accordingly.

The sternocleidomastoid muscle is an example of a muscle where play can be easily examined (Fig 13–13). One must examine this muscle along its entire course, from its attachment to the mastoid process down to its attachments into the sternum and clavicle. The muscle must have free play along its entire length from the underlying structures just as its constituent muscle bellies must be free to move relative to one another. The sternocleidomastoid is generally thought of as having both a sternal and a clavicular head, but often more than two muscle bellies are apparent. In fact, Kapandji[32] states that this muscle has four distinct bands. The mobility of a muscle relative to its bony attachment is also important. An example is mobility of the upper trapezius muscle along its attachment at the superior nuchal line. These bony contours[27] must be addressed along with play movements along the belly of the muscle to ensure normal muscle play in its entirety.

Muscle Condition

Of particular importance is muscle condition. A variety of techniques can be used here, most of which fall into the category of pressures that are applied

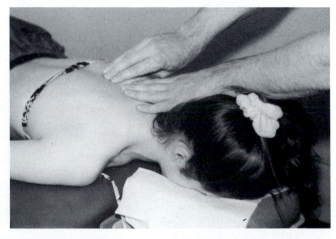

FIG 13–11. Soft tissue mobilization longitudinally to improve the muscle play of the thoracic paraspinal muscles.

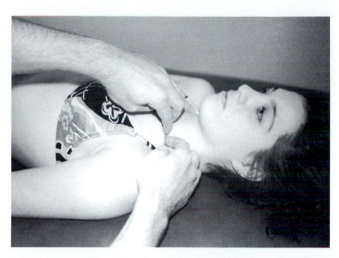

FIG 13–12. Soft tissue mobilization along the "bony contours" of the posterior border of the clavicle.

directly into the substance of the muscle. Rather than the emphasis on intertissue mobility as with muscle play techniques, with muscle condition techniques the emphasis is on intratissue mobility and condition. The goal of these pressures is to "break up" hardened, indurated, and edematous areas of the muscle interstitia and restore the muscle to its normal resilient, supple, and homogeneous condition. Travell and Simon's[56] trigger points fall into the category of abnormal muscle condition, and therefore some of these techniques are similar if not identical to the "ischemic compression" and "stripping massage" mentioned by these authors.[56] The pressures can be applied in a variety of forms including stationary sustained pressures and circular pressures, but most commonly the pressures will again be applied either longitudinally (in the direction of the muscle fibers) or perpendicularly (at right angles to the muscle fibers).

Longitudinally applied techniques can involve either focal or generalized pressures. Focal pressures can be applied as short repeated longitudinal strokes that resemble Travell and Simon's stripping massage[56] (Fig 13–14). The empha-

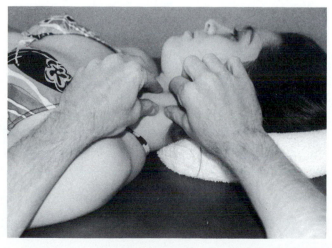

FIG 13–13. Evaluating and treating the muscle play of the sternocleidomastoid as a whole.

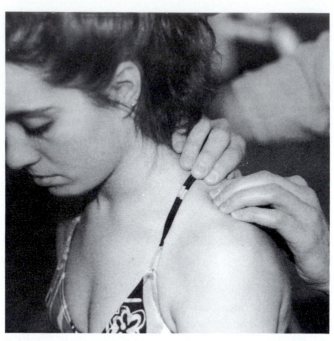

FIG 13–14. Focal longitudinally directed soft tissue mobilization improving the muscle condition of the upper trapezius.

sis with these techniques is on a very circumscribed area within the muscle. Larger areas of the muscle can be addressed with generalized techniques that employ broader contact areas and long, continuous, longitudinal strokes. These techniques have a more dynamic nature and can be performed in several ways. In one way, the patient is passive and the therapist applies "ironing" pressures to the muscle (Fig 13–15). Alternatively, the patient performs active physiologic movement while the therapist applies more or less stationary pressure against the muscle, guiding it in the proper direction and improving the "tracking" of the movement (Fig 13–16). This latter technique is derived from Rolfing.[46]

Perpendicular pressures can also be applied in a variety of forms. One form is known as strumming.[27] It is performed by sliding the fingers against the

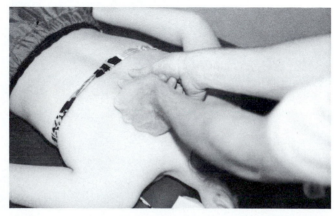

FIG 13–15. Inferiorly directed pressures to improve paraspinal muscle condition bilaterally.

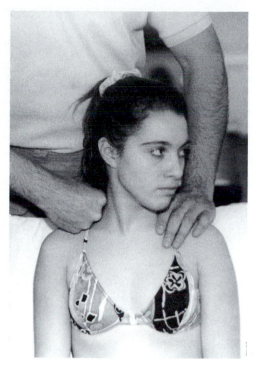

FIG 13–16.   Dynamic soft tissue mobilization involving posteriorly directed sustained pressure against the shawl muscles while the patient actively rotates to the left (pressure stationary but muscle moving).

muscle and then slipping on top of and over the muscle belly in a rhythmic fashion, perpendicular to the direction of its fibers (Fig 13–17). The site within the muscle which is addressed by this technique can be relatively constant and yet not quite fixed. This sounds paradoxical but involves the therapist constantly maneuvering the placement and angle of contact to give maximal access to the restrictions in muscle tone, play, and condition which can be addressed with this technique. While strumming can be used to treat muscle condition, play, and tone simultaneously, subtle variations in how it is performed usually shift the emphasis from one to the other. Strumming can be performed softly (as a hypostimulation technique) to mainly reduce tone, or it can be performed more vigorously (as a hyperstimulation technique) to produce an irritating response accompanied by a reactive production of neuroanalgesic substances.[58] When performed in this latter, more aggressive fashion, both muscle condition and muscle play are affected more. Perpendicular pressures can also be performed in a firm manner on a fixed site on the muscle (or tendon) to facilitate tissue analgesia and healing (Cyriax's transverse friction massage[7]).

Muscle Tonus

Muscle tonus can be addressed with a wide array of techniques designed to reduce hypertonicity. Hold or contract-relax techniques at minimal levels of activation can be used to eliminate excessive muscle tonus that the patient was often unaware of using (owing to the sensorimotor amnesia phenomena described by Hanna[23]). In addition to addressing tonus at the whole muscle level, sustained focal pressure can be used to direct the patient's awareness to specific points of elevated tonus within a particular muscle in a manner similar to

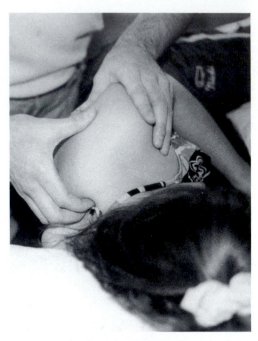

FIG 13–17.   "Strumming" on the levator scapulae near its insertion in the superome-dial angle of the scapula.

a tactilely directed "biofeedback"[27] (Fig 13–18). This useful procedure allows the patient to achieve improved muscle control and relaxation at a specific focal point within a muscle. Various adjunctive learning strategies involving visualization, imagery, breathing, and so forth can be used to assist in the development of this control.[27] Variations on this method can involve applying sustained pressure to a threshold of either pain or resistance and maintaining that pressure until the threshold changes, as demonstrated by a lessening of pain or a lessening of resistance.[8]

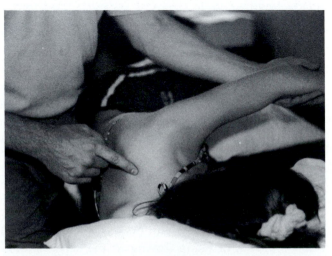

FIG 13–18.   Focal pressure technique directing the patient's awareness to redundant muscle activity in simulation of forward reaching movement.

The Feldenkrais method uses a variety of procedures to eliminate extraneous tone.[15] One is performing passive movements very slowly, smoothly, and gently, with frequent pauses and then repetition of the motion, so that the patient can become aware of and "turn off" any parasitic muscle activity. Another is to carefully shorten a muscle a very small amount through a variety of means (e.g., joint compression, support of a bony part against gravity, etc.). By doing so, the patient's central nervous system recognizes that the muscle effort previously required is no longer necessary for support and therefore reduces the muscle effort to the lowest essential level. This latter method is described as an effort substitution technique by Rywerant.[48]

The Trager® approach takes a different tack and uses gentle, flowing rhythmic oscillations of not only local and regional structures but also the whole body to achieve a lessening of both local and systemic tonus.[54] The way in which this effect is achieved is unclear but it may either be through peripheral mechanisms (such as stimulation of skin, joint, or muscle receptors) or it may be through a central mechanism (such as stimulation of the vestibular apparatus). The latter mechanism functions in much the same way that rocking soothes and calms a baby.

An additional approach is Aston's functional massage.[2] This unique technique involves the use of flowing massage strokes that are applied in an alternately counterdirectional manner and are "shaped" to the contours of the patient's body.[2]

Again, the reader must be reminded that when addressing restrictions in muscle play, condition, and tone, there is considerable overlap in these factors, and accordingly their respective techniques, since one tissue mobility factor is often closely linked to another. They are presented as totally distinct entities for teaching purposes only. Often one technique is combined with another such as using the oscillations from the Trager approach to enhance muscle play techniques (associated oscillations).[27]

Muscle Length and Extensibility

Muscle length can be restored with stretching techniques. Stretching can be specific for certain muscles or for certain directions and can be facilitated via activation of antagonists followed by activation of the agonists.[35] Considerations with stretching include (1) the anatomic direction of the preponderance of fibers, in particular, locating the precise three-dimensional direction of maximum perceived restriction, (2) the fact that most muscles have multiangular muscle fiber architecture (at times even involving a twist in the muscle) and therefore stretching in similar but slightly varied directions is often helpful, (3) attention to the "five S's," i.e., slow, small, soft, smooth, and sensitive[44] (these attributes are described in more detail under Sensorimotor Control, below), (4) after activation of the antagonists, allowance for a refractory period of at least several seconds for the muscle tonus to subside to baseline levels, and (5) release from the stretched position slowly and carefully to avoid rebound tightening.

Besides the traditional physiologic stretching, stretching can also be performed euthatactally with application of sustained, low-level, tensile forces (Fig 13–19). Variations include adding a spiral twist to the linear forces and employing hold and contract-relax variations[28] as well as including positional variations which facilitate stretching neuromeningeal elements. The myofascial release techniques described by Ward[59] fall into this category.

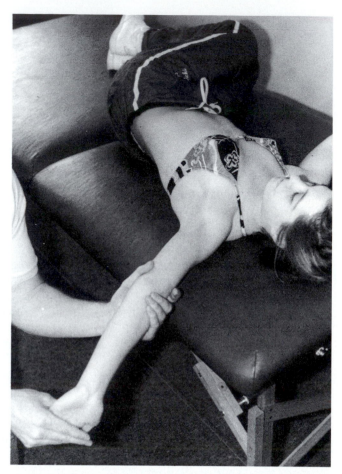

FIG 13–19. Stretching technique combining trunk rotation, shoulder external rotation and abduction, and wrist extension to achieve functional stretching of the pectoral muscles, upper extremity and forequarter fasciae, and neuromeningeal elements.

Neurosensorimotor Treatment Options

Any one of the methods which fall into this category encompasses a wealth of detail which goes beyond the scope of this chapter and therefore is mentioned here only in terms of general principles. Both traditional methods such as neurodevelopment treatment (NDT) and proprioceptive neuromuscular facilitation (PNF), as well as alternative methods such as those of Alexander,[30] Feldenkrais,[15] and Trager[54, 55] may be used.

A particular program that I have found useful in dealing with many cases of MPD consists of elements of the previously mentioned disciplines and includes the following strategies: (1) inhibiting redundant, dysponetic, or otherwise inappropriate muscle activity that would interfere with the desired movement, (2) selectively recruiting minimal muscle effort in an controlled fashion to achieve the desired movement with less effort and more efficiency, and (3) adding progressively graded resistance to smoothly amplify these minimal efforts into stronger ones, thereby facilitating the power and functionality of these desired movements. Depending upon the clinical situation, one or more of these strategies can be used, either in isolation or in sequential combination.

Inhibitory strategies can include (a) rhythmic oscillatory movement, (b) light sustained touch and handling having a directional intent and employing extremely low-load compressive or tensile forces, (c) a light exploratory touch that cultivates kinesthetic awareness, (d) very slow, smooth, gentle guided and supported movements, and (e) sustained and supported positions and postures.

The recruitment strategy utilizes many of the same techniques in a process of taking an unskilled, habitual movement, differentiating it into its component deliberate movements, and then reorganizing and integrating these deliberate movements back into a more efficient, skilled, and integrated movement.[5] This process can be achieved with gentle, slow, and precise "communicative" handling and the inclusion of a variety of nonhabitual movement patterns.

The resistance strategy involves taking the new, more efficient movement and progressively applying resistance in an incremental manner, maintaining the quality of movement, yet improving its power and quickness. With this strategy, it is desirable to develop muscle control through the full spectrum of facilitation, from minimal to maximal levels of muscle activation.

While the word *movement* has been used above, a more appropriate term may be the *neuromuscular organization* of the body. This latter term reflects both the more static aspects of posture and dynamic aspects of movement and avoids the tendency to view posture and movement as separate rather than interrelated entities. Certainly, all of the above strategies are applicable both to posture and movement.

An extremely common example of an aberrant neuromuscular pattern which can lead to MPD is the stiffening of the muscles of the neck that accompanies the initiation of movement. In time, this neuromuscular habit often progresses to a maintained co-contraction of the muscles of the neck which, in fact, is entirely unnecessary. This phenomenon is discussed in depth with regard to the Alexander technique under Sensorimotor Control. There is considerable overlap between manual therapy and the movement therapy since manual therapy is often needed to create the desired neuromuscular state, whereas movement therapy is required to train the patient to develop and maintain this state through practice with awareness.

Joint Mobilization Options

The role of joints in myofascial dysfunction must also be considered. Korr[34] has described the presence of somatosomatic and viscerosomatic reflexes in which both joint dysfunction and visceral dysfunction result in referred pain or even referred tenderness in the myofascial tissues.[6] While treating the myofascia can often result in temporary abatement or cessation of pain, ultimately the source of the problem must be addressed to avoid relapse. Thus *apparent* myofascial pain can arise from structures other than the myofascia and in instances where joint dysfunction is causing this pain, it is most effectively treated with joint mobilization or manipulation.[23]

Distinction between the different causes of *apparent* MPD is not easy and requires thorough evaluation and treatment of *all* the associated structures with the potential for contributing to the pain, particularly joints but also including such structures as the neuromeningeal elements.[4] These structures can be those located in the area of pain, those capable of referring pain into the area, and those which can adversely influence this area even though located outside of the immediate area. The assessment of the *response* to treatment will lend further corroboration to the source of the dysfunction and whether that source is in the condition of a structure itself or in the nature of the function(s) involving the structure.

Assistive Methods and Devices

While working on soft tissues, various assistive methods can be employed to facilitate normalization of these tissues. One such active-assisted method is the "sustained pressure" technique of Johnson,[27] which is actually the use of the therapist's finger to direct the patient's conscious awareness to focal areas of increased tone within a muscle. The area of increased tone is palpated and pressure is applied up to a certain critical amount and no more. This amount of pressure is determined by the patient's motor reflex threshold[36] with the therapist applying enough pressure so that his or her finger sinks down into the muscle without resistance but not so much pressure that a protective response is evoked whereby the muscle tightens against the pressure. At this point, various visualization and imagery strategies as well as directed breathing or focal muscle contraction and relaxation strategies can be used to bring about a local reduction of tonus.

More dynamic active-assisted methods can also be used. The patient can perform active physiologic movements of a body part while soft tissue mobilization is applied to the muscles involved in the movement. Other nonlocal isotonic movements such as eye movements or respiratory movements can be used to direct movement while simultaneous soft tissue mobilization is being applied to the muscles performing this movement. Eye movements are very useful in directing movements of the spine (most notably, the upper cervical spine), while respiratory movements are useful for directing movements of the trunk (particularly, the thoracic cage).

A valuable passive-assisted method is the use of "associated oscillations."[27] These are rhythmic, oscillatory, wavelike movements developed from the Trager® Approach of Psychophysical Integration[55] that the therapist applies to a local region or to the entire body. They can be used by themselves or in combination with soft tissue mobilization (Fig 13–20) for inducing both local muscular and systemic relaxation (via neural and possibly circulatory mechanisms), for using the momentum of the body to loosen restrictions, and for providing movement education in the form of creating a sensory experience of effortless movement.

Assistive devices such as specialized taping procedures[41] can be used to apply external tension (Fig 13–21). This tension can be corrective, i.e., the soft tissues are guided into a new position, thereby relieving stress on overloaded or overstretched tissues or applying a low-level stretch to overshortened and overtightened tissues, or by both. Tension can also serve as a simple behavioral reminder, regularly cuing the patient to assume a more optimal position. Rubber balls of various sizes and consistencies can also be used, as well as some recently developed specialized tools such as the J-bar,[49] to apply therapeutic pressure to dysfunctional areas. Foam or cardboard rollers can also be used in many ways including longitudinally along the spine in the supine position to teach more vertical alignment and horizontally across the spine to facilitate posterior segmental pressure over soft tissues and stretching of opposing anterior soft tissues (Fig 13–22).

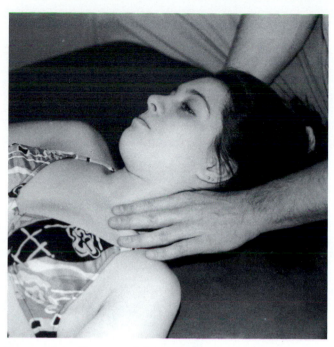

FIG 13–20.   Repeated oscillatory mobilization into cervical rotation with the therapist's right hand while the left hand encourages inhibition of the sternocleidomastoid by the supportive quality of contact.

Movement Therapy Options

Sensorimotor Control

A common error with application of movement therapy is to begin working on stretching, and particularly strengthening, prior to the patient developing fine motor control. The principles described by Miller[44] adapted from the Feldenkrais approach are instructing patients' to perform mobility exercises with emphasis on the five S's: (slow, small, soft, smooth, and sensitive). Moving as *slowly* and to the *smallest* degree possible (at least initially) allows the patient to perceive *every* step of the movement, to receive feedback *as* the movement is being done, and to do the movement with the lowest effort possible (and thereby have the greatest awareness of what is occurring as is physiologically dictated by the Weber-Fechner law[11]). Performing the movement *softly* means with as little effort as possible (again for the aforementioned reason), *sensitivity* meaning with maximum awareness of all facets of the movement, and *smoothly* meaning an absence of unnecessary acceleration or deceleration (again resulting in lower forces and higher sensitivity). Performing movements in such a manner creates a highly favorable environment for motor learning.

As an example, the head retraction exercise, which is often performed for reducing forward head position, is typically performed in an overly abrupt manner with redundant co-contraction and associated motions and some degree of flexion or extension rather than a more pure translational motion (Fig 13–23,A and B). Applying the five S's to the performance of this movement allows the person to refine that movement into a more fluid, beneficial one.

Loosening exercises[1, 9, 54] allow elimination of extraneous levels of muscle tonus, thereby allowing improved movement efficiency. For a person to stretch,

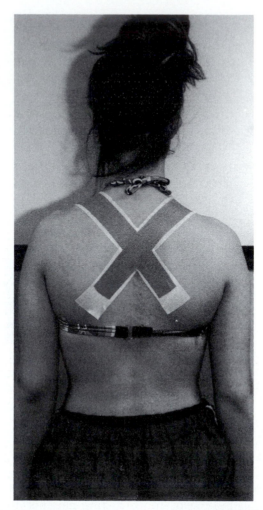

FIG 13–21.   Taping for postural correction and reeducation.

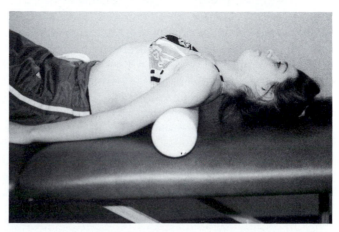

FIG 13–22.   Using foam roller as a fulcrum to obtain specific extension mobility.

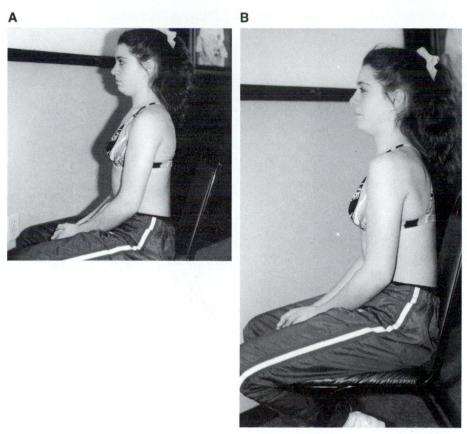

FIG 13–23. **A,** cervical retraction exercise performed as a translational glide with an emphasis on lengthening and utilizing minimal effort. **B,** cervical retraction exercise performed in a faulty manner with head extension, excessive effort, and undesired associated motions.

e.g., before relaxing his or her muscles to the baseline level of optimal tone is an exercise in futility and invariably results in minimal gains in range of motion (ROM) or unnecessary soreness from stretching. These rhythmic oscillatory exercises can be particularly useful for patients experiencing MPD largely from chronic muscle hypertonicity (Fig 13–24).

An example of a loosening exercise for the neck is slow, relaxed, rolling rotation of the head from side to side in the nonweightbearing position (to facilitate relaxation of the extrinsic cervical muscles) or soft left-and-right bouncing of the shoulder girdles alternately into elevation and depression (to relax and release tension in the shawl muscles).

Feldenkrais[12] developed hundreds of Awareness Through Movement lessons designed to reprogram habitually performed, inefficient movement patterns into more intelligent, skilled, and efficient movement. While many aspects of function are addressed in these lessons, a particularly important aspect is the correlation of movement in any one part of the body with movements in other parts of the body. Thus, in performing a motion such as cervical rotation, a sample lesson might introduce how movement from the eyes, the shoulder girdle, the rib cage, and the pelvis will enhance the comfort and ease of a movement, improving both its quantity and quality. For example, in rotating to look behind oneself, one will find this motion easier if there is a lateral weight shift

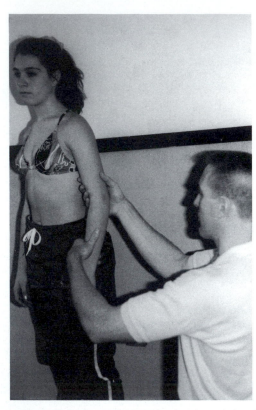

FIG 13–24.   Loosening mobilization to the arm to begin training in active inhibition of muscle hypertonus.

in the pelvis (in sitting) whereby the base of support shifts from being equally distributed on both ischial tuberosities more toward one tuberosity.

Among other things, the Alexander technique[30] teaches the patient how to dissociate the cervical muscles from the initiation and implementation of motor tasks involving other parts of the body, such as the stiffening of the neck which commonly occurs upon raising the arm. This inhibitory type of training can be applied to teaching someone to perform numerous functional tasks more efficiently, from light tasks such as writing and working at a keyboard to heavy tasks such as lifting and carrying. A light, guiding, directional touch with a "suggestive" quality can impart the necessary kinesthetic sensations to achieve this inhibitory effect. One can supplement the Alexander technique with generic postural reeducation employing various forms of auditory, visual, and kinesthetic cuing. For the patient who habitually holds the head in a slightly extended position, the patient can be told to imagine that there are eyes on the back of his or her head and to align them with an imaginary horizon. The patient who is tightly bracing with the neck muscles can be taught to visualize his or her head being like a gently floating balloon or a golf ball balanced on a golf tee. Obviously, a multitude of ideokinetic strategies can be employed.[32]

Stretching and Strengthening

Active stretching should follow the same general guidelines described under the passive technique. Again the point should be emphasized that stretching should be preceded by tonus reduction "exercises" to derive maximum benefit.

Strengthening is another area that is vast in its scope. One point that should be kept in mind is designing the exercise to match the demand placed upon a muscle. The best exercise for improved posture is working on improved posture via tonic activation as opposed to performing a few phasic exercises periodically throughout the day and then relapsing into one's previous poor postural patterns. However, the *way* in which one attempts to do this is critical. Typically patients attempt to hold a new posture until they tire or until they become so uncomfortable that they reject any further future attempts at assuming this posture. Rather, one should realize that much repetition is required and one should phase in and out of the "old" and "new" posture until the distinction between them blurs and either one (or any posture in between) can be assumed with equal ease.

Another important point is that posture should be improved through increasing efficiency via selective muscle inhibition rather than gross muscle facilitation. That means that using more muscle effort to overcome a poor posture is doomed to failure since it requires too much effort. Superimposing more tension upon preexisting tension only increases the total muscle effort and the resulting compressive and shearing forces imposed upon the osseoarticular system. In comparison, releasing or inhibiting the unnecessary and inappropriate muscle tone which pulls the patient out of the ideal position allows the automatic postural mechanisms of the nervous system to maintain an effortless upright stance with minimal opposition, thereby reducing stress on the system and greatly increasing patient compliance because of its more natural feel and effortless quality.

It is my opinion that only recently in physical therapy have we begun making the intelligent transition from emphasizing strength to emphasizing control (which in turn translates back into increased strength). A specific strengthening exercise in the neck involves activation of the deep flexors such as the longus colli and longus capitis and the rectus capitis anterior. These muscles are often inhibited by the overactivity of the posterior extensor muscles and the overaccentuated lordotic curve in the cervical spine is frequently a reflection of this.[15] To strengthen these muscles a slow sequential "curl-up" of the cervical spine (similar to that in the lumbar spine) should be performed with emphasis on maintaining the length of the cervical spine and avoiding shortening motions as would occur with protraction of the neck by excessive use of the sternocleidomastoid muscles (Figs 13–25,A, B, and C). An additional point in this exercise is to encourage the upper thoracic spine and rib cage to participate in the segmental motion.

In summary, intelligent and technically precise movement and exercise performance is a key factor in addressing MPD.

Behavioral and Cognitive Reeducation

Behavioral and cognitive reeducation is a valuable complement to kinesthetically implemented movement reeducation although the two often merge in practical application. The patient needs to be taught and then demonstrate back to the therapist various options for rest and work positions, especially prolonged positions such as those used when sleeping, reading, and performing station-

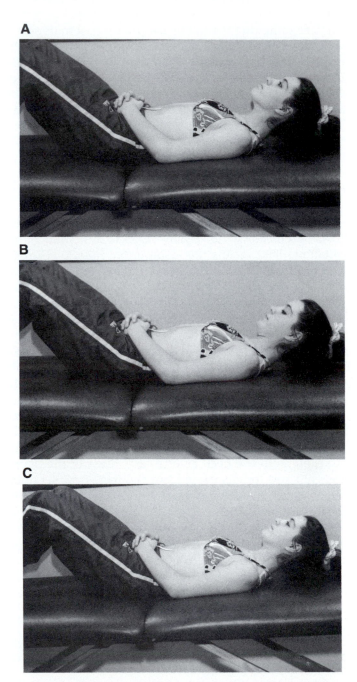

FIG 13–25.   A, faulty attempt to strengthen deep cervical flexors characterized by protraction or shortening of the cervical spine. **B,** faulty strengthening of deep cervical flexors characterized by excessive flexion of the lower cervical and cervicothoracic segments. **C,** correct strengthening of deep cervical flexors characterized by flexion distributed down into the upper thoracic spine with participatory action of the rib cage and abdominal muscles. Note that attempting to maintain the horizontal length of the cervical spine helps to minimize undesired sternocleidomastoid activity.

ary occupational tasks. The patient must also be taught problem-solving skills for optimizing functional posture and movements, both in the workplace and at home.

A particularly common fault is confusing organizational intent with movement intent. For any extended positioning or movement task (from working at a desk to walking), the body should be organized so that it assumes its maximum length (the "up" direction of the Alexander technique), and to a lesser extent its maximum width. This neuromuscular configuration constitutes the organizational intent of the body. The movement intent is the intent having to do with a desired direction of travel such as the forward direction when reaching or moving from one place to another. One can maintain an upward organizational intent of the body (an optimally aligned vertical posture) while still having a forward movement intent. However, the two are commonly confused during function. Hence, the person reaching forward to grasp an object frequently flexes in the lumbar spine, collapses through the thorax, excessively protracts the shoulder girdle, and compensatorily extends the neck to maintain level eye position. The result is that the person achieves forward movement but the body shortens (Fig 13–26,A). The more optimal version of the movement would involve maintaining the head, neck, torso, and shoulders in a near-neutral yet relaxed posture, achieving the forward movement with a simple hip flexion "hinging" at the hips (Fig 13–26,B).

Inappropriate and excessive use of accessory muscles of respiration can overload both those muscles and the joints in the region. While a person's unconscious breathing pattern is a deeply ingrained motor pattern and difficult to change, more superficial interferences to free, unconstrained breathing can be removed or inhibited thereby removing these subtle chronic myofascial stresses.

In addition, the therapist needs to educate the patient as to how chronic negative emotional states (anxiety, fear, anger, sadness, depression, etc.) can have an adverse influence on the neuromuscular configuration of the body, particularly the axial musculature. This circumstance is a commonly overlooked but widely pervasive perpetuating factor in MPD. It is one that may require psychotherapeutic consultation and major lifestyle change to rectify, and obviously

A   **B**

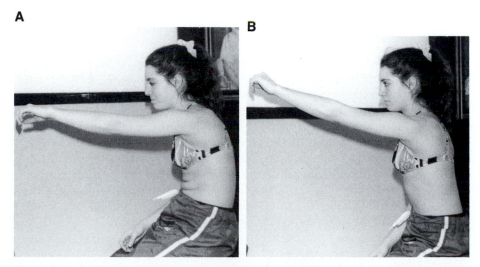

FIG 13–26. **A,** forward reaching accomplished by collapse of the spine into flexion. **B,** forward reaching initiated by hip flexion, maintaining the vertical integrity of the spine.

the patient's improvement rests heavily upon an acknowledgment of the problem and a desire to resolve it.

Nonmechanical Treatment Considerations

Although beyond the scope of this chapter, various physical therapy modalities can be utilized for their anti-inflammatory and healing action (see Chapter 16). If the patient is unresponsive to therapy that is normally successful, and especially if the therapist notes any unusual quality of the myofascial tissues or atypical behavior, it is important to consult with the referring physician. At this point a decision can be made by the physician to reexamine the patient or refer the patient to a specialist. Referral to other specialists, either to facilitate ongoing physical therapy or as a precursor to further physical therapy, can often provide the key to a patient's progress.

As an example, psychotherapeutic intervention may be indicated for MPD. I and a number of my colleagues have encountered patients that were marginally responsive to physical therapy. These patients did, however, demonstrate symptoms and objective signs of MPD. Either in the course of the rapport developed with sensitive and considerate manual therapy or through some other means, it was revealed that a large percentage of these patients were childhood or sometimes adult victims of physical, sexual, or psychological abuse. The distinction between the somatic and the psychological component of dysfunction in these cases is blurred and the therapist needs to inform the physician of these findings so that arrangements can be made for psychotherapeutic help. It should be emphasized that while a therapeutic relationship often involves counseling the patient in many aspects of his or her life, in no way should the physical therapist attempt to address the psychological problems. To do so can rightfully be construed as unprofessional, unethical, and illegal.

Nutritional counseling can also be invaluable, as pointed out by Travell and Simons.[55, 56] I have seen profound alterations in soft tissue quality after several weeks of dietary modification. Whereas prior to the dietary changes, the patient was refractory to physical therapy, afterward she responded in a positive fashion.

Possible Treatment Reactions

Soft tissue mobilization is normally a very safe procedure. The majority of adverse reactions can be avoided or minimized by refining communication and treatment skills. Soreness following treatment, however, is not uncommon. This soreness is most likely to occur after the initial treatments, especially in a case of longstanding dysfunction. Soreness may be immediate but is more often delayed. Warning of possible exacerbation prepares the patient for this contingency and avoids any possible "panic" reaction in which the patient's *fear* of the pain provokes a secondary reaction which is often more intense and long-lasting than the initial reaction. The proper development of patient rapport minimizes the likelihood of this development. An ideal treatment would result in minimal soreness to soreness lasting several hours. Soreness lasting beyond 24 hours usually indicates that the treatment was excessive in terms of its vigor, duration, or amount of work done, or that the patient is more sensitive than the normal patient and needs to be treated with extra caution.

Patients with congenitally loose or fragile connective tissue might experience bruising if the treatment is vigorous. Relative contraindications that would compromise tissue integrity such as anticoagulant and steroid use should tip the therapist to being especially careful with manual treatment. The rare occurrence of an autonomic reaction and how to deal with it was mentioned previously. Another unusual reaction is a somatoemotional episode. In cases mentioned previously where there was a history of abuse, it is not rare for the patient to experience flashbacks either in a conscious waking state or in a dream of the episode(s) or to experience an emotional release associated with the triggering of this memory. The therapist should be supportive and understanding at this juncture since the patient is often embarrassed by these episodes. Again, directing the patient toward appropriate counseling sources may be indicated in these situations. This situation should, of course, be managed with tact, kindness, and understanding.

Positive reactions will include looseness, lightness, and ease of movement, reduction or abolition of pain, and sometimes evidence of reduced sympathetic activity such as a general feeling of well-being or of sleepiness.

Special Considerations

The treatment of MPD should be considered as different from the treatment of fibromyalgia although many of the same general principles apply. Owing to a general lack of understanding at the present time as to the exact cause of fibromyalgia, there is no consensus on the best way of managing it. While exercise can be helpful, the acute pain present during stages of exacerbation often make it intolerable for the patient to perform any but the gentlest of exercises. Similarly, manual therapy must be gentle, avoiding hyperstimulation modes of treatment. Primary emphasis should be placed on optimizing movement efficiency so as to minimize the stresses on the myofascial tissues. Again, during stages of exacerbation, manual therapy may need to be avoided altogether with treatment shifting away from corrective therapy and more toward palliative therapy and medical management. Much research remains to be done is this area.

Reassessment Following Treatment

Following treatment, the therapist should look for a change in subjective findings such as tenderness to palpation, local pain, and referred pain. The therapist would also examine for objective alteration in function. Motion would be reexamined noting both range of motion and resistance to motion (the latter including end feel and through-range feel). Structural restriction could be differentiated to some degree from functional restriction with hold-relax techniques. Changes in tissue quality would also be noted with palpation. Lastly, one would observe how these changes carry over into changes in posture and movement habits.

CONCLUSION

Treatment of myofascial pain and dysfunction by manual means has been performed as far back as history records. Only in recent decades, as high tech machinery for the application of therapeutic modalities and elaborate but often nonphysiologic exercise regimens came into vogue and as "massage" fell into disfavor, has this therapeutic means been deemphasized and neglected. Fortunately, in recent years, there has been a resurgence in its popularity (owing to its demonstrated effectiveness) and an evolution in its sophistication. Various forms of manual therapy have been integrated and are now being applied in conjunction with various forms of movement therapy and more enlightened educational procedures. This integration is vital in making the transition from a passive treatment modality that may be effective but often has limited carryover to a comprehensive treatment program which has as its ultimate goal "educating" the patient, both kinesthetically and behaviorally and cognitively, so that he or she may progress to self-management.

The drawbacks to this approach are that it requires time—considerable time for effective training of the therapist and much time spent with the patient in a one-on-one relationship. With the increased emphasis on cost-effectiveness, time spent with the patient is threatened. One should remember, however, not to confuse cost-effectiveness with results-effectiveness. In the long term, only methods which produce results satisfactory to the patient (and not necessarily to third parties) are truly cost-effective.

Acknowledgments

The author expresses his indebtedness and gratitude to Gregory S. Johnson, P.T., who has developed and organized many of the concepts presented here and contributed immeasurably to the advancement of clinical treatment of MPD as well as to musculoskeletal treatment in general.

REFERENCES

1. Aston J: Overview of Aston patterning, course notes, Omega Institute, Rhinebeck, NY, July 7–11, 1986.
2. Aston J: Aston patterning functional massage, course notes, Mill Valley, Calif, April 16–24, 1987.
3. Boers T: Arthropraxis: Lumbar spine and sacroiliac joint evaluation and specific joint manipulation, course notes, Columbus, Ga, April 5–7, 1990.
4. Butler D: *Mobilisation of the nervous system*, New York, 1991. Churchill Livingstone.
5. Chaitow L: *Neuromuscular technique*, New York, 1980, Thorsons.
6. Cyriax J: *Textbook of orthopaedic medicine*, ed 7, London, 1978, Baillière Tindall.
7. Cyriax JH, Cyriax PJ: *Illustrated manual of orthopaedic medicine*, Boston, 1983, Butterworths.
8. Diehl B: Personal communication, 1990.
9. Eitner D: In Kuprian W, editor: *Physical therapy for sports*, Philadelphia, 1981, WB Saunders.
10. Evjenth O, Hamberg J: *Muscle stretching in manual therapy. A clinical manual: The spinal column and the TM joint*, vol 2, Sweden, 1985, Afta Rehab Forlag.
11. Feldenkrais M: *Body and mature behavior: A study of anxiety, sex, gravitation, and learning*, New York, 1949, International Universities Press.
12. Feldenkrais M: *Awareness through movement*, New York, 1977, Harper & Row.
13. Feldenkrais M: *The elusive obvious*, Cupertino, Calif, 1981, Meta.
14. Feldenkrais M: *The potent self: A guide to spontaneity*, San Francisco, 1985, Harper & Row.
15. *Feldenkrais method (practitioner training)*, Mia Segal, New York, NY, 1986–1988.
16. Fricton JR, Awad EA: *Advances in pain research and therapy*, vol 28, New York, 1990, Raven Press.
17. Garlick D, editor: *Proprioceptive, posture, and emotion.* Kensington, NSW, Australia,

Committee in Post-Graduate Medical Education, The University of New South Wales, 1982.

18. Greenman PE, editor: *Concepts and mechanisms of neuromuscular functions,* New York, 1984, Springer-Verlag.
19. Greenman PE: *Principles of manual medicine,* Baltimore, 1989, Williams & Wilkins.
20. Grieve GP: *Common vertebral joint problems,* ed 2, New York, 1988, Churchill Livingstone.
21. Headley BJ, North BA: *Myofascial exams and biofeedback.* St Paul, Minn, 1990, Pain Resources.
22. Hanlon WH: *Taproots: underlying principles of Milton Erickson's therapy and hypnosis,* New York, 1987, WW Norton.
23. Hanna T: *Somatics,* Reading, Mass, 1988, Addison-Wesley.
24. Herbert F: *Dune,* Berkeley, Calif, Berkeley Books.
25. Janda V: North American Academy of Manipulative Medicine Meeting on manipulative medicine in the management of soft tissue pain syndromes, Alexandria, Va, Oct 19–21, 1983.
26. Janda V: In Grant R, editor: *Clinics in physical therapy: Physical therapy of the cervical and thoracic spine,* New York, 1988, Churchill Livingstone.
27. Johnson GS: *Functional orthopaedics,* San Anselmo, Calif, 1985, Institute for Physical Art.
28. Johnson GS: Personal communication, 1986.
29. Johnson GS: In White AH, and Anderson R, editors: *Conservative care of low back pain,* Baltimore, 1991, Williams & Wilkins.
30. Jones FP: *Body awareness in action: A study of the Alexander technique.* New York, 1970, Schocken.
31. Juhan D: *Job's body—A handbook for bodywork,* Tarrytown, NY, 1987, Station Hill Press.
32. Kapandji IA: *The physiology of the joints,* vol 3: *The trunk and vertebral column,* New York, 1974, Churchill Livingstone.
33. Kendall HO, Kendall FP, Boynton DA: *Posture and pain,* Malabar, Fla, 1952, Robert E Krieger.
34. Korr I: *The collected papers of Irvin M. Korr,* Colorado Springs, Colo, 1979, American Academy of Osteopathy.
35. Knott M, Voss DE: *Proprioceptive neuromuscular facilitation: Patterns and techniques,* ed 2, New York, 1968, Harper & Row.
36. Lee D: In Grieve GP, editor: *Modern manual therapy of the vertebral column,* New York, 1986, Churchill Livingstone.
37. Lewit K. In Fricton JR, Awad EA, editors: *Advances in pain research and therapy,* vol 28, New York, 1990, Raven Press.
38. Lewit K: *Manipulative therapy in rehabilitation of the locomotor system,* ed 2, Boston, 1992, Butterworths.
39. Maitland GD: *Vertebral manipulation,* ed 5, Boston, 1986, Butterworths.
40. Maitland GD: In Grant R, editor: *Clinics in physical therapy: Physical therapy of the cervical and thoracic spine,* New York, 1988, Churchill Livingstone.
41. McConnell J: McConnell patellofemoral treatment plan, course notes, Kailua-Kona, Hawaii, Nov 30–Dec 1, 1990.
42. McGeary MP: Personal communication, 1992.
43. McKenzie RA: *The cervical and thoracic spine: Mechanical diagnosis and therapy,* Waikanae, New Zealand, 1990, Spinal Publications.
44. Miller B: Somatokinetic approaches, course notes, Somerset, NJ, 1990.
45. Miller B: In White AH, Anderson R, editors: *Conservative care of low back pain,* Baltimore, 1991, Williams & Wilkins.
46. Rolf IP: *Rolfing: The integration of human structures,* New York, 1977, Harper & Row.
47. Ruth S, Keggereis S: Facilitating cervical flexion using a Feldenkrais method: Awareness through movement, *J Spinal Phys Ther* 16:1, 1992.
48. Rywerant Y: *The Feldenkrais Method,* San Francisco, 1983, Harper & Row.
49. Sellers LS: Personal communication, 1991.
50. Selye H: *The stress of life,* New York, 1978, McGraw-Hill.
51. Sweigard LE: *Human movement potential: Its ideokinetic facilitation,* New York, 1974, Harper & Row.

52. Tengwall R: Toward an etiology of malposture, *Somatics*, vol 3: autumn/winter 1981–1982.
53. Todd ME: *The thinking body*, Brooklyn, NY, Dance Horizons.
54. Trager M: *Trager Mentastics movement as a way to agelessness*, Tarrytown, NY, 1987, Station Hill Press.
55. Trager practitioner training, Betty Fuller, New York, NY, Oct 30–Nov 1, 1986.
56. Travell JG, Simons DG: *Myofascial pain and dysfunction: The trigger point manual*, Baltimore, 1983, Williams & Wilkins.
57. Travell JG, Simons DG: *Myofascial pain and dysfunction: The trigger point manual*, vol 2: *The lower extremities*, Baltimore, 1992, Williams & Wilkins.
58. Tsujii Y: Myotherapy of the upper quarter, in LaCrosse, Wisc, Feb 27–29, 1992.
59. Ward R: Myofascial release, course notes, East Lansing, Mich, Michigan State University College of Osteopathic Medicine, April 13–15, 1984.
60. Whatmore GB, Kohli DR: *The physiopathology and treatment of functional disorder*, New York, 1974, Grune & Stratton.
61. White AA, Panjabi MM: *Clinical biomechanics of the spine*, Philadelphia, 1978, JB Lippincott.
62. Witt PL: *Trager psychophysical integration: An additional tool in the treatment of chronic spinal pain and dysfunction, Whirlpool* summer 1986.
63. Wyke B: Seminar on articular neurology, New York, Feb 1981.

Chapter 14

Therapeutic Massage in the Treatment of Myofascial Pain Syndromes and Fibromyalgia

Isabel Rachlin, P.T.

Massage is an excellent tool in the treatment of myofascial pain syndromes and at times the sole treatment necessary. A reasonable course of therapeutic massage along with other modalities may be tried before an invasive procedure such as injection is pronounced necessary. Two attributes not present in mechanical modalities are:

1. The ability of the practitioner to feel the exact tissue quality and the degree to which it responds during every moment of the treatment.
2. The well-known therapeutic effect of touch, whether for medical conditions or relaxation purposes.

PHYSIOLOGIC EFFECTS OF MASSAGE

The scientific community has documented the physiologic effects of massage, providing understanding of the mechanisms by which massage causes therapeutic results. Deep or kneading massage strokes, like muscle contraction, have been found to mechanically aid blood and lymph movement thereby increasing blood supply and nutrients in an area and speeding up the removal of metabolic waste products.[10, 23] The stretching force of massage on muscle fibers or across muscle fibers (as in deep friction massage) can mechanically break down adhesions and increase normal movement and flexibility of the tissues.[17, 19]

Pain relief as a result of massage has a number of physiologic explanations. One is the removal of metabolic waste products which can be responsible for cramping and soreness in muscles. Another reason pain is reduced is due to the stimulation of non-nociceptive nerve endings by pressure and movement. It is also thought that massage can contribute to the release of endorphins, a neurotransmitter which acts as a "central pain suppressant."[24]

MASSAGE TECHNIQUES

The massage techniques discussed in this chapter are those which specifically address the following myofascial pain conditions: trigger points, muscle spasms, and fibromyalgia.

Dozens of massage strokes from around the world have been defined and there is much overlapping in the techniques named. I will describe one specific technique called *stripping massage* and six broad categories: (1) stroking, (2) kneading, (3) friction, (4) compression, (5) shiatsu and acupressure, and (6) ice massage. These categories are intended to expose the reader to some possibili-

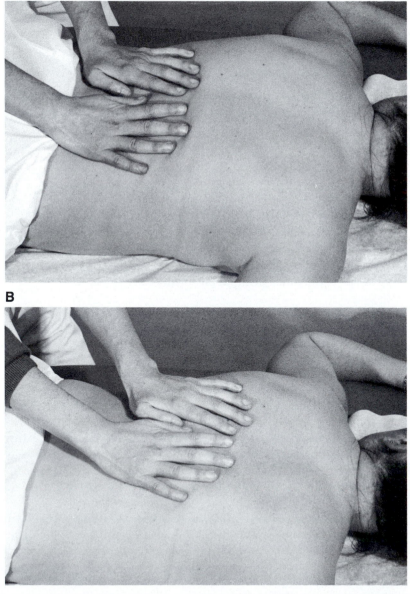

A

B

FIG 14–1.   A–D, stroking technique—gentle strokes gliding over and superficially into the tissue.

C

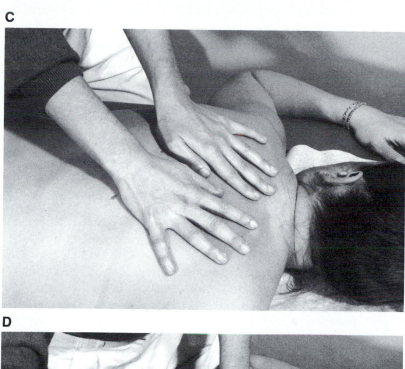

D

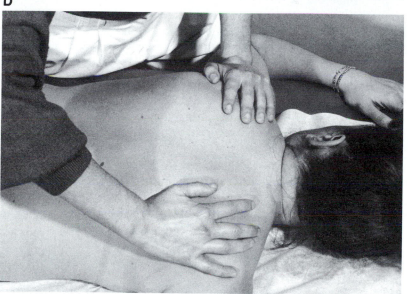

FIG 14–1.—(cont.). For legend see opposite page.

ties for therapeutic touch. Like any hands-on approach massage cannot fully be learned from a book. It is assumed that the practitioner will seek other sources and hands-on guidance or practice in massage techniques.

Stroking

Stroking employs gentle strokes gliding over and into the tissue. It is a superficial massage technique and is utilized to warm up an area for deeper strokes, to use as periodic rests during deeper work, and for calming and relaxation at the end of the treatment.[19, 24] (Fig 14–1,A–D).

Kneading

Kneading can be a moderately deep massage technique performed by contouring or "sinking" the hands into the underlying tissues and firmly gliding into or across the length of the muscle creating a squeezing or "milking" of the tissues[6, 19] (Figs 14–2 and 14–3). Kneading may be used to warm up muscles for deeper massage work, to decrease soreness in an area (due to the increased blood flow and removal of metabolic waste), increase muscle flexibility, decrease muscle spasm, and facilitate relaxation. Stroking and kneading are both applied with slow rhythmic strokes.

Friction Massage

Friction massage uses deep strokes on small specific locations such as trigger points (which may be palpated as "knots" in muscles), scarred or hardened areas, and other entities such as tendinitis which do not fall under the category of myofascial pain syndrome and therefore are not discussed in this chapter.

Friction massage is performed with the intent of using finger pressure to move the patient's skin and subcutaneous fascia rather than simply stroking over the skin. If the practitioner merely moves the fingers back and forth over the patient's skin instead of moving *with* the skin, blistering may occur and no therapeutic results will be achieved. A back-and-forth motion of the fingers is advocated by Cyriax[3] while a circular motion is described by Menell.[6] Friction massage is performed transversely across the muscle fibers in an effort to break down adhesions between the fibers and restore normal tissue mobility (Figs 14–4 and 14–5).

Compression

A number of practitioners advocate applying sustained compression in an effort to "inactivate" a trigger point.[2, 17, 22] Generally, compression is performed

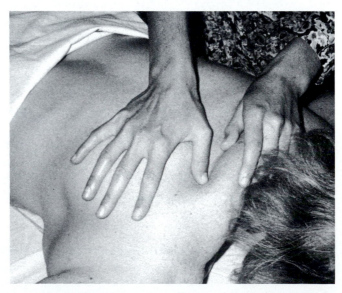

FIG 14–2.   Kneading technique—"milking" of the upper trapezius muscle.

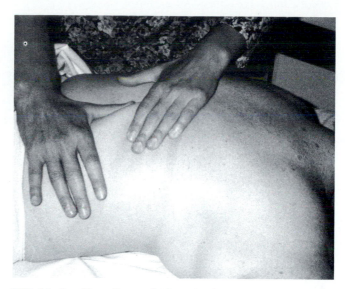

FIG 14-3.   Kneading technique in the midback.

with the patient's relaxed muscle stretched "to a point of discomfort"[22] while the practitioner administers deep pressure directed on the trigger point using thumb, finger, knuckles, or elbow depending on the area addressed (Figs 14-6 and 14-7). The initial pressure should be enough to cause tolerable pain and then pressure is gradually increased as the pain lessens. The pressure can be held for 5 to 25 seconds and repeated after approximately 1-minute rest until the pain of the trigger point cannot be reproduced. It should be mentioned here that I do not necessarily recommend forceful compression techniques because patients receiving this type of treatment often complain of excessive posttreatment soreness and ecchymosis *without* the benefit of therapeutic results.

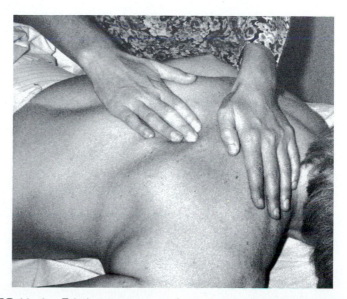

FIG 14-4.   Friction massage performed with the right fingertips.

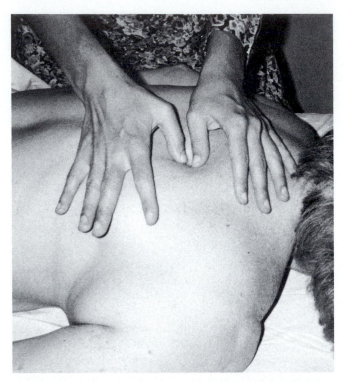

FIG 14–5.   Friction massage performed with the thumbs.

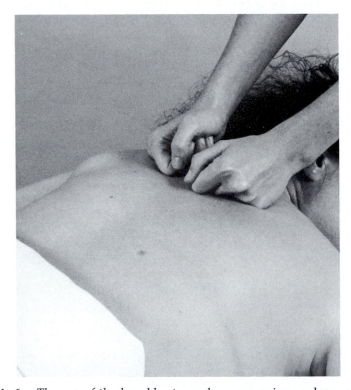

FIG 14–6.   The use of the knuckles to apply compression or deep massage.

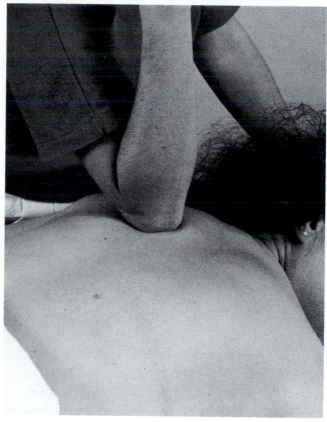

FIG 14–7. The use of the elbow to apply compression or deep massage.

Stripping Massage

Stripping massage is used in the treatment of trigger points. This technique, as described by Travell and Simons,[22] employs slow, progressively deeper strokes using full hand contact beginning at the distal end of the muscle, sliding up toward the trigger point and beyond it. The practitioner is able to feel the area of the trigger point as a "nodular obstruction"[22] and repeats the strokes until the lump decreases and the patient no longer experiences referred pain or tenderness when pressure is applied.

Shiatsu and Acupressure

Shiatsu and acupressure are two types of massage which utilize hand pressure to specific points on the body.[19] Although the theory behind these techniques is based on an ancient Oriental view of the body quite different from the model accepted by Western medicine, the points used in treatment have a high rate of correspondence to the points defined as trigger points.[22] As shiatsu and acupressure are very involved and are based on an entirely different medical model I will not give instruction in, but rather acknowledge, these techniques and propose further study and practice of them.

Ice Massage

Ice massage, though not formally massage, but rather a technique of ice application, is discussed here because of its use in the treatment of muscle spasms.[8] Many physical therapy departments keep paper cups of ice in their freezers so that the cup can be held upside down by the practitioner and peeled away as the ice melts. The practitioner should *keep the ice moving* so no one area becomes too cold. Circular motions may be used, covering the affected area. When the muscle is numbed, cold to the touch, and pink in color enough ice has been applied for therapeutic purposes. This may take approximately 5 minutes depending on the size and depth of the area as well as the patient's individual tolerance and response to cold. Lehman and Delateur write that cold therapy relieves pain "by elevating the pain threshold as a direct effect of temperature reduction on nerve fibers and receptors."[11] Other beneficial physiologic effects of cold treatment include local hyperemia due to reflex vasodilation of the vascular system after following an initial constriction of the vessels. Cold also lowers tone in muscles as a result of its effect on the autonomic nervous system.[16] Contraindications to the use of ice massage include poor circulation, allergy to cold, and extreme discomfort or aversion to cold.

APPLICATIONS OF MASSAGE

Therapeutic Massage for Trigger Points

Trigger points, palpated as tender "knots" or "taut bands" in muscles or ligaments may cause local as well as referred pain in a predictable and reproducible pain pattern.[9, 21] Some trigger points may cause symptoms only when excessive physical or emotional stress is present; other trigger points may create symptoms while the patient is at rest. I have found that more often than not a combination of massage techniques are utilized when treating trigger points. As with any condition the practitioner must be attentive to the needs of the particular patient and how those needs change during the course of treatment. The practitioner cannot mindlessly rub a patient's muscle and consider this treatment. The quality, texture, temperature, and color of the tissue will change in response to massage and the practitioner can use this feedback to guide him or her in the technique appropriate at each moment. The area to be treated must be warmed up with gentle stroking, progressing to kneading. Do not begin the treatment by working too deeply. If pain is caused, muscle spasm may occur. As the tissues become warmer and more elastic the practitioner is able to sink deeper into the muscles without hurting the patient and may then employ deeper strokes such as friction massage. Often a trigger point is palpable with superficial pressure at the onset of treatment; at other times it is not until the superficial layers have been relaxed with stroking, kneading, or stripping that a trigger point is revealed in the deeper layers of tissue. One must also keep in mind that the patient's reported site of pain may be referred from the trigger point and that massaging the area of reported pain without finding and trying to eradicate the trigger point will not provide the patient with lasting relief. Fibrositis (a diffuse hardening of muscles) may obscure trigger points. A "pinching" and "rolling" massage of the tissues can be used in conjunction with kneading massage to soften these areas and only then will trigger points, if present, be revealed.[9] The deep massage techniques such as friction massage, used to try and break down trigger points and adhesions in muscle or ligament fibers, may be painful to the patient. Kneading strokes which gently "milk the muscle" may be used periodically to soothe the area, facilitate circulatory exchange to speed up evacuation of metabolic waste products, and to rest the practitioner's hands. Gentler, lighter strokes should also be used to conclude the treatment for similar reasons: to encourage increased blood exchange to prevent soreness and to promote relaxation. Stripping massage can also be used with the above-named techniques. Overall, I recommend a combination of deep concentrated attention to the trigger point and milking of the muscles in general. The practitioner will, with practice, find a rhythm of making transitions smoothly from one technique to another.

Trigger points in the midscapulae, and upper trapezius and levator scapulae muscles are probably the most frequently treated trigger points by physical therapists. The techniques described above are commonly used on these areas. Another method which effectively addresses the midscapulae and upper trapezius regions is to have the patient lie supine on the treatment table with the practitioner positioned either seated in a chair, seated on (straddling) the treatment table, or standing, at the head of the patient. From these positions the practitioner can place his or her hands under the patient's back with fingers pointing up into the back musculature. The practitioner's entire forearm and elbows should be resting on the table to avoid unnecessary stress on the arm and wrist muscles. This position is advantageous because the supine position enables the patient's upper back muscles to stay very relaxed so that tight areas and trigger points are easily palpated. When a trigger point is found, the practitioner can either stay on that spot with constant pressure for a couple of minutes at a time, or do friction massage. The practitioner does not have to exert force to work deeply in the muscles; the weight of the patient's body provides this force. I have found that patients respond well to treatment in this position, and more often than any other type of treatment will enthusiastically exclaim, "Yes! Yes! That's the spot!" or, "That's what my back needed." The possible disadvantage to this position is that the practitioner's fingers and hands can become quickly fatigued. The practitioner must be sure to take breaks when necessary to rest his or her hands.

A massage may need to address multiple areas besides the area harboring the primary pain or trigger point. It is common that once the primary trigger point has been treated, trigger points in neighboring muscles or antagonistic muscles will become more obviously symptomatic. Often patients with pain and trigger points in the mid-and upper back or neck area have a forward-head and rounded-shoulder posture. The anterior muscles (i.e., pectoralis and sternocleidomastoid muscles) should be treated to achieve normal muscle length and long-lasting results.

The type of massage treatment that I have described may take 20 to 60 minutes depending on the endurance of the practitioner and the patient's response to treatment. Some trigger points may not produce referred pain after only a few minutes of treatment. Others may take multiple treatments of 30 to 60 minutes. Regardless of the time spent, postmassage passive and active stretching of the involved muscles is ideal to further increase the elasticity and normal length of the muscle fibers. Vapocoolant spray (or ice) and stretch (a technique discussed in the modality section of this chapter) can be used after the massage to facilitate stretching of shortened muscles. Patients should schedule two to three appointments per week so that there is time for the tissues to respond to the last treatment before the next is administered. The practitioner should tell the patient that soreness may occur 24 to 48 hours following treatment owing to direct stimulation of the trigger point area, but this soreness should subside without ill effects. (If the soreness does last longer the practitioner may have overworked the area and should move more slowly with this patient.)

Massage for Patients With Fibromyalgia

Fibromyalgia is a chronic pain syndrome characterized by a history of widespread pain for a minimum of 3 months. It usually includes low back pain as well as palpable pain in 11 of 18 defined tender points. Many people who have fibromyalgia find exercising or even activities of daily living too uncomfortable and strenuous and have difficulty finding pain relief.[1, 14] Massage, however, may provide some welcome relief from that chronic pain. The massage should be gentle and general, focusing on relaxation; it should not create pain. Patients with fibromyalgia may not be able to tolerate deep pressure on specific areas owing to the tender points which characterize the illness. Stroking and kneading are usually appropriate always applying pressure within the patient's pain tolerance. Because many people with fibromyalgia have difficulty exercising and moving in general the increased circulation to muscles provided by massage will help maintain healthy tissues as well as increase comfort.[23]

Special attention to positioning is often warranted for these sensitive patients; be flexible about treating patients in their position of maximum comfort. For some this position may be side-lying with a pillow between the knees for comfort (Fig 14–8). For others it may mean an extra pillow under the stomach, chest, or ankle in the prone position. If a patient cannot tolerate the head turned to one side while lying prone, try placing a folded towel or very small pillow under the side of the head pressing on the table; this bolstering will decrease torque on the neck. For some elderly or differently abled patients, climbing on and off the treatment table is too big an ordeal or impossible. Massage, therefore, can be performed with the patient sitting in a chair with attention to proper

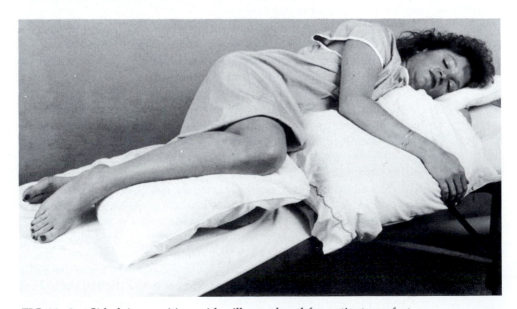

FIG 14–8.   Side-lying position with pillows placed for patient comfort.

lumbar support (Fig 14–9). From this position the therapist may still reach the patient's face, neck, upper back, arms, hands, legs, and feet.

Another consideration in the case of sensitive patients is the advantage of working on areas distant from reported sites of pain. For example, if the patient complains of pain in the upper trapezius but can tolerate little touching of this area, massaging the pectoralis muscles, neck, and midback will help relax the patient and often helps to decrease pain in the shoulder or problem area. Similarly, if a patient complaining of low back pain cannot comfortably attain or maintain the prone or side-lying position, massage of the feet, legs, psoas muscles, and neck in the supine position (with a pillow placed under the knees) may still provide the patient with an overall feeling of decreased pain.[24]

When treating chronic pain patients with syndromes such as fibromyalgia, the practitioner must sometimes be satisfied with achieving a lower level of the patient's pain; the goal of abolishing the patient's pain may still be reasonable but the practitioner should not blame himself or herself (or the patient) if this goal is not reached, even after many sessions. Remember,

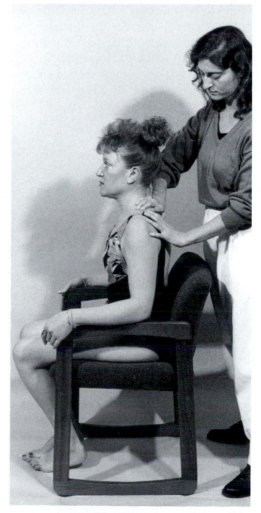

FIG 14–9. Massage may be performed with the patient seated in a chair. Pillows placed on the patient's lap may act as armrests to decrease stress on the shoulders and neck.

frustration can lead to burnout and most chronic pain patients are grateful for *any increased comfort gained.* Many people with chronic pain have lost sight of ever attaining a pain-free state. Until the patient is able to believe that he or she *can* live without pain it is unlikely that such an outcome will be reached. As the course of treatment progresses and the patient is experiencing greater pain relief, the ultimate goal of "zero" pain becomes more possible. Massage, even after the first treatment or two, may create enough pain relief needed for the patient to do some active exercises or activities of daily living that he or she was otherwise unable to perform. Stretching exercises, and active range-of-motion, and in particular, cardiovascular exercises as tolerated should be included in the physical therapy programs of these patients (as with other physical therapy patients).[14]

Massage for Muscle Spasms

The cause of a muscle spasm must be addressed before massage is considered as treatment. If the cause of a muscle spasm is, e.g., a facet joint impingement, obviously massage will not suffice as treatment of the underlying problem. In many cases, though, the muscle spasm masks the underlying problem and until the muscles are relaxed the causative problem is not apparent. Ice massage is known to help decrease pain and can be used to help "break a vicious cycle of secondary muscle spasm with ischemia and pain and more muscle spasms."[11] Stroking and kneading are also used to increase blood flow to an area and aid in relaxation. In the case of muscle spasm the practitioner should proceed very slowly and gently, progressively deepening the strokes as the muscle spasm decreases. Often other modalities such as tetanizing electrical stimulation, hot packs, contract-relax, or postisometric relaxation exercises may be used instead of or prior to massage.[12, 25]

CONTRAINDICATIONS TO MASSAGE

The presence of the following conditions are regarded as contraindications to massage treatment.

1. Inflammation secondary to bacterial infection.
2. Calcification of soft structures where myositis ossificans may be a consideration.
3. Hematoma.
4. Rheumatoid and gouty arthritis.
5. Traumatic arthritis at the elbow.
6. Bursitis. (Do not massage the bursa itself. Massage of muscles thought to be contributing to the bursitis may be indicated, such as massage of the gluteal and lateral thigh muscles in cases of greater trochanteric bursitis.)
7. Pain due to nerve entrapment, e.g., with carpal tunnel syndrome.
8. Phlebitis and cellulitis.
9. The presence of metastatic cancer.
10. Infectious skin diseases.[7, 23]

Lubrication

Choosing to use lubrication for massage purposes will be determined by the technique used, the practitioner's preference, and the sensitivity or preference of the patient. Lubrication is used to decrease friction between the practitioner's hands and the patient's skin, thereby decreasing uncomfortable pulling of skin or body hair and allowing the practitioner's hands to stay relaxed.

Many brands of oils and lotions are marketed specifically for massage use and can be found in drugstores, health food stores, and medical supply stores and catalogues. Popular oils are almond oil, coconut oil, arnica oil, mineral oil, glycerine oil, and combinations of these and other oils. Solid lubricants are generally less slippery; common ones used are cocoa butter, lanolin, and Aboline cream.[24] A variety of lotions exist and offer a consistency between an oil and a solid lubricant. A lotion manufactured for the purposes of dry skin may be absorbed too quickly for therapeutic massage treatment. I have found that ultrasound media such as ultrasound gel and lotion are frequently used as massage lubricants in physical therapy departments. I believe that these are inferior lubricants *for the purpose of massage;* they are too slippery or sticky for good hand-tissue contact and therefore cause decreased sensitivity and increased tension in the practitioner's hands.

Generally, some type of lubricant is used with stroking and kneading techniques because of its ability to reduce surface friction. For the same reason friction massage (when performed alone) and compression are performed without lubrication. In the case of these approaches nonslippery skin contract is desired; the practitioner wants the fingers to move "as one"[22] with the patient's skin, not on or over the skin.

Powder may also be used as a medium for massage. It can actually decrease slipping on skin when that is desirable as in the case of sweaty hands on a hot day.

Only nonscented lubricants should be used in the clinical setting. Many people have sensitivities or allergies to perfumes and scents. Similarly, there are people who have sensitivities or allergies to oils and lotions in general and this must be assessed before a lubricant is applied.

The practitioner should try a variety of media to find which ones work best for him or her. I prefer using small amounts of almond or arnica oil, or both, or cocoa butter—just enough to decrease surface friction but still allow firm nonslippery hand contact. I have found that this type of lubrication is suitable for trigger point treatment that includes stroking, kneading, stripping, or friction techniques. The practitioner must not be sliding over the muscles to the extent that the tissue quality cannot be sensitively assessed throughout the treatment; too much oil or lotion or the use of ultrasound media will not allow this level of sensitivity.

The medium to be used should be applied onto the practitioner's hands rather than poured directly onto the patient. This enables the practitioner to better control the amount applied and to warm up the medium before it touches the patient's skin.

ADJUNCTS TO MASSAGE

Adjunctive modalities are often used to enhance the therapeutic effects of massage. Hot packs when used for 15 to 20 minutes prior to treatment warm up the area to be treated inducing pliability in the tissues and allowing the practitioner to use deep pressure earlier in the treatment. Hot packs or ultrasound treatment may be helpful after the massage to prevent or decrease possible post-massage soreness and to further relaxation and increased blood flow to the area; this is particularly recommended following trigger point therapy when friction massage has been used. The use of vapocoolant spray or ice with stretch can be important adjuncts in the treatment of trigger points, muscle spasm, or shortened muscles in general. The use of the quick cold stimulus applied by a stroke of ice or vapocoolant spray (fluorimethane or ethyl chloride) causes an anesthetizing effect allowing increased stretching of a muscle.[20] Electrical stimulation is used to induce muscle relaxation and pain relief and is often used in combination with ultrasound in the treatment of trigger points. (See Chapter 13 on physical therapy modalities.) Numerous manual techniques employing the use of muscle contraction and reflex relaxation are used in conjunction with massage. Contract-relax, isometric relaxation, proprioceptive neuromuscular facilitation, and muscle energy technique are some of the methods used.[12, 22, 25]

POSITIONING THE PATIENT

Patient comfort is essential during massage therapy. The patient's body or body part must be fully supported so that the patient is able to completely relax. Tension in the muscles is counterproductive. Proper bolstering can aid in positioning, so it is wise to have pillows, bolsters, and towel rolls available for this purpose (see also discussion of massage for fibromyalgia). In the supine position a pillow under the knees removes stress on the low back (Fig 14–10) and a towel roll under the neck may be helpful to remove stress off the neck. The prone position can be made more comfortable by placing a pillow or low

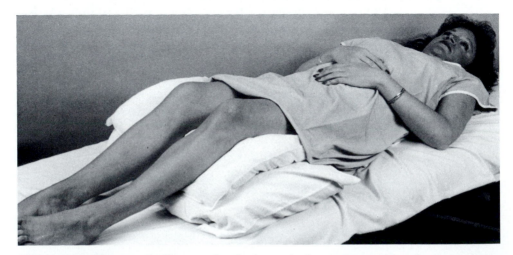

FIG 14–10. The use of pillows under the knees in the supine position decreases stress on the low back.

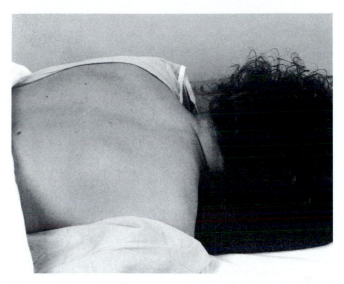

FIG 14–11.   The use of a small pillow or towel roll under the side of the head decreases torque on the neck.

bolster under the ankles and a pillow under the stomach or chest when necessary. As mentioned earlier, if a patient in the prone position cannot tolerate lying with the head turned to one side, try placing a folded towel or a very small pillow under the side of the head touching the table; this will decrease torque on the neck (Fig 14–11). (Some treatment tables have face cradles which allow the neck to stay straight instead of turned to the side.) If the patient is receiving massage seated in a chair, be attentive to the posture and support of the entire patient, not only the part being treated (see Fig 14–9). One or two pillows on the patient's lap can act as an arm support and take stress off the neck, shoulders, and arms. A lumbar support will take stress off the neck and back. Proper draping will also facilitate comfort and relaxation. Only those areas being worked on should be exposed; clothing or a sheet can cover the rest of the body to prevent unnecessary embarrassment or chill. Extra lightweight blankets should be on hand; cold will cause muscles to tighten.

POSITIONING AND SELF-CARE FOR THE PRACTITIONER

Practitioner comfort is equally as important as patient comfort. The practitioner who is a martyr and strains all day will suffer injury and have nothing to give the next day. The table height should be low enough so that the practitioner can use his or her body weight to lean into the massage; if the table is not adjustable in height, some low platforms or step stools may be necessary. Standing with the feet shoulder width apart will enable the practitioner to shift weight easily with the direction of the massage. Proper posture must also be maintained to avoid back and neck strain; do not hunch over the patient. Keep knees, shoulders, and back relaxed. Comfortable supportive shoes should be worn. Many practitioners prefer to sit when performing massage on small areas such as a limb or trigger point in the upper back. If choosing to sit one must still be aware of keeping the body weight over the area being treated so as not to overstress the hands. Massage of the forearm and hand can be performed with the patient and practitioner seated opposite each other with the affected extremity resting on the treatment table. The main concerns for practitioner comfort are keeping the back relatively straight and making sure that body weight, not hand or arm strength, is the force behind the massage.

Practitioners who do massage must be careful to prevent hand and wrist injuries due to improper use and overuse. Many physical therapists and massage therapists develop thumb and wrist strains, tendinitis or tenosynovitis, as well as carpal tunnel syndrome. Correct practice includes keeping the hands and wrists relaxed while working. If they become tense or cramped, gently shake them out and come back to the patient with relaxed hands. *Relaxed hands will also allow the practitioner to better appreciate the quality of the underlying tissues.* The wrists should remain relatively straight to prevent wrist strain and carpal tunnel syndrome. Do not overuse the thumbs! An invitation to strain and eventual arthritis is to continually use the thumbs as the main tools of massage treatment. Instead of using the thumbs, allow the force of the movement to come through the entire arm (not the finger or wrist joints) and lean body weight into the movement. Substitute knuckles, elbow, or other fingers if a lot of force is required on an area. A great way to prevent thumb injury is to NOT USE THE THUMBS AT ALL. I have adopted this policy as a result of having misused and overused my thumbs and wrists early in my career when ignorant about proper techniques and self-care.

Another way to prevent overuse injury is to avoid scheduling two or more patients consecutively who require deep massage work; have rest time between these patients.

The primary thought to remember about massage is that the practitioner should be comfortable and find what works best for him or her. Be creative! Use ideas from this chapter and other books, articles, and courses. Adapt or make up new techniques as needed. Although the physiologic and clinical effects of massage can be researched and documented, it will always remain more art than science.

FOLLOW-UP CARE AND CONSIDERATIONS

Massage treatment or treatment by any modality is worthless in the long run if causative factors and follow-up care are not addressed. Instruction in proper posture is essential in the case of any neck or back problem. It is pointless to give a 45-minute trigger point treatment to someone who then drives home with a slumped, forward-head posture. Specific stretching and strengthening exercises must be performed by the patient when shortened or weak muscles are contributing factors. The necessity for arch supports or corrective footwear may need to be assessed when muscular and postural imbalances are present. When possible, patients should be encouraged to do aerobic exercise. Aerobic exercise promotes general health and well-being, increases circulatory flow promoting healthy tissues, and helps reduce muscular and emotional tension.

The effect of emotional tension on myofascial problems cannot be overemphasized. Just as in the case of poor posture, a trigger point, e.g., can be treated for 45 minutes, but if the patient has problems which cause him or her to be constantly tense or angry, the physical therapy will probably have little long-term effect. Insufficient sleep and poor diet can also contribute to myofascial pain syndromes and should not be neglected.

There are other manual therapies which do not employ massage and show a high rate of clinical success. Some patients do not like or cannot tolerate massage. Some respond better to one treatment, while others respond better to another. For these reasons, I recommend three techniques which employ gentle movement (as opposed to pressure which is used in massage): Trager® Psychophysical Integration and Mentastics® Movement Education,[5] the Feldenkrais Method of Functional Integration and Awareness Through Movement,[4] and the Alexander Technique.[13, 15] Each of these methods is unique and noteworthy, but for convenience they are grouped together here because of their commonalities. Each of these techniques has a "hands-on" component in which the therapist uses touch and passive movement, and a second component composed of self-care "exercises" taught to the patient to be performed at home.[5, 18] These techniques promote increased pain-free movement, increased body awareness, and improved posture; they are excellent adjuncts in the treatment of myofascial pain conditions and fibromyalgia (see Chapter 13).

A practitioner rarely "cures" a myofascial pain syndrome. Successful results are gained only when therapy by a health professional is one tool in the patient's active attempt to take care of himself or herself. It is a disservice to massage patients and create a situation where patients are merely passive recipients of treatment and feel they must rely on someone else to "fix" them. As a physical therapist, it is my practice to try and empower all patients by first teaching them what they can do for themselves; secondly, to encourage and guide patients in carrying out their home program; thirdly, applying hands-on treatment and modalities when self-care treatment is not enough; and finally, referring them to other health professionals when necessary.

REFERENCES

1. Backstrom G: *When muscle pain won't go away*, Dallas, 1992, Taylor.
2. Chaitow L: *Osteopathic self-treatment*, Wellingborough, England, 1990, Thorsons, p 43.
3. Cyriax J: *Textbook of orthopaedic medicine*, vol 2, ed 8, Baltimore, 1971, Williams & Wilkins.
4. Feldenkrais M: *Awareness through movement*, New York, 1977, Harper & Row.
5. Guadagno-Hammond C: *Trager Mentastics: Movement as a way to agelessness*, New York, 1987, Stanton Hill Press.
6. Hofkosh JM: Classical massage. In Basmajian JV, editor: *Manipulation, traction and massage*, ed 3, Baltimore, 1985, Williams & Wilkins.
7. Knapp ME: Massage. In Keottke FT, Stillwell GK, Lehman JF, editors: *Krusen's handbook of physical medicine and rehabilitation*, Philadelphia, 1982, WB Saunders Company.
8. Kraus H: *Clinical treatment of back and neck pain*, New York, 1970, McGraw-Hill.
9. Kraus H, editor: *Diagnosis and treatment of muscle pain*, Chicago, 1988, Quintessence Books.
10. Kuprian W, editor: *Physical therapy for sports*, Philadelphia, 1982, WB Saunders.
11. Lehmann JF, DeLateur BJ: Cryotherapy. In Lehman JF editor: *Therapeutic heat and cold*, Baltimore, 1982, Williams & Wilkins.
12. Lewit K: *Manipulative therapy in rehabilitation of the motor system*, London, 1985, Butterworths.
13. Maisel E, editor: *The resurrection of the body; The essential writings of F. Matthias Alexander*, New York, 1980, Delta Books.
14. McCain GA: Management of fibromyalgia syndrome. In Fricton JF, Awas EA, editors: *Advances in pain research and therapy*, New York, 1990, Raven Press, p 297.
15. Miller B: Alternative somatic therapies. In White A, Anderson R, editors: *Conservative care of low back pain*, Baltimore, 1991, Williams & Wilkins.

16. Ork H: Uses of cold. In Kuprian W, editor: *Physical therapy for sports*, Philadelphia 1982, WB Saunders.
17. Prudden B: *Pain erasure: The Bonnie Prudden way*, New York, 1980, Ballantine Books.
18. Rickover R: *Fitness without stress: A guide to the Alexander technique*, 1988, Metamorphous Press.
19. Tappan F: *Healing massage techniques. A study of Eastern and Western methods*, Va, 1978, Reston Publishing.
20. Torg J, Vegso J, Torg E: *Rehabilitation of athletic injuries. An atlas of therapeutic exercises*, St Louis, 1987, Mosby–Year Book, p 6.
21. Travell JG, Simons DG, *Myofascial pain and dysfunction. The trigger point manual*, vol 1, Baltimore, 1983, Williams & Wilkins.
22. Travell JG, Simons DG: *Myofascial pain and dysfunction. The trigger point manual*, vol 2 Baltimore, 1992, Williams & Wilkins.
23. Wakim K: Physiologic effects of massage. In Basmajian JV, editor: *Manipulation, traction and massage*, ed 3, Baltimore, 1985, Williams & Wilkins.
24. Wook EC, Becker PD: *Beard's massage*, ed 3, Philadelphia, 1981, WB Saunders.
25. Voss DE, Ionta MK, Myers BJ: *Prioprioceptive neuromuscular facilitation*, ed 3, Philadelphia, 1985, Harper & Row.

Chapter 15

Electrical Modalities in the Treatment of Myofascial Conditions

Joseph Kahn, Ph.D., P.T.

The administration of electrical modalities to patients with myofascial conditions presents few problems for the physical therapy clinician. Most tissues involved lie within the superficial layers and are especially favorably suited to this approach. Electrical stimulation (impulses) travels along the first moist conductor encountered and so the depth of penetration becomes less of a factor than direction and fiber recruitment. Increased penetration may be obtained with higher frequencies, following the laws of electrophysics which indicate "the higher the frequency (or shorter wavelength), the deeper the penetration." Increased intensities (voltage, amperage) may also be utilized to increase the depth of penetration, but dermal irritation, burns, and discomfort accompany higher electrical amplitudes. Present equipment employs differential frequency control for increased depth. It should also be noted that not every fiber responds to the same frequency, and that a unit offering variable frequencies is desired in order to provide a wide spectrum of fiber stimulation and maximum recruitment.

Electrode placement is an essential factor in success. Size and conformity of electrodes are also important. With myofascial stimulation, it is recommended that the electrodes parallel the shape of the target tissue as closely as possible. In specific cases, however, a transarthral approach may be preferred to insure stimulation *around* an entire joint or target tissue, since, as mentioned previously, the current will follow a good conductor between electrodes rather than *across* a highly resistant region. Stiff, or nonflexible electrodes do not make good skin contact, leaving air spaces with high resistance, which leads to discomfort, and often burns. Well-moistened electrodes are essential for good transmission, comfort, and recruitment. Flexible commercial electrodes, paper towel or aluminum foil electrodes (requiring "alligator clips"), and self-adhering electrodes are recommended.

With two electrodes on the same muscle, maximum recruitment may be obtained. This has traditionally been termed "bipolar" placement, even though it has nothing to do with polarity! With only *one* electrode on the target muscle, i.e., motor point stimulation, the correct term is *unipolar* placement. With *low-volt* procedures, two electrodes complete the circuit, or four with dual channel operations. With *high-volt* apparatus, three electrodes (or more) complete the circuit(s), using a large reference electrode and smaller active pads. This arrangement facilitates reciprocal techniques, possible only with low-volt dual channel apparatus and special parameter controls. Interferential currents require four electrodes in a crossed pattern over the target area for maximal effectiveness. Microampere stimulation may be administered via pad electrodes, probes, or manually, with the physical therapist in the circuit (explained elsewhere in this chapter). Transcutaneous electrical nerve stimulation (TENS) electrode placements include nerve roots, trigger points, points of pain, and, of course, acupuncture points. With iontophoresis, yet another requirement is recommended and is explained under Iontophoresis

ELECTRICAL STIMULATION

Electrical stimulation comes in many forms. Each mode and waveform is individualized for specific therapeutic purposes. The three main divisions of electrotherapeutic stimulation are: (1) continuous or tetanizing, (2) surged or ramped, and (3) pulsed or interrupted modes. These forms apply to ac, dc, and when offered, faradic current. Alternating current consists of a biphasic waveform with variable polarity changes ("frequency") in waveform. Direct current is represented by a monophasic (unipolar) form. Faradic current is a form of ac current with sharply defined phases, not generally offered on American-made equipment.

With the continuous or tetanizing mode, so long as the frequency is greater than 50 Hz (although the range is 30–100 Hz), smooth, tetanic contractions will be elicited. This mode is advantageous in producing relaxation to tense myofascial tissues, as well as enhancing production of β-endorphins for mild analgesia. This optimal frequency may be obtained from ac at 50 Hz, pulsed dc at 50 pulses per second (pps), or other carrier frequencies pulsed at 50 pps. Clinical experience suggests this continuous mode prior to exercising modes, i.e., ramped or pulsed, or both.

The ramped or surged modes reach peak intensity over a short duration, usually in milli- or microseconds, and are primarily used to produce contractions with (mainly) "slow-twitch" fiber involvement. Pulsed or interrupted modes reach peak intensity instantaneously and are utilized to produce contractions with (mainly) "fast-twitch" fiber involvement.

With each of these three modes, *amperage* will determine the intensity of contractions, while the *duty cycle* will establish the on/off relationship. Current amplitudes usually run in the low to mid-amperage range, e.g., 1 to 75 mamp. *Pulse durations* provide relative comfort and are measured in milliseconds in the 1 to 300 ms range. Many clinicians utilize all three modes in a general treatment session: tetanizing for relaxation, followed by the ramped or pulsed mode for exercising.

The advantages of electrical stimulation are: relatively weight-free exercise, increased fiber recruitment, enhanced reticuloendothelial waste removal, increased circulation, and endorphin-release analgesia. It should be noted that electrical stimulation is far from "passive," since the target myofascial tissues contract! The work of Dr. Rosemary Jones, in England,[6] indicates the possibilities of changing slow-twitch fibers to fast-twitch fibers, and the reverse, by selected differential frequency stimulation. Truly, a form of bioengineering! (It is interesting to note that two other Britishers report success with specialized elec-

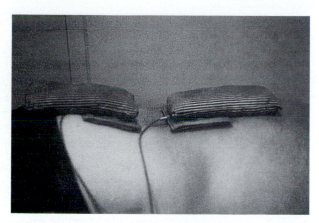

FIG 15–1. Low-volt ac stimulation to the lumbosacral region. (Courtesy of Preston Corp., Jackson, Mich.)

trical stimulation with specific conditions: Nobuku Shindo[13] reports obtaining active contraction and relaxation with spastic paraplegics using low-volt parameters; and Diane Farragher[5] administers low-volt pulsed dc with physiologically matched parameters for chronic Bell's palsy.)

Traditional low-volt stimulation utilizes both ac and dc to produce contractions in normally innervated musculature (and the associated myofascial tissues). However, in the presence of nerve damage (reaction of degeneration, or "RD" to physical therapists), the ability to respond to ac (and faradic) is lost, and *only pulsed dc will be effective*. Low-volt procedures usually fall below 100 V and 1 kHz. Current amplitudes lie in the 1 to 75-mamp range. (Figs 15–1 and 15–2).

IONTOPHORESIS

Iontophoresis is not a form of electrical stimulation per se, although the current used may offer some stimulatory effects indirectly. The continuous low-volt dc mode is utilized for ionic transfer, or iontophoresis, and is the *sole* current form for this purpose. Despite the dc characteristics of high-volt pulsed dc, it is not used for iontophoresis owing to the extremely short duration of the

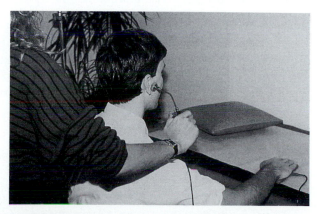

FIG 15–2. Low-volt stimulation for nerve degeneration using pulsed dc. (Courtesy of Preston Corp., Jackson, Mich.)

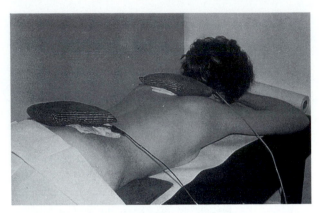

FIG 15–3.   Double iontophoresis, administering two ions of different polarities simultaneously with a standard dc generator. (Courtesy of Teca Corp., Pleasantville, N.Y.)

pulses (in the microsecond range) and low microamperage involved. The formula for ionic transfer requires amperage over a period of time, negating the effectiveness of any *pulsed* waveforms. The successful introduction of chemical substances into the body is accomplished via the continuous polarity of dc (Fig 15–3).

Electrode placement with iontophoresis becomes a most important aspect of technique. Since the cathode (−) is considerably more irritating to the skin because of the sodium hydroxide formed at the skin-electrode interface with dc, it is advised to keep the cathode at least twice the size of the anode (+) at all times, *even if the cathode is the active electrode. This reduces current density on the cathode and lessens the chance of burns.* One commercial source[3] now offers "buffered" electrodes for iontophoresis which are claimed to be effective in reducing the chemical irritation formed at the cathode as well as the weak hydrochloric acid formed at the anode. Consequently, their electrodes are almost of equal size. Whether the buffering substance or mechanism affects the ionic transfer *itself* remains to be seen. (Figs 15–4 and 15–5).

HIGH-VOLTAGE STIMULATION

High-volt pulsed dc was originally considered for deeper penetration than obtained with low-volt. The extremely short pulse durations in the microsec-

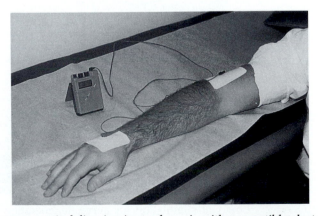

FIG 15–4.   Compact unit delivering iontophoresis with compatible electrodes. (Courtesy of Empi Inc., St. Paul, Minn.)

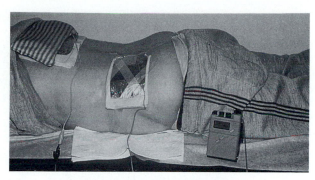

FIG 15–5. Compact unit with traditional electrodes. (Courtesy of Empi Inc., St. Paul Minn.)

ond range, as well as the microamperage attained, necessitate increased power up to 500 V in order to obtain muscular contractions. This neatly falls under the aegis of the traditional strength-duration curve phenomenon, so familiar to physical therapy students. The relative comfort of this mode is a matter of individual sensitivities. The quality of the contractions, however, remains similar to those with traditional low-volt techniques. The typical waveform is a twin-spiked dc, 7 to 20 μs duration, pulsed at 1 to 100 pps. at microamperage levels, with selected active electrode polarity.[1] (Fig 15–6).

INTERFERENTIAL CURRENTS

Interferential currents utilize the penetrating quality of the medium frequencies, i.e., 4,000 Hz, to reach greater depths than with low-volt equipment. Here, two different medium frequencies are "crossed" to produce "beat" frequencies in the optimal range of 50 to 100 Hz *deeper than what is available with low-volt procedures at the same frequencies.* By maintaining one of the two frequencies constant (4,000 Hz), and taking the second through a range of frequencies (4,001–4,100 Hz), a broad spectrum of beat frequencies are obtained, stimulating a wide number of fibers with differential frequency response capabilities. Thus, a greater recruitment possibility is realized, as are diagnostic clues regarding stronger responses to the lower beat frequencies where partial denervation is present. Since the interferential currents are normally biphasic (ac), near-normal innervation is necessary. Power runs in the 1- to 100-V range, with continuous

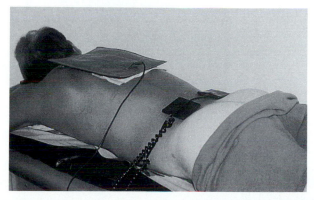

FIG 15–6. Typical high-volt pulsed dc for a low back syndrome (sandbags removed). (Courtesy of Dynamax Corp. [Preston Corp.], Jackson, Mich.)

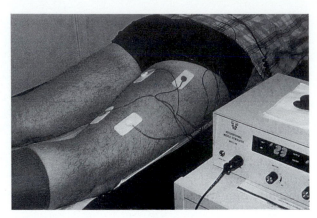

FIG 15–7. Interferential current stimulation with circuits crossed over the hamstring musculature. (Courtesy of Birtcher Corp., El Monte, Calif.)

and variable beat frequencies used singularly or in a "sweep" mode, covering many frequencies. "Vectoring" is also available on many models, and is a method of pinpointing the exact location of the crossing point and permitting variation of frequency ranges and targeting. (Fig 15–7).

RUSSIAN STIMULATION

So-called Russian stimulation is usually 2,500 Hz, pulsed at variable rates from 1 to 100 pps, with an asymmetric biphasic waveform. Here again, patient comfort is determined by individual sensitivities. At the 2,500-Hz frequency, higher voltages are again required, i.e., 300 to 500 V (Fig 15–8).

MICROAMPERE STIMULATION

The latest entry into the field are the microampere stimulation devices. The mnemonic MENS is incorrect, since the N (neural) is out of place. Stimulation here is to the "second circuit" in the body, advocated by Dr. Bjorn Nordenstrom[12] and others. The microamperage is hardly sufficient to affect the primary

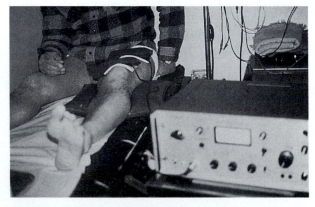

FIG 15–8. "Russian" stimulation to the quadriceps muscle groups. (Courtesy of Promotek Corp., Joliet, Ill.)

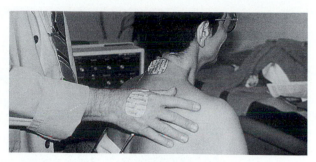

FIG 15–9. Manual technique with microampere stimulation. (Courtesy of Monad Corp., Pomona, Calif.)

neural system. It is designed to reach the circulatory ionic transfer routes within the capillaries, rather than the sensory or motor nerve circuitry. Microampere stimulation is programmed to enhance healing of damaged tissues by bringing bloodborne nutrient materials to the target zone. The naturally high resistance of damaged tissues is overcome by the addition of microcurrents to the ion transport system in the capillaries, simulating the intrinsic microcurrents of the body's own system. Polarity is obtained via square wave dc, with alternating polarity capabilities of the symmetric square waveform. Frequency capabilities range from less than 1 Hz through 100 Hz. Amplitude range is up to 500 μamp. In many instances, microampere stimulation provides a modicum of analgesia. Little or no sensation or contractions are noted by the patient, since neither sensory nor motor points are stimulated with these parameters (Fig 15–9).

TRANSCUTANEOUS ELECTRICAL NERVE STIMULATION

TENS is designed to block the pain sensation's pathway along the ascending neural tracts. Explained in Melzack and Wall's "gate theory"[10] and by the endorphin release phenomena, this modality has gained in popularity in the past two decades despite unjustified criticism. Most TENS devices today utilize an asymmetric biphasic waveform, with frequency ranges from 1 to 150 Hz, pulse widths from 50 to 300 ms and amplitudes through 75 mcmp. Frequency and pulse width modulation are usually available to minimize accommodation. Several models also offer a "burst" mode, with stimulation in a pulselike form, found by some clinicians to be an effective temporary analgesic mode. Very few,

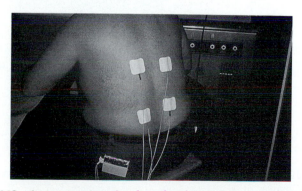

FIG 15–10. TENS administered to the dorsolumbar region. (Courtesy of Minnesota Mining and Manufacturing Co., St Paul, Minn.)

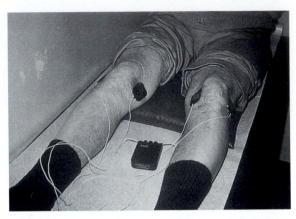

FIG 15–11. TENS shown in the transarthral mode for bilateral knees. (Courtesy of Dynex Corp., St. Paul, Minn.)

if any, TENS models offer the polarity found with square waves. An asymmetric biphasic waveform will indicate a slight polar phenomenon, but not at clinically significant or detectable levels. This would explain the differential color coding on lead wires, i.e., red (+) and black (−) (Figs 15–10 and 15–11). TENS has also been found effective in osteogenic enhancement for nonunited fractures.[8] (Fig 15–12).

ULTRASOUND

Ultrasound, although not electrical in nature, behaves much like electrical phenomena. Household current, 110 V at 60 Hz, is amplified to 500 V at 1 MHz, and is imposed on a piezoelectric crystal (usually PZT: lead-zirconium-titanate) to produce sound waves at 1 Mc for therapeutic purposes. Currently there are units available which operate at 3 Mc. Unlike electromagnetic phenomena, increased absorption levels are obtained with *lower* frequencies with ultrasound. The 1-Mc units, therefore, are utilized for deeper penetration, while the 3-Mc

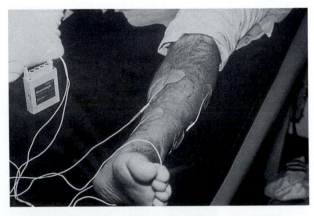

FIG 15–12. TENS administered for osteogenic enhancement with a nonunion fracture. (Courtesy of Neurologix Corp., Franklin Square, N.Y.)

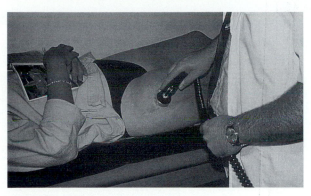

FIG 15–13. Ultrasound administered over a painful, tight scar. (Courtesy of Birtcher Corp., El Monte, Calif.)

units are suggested for superficial tissues, i.e., myofascial (Fig 15–13). Subaqueous techniques with ultrasound are recommended for anatomic problem areas (Fig 15–14).

PHONOPHORESIS

The introduction of chemical substances into the body with sound waves, i.e., *phonophoresis,* offers clinicians a convenient, noninvasive procedure to obtain the benefits of specific therapeutic chemical agents. There should be no confusing phonophoresis with iontophoresis, however. They are two distinctly different concepts. Phonophoresis is the introduction of entire *molecules* into the tissues, which then must be broken down into usable components by the body's systems. Iontophoresis is the introduction of *ions,* which are chemically active and ready for recombination. Ultrasound provides slightly deeper penetration than the 1 mm offered by iontophoresis. At deeper levels, however, the circulating blood washes away the introduced molecules sooner than the ions deposited at a shallower level where there are fewer blood vessels. Many clinicians take advantage of these phenomena by utilizing *both* procedures when-

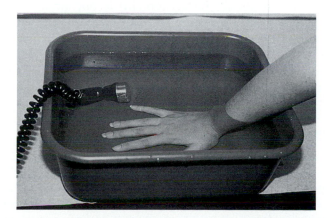

FIG 15–14. Subaqueous ultrasound. (Courtesy of Birtcher Corp., El Monte, Calif.)

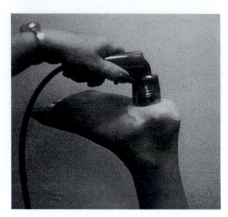

FIG 15–15.   Phonophoresis administered with hydrocortisone ointment for a painful heel. (Courtesy of Mettler Corp., Anaheim, Calif.)

ever possible. (Solutions may be used with iontophoresis, as well as ointments, as ion sources.) Phonophoresis is not recommended with solutions, only ointments. If an ointment is used as an ion source, the treatment may be followed by application of ultrasound with the usual gel or other transmission medium superimposed over the remaining ointment (Fig 15–15).

Simultaneous ultrasound with electrical stimulation has been a popular procedure for many years. Unfortunately, there is little in the literature to document the advantages of this technique other than the saving of time. After all, ultrasound is utilized to obtain muscle relaxation, while electrical stimulation favors contraction! It is difficult to conceive maximum benefit of *either* if administered simultaneously! Ultrasound treatments usually require a much shorter time than effective electrical stimulation procedures. Pulsing the ultrasound in order to use a longer treatment time has satisfied some practitioners, but not the die-hards!

SHORTWAVE DIATHERMY

Shortwave diathermy remains in our armamentarium as the single modality able to produce heat *deep* within the tisues without heating the superficial layers. It becomes a very valuable procedure when the target tissues are within the thorax, abdominal cavity, sinuses, and joint capsules, inaccessible by other means. With myofascial targets at *deeper* levels, shortwave diathermy becomes a modality of choice. (Fig 15–16).

COLD LASER

The helium-neon COLD LASER offers the clinician a unique opportunity to penetrate the cell membrane in order to facilitate healing. The selected wavelength of 632.8 nm, obtained from a helium-neon mixture, has been shown to penetrate the cell membrane and effectively stimulate the mitochondria responsible for production of DNA, adenosine triphosphate (ATP), etc. Operating at

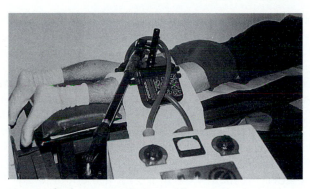

FIG 15–16. Shortwave diathermy applied over the popliteal region. (Courtesy of Burdick Corp., Madison, Wis.)

only 1 mW, the cold laser also serves as a point stimulator over known acupuncture points, trigger points, and inflammatory sites. (A familiar analogy is often made by practitioners to the laser as "acupuncture with a beam of light instead of a needle!") Recent developments have led to the addition of units operating at higher milliwatt levels. Canadian and European models utilize milliwattage *considerably higher* then domestic models. At the time of this writing, the helium-neon cold laser is still under "clinical investigation" status, requiring much paperwork, statistical submissions, and administrative protocols. Those physical therapists currently working with the cold laser are extremely enthusiastic over their results, and are anxiously awaiting premarket approval by the Food and Drug Administration (FDA) so that studies and clinical applications may be expanded.[2, 7, 9, 11, 14] (Fig 15–17).

TRIGGER POINTS

Special attention to trigger points is warranted here. These mysterious points, when stimulated, elicit reactions at distant points. Generally, these reactions lie within dermatomes, myotomes, or the oriental "meridians" familiar to acupuncturists. The ideal practitioner to treat trigger points is the physical

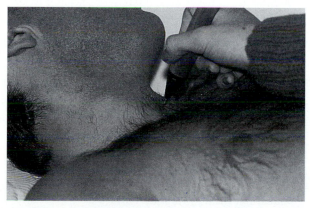

FIG 15–17. Helium-neon cold laser directed at a contracted tracheostomy scar with a postcoma patient. (Courtesy of Dynatronic Corp., Salt Lake City, Utah)

therapist, since much of his or her training is at the "hands-on" level of care. Manual palpation remains the best method of locating trigger points. Once located, however, the method of stimulation becomes a matter of choice, experience, and training for the clinician. There is an extensive menu for the clinician: heat (moxibustion), cold (cryotherapy), digital pressure (shiatsu), ultrasound (sonopuncture), electricity (TENS and microampere stimulation), light (cold laser), and, of course, invasive techniques (injections and acupuncture). For the average physical therapist, the choices usually are limited to TENS, cold laser, ultrasound, or manual pressure, individually or in varied combinations. With the exception of TENS, the others are clinical or office procedures. TENS, however, is mainly designed for use at home, by the patient, *after* clinically ascertaining efficacy. Manual techniques may be included during massage or mobilization, as well as during the initial evaluation procedures. Ultrasound, since it is a short procedure, may be added to and included in any of the scheduled treatment sessions. Heat has been used to reduce pain for decades in the form of diathermy, microthermy, moist heat, and infrared radiation. Cold has been used in acute conditions but has also been utilized over trigger points for temporary analgesia. Electric stimulation, in the form of TENS, is widely used for analgesia, with electrode placements including trigger points, nerve roots, and known acupuncture points. Neither the motor nor sensory circuitry in the body will respond readily to microamperage. The healing characteristics and polar phenomena with microamperage apparently account for its efficacy.

In summary, the physical therapist's noninvasive approach to trigger point treatment is a matter of selective, personal experience, and expertise with each of the listed modalities, leaving invasive methods by physicians and acupuncturists as a last resort.

REFERENCES

1. Alon G: *High voltage stimulation,* Chattanooga Corp., Chattanooga, 1984, Chattanooga Corp.
2. Barnes JF: Electro-acupuncture and cold laser therapy as adjuncts to pain treatment, *J Craniomandibular Pract* 2:148, 1984.
3. Empi Inc: Dupel System, St Paul, Minn.
4. Enmeweka C: Laser biostimulation of healing wounds: specific effects and mechanisms of action. *J Spinal Phys Ther* 9:333–338, 1988.
5. Farragher Diane: Personal communication, 1985.
6. Jones Rosemary: Personal communication, 1985.
7. Kahn J: Open wound management with the HeNe cold laser, *J Spinal Phys Ther* 6:203, 1984.
8. Kahn J: *Principles and practice of electrotherapy,* ed 2, New York, 1991, Churchill Livingstone.
9. Kleinkort J, Foley RA: *The cold laser, Clin Manage* 2:30, 1982.
10. Melzack R, Wall PD: *Pain mechanisms, a new theory, Science* 150:971, 1965.
11. Mester E: The effect of laser rays on wound healing, *Am J Surg* 122:532, 1971.
12. Nordenstrom B: An electrifying possibility, reviewed by Gary Taubes in *Discovery,* April 1986, pp 22–27.
13. Shindo Nobuko: Personal communication, 1985.
14. Snyder L, Meckler C, Borc L: The effect of cold laser on musculoskeletal trigger points, *Phys Ther,* 745, May 1984.

SUGGESTED READING

Gersh MR: *Electrotherapy in rehabilitation*, Philadelphia, 1992, FA Davis.

Kaplan PG, Tanner E: *Musculoskeletal pain and disability*, East Norwalk, Conn, 1989, Appleton & Lange. pp 291–303.

Low J, Reed A: *Electrotherapy explained*, London, 1990, Butterworth-Heinemann.

Scully M, Barnes MR: *Physical therapy*, Philadelphia, 1989, JB Lippincott, pp 876–900.

Wilder E: *Obstetric and gynecologic physical therapy*, New York, 1988, Churchill Livingstone, pp 113–129.

Chapter 16

The Role of Ergonomics in the Prevention and Treatment of Myofascial Pain

Tarek M. Khalil, Ph.D., P.E.
Elsayed Abdel-Moty, Ph.D.
Renee Steele-Rosomoff, R.N., M.B.A.
Hubert L. Rosomoff, M.D., D.Med. Sci.

ERGONOMICS: SCIENCE AND PRACTICE

Over the centuries, humans have designed tools and equipment with the purpose of increasing productivity and making tasks and life easier. With the advancement of technology, task demands increased and tools and equipment became complex and sometimes hazardous to the users. Soon developed the need to consider human factors (body size, strength, etc.) in the design and development of "things" in order to preserve health and safety and improve the quality of life. The term "fitting the man to the job" was then used to describe the process of selecting and training military personnel. The objective was to increase accuracy, safety, and efficiency of individuals through matching human characteristics with the task demands as well as designing equipment that best meet human expectations. Shortly after World War II the field of human factors became more defined and ergonomics became recognized.

Derived from the Greek *ergon*, "work," and *nomos*, "law," ergonomics is the scientific study of work and of the relationship between people and their working (or living) environment. This relationship entails people, equipment, environmental conditions, and tasks. On the one hand, humans have certain capabilities. These can be described in terms of anatomic (structural), physiologic (functional), and psychological (behavioral) attributes. Humans also have limitations arising from factors such as gender differences, aging, physical fitness, diet, stress, as well as pain and injury. Our abilities (and limitations), combined with the necessary acquired skills, determine how well we perform daily tasks. Ergonomics help people recognize their abilities and limitations for safe and effective performance within the environment.

A major dilemma facing ergonomists and occupational health and safety specialists has been that the work environments are often designed without adequate consideration for the people who must use them. It has been realized that inadequate workplace design can contribute to stress, injury, pain, job-related disabilities, and subsequently lost productivity. If products are designed with the human factor in mind, a high level of performance may be expected. If products are designed without considering the human factor, health and safety hazards can be expected.

Ergonomics is an interdisciplinary field of study that integrates engineering, medical, physical, and behavioral sciences to address issues arising from the existences of humans in an increasingly technological society. As a field of study, ergonomics deals with many areas, including job design, work performance, health and safety, stress, posture, body mechanics, biomechanics, anthropometry, manual material handling, equipment design, quality control, environment, worker's education and training, and employment testing.

The Basis of the Ergonomic Approach—The Human-Machine System: Our Interaction With What We Use

The basis of the ergonomic approach to the management of musculoskeletal injuries in general, and to myofascial pain in particular, is based on the model of the human-machine system (HMS). This system has three main elements (Fig 16–1): (1) humans, (2) machines, and (3) the environment.

The main interest is the human and how he or she interacts with tools, machines, and environments (whether at work, in a rehabilitation setting, at home,

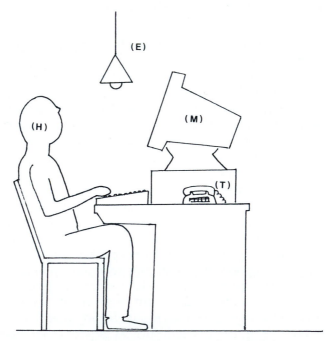

FIG 16–1. The basis of the ergonomic approach to the management of myofascial pain is the study of the "human-machine system." The components of this system are: humans *(H)* having certain capabilities and limitations; machines *(M)* and tools *(T)* having specific design and layout characteristics; and environment *(E)* being physical (light, heat, etc.) as well as social (family, job satisfaction, etc.).

or on the golf course). A mismatch between human characteristics and the environment can create stresses on human anatomic, physiologic, and psychological systems that can result in acute or chronic health problems in general and to soft tissue injury and myofascial syndromes in particular.

The goal of ergonomics is to establish an HMS that insures a proper match between people and their surroundings and reduces the levels of stresses imposed by machines and the environment. These goals may be summarized as follows:

- Help people recognize their abilities and limitations.
- Increase knowledge and safety awareness.
- Reduce fatigue.
- Reduce stress.
- Improve performance.
- Increase job satisfaction.
- Match people to tasks.
- Adjust environments to people.
- Design products for people.
- Reduce human errors.
- Improve work habits.

- Improve safety.
- Reduce health hazards.
- Control injury.
- Reduce accidents.
- Reduce cumulative trauma.
- Simplify work methods.
- Modify tasks and jobs.

- Decrease work lost time.
- Help the injured person to return to work.
- Prevent reinjury.

- Reduce absenteeism.
- Reduce labor turnover.
- Reduce health and disability costs.
- Improve quality at work.
- Improve productivity.
- Improve quality of life.

These goals, in turn, involve recognizing and solving problems inherent in the HMS. In doing so, ergonomics recognizes four important facts:

1. Machines and equipment should be designed and prescribed based on recognized human characteristics.
2. Tasks should be structured to enhance ease, efficiency, and safety.
3. Job demands and human capabilities should be matched.
4. People must be made aware of the environment within which they perform.

ERGONOMIC CONTRIBUTIONS

The management of work-related stress and injury can be viewed as consisting of three main components. These can be classified according to the stage of injury or pain occurrence. The first component represents efforts in the prevention and avoidance of injury and pain *(injury prevention stage)*. Once an injury takes place, the second component is pain management, rehabilitation, and treatment *(rehabilitation stage)*. The third component follows rehabilitation, where efforts are directed to insure the patient's safe return to a productive lifestyle while minimizing the chances of reinjury *(postrehabilitation stage)*. The contributions of ergonomics to each of these stages are described below.

Ergonomics in the Injury Prevention Stage

Ideally, the thrust of the ergonomics approach is to control the risk factors that can contribute to injury rather than take corrective actions after a mishap. In this stage of prevention (also known as the *primary prevention stage*), the implementation of established ergonomics guidelines for safety and accident prevention reduces the individual's exposure to risk factors. Some of these guidelines are summarized in Table 16–1. Following the theme of the HMS, these guidelines deal with: (1) the human; and (2) the environment.

Human Safety

It has been recognized that safety is everyone's responsibility (Fig 16–2). For this purpose, engineering design for safety is the primary line of defense. However, people should also be made aware of the stresses imposed by the work (or home) environment and by the biomechanical principles of posture and task performance. Workers should be trained to recognize their abilities and limitations. Increasing safety knowledge and practice should be individualized for the person and for the job with a sufficient degree of generalization since the same concepts must be transferred to the home and to recreational activities, and become an integral part of daily activities.

Workplace Safety

Safety in the workplace has been a main area of interest to engineers, human factors, and occupational health and safety specialists. In order to

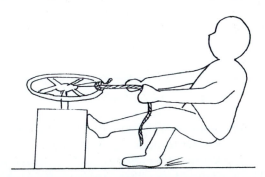

FIG 16–2. Safety is everyone's responsibility. Careless acts, whether resulting from poor safety awareness, human error, or problems in the engineering design of tools and equipment, can be detrimental to health and can become very costly to the individual and the organization.

TABLE 16–1.

Ergonomic Safety Guidelines for the Prevention of Injuries

Designing for people
    Accommodate population percentiles: do not design for an average person
    For space requirements, accommodate the large person
    For reaches, accommodate the small person
    Provide adequate space for movement
    Consider the limits of muscular force and strength
Making workstations safe and comfortable
    Educate and train workers
    Design adjustable workstations
    Select appropriate seating for the individual and the task
    Design tools to facilitate task performance
    Lay out work areas within easy access (Fig 16–3)
    Keep equipment and supplies for immediate use
    Locate control switches within easy reach
    Allow sitting and standing
    Take note of the visual attributes of the individual
    Provide good environmental conditions
Posture is as important as equipment
    Maintain proper posture: keep joints in the neutral position (Fig 16–4)
    Avoid unnatural posture (Fig 16–5)
    Provide a wide balanced support on the feet while standing
    Avoid prolonged periods of static posture
    Stand straight without slumping
    Alternate the sides of the body (Fig 16–6)
    Both sitting and standing are preferred
    Support the arms and the back while sitting
    Analyze posture to pinpoint cause of pain
    Practice perfect posture
    Reclined postures are acceptable provided there is good support
    Maintain knees at optimal level
    Distribute weight uniformly
Lifting safely
    Think! Plan the lifting job ahead—size it up!
    Test the "object"—examine it!

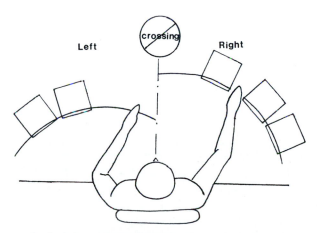

FIG 16–3. Human body joints are not functionally structured to move in straight lines. The layout of work tools must allow natural movements while minimizing repetitive twisting and excessive turning. In this case, work tools should be arranged within the area defined by the "maximum" and "comfortable" reaches of the operator. Excessive "crossing" of the imaginary midline should be minimized, as well as the resulting twisting action.

TABLE–1.(cont.).

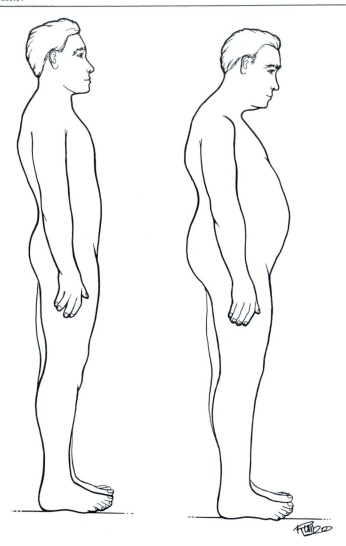

FIG 16–4.   Poor posture can be the result of obesity, poor work habits, structural deficiencies, poor self-esteem, muscle weakness, as well as a variety of other factors. Good posture should be consciously practiced and maintained.

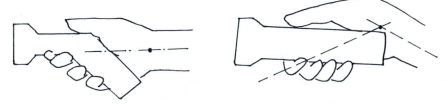

FIG 16–5.   In some instances *(right)* the design of tools and equipment does not allow proper natural alignment of body joints, thus placing unnecessary stress on the soft tissue. Whenever possible, better engineering designs *(left)* should be provided. People should be made aware of this type of condition and learn corrective methods.

TABLE—1.(cont.).

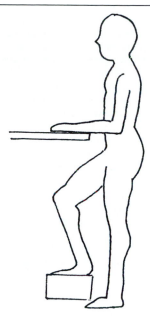

FIG 16–6. By providing a step stool, standing tolerance can be increased. Allowing weight shifting reduces static loading on muscle groups.

    Position yourself—have a stable lift position
    Grasp firmly
    Choose a proper lifting technique (Fig 16–7)
    Prepare your muscles for action
    Lift smoothly
    Move with the object
    NEVER lift beyond YOUR capacities
Practicing good body mechanics
    Work within the viewing area
    Bring objects close to your focus without crouching

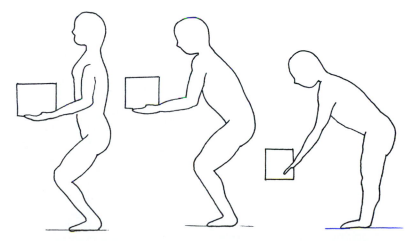

FIG 16–7. Lifting an object far away from the body *(right)* places higher stresses on the body than if the object is held closer to the body's center of gravity *(middle* and *left)*. A hot or greasy object, on the other hand, may be difficult to handle while applying proper lifting techniques. In this case, other ergonomic solutions should be investigated.

TABLE–1.(cont.).

Shift weight
    Avoid holding the telephone between the head and the shoulder (Fig 16–8).
    Avoid carrying too much in one hand (Fig 16–9)
    When pulling, switch hands to avoid straining muscles
    Don't hunch the trunk over your desk
    Don't slouch when reading in a chair
    Avoid prolonged hyperextension and hyperflexion
    Get as close to the work area as possible
    Avoid twisting and sudden turning
    Avoid abrupt reflex movements
    Minimize repetitive movements
    Avoid working overhead for extended periods of time
    Minimize overreaching as well as reaching behind the head
    Make use of stronger muscles to perform the same task
    Modify sleeping habits or reevaluate bed and pillows
    Exercise for stretching and strengthening
    Sit better to drive better (Fig 16–10)
Choosing the right chair
    Back and seat supports should be contoured
    The chair should be upholstered
    Flexible tilting is desirable
    Adjust the seat and the backrest independently
    A high backrest is preferable

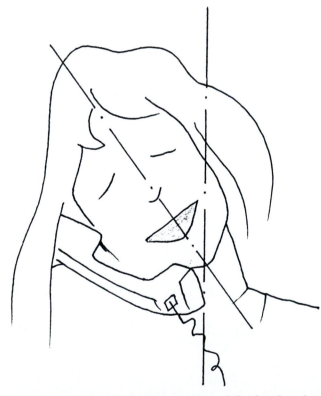

FIG 16–8.   A very common, yet incorrect, posture of the head and neck while using the telephone. Such severe deviations from the neutral posture place a significant amount of stress on the neck muscles and can result in myofascial pain. This posture violates the ergonomic principal of "efficiency in muscle use."

TABLE–1.(cont.).

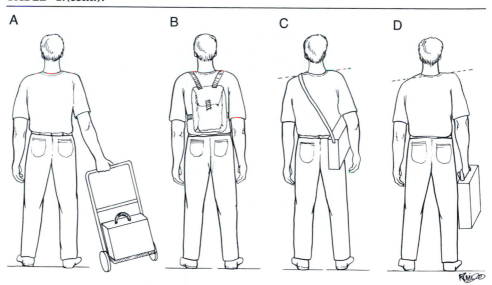

FIG 16–9.   There are many ways to perform a single-handed carrying task. Ergonomically, some postures are preferred (**A** and **B**) since the resulting biomechanical stresses are lower or are distributed on the body. For some patients who experience recurrent pain on one side, the posture shown in **C** may be preferred. In this case, weight distribution is shared by the body with some concentration on the nonpainful side. Carrying a heavy load in one hand without alternating sides, as in **D,** is the least desirable and should be avoided. In all cases, good postural habits should be maintained.

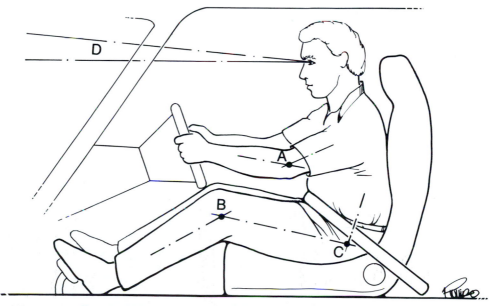

FIG 16–10.   Driving postures vary depending on the type of car, the space allowed, and the dimensions of the individual driver. In general, angulation is recommended at the elbows, knees, and hips to allow for comfortable reaching to all controls, sufficient force to apply the brakes safely, and comfortable viewing of the rear-view-mirror and the side mirrors.

TABLE–1.(cont.).

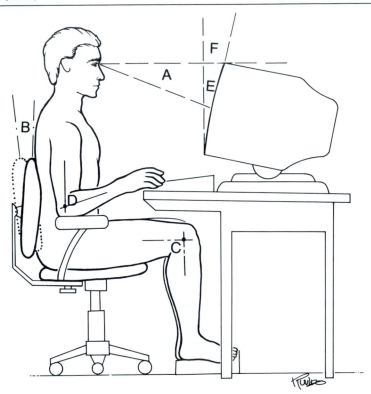

FIG 16–11. The complexity in designing computer workplaces is largely due to the number of variables involved. Recommendations call for a slightly tilted backrest *(b)*, about a 90-degree angle at the elbows *(d)*, knees slightly higher than the hips *(c)*, the VDT within the viewing area *(a)*, and the VDT screen at an angle that minimizes glare and light reflections *(f)*. The magnitude of these parameters should be individualized for the workplace user.

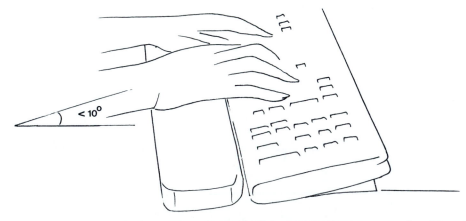

FIG 16–12. By providing a soft support to this computer operator, a comfortable wrist angle can be maintained and shoulder stress resulting from the unsupported weight of the arms can be minimized. Chair arm supports, keyboard holders, and adjusting the chair height may provide a similar effect.

TABLE–1.(cont.).

The backrest should be angled about −10 degrees
The seat height should be easily adjustable
An adjustable seat depth is desirable
The front edge of the chair should be contoured
Seat width should allow movement
Provide adjustable arm supports
Casters are desirable
Provide a five-spur pedestal
Provide swivel chairs
Guidelines for working with computers
The VDT screen should be 5–10 degrees below the horizontal (Fig 16–11)
The primary viewing areas should be less than 60 degrees
The keyboard should fall directly below the hands
Gentle resting of the palms and forearms is recommended (Fig 16–12)
Having a stand for reference material is essential
The workstation desktop should have two levels
Provide appropriate seating for the job
The angle between the upper arm and forearm should be less than 135 degrees

implement human factor considerations in design, ergonomic guidelines published in the general literature[48, 66] as well as industry standards (American National Standards Institute, ANSI, 1981) must be followed. The focus of these guidelines is reducing stress on human systems. These recommendation are to be implemented by suitably trained and knowledgeable persons. In order to insure the comprehensiveness of safety implementation, a checklist can be developed (an example is given in Table 16–2) and used. Addressing the issues in the checklist helps in identifying risk factor(s) and documenting actions taken to insure proper implementation of subsequent interventions.

Ergonomics in the Rehabilitation (Postinjury) Stage

Until the early 1980s, the management of myofascial pain was considered the sole domain of medical professionals. In 1982, the concepts of "technology rehabilitation" and "clinical ergonomics" were introduced at the University of Miami Comprehensive Pain and Rehabilitation Center (CPRC).[36, 40, 42, 44, 56, 57] Technology intervention implies the use of prosthetic, orthotic, and ergonomically inspired equipment and techniques to restore performance of patients with chronic injuries to a state of wellness.

At the CPRC, ergonomists work jointly with physicians, therapists, and other health care professionals in a rehabilitation environment (Fig 16–13). This interaction has provided an excellent intervention forum for recognizing and solving many complex problems related to myofascial pain and musculoskeletal injury.

Once injury and pain occur, the ergonomic approach to the management of the problem is hierarchial and can be identified under three steps: (1) identification of the problem and its source (s) or origin(s); (2) evaluation of the effect of the injury and pain on its victim; (3) implementation of intervention strategies to deal with the problem and its effects.

TABLE 16–2.

An Ergonomic Checklist

Operator	
Age	Strength
Flexibility	Mobility
Alertness	Skills
Fitness level	Diet
Behaviors	Attitudes
Workplace	
Reach	Space
Location	Chair
Work surface	Pedals
Gloves	Stairs
Ladders	Computer
Physical demands	
Lifting	Carrying
Reaching	Walking
Standing	Sitting
Climbing	Fingering
Handling	Squatting
Kneeling	Crouching
Crawling	Seeing
Hearing	Talking
Environment	
Illumination	Contrast
Glare	Color perception
Optical aids	Instruments placement
Warning signals	Noise level
Air circulation	Temperature
Humidity	Dust
Mist	Shock hazards
Smell	Even floors
Wet floors	Hot surface
Protective devices	Radiation
Task	
Variety	Complexity
Equilibrium	Flexibility
Mental load	
Speed	Quantity
Rate	Memory
Choice	Feedback
Monotony	Tolerance for error

Identification of the Problem

It is important to identify, as early as possible, the cause of the problem. During this process, the origins of the problem are searched and pinpointed from the following perspectives:

1. Medical (e.g., symptoms and presence of other illnesses).
2. Physical (e.g., strength, body dimensions).
3. Physiologic (e.g., lack of fitness, aging).
4. Functional (e.g., limitations in performance).
5. Occupational (e.g., workload, poor posture).
6. Behavioral (e.g., job dissatisfaction).

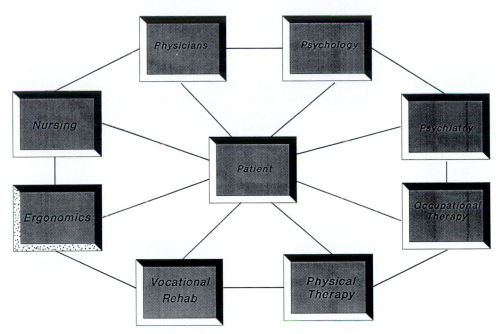

FIG 16–13. At the University of Miami Comprehensive Pain and Rehabilitation Center, ergonomists work jointly with physicians, therapists, and other health care professionals in a multidisciplinary rehabilitation setting to provide the patient with the necessary tools for functional restoration.

The underlying assumption in this approach is that the majority of disorders may be induced environmentally or occupationally or through a combination of one or more of the above factors. The scientific ergonomic approach does not subscribe to the notion that people who claim to have injuries or pain are malingerers or that they have the so-called compensation neurosis. Searching for the origin of the problem is therefore considered the most important prerequisite to intervention.

There are health concerns regarding the musculoskeletal response to daily demands in activities of daily living (ADL) and at work. Disorders such as muscle strain, carpal tunnel syndrome, tendinitis, and tenosynovitis have been linked to work tasks. Pain and injury to the soft tissues (muscles, tendons, ligaments) in particular due to work situations is an increasing problem for industrialized societies. Soft tissue injuries (STIs), in general, can result from: (1) a single event of high magnitude of stress (acute injury or traumatic incident); (2) cumulative events of low magnitude of stress (a series of events resulting in microtrauma).

Some traumatic accidents (e.g., slips and falls and car accidents) will continue to occur. However, safety education and awareness may help reduce the chances of accidental injuries. Cumulative trauma disorders (CTDs), also known as cumulative trauma injuries, repetitive stress disorders, overuse motion strain are the industrial disease of modern age. They are the most frequently reported on-the-job ailment. CTDs accounted for 18% and 48% of all occupational injuries in 1981 and 1988, respectively. By the year 2000, over half the work force could be vulnerable to CTDs (US News & World Report, 1990). In terms of medical cost, $27 billion a year is spent on medical bills and lost days. (American Academy of Orthopaedic Surgeons).

Risk Factors Associated With STIs. Many factors have been linked to the onset or development of STIs. Among these are:[48, 64, 67]

1. Physical factors (e.g., posture, strength, flexibility, body build, reflexes, aerobic capacity).
2. Individual factors (e.g., age, medical history, body weight, height, degeneration, education, alcohol misuse, fitness level, nutrition).
3. Psychological factors (e.g., depression, marital discord, family problems, anxiety, job dissatisfaction, personality traits, attitudes toward work).
4. Environmental and work factors (e.g., lifting, prolonged sitting, accidents, vibration, years on job, driving, slips and falls, climate).

There are many types of daily tasks and jobs which can eventually cause cumulative trauma leading to an STI. Among these are: passing thousands of groceries over a checkout scanner, supermarket checking, typing at a computer keyboard, assembly line work, manufacturing, meat processing and butchering, hairdressing, sewing and knitting, packing, stapling, tight grasping of the steering wheel, polishing and buffing, welding, surface grinding, painting, dentistry, interpreting, postal work, milking cows, use of a spray gun, stirring, and sports.

While it has been thought that the highest incidence of pain is seen in heavy physical work,[32] recent data[35] suggest that people performing light jobs are as likely to experience musculoskeletal injury and pain as those involved in heavy jobs (Table 16–3). There are certain industrial jobs, however, that have been associated with musculoskeletal problems, e.g., welding,[63] which involves a high degree of working above shoulder level, static stress, and fatigue. These problems of the shoulders manifest themselves in the form of tendinitis, muscle atrophy, limitation in the range of joint motion, and pain,[28] not only in the shoulders but also in the neck, arms, and knees.[64]

Another factor that has been associated with workers' complaints or work-related injuries are activities involving repetitive movements, especially those of the hands and wrists. This phenomenon has been widely publicized, especially in computer keyboard operations such as word processing.

TABLE 16–3.

Descriptive Data of 265 Low Back Pain Patients

No. of males	179
No. of females	86
Average age (yr)	41.7
Occupation	
Heavy work	34.8%
Moderate work	29.8%
Light work	36.4%
Cause of injury	
Falls	41.5%
Lifting and carrying	24.9%
Accidents	7.9%
Simple bending	4.9%
Struck by an object	4.9%
Pushing or pulling	7.9%
Others	7.5%

Studies on the relationship between the incidence of CTDs and task variables have been reported in the literature. While finding *the* factor that is clearly responsible for a CTD is not an easy task, a combination of the following variables has been thought to contribute to the problem:

1. *High frequency:* the repetitiveness of the motion or the cycle time for performing the specific task (Fig 16–14).
2. *High force:* the high forcefulness of muscular exertion.
3. *Poor posture:* in the form of continuous, repeated, and excessive extreme angulation or restriction of a body joint; also, tasks resulting in constrained movements where isometric muscle contraction is sustained.
4. *Long duration:* the length of the task potentially resulting in fatigue and deterioration of neuromuscular performance.
5. *High speed:* where in general faster actions create situations with greater chance for injury.
6. Other factors include, e.g., mechanical vibration (Fig 16–15), cold, mental stress, use of gloves.

In addition to the above physical variables, it has been suggested that a great deal of the CTD phenomenon is behavioral. Some believe that CTD is not an injury but a form of epidemic hysteria[47] in which psychological conflict is subconsciously converted into pain symptoms.[30] Other investigators cite the organized labor movement and its concern with occupational health and safety is-

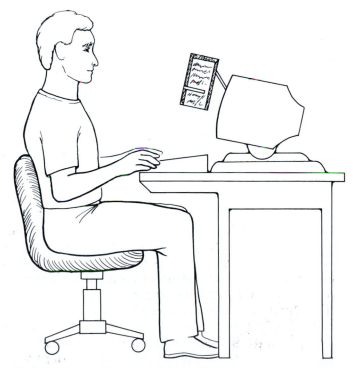

FIG 16–14.   Tasks performed with prolonged high repetition, such as keyboard operations, have been associated with musculoskeletal complaints. In this case, the location of the document holder, the VDT, and the operator, as well as the chair parameters, may contribute to the problem.

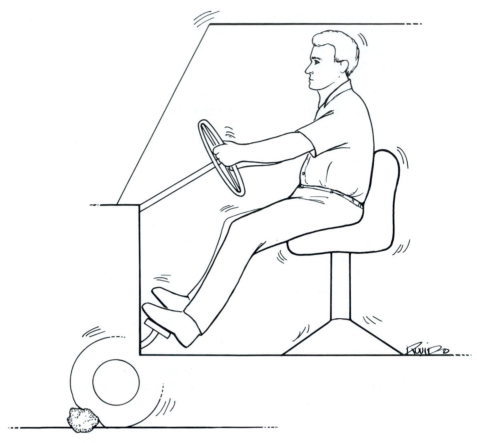

FIG 16–15. Vibration and poor road conditions while driving heavy equipment are a source of discomfort to people with pain. Recent advancements in car design provide "damping" to this type of vibration.

sues[65] and poor work environment,[30] including stress, boredom, and lack of job satisfaction. Still other investigators argue that there is a biomechanical origin to the health problems arising from repetitive movements. The chances are that the explosion in CTD cases has been caused by many of the aforementioned elements.

Manual Lifting and STI. Repetitive material handling (including lifting and carrying) increases vulnerability to myofascial injuries. There have been attempts to control this type of injury through: (1) workers' evaluation, (2) education of proper methods of lifting, and (3) task engineering and design. Various approaches to evaluate the capacity for manual handling tasks have been developed. The most popular of these has been the "psychophysical approach" for determination of lifting capacity[62] in which subjects are allowed to adjust the weight lifted in order to reach what is perceived as the "maximum acceptable weight of lift." Based on this approach, guidelines have been developed for the evaluation and design of tasks involving manual handling of materials.[60, 61] The amount that a person can lift depends on many variables. Any evaluation aimed at establishing the lifting capacity of an individual should take these factors into consideration:

- The distance to load (horizontal).
- The handles (vertical distance, hand spread).

- Task frequency (the weight lifted decreases as frequency increases).
- Load factors (weight distribution, load stability).
- Plane of lifting (e.g., in front of the body).
- Body posture (e.g., twisting, restricted lifting).
- Pattern of lift (e.g., one-handed vs. two-handed lift; smooth, jerking, lifting technique).
- Coupling (e.g., handles, floors, and shoes).
- Ambient environment (space constraints, stairs, altitude).
- Container shape and size.
- Task variables (e.g., distance load is to be carried, rest between lifts, time of day, unexpected motions, duration of lift).
- Human variables (age, gender, fatigue, employee capabilities, employee weight and height, employee skills, past medical history, stress, diet).

Current evidence suggests that training which only stresses approaches of "proper and safe lifting techniques" is not effective in reducing injuries. Most often task demands, environmental conditions, worker awareness, fatigue, and so forth do not permit applying "safe techniques." Programs to teach employees "proper lifting" may not be an effective substitute for a well-engineered workplace and a fit worker. Proper lifting may not be as safe as previously assumed. Loads which can be lifted with the legs can easily exceed the capacity of the low back.

Therefore, in the process of identifying the factors causing or leading to myofascial pain and how to manage it, one should consider the patient in relation to the job factors and the environmental variables. Failure to do so can result in ergonomic misdiagnosis of the problem or misapplication of the solution.

Evaluation

Once the origin of the problem has been identified, the objectives of the ergonomic approach are to: (1) document the effect of pain on the functional abilities of the patient through the use of a quantitative battery of measures describing human abilities; (2) analyze the job and its demands (physical, mental, and environmental). In order to accomplish these objectives, human abilities are measured, job descriptions are analyzed, and environmental factors are determined. Engineering methods are used to analyze jobs and screen work elements through the use of well-established industrial engineering procedures of motion and time study. A combined approach is used to comprehensively review the data collected with respect to the operator's capabilities, work demands, and environmental conditions. Also, alternative methods for performing critical tasks are evaluated.

The quantitative evaluation of patients' abilities is an important undertaking in rehabilitation. In this area, patients' capabilities and limitations are described in terms of the human performance profile (HPP). This profile can consist of physical, physiologic, functional, or work-related measures, or any combination of these.[1, 2, 14–16, 19] The evaluations of physical and physiologic characteristics of human systems (e.g., muscular, skeletal, cardiovascular) yield measurements of strength (Fig 16–16), flexibility, endurance, walking pace, posture, and so forth. Functional evaluations result in measures describing human performance in ADL (e.g., sitting, standing, walking, lifting, etc.). Work-related

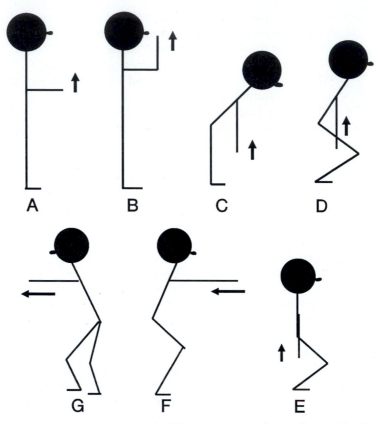

FIG 16–16. Illustrative examples of different postures for testing static strength: arms *(A)*, shoulders *(B)*, stooping *(C)*, squatting *(D)*, legs *(E)*, pulling *(F)*, and pushing *(G)*. Standardization of testing postures, instructions to the subject, test protocols, and measurement methods are of ultimate importance.

measures describe human abilities to perform "specific job" tasks under prescribed conditions.

Human Performance Analysis in Patients With Myofascial Pain. Human performance can be described either in terms of capacities (tolerance limits such as maximum voluntary contraction) or abilities (acceptable levels of performance). For the evaluation of patients with pain conditions, measuring abilities is the most appropriate and realistic.[35] Once an HPP is established for a pain patient, it can then be compared to profiles of healthy persons of equivalent age, sex, and work category in order to determine limitations. Rehabilitation usually involves efforts to restore the patient to the target range of scores for healthy persons. The HPP can then be reestablished to document progress during rehabilitation. When combined with medical and behavioral examinations, the HPP provides a sound basis for evaluation of rehabilitation outcome.

At the University of Miami CPRC, the ergonomics division utilizes these approaches with patients for the purpose of evaluating function[19, 25, 39], monitoring progress during rehabilitation, and quantifying outcome to determine ability to return to work.[10–13, 17, 18, 68] This information is also used to determine patients' daily performance during treatment through computer-generated daily goals.

The interpretation of findings from the HPP in pain patients should be based not on pain factors alone but also on a clear understanding of the factors influencing human performance. Pain factors may include suboptimal muscle performance[51] and muscle wasting.[54] Other factors that may influence performance are anthropometric differences between individuals, gender differences, presence of surgery, behavioral factors, and so on. For instance, in the evaluation of posture, it should be realized that variations in spinal posture may be an attempt to compensate for specific anthropometric and gender differences.[55] There are also differences among patients which arise due to factors such as spinal surgery. Postsurgical patients demonstrate reduced muscle density, fatty replacement, and muscle atrophy,[23, 51] each of these may affect performance. While the exact cause-effect relationship for all the variables involved may not be totally clear, their effect on performance should be investigated medically in order to increase treatment efficiency, as well as investigated ergonomically for the purpose of designing job tasks for safe performance.

Electromyographic Evaluations.   Functional electromyography (EMG) using surface electrodes is often used for the evaluation of muscular function.[4, 53, 58, 59] Other applications of EMG in pain management include:

- Evaluating muscular response to injury and pain (e.g., trigger points).
- Evaluating the neuromuscular response to a treatment modality.
- Assessing posture.
- Evaluating the effects of workplace factors on patients' performance (e.g., equipment design, mechanical vibration).
- Rationalizing body mechanics principles (Fig 16–17, A and B).
- Validating biomechanical models as they apply to pain patients.
- Maximizing muscle work while controlling pain and modifying behaviors (the process of muscle reeducation).

Biomechanical Modeling in Evaluation.   Biomechanical models are used for the theoretical evaluation of stresses on joints or muscles. These models provide a gross estimation of the amount of mechanical stress placed on a body segment, especially in terms of muscle force, joint reactions, and compression forces. Biomechanical models can also be useful for the analysis of job tasks. The development of biomechanical models is rather complex and requires the use of specially developed techniques using computerized systems. Biomechanical models have been utilized repeatedly for the evaluation of the effects of manual handling of materials on the lower back area. Based on the results, guidelines for safe lifting limits have been developed and industrial tasks have been evaluated based on such guidelines (NIOSH, 1981).

In pain management, we use biomechanical models as an educational tool and in determining postural stress in response to certain activities such as sitting and lifting[46] (Fig 16–18). While static and dynamic strength testing methods provide useful information, e.g., about the amount of weight a patient can handle, biomechanical analysis of motion adds a valuable dimension regarding the "manner" in which an activity is performed. Thus it provides a comprehensive view of the quantitative and qualitative performance parameters. Methods of motion analysis are being used to analyze work tasks, sports activities, and walking patterns in order to evaluate the effect of injury, and the response to treatment, and to modify performance in a way that produces less biomechanical stress. Biomechanical methods are also used to study body sway and bal-

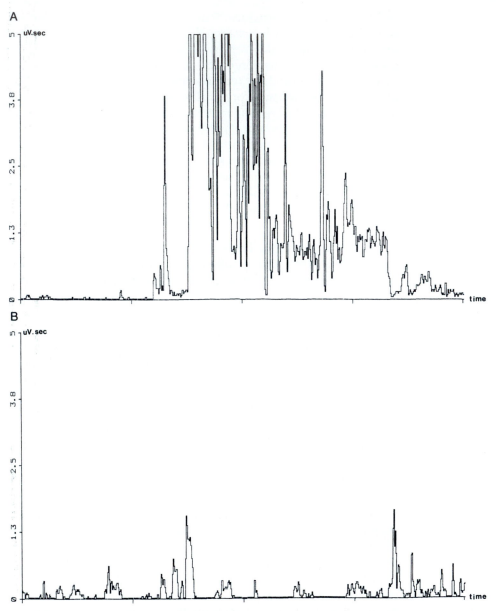

FIG 16–17. Integrated electromyographic (EMG) recording of the right shoulder muscles of a patient performing a selected number of desk tasks. **A** shows saturation at this level of amplification. **B** shows EMG of the same patients while performing the same activity following appropriate interventions. EMG was effective in documenting the effect of intervention on muscle tension reduction.

ance.[37] Sway analysis can be useful in clinical evaluations and in the study of environmental and work factors.

It should be mentioned that the use of biomechanical models has been criticized since they depend on scaled anatomic drawings, thus providing only semi-quantitative data. Biomechanical models lack the anatomic accuracy and faithful representation of the real human system. They also do not account for factors such as fatigue, pain, behaviors, etc. For the clinician, such factors should

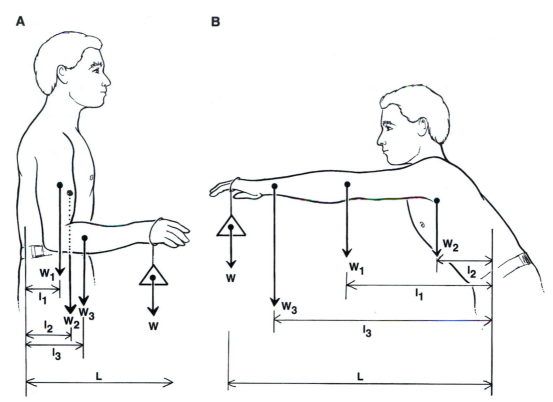

FIG 16–18. Biomechanical analysis can be used to rationalize body mechanics and demonstrate the effects of changing body posture while handling an object weighing W on the lower back. It can be clearly demonstrated that the quantity $[(W \cdot L) + (w_1 \cdot l_1) + (w_2 \cdot l_2) + (w_3 \cdot l_3)]$ is much greater for posture **B** than for posture **A**. In biomechanical analysis the estimated weight of body segments and their lengths provide individualization of the analysis.

be considered in the interpretation of reports provided by motion analysis and lifting evaluation "machines" currently available in the market.

Intervention

Intervention is the actual implementation of the solutions and suggestions derived from previous steps. In most cases, this is a joint effort involving the patient, the health care professional, the ergonomist, and the keeper or administrator of the environment to which the patient will return upon completion of rehabilitation (i.e., the employer). The general categories under which interventions can be identified follow:

Physical Interventions. These interventions represent the effort made to design effective methods for the physical and functional restoration of human abilities. These include methods of biofeedback, muscle reeducation, and functional electrical stimulation. The objective here is to increase human abilities up to a level which matches or exceeds job demands.

Intervention Through Muscle Reeducation. Muscle reeducation (MR) is a therapeutic modality where patients combine the "physical" progressive resistance exercise methods with the "behavioral" EMG biofeedback principles in order to overcome neuromuscular inhibition caused by pain or injury, thereby facilitating muscle performance.[20, 26, 41]

Intervention Through Functional Electrical Stimulation.   Owing to muscle weakness, some patients may experience difficulty while performing physical therapy strengthening exercises. Since many patients with soft tissue changes may suffer loss of muscle mass and bulk owing to disuse, their voluntary effort may be reduced, thus requiring a longer time to improve muscle strength. It is, therefore, desirable to provide pain patients with alternative passive methods of muscle strengthening such as the use of functional electrical stimulation (FES) (see Chapter 15). In FES, electrical stimulation is used to induce muscle contraction involuntarily. With the addition of graded resistance (such as weights) to the affected limb, muscle strength can then be increased. FES has been shown to provide reconditioning and restoration of function of weak muscles in a variety of conditions.[10, 11, 34, 41, 45] As an add-on modality during pain treatment,[43] FES can help to accelerate muscle strength recovery. This process may be especially useful in the presence of medical conditions that do not allow the patient to perform his or her "regular" exercises.

Engineering Interventions.   This set of interventions includes the design of work objects, equipment, and tools, and designing tasks that allow safe performances. The interventions can range from simple accommodations to changing work tools.

Workplace and Task Design and Reengineering.   Pain related to work situations is a complex modern problem in industrialized countries. While it is generally agreed that work may be considered to be a stress, elements of the work (task, tools, etc.) have been identified as being contributors to stress and health problems in the workplace (Fig 16–19). Meanwhile, the proper design of the same tools and equipment has been linked to good health habits. For example, the shape of a chair is important for good sitting posture.[24] Adjustability, good armrests, good lumbar support, an inclined backrest, and compatibility between the chair and the task have been shown to reduce neck and low back tension significantly. It should, however, be noted that, contrary to common belief, providing patients with ergonomically designed workstations does not necessarily insure a stress-free situation (Fig 16–20). It is the combination of good health, good postural habits, and proper body mechanics that augments an ergonomically designed workplace (Fig 16–21, A and B).

Computer-Aided Design of the Workplace.   Ergonomics can provide engineering solutions that reduce musculoskeletal stresses resulting from the environment, the task, the tools, and the workplace in general. As presented earlier, ergonomics guidelines are numerous and should be interpreted carefully. In order to facilitate the implementation of these guidelines in design and modification of workplaces, we have utilized artificial intelligence (known as expert systems) technology to developed a software to assist in solving workplace design problems. This SWAD (*s*itting *w*orkplace *a*nalysis and *d*esign) program combines anthropometric data, workplace information, and recognized principles and considerations to produce an optimal sitting workplace.[3-6] Using this computer-aided design method, workplaces are designed, analyzed, or modi-

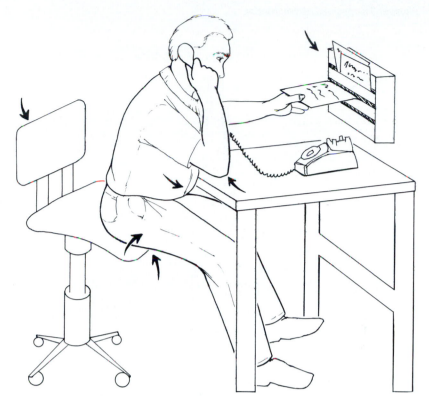

FIG 16–19. It is estimated that more than half of office workers sit either forward or in the middle of the chair. Ergonomics analyzes not only sitting habits but also chair design, individual characteristics, and workplace layout in relation to the task demands.

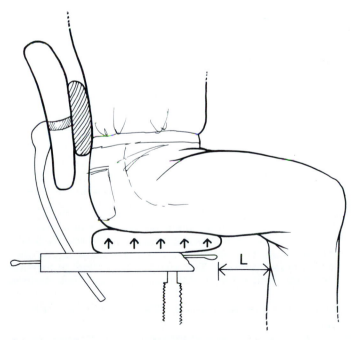

FIG 16–20. Recommending a rounded cushion for this person while using this chair may not be beneficial at all. The added cushion reduces the effective seating area thus increasing the static pressure under the thighs. The ergonomic approach to this and similar situations relies on fitting equipment to individuals within the constraints of the environment and the requirements of the task.

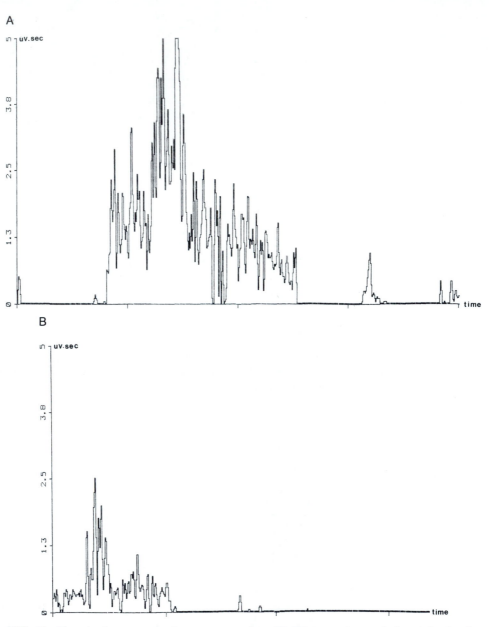

FIG 16–21.   **A,** integrated electromyographic (EMG) recording of the right lumbar paraspinal muscles of a patient performing a lifting and lowering task. **B** the EMG of the same patient while performing the same activity following appropriate ergonomic interventions. The effectiveness of intervention can be shown in the significant reduction in muscle tension. This also becomes a tool to increase patients' awareness of the importance and value of utilizing proper ergonomic methods.

fied and proper furniture is determined on an individual basis (Figs 16–22 and 16–23).

Adjustability and Flexibility of Workplace Design.   In order to reduce musculoskeletal stresses at work, adjustability has been recommended. Relatively new concepts such as tiltable chairs,[22, 50] slanted desktops,[21] and arm and tool support[31] have been introduced. These features have been shown to induce

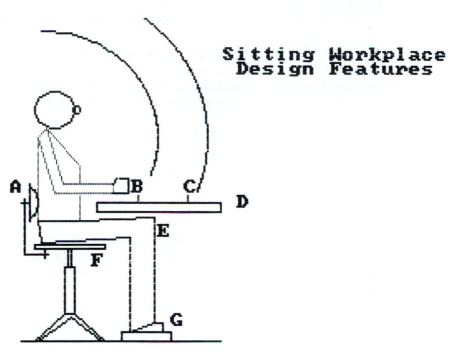

FIG 16–22.   Computer printout of SWAD (sitting *w*orkplace *a*nalysis and *d*esign) output showing workplace parameters individualized for its user. The dimensions are produced following automated computerized analysis.

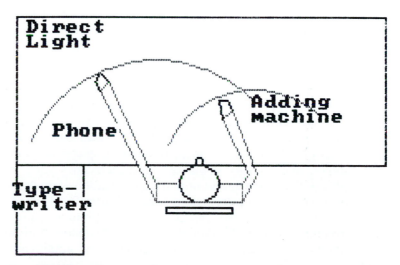

FIG 16–23.   SWAD produces a schematic presentation of the recommended layout of the workplace based on inputs to the model combined with rules and principles programmed into the software.

more mobility, improve posture, facilitate leg movement, and significantly reduce muscle tension. Recently, DeWall et al.[24] showed that inclined desks for reading and writing appear to have a positive effect on posture. It should be emphasized here that these concepts must not be generalized to all activities or tasks without careful analysis. For example, while a slanted work surface may be preferred for reading tasks, the same surface will not be recommended for writing activities. The same is true for "mobile" chairs where a stationary position is certainly recommended in tasks involving fine motor coordination and activities requiring precision. In a recent report, Jensen and Bendix[32] indicate that subjects did not prefer a tiltable chair over an "ordinary chair." The authors found "no conclusive evidence for an improved posture when using tiltable seats compared to fixed seats."

Computer Workplaces.   In this information age, millions of computers are being used for a variety of purposes ranging from data manipulation in offices to video games at home. The introduction of computers has brought about a new set of health problems. While facilitating work and aiding productivity, using computers requires a considerable amount of physical effort, especially of the eyes, head, fingers, and hands. While being credited for increased productivity, computers have been accused of causing distress to humans. Eye fatigue and strain, sensitivity to light, blurred vision, changes in color perception, numbness of fingertips, headache, neck strain, back discomfort, skin problems, poor pregnancy outcomes, and stress are but some of these accusations! Some think this is due to increased repetitious movement, straining of tendons, hyperextension of wrists, and restricted static postures (as compared to using a typewriter, which requires manual adjustment of margins and frequent paper changes).

Ergonomics recognizes that computers themselves are a minor contributor to the majority of these symptoms. Many of the reported health problems are a result of improper task design, poor workplace design, poor conditions in the general environment, as well as operators' lack of knowledge of safety issues when dealing with computers. The identification of the origin of the problem is essential for the development of appropriate intervention.

Ergonomic Job and Task Analysis.   Ergonomic job analysis (EJA) follows the theme of the HMS discussed earlier which addresses job demands in relation to environmental conditions and human functional characteristics. In EJA, job demands are those required to perform each task. These are determined through observations, measurement of physical parameters (motion, time, forces, and sensory demands), and interviews with the worker and the employer. The work environment and conditions are also assessed for their effect on performance. Information obtained from EJA is used to determine work duties that an individual can assume, taking into account possible modification or accommodations. This approach is in compliance with the Americans with Disabilities Act (ADA) and its rulings related to employment.

Job Simulation in Rehabilitation.   In the determination of work demands and performance on the job, ergonomists in clinical settings develop realistic job simulations with the purpose of allowing patients to:

- Perform selected tasks under supervision.
- Review work activities.
- Execute job tasks while using proper methods of posture and body mechanics.
- Receive feedback.
- Implement recommendations in the simulated environment.
- Insure that they are capable of performing when they return to work following treatment.

For maximum benefit to the patient, job simulation activities should be performed as a joint effort between ergonomics, occupational therapy, vocational rehabilitation, and biofeedback since professionals in each of these fields have valuable input to this process.

Work Conditioning.   Properly designed work conditioning methods allow patients to progressively practice job tasks. Progression should be linked to patients' treatment goals. During this process, ergonomists assist the patient and the occupational therapists in further dealing with the increased physical demands resulting from increased weights, longer sitting, etc. Necessary modifications in body mechanics take place during activity. Performance in work conditioning should be evaluated and discussed with the medical team on a daily basis in order to assess task demand needs in relation to patients' abilities and orient treatment efforts toward functional restoration.

Behavioral Interventions.   The contribution of ergonomics here is through providing the knowledge, instructions, education, and training in proper postures, body mechanics, and work habits. An essential element in this process is insuring that the knowledge gained translates into increased awareness; i.e., the actual application of the knowledge.

Patient Education.   As can be seen, the thrust of the ergonomic approach puts people as the primary element of concern in pain management and functional restoration. Throughout all the interventions described above, patients' knowledge and awareness are developed. Patients with pain are taught to recognize their capabilities and limitations, to incorporate and follow ergonomics guidelines when performing virtually any activity. In this process, patients learn not to rely solely on "assistive" devices in order to function. They also learn to realize and identify commercial "gimmicks" directed at their pain and suffering.

Interventions Through Posture Correction.   The relationship between poor posture and discomfort is well established. Poor awkward postures cause fatigue, strain, and eventually pain, and should be corrected. Poor postures (Figs 16–24, 16–25, and 16–26) may result in anatomic deformation, pain, many irregularities in the body functions, loss of stability, and falls, slips, and other related accidents.[38] Faulty posture and poor body alignment develop slowly and may not be observed by the individual. Poor posture can develop due to obesity, weakened muscles, emotional tension, and poor postural habits in the workplace.

Postural fixity is commonly seen in today's offices. It has been indicated that the incidence of pain increases in predominantly sitting work activities as

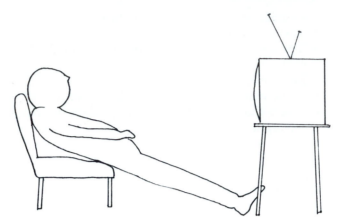

FIG 16–24. Comfortable postures are not necessarily good. Fatigue, pain, and poor habits cause poor postures. Ergonomics education and rationalization are essential in this regard. Principles must be generalized to all activities of daily living.

compared to work tasks allowing walking, standing, and sitting.[33, 49] Fixed postures were associated with circulatory disadvantage,[52] and diminished blood flow in the muscle giving rise to pain, reflex muscle contraction, or spasms and eventually tissue damage.[24] A work environment that facilitates movements may reduce the impact of this disadvantage.[32]

The specific effects of individual postural differences on health and functional activities remain unclear. It is recognized that postures that place static loading on muscles and place joints in awkward positions are not healthy. Prolonged forward bending of the head and trunk, stooped postures, forced postures, and postures causing constant deviation from neutral positions are but

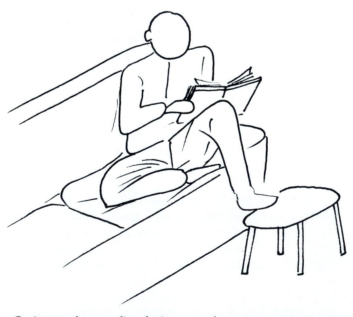

FIG 16–25. Owing to the peculiar design, people assume many postures while on a sofa in their attempt to obtain comfort. Ergonomics can aid in the design and use of sofas as well as in the selection of which activities they should be used for (e.g., reading, watching TV).

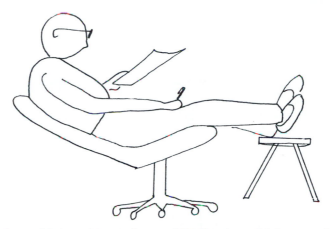

FIG 16–26.   An accident waiting to happen! Neck pain and injury resulting from mechanical failure of the chair are possibilities. Ergonomics can intervene for education and task modification to correct this situation.

few examples of poor postures. Many causes of poor postures can be easily identified. Among these are: body structural abnormalities such as scoliosis; poor postural habits, including slouching when sitting; and poor design of chairs and furniture.

Ergonomics addresses the factors contributing to poor postures from both the physical as well as the engineering perspective. On the physical level, deficiencies in human structural capabilities can be considered in the design and selection of products and tools. Human knowledge and awareness of proper posture can be increased through education and training. Also, products that encourage poor posture must be modified or replaced whenever feasible. Stress and its physiologic consequences can also lead to poor postural habits. People need to be aware of stress as a source of musculoskeletal strain.

In the rehabilitation of low back pain, posture correction is a key element in functional restoration. Patients are taught, through practice and the use of biofeedback, to maintain proper posture, to choose proper equipment, to modify their working environment to encourage good postural habits, and to alternate activities to avoid postural fatigue.[10, 11, 13, 17, 18]

Body Mechanics Interventions.   Body mechanics is the manner by which an activity is carried out. Proper body mechanics provides the basis for the safest way to perform functional ADL (Figs 16–27 through 16–31). Ergonomics intervention in this area consists of education as well as observation during practice. Proper ways to sit, stand, walk, lift, carry, and so forth and their rationale are taught to patients. In order to insure effective implementation, patients must be observed while performing the activity. Feedback can then be offered as patients increase their tolerances to perform the activity. Most often, ergonomics utilizes biofeedback principles to assist patients in learning proper body mechanics and to demonstrate that proper techniques do indeed reduce muscular tension and increase work efficiency.[13, 18, 27] It is important that body mechanics techniques be taught with sufficient generalization. This will allow patients to accommodate the specific body mechanics technique in the presence of conditions other than pain and as the task demands change. In other words, while it may be advisable to bend the knees and keep the back straight while lifting, this rule may be modified in the presence of knee precautions or as the amount

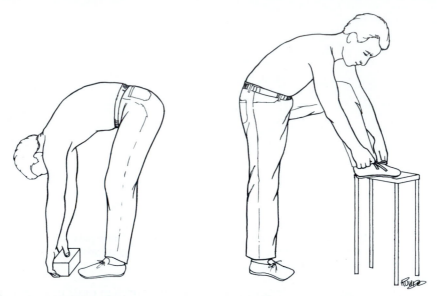

FIG 16–27. Improper body mechanics in performing activities of daily living can cause or lead to injury and pain. Alternative ways should be studied while considering the capabilities and limitations of the individual.

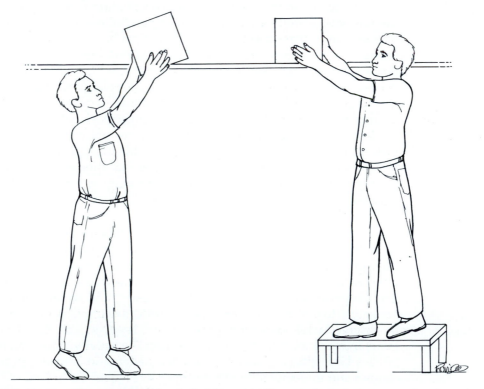

FIG 16–28. The use of mechanical aids can facilitate task performance and reduce the potential of serious injuries.

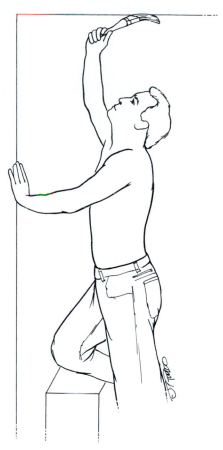

FIG 16–29. Working overhead is one of the most stressful activities involving the shoulder, neck, and arms. Caution must be exercised in such cases and the use of alternative methods must be investigated.

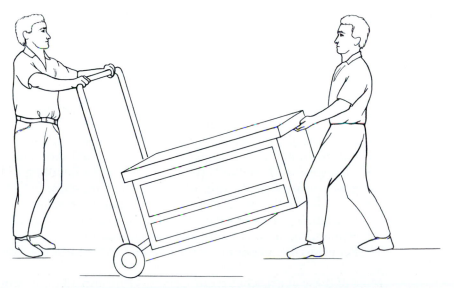

FIG 16–30. The use of mechanical aids and help from co-workers are strongly recommended in tasks involving bulky and heavy objects.

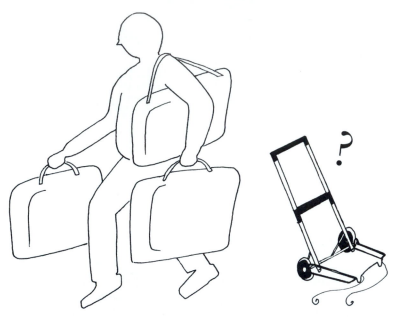

FIG 16–31. Wheeled carts are very useful for daily activities involving handling heavy or bulky objects, provided that there are no stairways or escalators.

of weight lifted increases beyond a certain value or when the object lifted is of a large size that can not fit between the legs.

   Managerial and Administrative Interventions.   Ergonomics contributes in this area through these recognized methods:

- Work diversification.
- Relieving workers.
- Rest pauses.
- Employment and preemployment screening.
- Reducing workload.
- Automation.
- Mechanization.
- Enlargement of work team (i.e., getting two people to do the job instead of one).
- Job rotation (allowing the worker to alternate hands, or rotating jobs among workers as an option).
- Providing the proper work tools at home or on the job (e.g., sharper knives, thumb or stop triggers, tools with good mechanical balance).
- Changing work methods (e.g., avoiding tight handling of tools, changing grasp, using a power grip instead of the flat palm).
- Considering the use of mechanical restraints for safety.
- Rearranging the workplace to preserve neutral postures.
- Minimizing or eliminating awkward deviations.
- Reducing the amount of force required to perform the task.

Most of these approaches require engineering and administrative collaboration. While the efficacy of some of these methods is yet to be established, their biomechanical rationale appears sound. In some instances an approach consisting of a combination of the above factors may be necessary.

Ergonomics in the Postrehabilitation Stage

Effective pain rehabilitation approaches can succeed in achieving the goal of functional restoration and return to work or a productive lifestyle. However, if no effort is made to insure that functional gains obtained during rehabilitation are maintained following discharge from treatment, reoccurrence of pain or disability may result.

In this stage, ergonomics' emphasis is on the reengineering of the task and the environment to permit a more compatible and safer relationship between the person with pain and his or her working or living environment. During this stage ergonomics contributes by:

1. Designing effective programs for continued health following hospitalization to insure that the rehabilitated person continues to be active. A properly designed home program (physical, avocational, etc.), that incorporates good body mechanics, relaxation, pacing, and so forth should become an integral part of the patient's daily routine indefinitely, even if there is no pain.
2. Reengineering of the work and home environments. If the patient returns to the same poorly designed environment where, in many cases he or she sustained the injury, there is a good possibility that reinjury may occur. Therefore, it becomes a priority to analyze and study the working or living environment (as well as the task) to insure that the rehabilitated person will be able to perform productively without risk of reinjury. Many forms of intervention have been suggested in this process. Among these are:
   a. Redesigning of the workplace and finding ways to adapt the workplace or working conditions to the worker.
   b. Adjusting workplace parameters together with the environmental conditions according to the task being performed.
   c. Using work aids (such as a document holder to keep documents at the same level and proximity as the computer screen and using eyeglasses of correct focal length for computer tasks).
   d. Using proper workplace tools and furniture (e.g., a comfortable adjustable chair).
   e. Realizing that, ergonomically, a good workplace does not necessarily have to be an expensive one.

SUMMARY

The management of myofascial pain is far from simple. The contributions of ergonomics to the management of myofascial pain are many and should be integrated in all efforts aimed at the prevention and management of the problem. The utilization of ergonomics at the University of Miami CPRC has resulted in valuable approaches that are clinically based. These approaches originate from actual applications of ergonomics methods with patients presenting with myofascial pain. Not only does ergonomics benefit treatment, its benefits in the prevention of injury (or reinjury) are apparent. Successful ergonomic intervention strategies have demonstrated that pain management should be comprehensive and multidisciplinary. The inclusion of human engineering principles is therefore needed, especially where the objective is functional restoration, reduction of pain, and return to a productive lifestyle.

REFERENCES

1. Abdel-Moty E, Diaz E, Khalil TM, et al: Ergonomic job analysis for patients with cervical trauma during rehabilitation. In Kumar S, editor: *Advances in industrial ergonomics and safety* IV, London, 1992, Taylor & Francis, pp 1195–1200.
2. Abdel-Moty E, Field E, Miles N, et al: Center of pressure reproducibility of comfortable and predetermined stances in healthy subjects, *Phys Ther* 71(suppl):S54, 1991.
3. Abdel-Moty E, Khalil TM: Computerized design of the sitting workplace. *Comput Ind Eng* Suppl 1, 22–26, 1986.
4. Abdel-Moty E, Khalil TM: Computerized electromyography in quantifying the effectiveness of functional neuromuscular electrical stimulation. In Asfour SS, editor: *Trends in ergonomics/human factors IV*, vol B, Amsterdam, 1987, Elsevier, pp 1057–1066.
5. Abdel-Moty E, Khalil TM: The use of personal microcomputers in the design and analysis of the VDT sitting workplace. In Asfour SS, editor: *Trends in ergonomics/human factors IV*, vol A, Amsterdam, 1987, Elsevier, pp 113–120.
6. Abdel-Moty E, Khalil TM: A computerized expert system for work simplification and workplace design. In Botton NA, Raz T, editors: *Expert systems*, Norcross, Ga., 1988, Industrial Engineering and Management Press, IIE, AIIE, pp 221–226.
7. Abdel-Moty E, Khalil TM: Computer-aided design and analysis of the sitting workplace for the disabled, *Int Disabil Stud* 13:121–124, 1991.
8. Abdel-Moty E, Khalil TM: Computer-aided design and analysis of the sitting workplace for the disabled. In Mital A, editor: *Advances in industrial ergonomics and safety*, New York, 1989, Taylor & Francis, pp 863–870.
9. Abdel-Moty E, Khalil TM: Computer-aided design and analysis of the sitting workplace for the disabled, *Int Disabil Stud* 13:121–124, 1991.
10. Abdel-Moty E, Khalil TM, Asfour SS, et al: Ergonomics considerations for the reduction of physical task demands of low back pain patients. In Afaghazedh F, editor: *Trends in ergonomics/human factors V*, vol 4, Amsterdam, 1988, Elsevier, pp 959–967.
11. Abdel-Moty E, Khalil TM, Asfour SS, et al: Functional electrical stimulation in low back pain patients, *Pain Manage* 258–263, 1988.
12. Abdel-Moty E, Khalil TM, Asfour SS, et al: Effects of low back pain on psychomotor abilities. In Mital A, editor: *Advances in industrial ergonomics and safety*, New York, 1989, Taylor & Francis, pp 465–471.
13. Abdel-Moty E, Khalil T, Asfour S, et al: On the relationship between age and responsiveness to rehabilitation. In Das B, editor: *Advances in industrial ergonomics and safety* II, New York, 1990, Taylor & Francis, pp 49–56.
14. Abdel-Moty E, Khalil TM, Asfour SS, et al: Workers' compensation and non-workers' compensation chronic pain patients' responsiveness to rehabilitation. In Karwowski W, Yates JW, editors: *Advances in Industrial Ergonomics and Safety* III, New York, 1991, Taylor & Francis, pp 467–474.
15. Abdel-Moty E, Khalil T, Diaz E, et al: Ergonomic job analysis for patients with chronic low back pain during rehabilitation. In Queinnec, Y, Daniellou F editors: *Designing for everyone*, London, 1991, Taylor & Francis, pp 1638–1640.
16. Abdel-Moty E, Khalil TM, Fishbain D, et al: Functional capacity assessment of low back pain patients. In Karwowski W, Yates JW, editors: *Advances in industrial ergonomics and safety III*, London, 1991, Taylor & Francis, pp 475–482.
17. Abdel-Moty E, Khalil T, Goldberg M, et al: Posture and pain: Health effects and ergonomics interventions. In Das B, editor: *Advances in industrial ergonomics and Safety* II, London, 1990, Taylor & Francis, pp 117–124.
18. Abdel-Moty E, Khalil TM, Rosomoff RS, et al: Ergonomics considerations and interventions. In Tollison CD, Satterthwaite JR, editors: *Painful cervical trauma: Diag-*

nosis and rehabilitative treatment of neuromusculoskeletal injuries, Baltimore, 1990, Williams & Wilkins, pp 214–229.

19. Abdel-Moty E, Khalil TM, Sadek S et al: Functional capacity assessment: A test battery and its use in rehabilitation. In Kumar S, editor: *Advances in industrial Ergonomics and Safety IV*, London, 1992, Taylor & Francis, pp 1171–1178.
20. Asfour S, Khalil T, Waly S, et al: Biofeedback in back muscle strengthening, *Spine* 15:510–513, 1990.
21. Bendix T, Hagberg M: Trunk posture and load on the trapezius muscle whilst sifting at sloping desks, *Ergonomics* 27:873–882, 1984.
22. Bendix T, Jenssen F, Winkel J: An evaluation of a tiltable office chair with respect to seat height, backrest position, and task, *Eur J Appl Physiol*, 55:30–36, 1986.
23. Cooper RG, Freemont AJ, Alani SM, et al: Anthropometric assessment of paraspinal muscles in patients suffering low-back pain, *Br J Rheumatol* 28:69, 1989.
24. DeWall M, Van Riel MPJM, Snijders CJ: The effect of sitting posture of a desk with a 10-degree inclination for reading and writing, *Ergonomics* 34:575–584, 1991.
25. Field E, Abdel-Moty E, Khalil T, et al: Postural proprioception in healthy and back injured adults, *Phys Ther* 71(suppl):S104, 1991.
26. Fishbain DA, Goldberg ML, Khalil TM, et al: The utility of electromyographic feedback in the treatment of conversion paralysis, *Am J Psychiatry* 145:1572–1575, 1988.
27. Goldberg ML, Orozco M, Arejano J, et al: Use of electromyographic biofeedback in the rehabilitation of low back pain patients: Body mechanics instruction. Proceedings of the 21st Annual Conference of the Human Factors Association of Canada, Edmonton, Alta, 1988.
28. Herberts P, Kadefors R, Andersson G, et al: Shoulder pain in industry: An epidemiological study on welders, *Acta Orthop Scand* 52:299–306, 1981.
29. Holm S, Nachemson A: Variation in the nutrition of the canine intervertebral disk induced by motion, *Spine* 8:866–974, 1983.
30. Hopkins A: Stress, the quality of work, and repetition strain injury in Australia, *Work Stress* 4:129–138, 1990.
31. Jarvhol U, Palmerud G, Kadefors R, et al: The effect of arm support on paraspinatus muscle load during simulated assembly work and welding, *Ergonomics* 34:57–66, 1991.
32. Jensen CV, Bendix T: Spontaneous movement with various seated-workplace adjustments, *Clin Biomech* 7:87–90, 1992.
33. Kelsey J: An epidemiological study of the relationship between occupations and acute herniated lumbar intervertebral discs, *Int J Epidemiolol* 4:197–205, 1976.
34. Khalil TM, Abdel-Moty E, Asfour SS, et al: Functional electric stimulation in the reversal of conversion disorder paralysis. *Arch Phys Med Rehabil* 69:545–547, 1988.
35. Khalil TM, Abdel-Moty E, Asfour SS: Ergonomics in the management of occupational injuries. In Pulat BM, Alexander DC, editors: *Industrial ergonomics: Case studies*, Norcross, Ga, 1990, Industrial Engineering and Management Press, pp 41–53.
36. Khalil TM, Abdel-Moty E, Rosomoff RS, et al: *Ergonomics in back pain: a guide to prevention and rehabilitation*, New York, 1993, Van Nostrand Reinhold.
37. Khalil TM, Abdel-Moty E, Sadek S, et al: Postural sway and balance in healthy subjects and in patients with chronic pain. In Kumar S, editor: *Advances in industrial ergonomics and safety IV*, London, 1992, Taylor & Francis, pp 925–932.
38. Khalil TM, Abdel-Moty E, Zaki AM, et al: Reducing the potential for fall accidents among the elderly through physical restoration. In Kumar S, editor: *Advances in industrial ergonomics and safety IV*, London, 1992, Taylor & Francis, pp 1127–1134.
39. Khalil TM, Abdel-Moty E, Zaki AM, et al: Effect of secondary gain issues on performance and response to rehabilitation of workers' compensation chronic low back pain patients. In Kumar S, editor: *Advances in industrial ergonomics and safety IV*, London, 1992, Taylor & Francis, pp 1187–1194.
40. Khalil TM, Asfour SS, Abdel-Moty E, et al: New horizons for ergonomics research in low back pain. In Eberts RE, Eberts CG, editors: *Trends in ergonomics/human factors*, Amsterdam, 1985, Elsevier pp 591–598.

41. Khalil TM, Asfour SS, Moty EA, et al: Ergonomics contribution to low back pain rehabilitation. *Pain Manage* 225–230, 1987.
42. Khalil TM, Asfour SS, Moty EA: Clinical ergonomics: Ergonomic practice in health care setting. In Queinnec Y, Daniellou F, editors: *Designing for everyone*, London, 1991, Taylor & Francis, pp 314–316.
43. Khalil T, Asfour S, Martinez L, et al: Stretching in the rehabilitation of low back pain patients, *Spine* 17:311–317, 1992.
44. Khalil T, Ayoub M, Snook S, et al: Ergonomic issues in low back pain: Intervention strategies. Proceedings of the Human Factors Society 35th Annual Meeting, San Francisco, Sept 2–6, pp 834–837.
45. Khalil TM, Goldberg ML, Asfour SS, et al: Acceptable maximum effort (AME): A psychophysical measure of strength in low back pain patients, *Spine* 12:372–376, 1987.
46. Khalil TM, Ramadan MZ: Biomechanical evaluation of lifting tasks: A microcomputer-based model, *Comput Ind Eng* 14:1, 1987.
47. Lucire Y: Social iatrogenesis of the Australian disease RSI. *Community Health Stud* 12:146–150, 1988.
48. Maeda K: Occupational cervicobrachial disorders and its causative factors, *J Human Ergol* 6:193–202, 1977.
49. Magora A: Investigation of the relation between low back pain and occupation. 3. Physical requirements: Sitting, standing, and weight lifting, *Scand J Rehabil Med* 41:5–9, 1972.
50. Mandal AC: Work-chair with tilting seat, *Ergonomics* 19:157–164, 1976.
51. Mayer TG, Vanharanta H, Gatchel R, et al: A comparison of CT scan muscle measurements and isokinetic trunk muscle strength in postoperative patients, *Spine* 14:33–36, 1989.
52. Milner-Brown H, Stein R: The relation between the surface electromyogram and muscle force, *J Physiol*, 246:549–569, 1975.
53. Moty EA, Khalil TM: Computerized signal processing techniques for the quantification of muscular activity, *Comput Ind Eng* 12:193–203, 1987.
54. Nicholaisen T, Jorgensen K: Trunk strength, back muscle endurance and low-back trouble, *Scand J Rehabil Med* 17:121–127, 1985.
55. Pearsall DJ, Reid JG: Line of gravity relative to upright vertebral posture, *Clin Biomech* 7:80–86, 1992.
56. Rosomoff HL: Comprehensive pain center approach to the treatment of low back pain. In *Low back pain, Report of a workshop*, 1987 Rehabilitation Research and Training Center, Department of Orthopedic Rehabilitation, University of Virginia, Charlottesville, pp 78–85.
57. Rosomoff HL, Green C, Silbert M, et al: Pain and low back rehabilitation program at the University of Miami School of Medicine. In Lorenzo KY, editor: *New approaches to treatment of chronic pain: A review of multidisciplinary pain clinics and pain centers*, US Department of Health and Human Services, National Institute of Drug Abuse Research Monograph 36.
58. Sigholm G, Herberts P, Almstrom C, et al: Electromyographic analysis of shoulder muscle load, *J Orthop Res* 1:379–386, 1984.
59. Sjogaard G, Jorgensen K, Kiens B, et al: Potassium and EMG changes in human skeletal muscle during low-intensity, long-term isometric contraction, *Acta Physiol Scand* 121:145, 1984.
60. Snook SH: Approaches to the control of back pain in industry: Job design, job placement, and education/training, *Spine* 12:45–59, 1987.
61. Snook SH, Ciriello VM: The design of manual handling tasks: Revised tables of maximum acceptable weights and forces, *Ergonomics* 34:1197–1213, 1991.
62. Snook SH, Irvine CH: Maximum acceptable weight of lift. *Am Ind Hyg Assoc J* 28:322–329, 1967.
63. Torner M, Zetterberg C, Anden U, et al: Workload and musculoskeletal problems: A comparison between welders and office clerks, *Ergonomics* 34:1179–1196, 1991.
64. Weisman G, Pope M, Johnson R: Cyclic loading in the knee ligament injuries, *Am J Sports Med* 8:24–30, 1980.
65. Willis E: Commentary: RSI as a social process, *Community Health Stud* 10:210–218, 1986.

66. Woodson W: *Human factors design handbook*, New York, 1981, McGraw-Hill.
67. Yang K, King A: Mechanism of facet load transmission as a hypothesis for low back pain, *Spine* 9:557–565, 1984.
68. Zaki AM, Khalil TM, Abdel-Moty E, et al: Profile of chronic pain patients and their rehabilitation outcome. In Kumar S, editor: *Advances in industrial ergonomics and safety IV*, New York, 1992, Taylor & Francis, pp 1179–1186.

Appendix

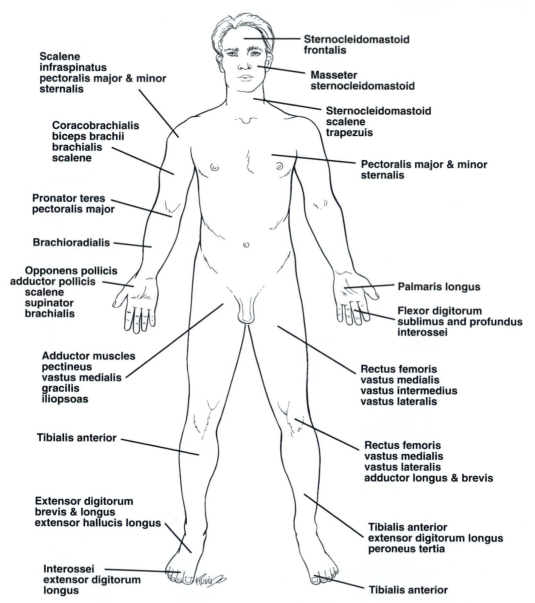

FIG A-1.   Common myofascial trigger points that may be responsible for local or referred pain patterns to the indicated pain areas.

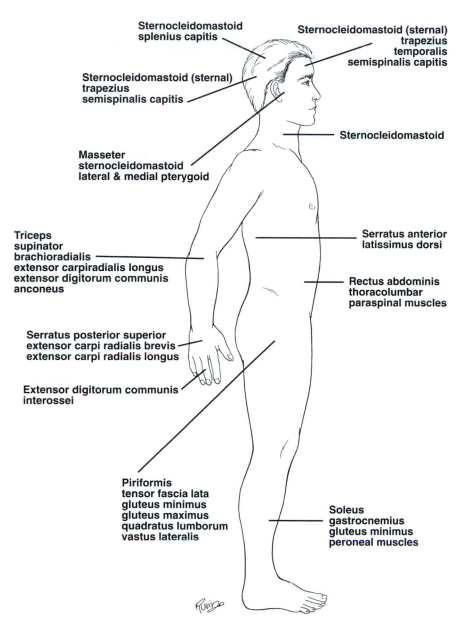

FIG. A-2. Common myofascial trigger points that may be responsible for local or referred pain patterns to the indicated areas.

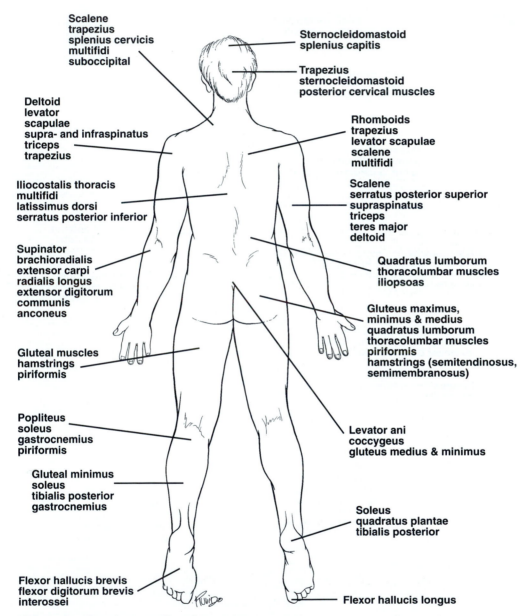

FIG A–3. Common myofascial trigger points that may be responsible for local or referred pain patterns to the indicated body areas.

Index